Current Orthopaedic Practice

Sanjeev Agarwal
Editor

Current Orthopaedic Practice

Second Edition

Springer

Editor
Sanjeev Agarwal
University Hospital of Wales
Consultant Orthopaedic Surgeon
Cardiff
UK

ISBN 978-3-030-78528-4 ISBN 978-3-030-78529-1 (eBook)
https://doi.org/10.1007/978-3-030-78529-1

This Springer imprint is published by the registered company Springer Nature Switzerland AG
The registered company address is: Gewerbestrasse 11, 6330 Cham, Switzerland

To my parents—Dr Ramesh Chandra and Dr Padam K Agarwal for making me what I am

To my wife—Jyoti for her love and support

To my children—Suyash and Harshita for making it all worthwhile

Sanjeev Agarwal

Preface

The purpose of a book is to give its reader the information he or she seeks in an easily understandable and retainable format. With this in mind, we are pleased to present this second edition of 'Current Orthopaedic Practice'. It builds on the success of the first edition, and at the same time, a quantum leap forward in the manner of presenting the information.

Change is the only constant (Heraclitus).

Orthopaedics is constantly changing as researchers challenge existing concepts and beliefs. It is amazing to see how much updating was needed in the 8 years since the first edition of this book. Almost the entire text has been updated and re-written. The sports medicine chapter has been split into two chapters of adult pathology—hip and knee. A lot of drawings have been added which makes the information easier to absorb, relying on eidetic memory of the reader. We have tried to include tables to highlight important classification systems and done away with a lot of bullet points. Having a relatively fewer number of contributors has minimised duplication of text.

The core value of 'keeping it simple' stays ever close to heart for us, as it was in the first edition. The references have been updated and have been kept in continuity with the main text instead of a bibliography at the end.

Many new contributors have joined the team, each and every one of whom has added so much value while making this project a delight to work on. This is not intended to be a fully comprehensive textbook. It does not, in any way, reduce the importance of the regular teaching and clinical skills, which remain integral to understanding orthopaedics.

The task of an author is to facilitate the information transfer to the reader, taking as little time from the reader as possible in the process. We aim to make Orthopaedics simple, easy and fun for everyone. We hope the readers around the world enjoy this book.

On behalf of all contributors

Cardiff, UK Sanjeev Agarwal

Acknowledgement

I am deeply indebted to the contributors of this book, who set time aside from their busy schedules and clinical practices to make this project possible. Each is an expert in their chosen fields and their experience and knowledge has greatly enriched this book.

The orthopaedic residents, fellows and junior surgical trainees who work in our orthopaedic department are a constant academic stimulus. I am thankful to them for challenging the teaching and pushing us to do better. They will surely be pushing the boundaries of surgical expertise in years to come.

I must record my gratefulness to the staff at Springer—Felina Francois and Melissa Morton who provided guidance and were instrumental in getting us over the finishing line.

I am grateful to Harshita Agarwal for her help with many drawings in the book. I am also indebted to Dr Ramesh Chandra and Dr Padam Agarwal for proofreading the manuscript. They are highly experienced teachers, researchers and authors. They weeded out a lot of oversights and helped edit the book to reach its current form. All remaining errors are entirely mine.

Sanjeev Agarwal

Contents

List of Contributors

Rishi Agarwal, M.R.C.S. All Wales Orthopaedic Program, Cardiff, UK

Sanjeev Agarwal, F.R.C.S. Orth. University Hospital of Wales, Consultant Orthopaedic Surgeon, Cardiff, UK

Robert Ashford, F.R.C.S. Orth. East Midlands Sarcoma Service and Leicester Cancer Research Centre, University Hospital of Leicester, Leicester, UK

University Hospital of Leicester, Leicester, UK

Randeep S. Aujla, F.R.C.S. Orth. University Hospital of Leicester, Leicester, UK

Jyoti Bansal, M.R.C.P., F.R.C.R. University Hospital of Wales, Cardiff, UK

Clare Carpenter, F.R.C.S. Orth. University Hospital of Wales, Cardiff, UK

Iqroop Chopra, F.R.C.S. (S.N.) University Hospital of Wales, Cardiff, UK

Oliver Donaldson, F.R.C.S. Orth. Consultant Orthopaedic Surgeon, Yeovil District Hospital, Yeovil, UK

Gavin John Heyes, F.R.C.S., M.Sc. Liverpool University Hospitals NHS Foundation Trust, Aintree University Hospital, Liverpool, UK

J. S. Jayadeep, F.R.C.S. Orth. Consultant Orthopaedic Surgeon, North Cumbria NHS Foundation Trust, Cumbria, UK

Alastair Jones, F.R.C.S. Orth. Consultant Orthopaedic Surgeon, Taunton, UK

Sridhar Kamath, F.R.C.R. University Hospital of Wales, Cardiff, UK

Wasim Khan, F.R.C.S. Orth. Addenbrooke's Hospital, Cambridge, UK

Lyndon Mason, F.R.C.S. Orth. University of Liverpool, Liverpool, UK

Khitish Mohanty, F.R.C.S. Orth. Consultant Orthopaedic Surgeon, University Hospital of Wales, Cardiff, UK

Abdul Nazeer Moideen, F.R.C.S. Orth. University Hospital of Wales, Cardiff, UK

Anurag Negi, M.R.C.P. University Hospital of Wales, Cardiff, UK

Kaushik Rajamani, M.R.C.P. University Hospital of Wales, Cardiff, UK

Matthew Seah Addenbrooke's Hospital, Cambridge, UK

Julia Street, F.R.C.S. Orth. Wales Orthopaedic Program, Cardiff, UK

Contributors to First Edition

Sharon M. Jones, B.M., M.D., F.R.C.P. University Hospital of Wales, Cardiff, UK

Andy Logan, F.R.C.S. Orth. University Hospital of Wales, Cardiff, UK

About the Author

Sanjeev Agarwal is a consultant orthopaedic surgeon at the University Hospital in Cardiff, UK. He specialises in hip and knee arthroplasty, for which he is fellowship trained from the Massachusetts General Hospital, Boston.He has trained orthopaedic residents and fellows for over 12 years and is an examiner for the FRCS Orth examination in the UK.

Trauma

1

Khitish Mohanty and Rishi Agarwal

Major trauma is the commonest cause of mortality in patients under the age of 40 years. Road traffic accidents account for over 5000 deaths in the UK every year. Major trauma is defined as an Injury Severity Score (ISS) over 15. Trauma networks were set up in England from 2012 onwards and are designed to provide specialist trauma care. Transfer time to a major trauma centre is expected to be within 45 minutes of injury, and patients in need of specialist trauma care bypass other nearby hospitals.

Major trauma centres are able to provide resuscitation, emergency surgery, interventional radiology, consultant led trauma team, massive transfusion protocols, immediate access to CT scans, MR scans and operation theatre, along with dedicated major trauma beds, intensive care support and comprehensive treatment and rehabilitation.

Calculation of Injury Severity Score (ISS)

$$ISS = A^2 + B^2 + C^2$$

A, B, C are the AIS (Abbreviated Injury Score) of the three most injured body regions

AIS is individually calculated (Table 1.1) for each of the six body regions—head and neck, face, chest, abdomen, extremity and external.

Primary assessment follows ATLS (Advanced Trauma Life Support) guidelines. Life threatening injuries are identified and managed. Airway control may require intubation. Intravenous access is established at scene of injury.

Haemorrhage is second commonest cause of mortality in major trauma after brain injury. The degree of shock is categorized as shown in Table 1.2.

Aggressive fluid resuscitation may be counter-productive as it can increase intraluminal pressure, dislodge clots, cause hypothermia and dilute coagulation factors. 'Permissive hypotension' allows adequate tissue perfusion, but is contraindicated in brain and spinal cord injury patients.

Trauma induced coagulopathy (TIC) was considered to be the result of acidosis, hypothermia and dilution of coagulation factors (Fig. 1.1).

The cell based concept of TIC proposed excess activation of protein C in response to thrombo-

Table 1.1 AIS (Abbreviated injury score)

Injury severity	Score
Minor	1
Moderate	2
Serious	3
Severe	4
Critical	5
Maximal (untreatable)	6

K. Mohanty (✉)
Consultant Orthopaedic Surgeon, University Hospital of Wales, Cardiff, UK

R. Agarwal
All Wales Orthopaedic Program, Cardiff, UK

S. Agarwal (ed.), *Current Orthopaedic Practice*, https://doi.org/10.1007/978-3-030-78529-1_1

Table 1.2 Degree of haemorrhagic shock

Class	Blood volume loss	Heart rate	Blood pressure	Urine output	Treatment
I	Up to 15%	<100	Normal	>30 ml/hr	Fluids
II	15–30%	>100	Decreased	20–30 ml/hr	Fluids
III	30–40%	>120	Decreased	5–15 ml/hr	Fluids and blood
IV	Over 40%	>140	Decreased	minimal	Fluids and blood

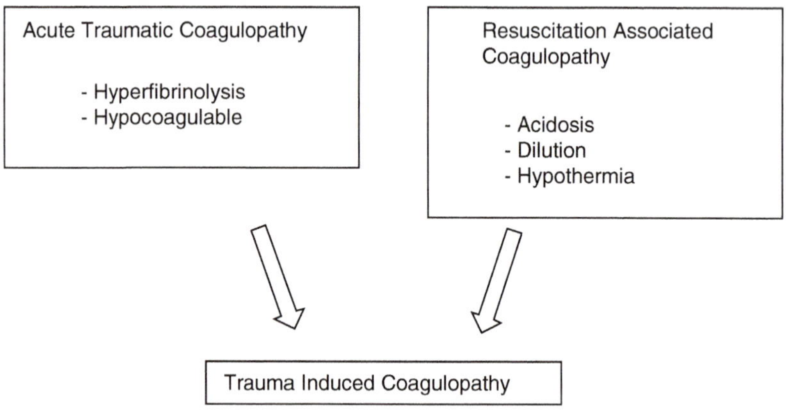

Fig. 1.1 Mechanism of TIC

modulin bound thrombin complexes on endothelial cells. Activated protein C inactivates Factor V and VIII. Early platelet dysfunction may also be related to TIC.

PT (Prothrombin time) and aPTT (Activated partial thromboplastin time) are unreliable markers for TIC. Thromboelastography (TEG) and Rotational thromboelastometry (ROTEM) is gaining popularity as a quick and effective guide to TIC.

The CRASH-2 trial evaluated the use of Tranexamic acid 1 g i.v. given within 1 h of injury in patients with severe haemorrhage and found a slight reduction in mortality.

Massive transfusion protocol is transfusion of over 10 units of packed RBC within 24 h or replacement of total blood volume in 24 h or >50% blood volume in 3 h. This follows the local guidelines in trauma centres.

CT scan (Pan scan) from vertex to ischial tuberosity as soon as the patient is stable enough is the current imaging of choice for polytrauma patients. Many resuscitation rooms have a CT scan gantry along the resuscitation bay avoiding transfer of patient to the scanner. If CT not available, imaging of polytraumatised patient involves a chest and pelvis x ray. Lateral C spine x ray is no longer routine.

Damage control surgery was first proposed in 1983 for abdominal trauma. The idea is to control bleeding, correct coagulopathy and physiological abnormalities before definitive surgery. Trauma results in surge of inflammatory mediators, which in turn leads to leukocytes susceptible to activation in the event of further trauma or surgery. This can lead to ARDS (Acute Respiratory Distress Syndrome) or multi organ failure. Damage Control Orthopaedics (DCO) should be considered in major trauma patients who are haemodynamically unstable. Patient with associated severe brain/chest/abdominal injuries unresponsive to initial resuscitation also qualify for DCO.

DCO involves external stabilisation of unstable fractures, revascularization of limbs, compartment decompression and debridement of open wounds. Only life threatening injuries are treated acutely. Definitive stabilization is carried out once physiological stability is achieved—usually a few days after major trauma.

Current evidence suggests that with aggressive resuscitation and correction of acidosis, early appropriate care (EAC) can be administered with definitive fracture fixation as long as there are no associated severe chest injuries and the serum lactate remains less than 4 mmol/L.

Vallier HA, Wang X, Moore TA, Wilber JH, Como JJ. Timing of orthopaedic surgery in multiple trauma patients: development of a protocol for early appropriate care. J Orthop Trauma. 2013;27(10):543–51.

Management of Open Fractures

An open fracture is a combined bone and soft tissue injury where the fracture hematoma communicates with the exterior through the skin or with a mucous membrane.

The management recommendations for open fractures were published in 2009 through a joint effort of the British Orthopaedic Association (BOA) and the British Association of Plastic, Reconstructive and Aesthetic Surgeons (BAPRAS) and were further updated in December 2017.

Classification

The Gustilo–Anderson system is most commonly used for classifying open fractures. It is applicable after initial wound debridement. The original classification was proposed in 1976 and had 3 types of injuries. This was based on the different infection rate in each of these types (Table 1.3)

Gustilo RB, Anderson JT. Prevention of infection in the treatment of one thousand and twenty-five open fractures of the long bones: retrospective and prospective analyses. J Bone Joint Surg Am 1976;58:453–8. Classification system for open fractures.

Table 1.3 The original gustilo anderson classification

Type I	Wound of less than 1 cm, clean, minimal contamination, minimal soft tissue injury
Type II	Wound of more than 1 cm without extensive soft tissue damage, flaps or avulsions
Type III	Open segmental fracture, open fracture with extensive soft tissue damage or a traumatic amputation. Special categories were gun shot wounds, farm injuries and open fracture requiring vascular repair

In 1984, the Type III injuries were divided into 3 further subtypes (Table 1.4).

It is important to note that the size of wound (10 cm) was not defined in the original classification, but was added in later modifications.

Mangled extremity severity score (MESS) was first introduced in 1990. It is a prognostic score to indicate the severity of limb injury and predict the limb which may eventually end up in amputation.

The mangled-extremity severity score (MESS) of Johansen (1990) is also used (Table 1.5).

Table 1.4 Subdivisions of Type III injuries

IIIA	Severe soft tissue injury, bone cover possible, irrespective of size of wound
IIIB	Extensive soft tissue injury with periosteal stripping and bone exposure. Associated with massive contamination
IIIC	Open fracture with vascular injury requiring repair

Table 1.5 The mangled-extremity severity score

Criteria	Description	Score
A. Skeletal soft tissue injury	Low energy (stab or simple fracture)	1
	Medium energy (open or multiple fractures, dislocation)	2
	High energy (close-range gunshot, crush injury)	3
	Very high energy (as above plus gross contamination)	4
B. Limb ischaemia[a]	Pulse reduced or absent, normal perfusion	1
	Pulseless, paresthesia, diminished capillary refill	2
	Cool, paralysed, insensate, numb	3
C. Shock	Systolic blood pressure always >90 mmHg	0
	Transiently hypotensive	1
	Persistent hypotension	2
D. Age	<30 years	0
	30–50 years	1
	>50 years	2

[a]The ischaemia score is doubled if the ischaemia time is >6 h

Principles of Management

Open fractures should be ideally managed at specialist centres with experienced plastic surgical and orthopaedic teams working together. These centres should have appropriate facilities for the required procedures, including theatre space and intensive care, microbiology, prosthetic and rehabilitation support.

The initial management is performed as an emergency following the ATLS guidelines. Resuscitation of the patient is the priority.

Broad-spectrum antibiotic prophylaxis (co-amoxiclav 1.2 g every 8 h or cefuroxime 1.5 g every 8 h) should be administered as soon as possible, ideally within 1 h of injury. Clindamycin is given to patients who are allergic to penicillin.

The patient's tetanus vaccination status should be ascertained and prophylaxis administered as appropriate.

A picture of the wound should be taken for the patient's records and to inform the multidisciplinary team. No irrigation or exploration is performed in the emergency department apart from removal of gross contaminants. Haemorrhage is controlled with direct pressure. Significant arterial bleeding requires vascular surgery support. The wound is dressed with a sterile dressing soaked in saline and the extremity is splinted. Appropriate radiographs are requested, making sure to include other injured areas.

The patient is moved to the operating suite after resuscitation for wound debridement and operative management of the fracture. Highly contaminated wounds (agricultural, aquatic or sewage) require immediate debridement. Urgent surgical exploration is needed for patients with gross contamination, multiple injuries, compartment syndrome or an ischaemic limb. High energy open fractures are debrided within 12 h and low energy wounds can be debrided within 24 h. Plastic surgeons should be involved at an early stage and vascular surgeons are consulted for major vascular injuries.

Management in the Operating Room

Thorough debridement and washout of the wound with normal saline is the key to a good outcome. All dead, devitalised tissue is excised, with the obvious exception of neurovascular structures. Small wounds are surgically extended to gain access and perform adequate debridement. An assessment is made regarding skin loss.

Bone debridement may be required. A bleeding bone is the best indicator of viability, hence a tourniquet should not be inflated for this part of the procedure. Loose fragments of bone and non-viable ends should be removed. Articular surface fragments are fixed back with rigid fixation. Pulse lavage is not recommended.

Bones can be stabilised at the time of debridement if there is no bone loss. In patients with bone loss, spanning external fixators or ring fixators are used. Internal fixation is performed when soft tissue cover can be achieved, which should be within 3 days (preferably) and usually within 7 days. Free flaps should be applied within 7 days.

Wounds with no Skin Loss

Following debridement, the fracture is managed with stable internal fixation. The wound is left open and surgical extensions, if any, are sutured. A second look is planned after 48–72 h, depending on the degree of contamination. At the second look procedure, a healthy and granulating wound can be sutured or covered with a skin graft or myocutaneous flap. Infected wounds are managed with further debridement, with follow-up after a further 48 h.

Wounds with Skin Loss

Thorough debridement and skeletal stabilisation is the first step. Once the fracture has been stabilised the wound can be covered with a flap, either at the same time as the initial debridement or as a staged procedure within 72 h, depending on the degree of contamination and adequacy of debridement. A vacuum-foam dressing (negative pressure dressing) may be applied until definitive surgery can be performed. Definitive soft tissue cover should be achieved at the same time as definitive internal fixation.

Evidence for the Management of Open Fractures

Antibiotics in open fractures reduce risk of infection.

Gosselin RA, Roberts I, Gillespie WJ. Antibiotics for preventing infection in open limb fractures. Cochrane database Syst Rev 2004; 1: CD003764. This review determined that antibiotics reduce the risk of infection by 59%.

Pulse lavage is not recommended for washout.

FLOW Investigators, Bhandari M et al. A Trial of Wound Irrigation in the Initial Management of Open Fracture Wounds. N Engl J Med. 2015 Dec 31;373(27):2629–41.

Hassinger SM, Harding G, Wongworawat MD. High-pressure pulsatile lavage propagates bacteria into soft tissue. Clin Orthop Relat Res 2005;439 27–31.

Scapular Fractures

The scapula is well covered by muscles on both surfaces, and fractures to the scapula are often high energy injuries, and may be associated with other injuries.

Classification

Four types of scapular fractures are described in the anatomic classification (Fig. 1.2). A number is ascribed to the different parts of the scapula and this is a purely descriptive system.

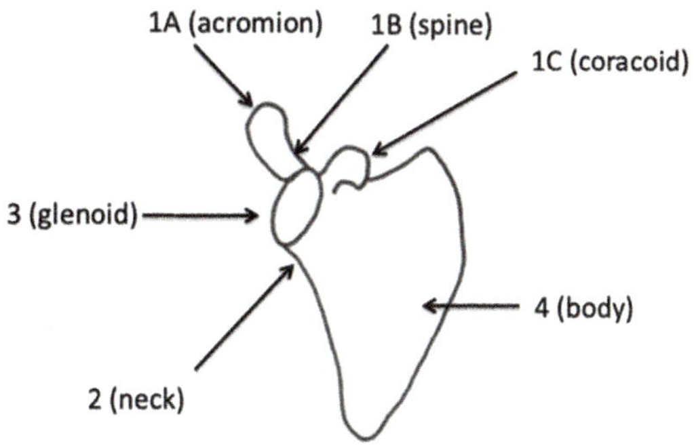

Fig. 1.2 Types of scapular fractures

Management

Most scapular fractures are managed with a sling and early mobilisation. Surgery is indicated for glenoid rim fractures and coracoid fractures with acromioclavicular joint (ACJ) separation (see below).

Glenoid Fractures

Classification

The classification of glenoid fractures was proposed by Ideberg. The original classification proposed in 1995 comprised 5 types of fractures (Fig. 1.3).

Ideberg R, Grevsten S, Larsson S. Epidemiology of scapular fractures. Incidence and classification of 338 fractures. Acta Orthop Scand 1995;66(5): 395–7.

Further modification to the system has been proposed (Fig. 1.4).

Management

CT scan is often helpful to define the fracture pattern. Displaced fractures of glenoid can lead to persistent pain, malunion, glenohumeral arthritis or shoulder instability.

Operative stabilisation is generally required to achieve shoulder stability for glenoid rim frac-

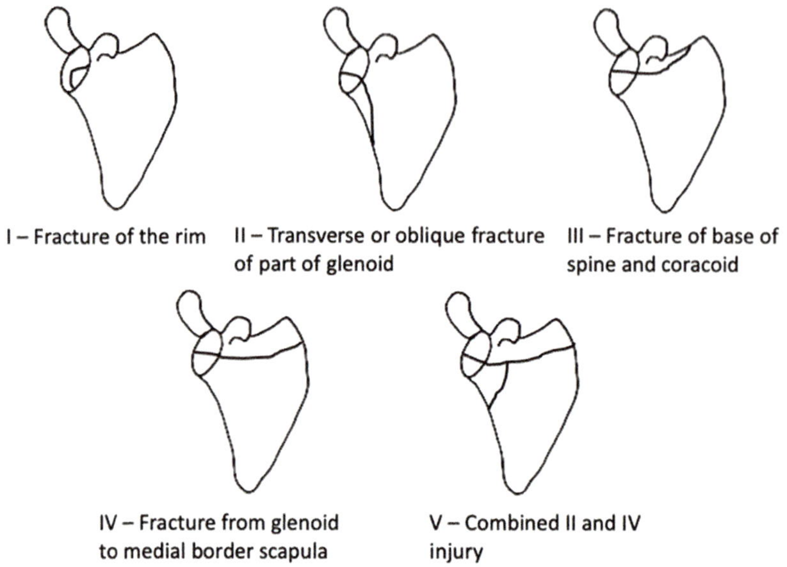

Fig. 1.3 The original Ideberg classification

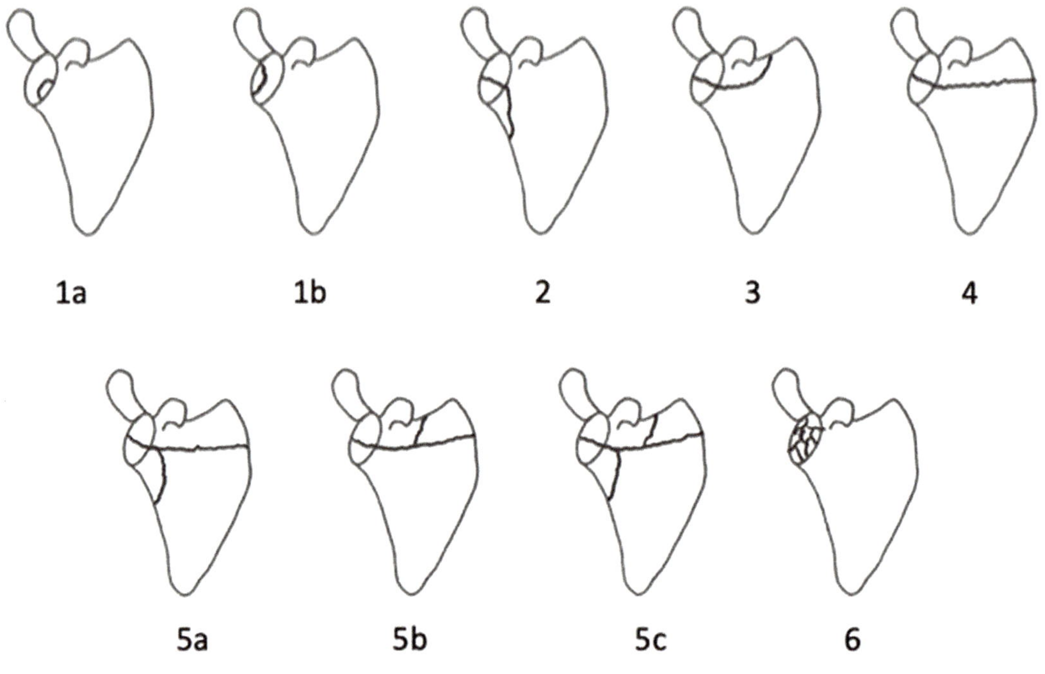

Fig. 1.4 Modified classification of glenoid fractures

tures. Fractures involving over 20% of the glenoid should be considered for operative intervention. An anterior deltopectoral or posterior Judet approach is used. Results are generally satisfactory.

Glenoid Neck Fractures

Glenoid neck fractures can be undisplaced (Type I) or displaced (Type II). Type II fractures can be Type IIa which are displaced over 1 cm or IIb which are angulated over 40 degrees.

Surgery is considered for glenoid neck fractures if the angulation is more than 40° or displacement is more than 1 cm. The Gleno-Polar angle (GPA) is the angle between the face of glenoid and lateral border of scapula (Fig. 1.5). It is normally 36 to 43 degrees. A GPA of less than 20 degrees is an indication for surgery.

Goss TP. Fractures of the glenoid neck. J Shoulder Elbow Surg. 1994;3(1):42–52. This study reported that type I fractures (90% of glenoid neck injuries) are not significantly displaced and can be managed non-operatively. Type II injuries have more than 1 cm displacement or over 40° angulation and should be reduced and fixed.

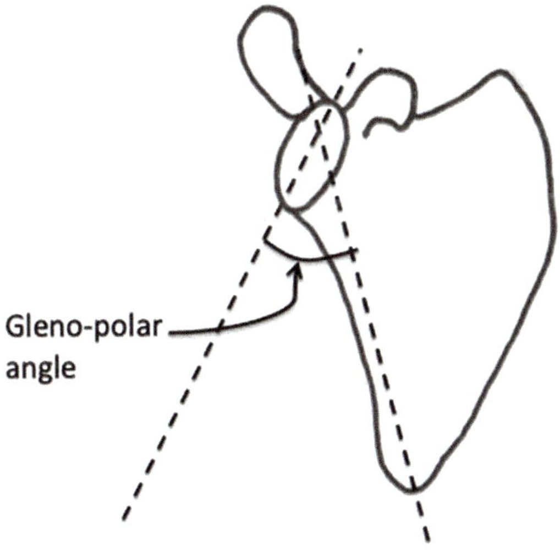

Fig. 1.5 Gleno-polar angle

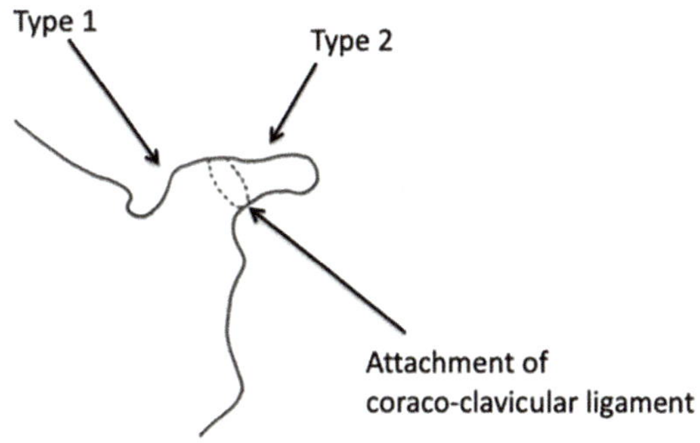

Fig. 1.6 Classification of coracoid fractures. (Figure modified from Ogawa 1997)

Coracoid Fractures

These are rare injuries and are often associated with acromioclavicular dislocation.

Classification

A clinically relevant classification was proposed by Ogawa in 1997 whereby two types were recognized based on the location of fracture in relation to the coraco-clavicular ligament (Fig. 1.6).

Management

Type 1 injuries are stabilised to restore the link between clavicle and scapula. A single partially threaded cancellous screw is used to stabilise the fracture.

Type 2 injuries do not require operative stabilisation. A sling and early physiotherapy results in a good outcome.

Ogawa K, Yoshida A, Takahashi M, Ui M. Fractures of the coracoid process. J Bone Joint Surg Br 1997;79(1):17–9. Review of 53 type 1 and 22 type 2 fractures. Type 1 fractures were managed operatively and type 2 fractures had good outcome with nonoperative measures.

Floating Shoulder

Although traditionally defined as a combination of clavicle and scapula neck fracture, current evidence suggests that scapular neck fracture with ligament disruption also equates to a floating shoulder. Floating shoulder implies an injury where the glenoid fossa has lost all osseoligamentous connection with the rest of the scapula.

A superior shoulder suspensory complex has been described by Goss. This comprises the superior part of glenoid, the coracoid process, coracoclavicular ligament, distal end of the clavicle, AC joint and acromion process as labeled in Fig. 1.7. Disruption of one part of this ring is often associated with injury to another part—so-called 'double disruptions'. Injuries to one component of the complex usually respond well to non-operative treatment, but double disruptions require operative stabilisation.

Goss TP. Double disruptions of the superior shoulder suspensory complex. J Orthop Trauma 1993;7(2):99–106.

Injuries to superior shoulder suspensory complex are considered less important for the diagnosis of floating shoulder in absence of glenoid neck fractures.

Bartonicek J, Tucek M, Nanka O. Floating shoulder: Myths and reality. J Bone Joint Surg review 2018;6(10). Injury of the superior shoulder suspensory complex without an associated fracture of neck of glenoid does not comprise floating shoulder.

Unstable fracture of the glenoid neck should be stabilised through a Judet approach. In general, significant displacement at any site of the superior shoulder suspensory complex should prompt consideration of open reduction and internal fixation.

Owens BD, Goss TP. The floating shoulder. J Bone Joint Surg Br 2006;88(11):1419–24. The authors recommended considering fixation of the clavicle, scapula or both if there is significant displacement.

Acromioclavicular Joint Injuries

The acromioclavicular joint (ACJ) couples glenohumeral and scapulothoracic movements. It allows 15 degrees of protraction, 21 degrees of upward rotation and 22 degrees of posterior tilting of the scapula in relation to the clavicle in shoulder abduction.

Classification

Three types were first described by Tossy, Mead and Sigmond. This was later expanded to six types by Rockwood (Fig. 1.8). In Type III vertical translation of the clavicle is up to the width of the clavicle. A Type VII has been described where there is total clavicular dislocation with disrupted AC and sternoclavicular joints.

Nguyen V, Williams G, Rockwood C. Radiography of acromioclavicular dislocation

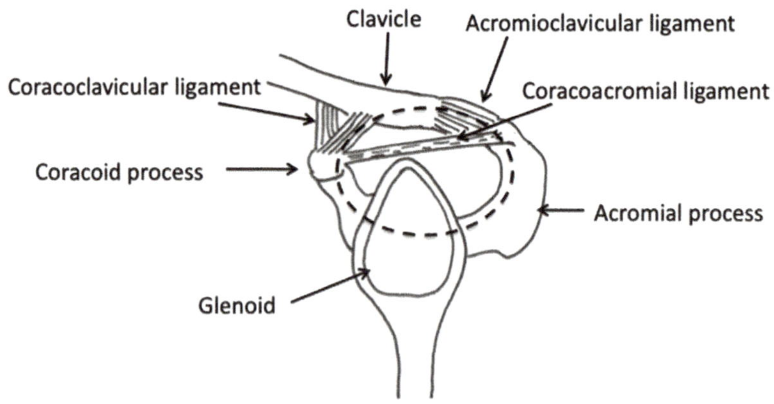

Fig. 1.7 Superior shoulder suspensory complex. The ring of the complex is indicated by the dashed line. All labeled structures are part of the complex

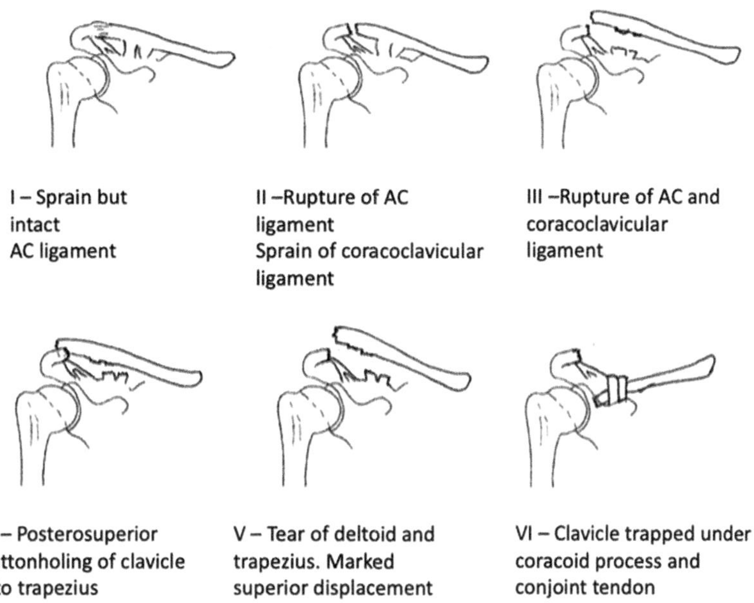

Fig. 1.8 Classification of ACJ injuries

and associated injuries. Crit Rev Diagn Imaging 1991;32(3):191–228.

Pathology

The coraco-clavicular ligament has a conoid and a trapezoid part, which helps to stabilise the ACJ. Double disruptions of the superior shoulder suspensory complex lead to instability and may be an indication to stabilise at least one of the two injuries.

Diagnosis

The clinical diagnosis is based on local swelling and tenderness. The distal end of the clavicle is prominent in types III and V. The clavicle feels mobile (piano-key sign).

In the scarf test, adduction of the arm across the chest reproduces the pain. O'Brien's test is done with the arm in 90 degree forward elevation, 10 degree adduction and with forearm pronated and then supinated. Examiner applies resisted downward pressure on the hand. Pain localised to the AC joint in pronation, but relieved in supination is also specific for injuries to the joint (see Chap. 17—shoulder examination).

Radiographs are normal in types I and II. A 10 degree cephalad view (Zanca view) helps in accurate estimation of displacement.

Management

For types I and II, non-surgical management is adequate, with a polysling to support the weight of the arm for comfort. Movements are allowed as comfortable.

The management of type III is debatable. Most patients respond well to non-operative management even in athletes. The prominence of clavicle persists, but restoration of function is adequate.

For types IV, V and VI, surgical treatment is generally recommended.

Phillips AM, Smart C, Groom AF. Acromioclavicular dislocation. Conservative or surgical therapy. Clin Orthop Relat Res 1998;353:10–7. This meta-analysis found no difference in the results of surgical and non-surgical management.

Spencer EE Jr. Treatment of grade III acromioclavicular joint injuries. A systematic review.

Clin Orthop Relat Res 2007;455:38–44. This review found that operative management was not better than non-operative management. In addition, operative management was associated with a higher complication rate, longer recovery and delayed return to work and sport.

Fixation methods include screws, cerclage wire or sutures (e.g. Tightrope). Other options include reconstruction of the coracoclavicular ligament and transfer of the tip of the coracoid to the clavicle to function as a dynamic transfer. Excision of the lateral end of clavicle is a further option.

Weaver and Dunn described the classic procedure of transfer of the coracoacromial ligament, whereby the ligament is detached from the acromion and transferred to the lateral end of the clavicle (Fig. 1.9). This is combined with excision of the lateral 5–10 mm of the clavicle. Various modifications have been described since. This procedure is associated with ongoing instability and only partial improvement in strength compared to the original coracoclavicular ligament.

Weaver JK, Dunn HK. Management of acromioclavicular injuries, especially complete acromioclavicular separation. J Bone Joint Surg Am 1972;54:1187–94. Description of transfer of the coracoacromial ligament

Coracoacromial stabilisation is an option and has been achieved using a wide variety of synthetic materials, endobuttons, as well as tendon grafts. The Bosworth screw stabilises the clavicle to the coracoid, although is technically difficult and prone to loosening and screw cut out. A hook plate was developed to maintain reduction of the joint but the plate has to be removed 8–12 weeks after insertion. It carries the risk of shoulder stiffness and pain, clavicular osteolysis and loss of reduction on removal of the plate.

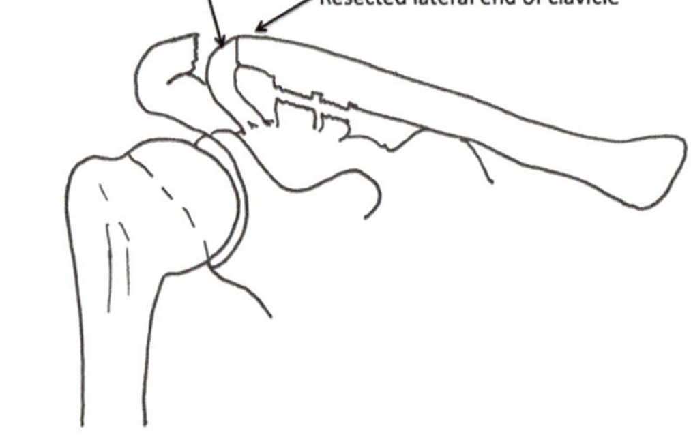

Fig. 1.9 Weaver Dunn procedure

Many techniques for reconstruction of the coracoclavicular ligament have been described. This can be open or arthroscopic. Hamstring graft can be used. The lateral half of the conjoint tendon can be used as a graft. Transfer of the tip of coracoid with the conjoint tendon to the clavicle allows bone to bone healing. The musculocutaneous nerve is at risk of injury due to close proximity to the conjoint tendon.

Clavicle Fracture

Clavicle fractures are one of the commonest bone injuries. Middle-third fractures account for most of clavicular fractures (85%), with the remaining fractures involving the medial third (5%) and the lateral third (10%) (Allman's classification).

Allman FL Jr. Fractures and ligamentous injuries of the clavicle and its articulation. J Bone Joint Surg Am 1967;49(4):774–84.

Non-operative management is generally adequate and, despite healing in an overlapped position, functional results are acceptable. More recently, there has been an increasing trend towards fixation of fractures displaced 100% and shortening over 2 cm in active, high-demand individuals. Displaced multifragmentary fractures of the mid portion of the clavicle carry a 10–15% risk of non-union.

Indications for open reduction and internal stabilisation include open fractures, neurovascular injury, non-union, fracture of the distal third with injury to the coracoclavicular ligament, soft tissue interposition and an unstable floating shoulder.

Robinson CM, Court-Brown CM, McQueen MM, Wakefield AE. Estimating the risk of nonunion following nonoperative treatment of a clavicular fracture. J Bone Joint Surg Am 2004; 86: 1359–65. A total of 581 middle-third clavicle fractures were treated non-operatively. Lack of cortical apposition and comminution correlated with a higher risk of non-union.

There have been many randomized trials comparing operative and non operative treatment of clavicle fractures. The Canadian Orthopaedic Trauma Society (COTS) trial was one of the first and the Clavicle trial from UK was one of the largest. Both favoured plate fixation for displaced midshaft clavicle fractures as there was a higher risk of nonunion in the non operatively managed patients. However, operative intervention was associated with risks of infection, prominent metalwork and mechanical failure. Clinical outcome of patients with a united fracture was similar in the operated and non-operated groups.

Canadian Orthopaedic Trauma Society. Nonoperative treatment compared with plate fixation of displaced midshaft clavicular fractures. J Bone Joint Surg Am 2007;89:1–10. 132 patients, the DASH and Constant score were better for the operated group. Faster healing and lower rate of nonunion was seen in the operated group.

Ahrens PM, Garlick NI, Barber J, Tims EM, Clavicle trial collaborative group. The clavicle trial: a multicentre, randomised controlled trial comparing operative with nonoperative treatment of displaced midshaft clavicle fractures. J Bone Joint Surg Am 2017;99(16):1345–1354. 301 patients, less rate of nonunion in the operated group, as well as better satisfaction and better score in the early post injury period only.

Options for internal fixation include threaded pin (Rockwood pin), reconstruction plate, or contoured locking clavicular plates. Threaded pins are rarely used as these are suitable in only for some fracture patterns. Reconstruction plates have a high risk of breakage. Contoured locking clavicular plates provide the most secure fixation. Anterior plating is increasingly popular compared to the traditional superior plating.

The surgical approach can be through two different incisions—along the subcuticular border of clavicle that gives easier access, or a vertical incision centred over the fracture site can be used to avoid injury to the supraclavicular cutaneous nerves.

Hill JM, McGuire MH, Crosby LA. Closed treatment of displaced middle-third fractures of the clavicle gives poor results. J Bone Joint Surg Br 1997;79(4):537–538. A total of 52 completely displaced fractures of the middle third in adults were studied. Fifteen percent resulted in non-union and the results were unsatisfactory in 31%. An initial shortening of more than 2 cm was associated with a higher risk of non-union and a final shortening of more than 2 cm was associated with a higher incidence of poor function.

Distal Third (Lateral Third) Fractures of the Clavicle

Classification

The Neer and Rockwood classification is commonly used (Table 1.6)

Neer CS 2nd. Fractures of the distal third of the clavicle. Clin Orthop 1968;58:43–50.

A modification was proposed by Jackson whereby type 2 injuries were divided into 2A and 2B (Fig. 1.10). In 2A injuries, the fracture is medial to the coracoclavicular ligaments and there is marked displacement of the proximal fragment. In Type 2B injuries, there is a bony avulsion of the coracoclavicular ligament with a small fragment of bone from the inferior surface of clavicle.

Treatment

Types I and III are treated non-operatively.

Type II injuries have marked deformity and displacement, and up to a 30% non-union rate. Surgery is often needed. Type 2A fractures are

Table 1.6 Classification of lateral third clavicle fractures

Type I	Fracture lateral to an intact coracoclavicular ligament
Type II	Fracture medial to the coracoclavicular ligament
Type III	An intra-articular AC joint fracture

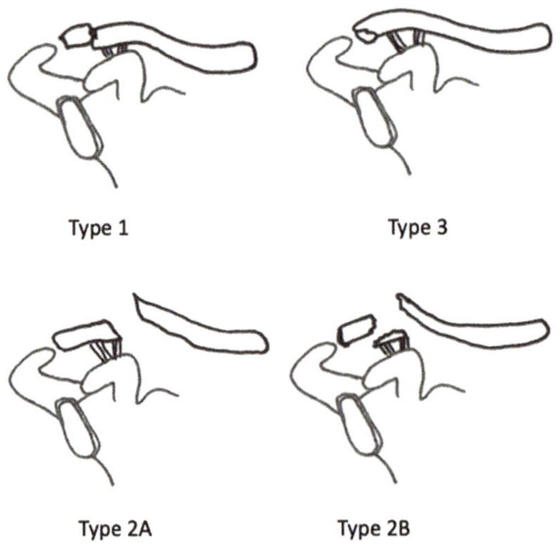

Fig. 1.10 Modified classification of lateral third clavicle fractures

managed similar to shaft fractures although often are more displaced and require surgical stabilisation using a locking plate.

Type 2B fractures can be managed by making 2 drill holes in the proximal fragment and repairing the avulsed fragment of the coracoclavicular ligament to the proximal fragment with non-absorbable sutures (5-0 ethibond). This restores continuity between the coracoclavicular ligament and the proximal fragment and keeps the fracture reduced.

Jackson WFM, Bayne G, Gregg-Smith SJ. Fractures of the lateral third of the clavicle: An Anatomic approach to treatment. J Trauma 2006; 61: 222–225. Description of the classification—2A and 2B fractures and surgical technique to repair 2B injuries.

A hook plate has been used for these injuries, but is associated with a high rate of impingement due to presence of metalwork in the subacromial space. Plate removal is required to resolve these symptoms.

Contoured locking plates allow multiple screw options in the lateral fragment and provide secure fixation if there is adequate bone stock in the lateral fragment.

Sternoclavicular Joint Dislocation

Sternoclavicular joint injuries are relatively rare. The joint is reliant on surrounding ligamentous structure for its stability. Dislocation can be anterior or posterior.

Posterior dislocation of the joint can be potentially life threatening. Atraumatic dislocation and subluxations are known to occur in collagen deficiency condition.

Anterior Dislocation

Anterior dislocation is evident clinically from a history of trauma and prominence of the medial end of the clavicle. 'Serendipity views' are the preferred radiographs. Computed tomography (CT) scanning is the best imaging modality for diagnosis. Closed reduction is possible and functional limitation is minimal even if the joint is irreducible or unstable. Most anterior dislocations are treated expectantly.

Posterior Dislocations

Posterior dislocations risk causing pressure on the mediastinal structures such as oesophagus, trachea and neurovascular structures with its incidence quoted as 30% with a mortality of 3–4%. Manipulation under anaesthetic and reduction by holding the fragment with a sharp towel clip or bone-holding forceps is needed. If unstable, soft tissue reconstruction can be planned. The reconstruction involves using a tendon graft from the semitendinosus or palmaris longus passed through the medial end of the clavicle and manubrium. More recently success has been reported using suture anchors combined with capsular repair.

Alternatively, the medial 1–2 cm of the clavicle can be excised and the remaining part stabilised to the first rib. The results of excision without soft tissue stabilisation are unsatisfactory.

Morell DJ, Thyagarajan DS. Sternoclavicular joint dislocation and its management: A review of the literature. World J Orthop. 2016:7(4):244–50.

Dislocation of the Glenohumeral Joint

Dislocation of the glenohumeral joint is a common injury. The underlying mechanism is an abduction and external rotation force that dislocates the humeral head anterior to the glenoid. The vast majority is anterior dislocation. Posterior dislocations are rare and are sometimes missed on radiographs. From a mechanistic point of view more than 95% of these dislocations are classed as 'traumatic', but a minority can occur without significant trauma and demonstrate glenohumeral laxity.

Almost 90% of patients with anterior dislocation have a Bankart's lesion. The inferior glenohumeral ligament (IGHL) is avulsed, usually from the glenoid. Occasionally the ligament may be detached from the humeral attachment. This is known as HAGL (humeral avulsion of the glenohumeral ligament). Other associated injuries include rotator cuff tears and SLAP (superior labral anterior and posterior) lesions.

Clinical Features

Patient with dislocation present with pain around the shoulder and a restricted range of motion. In anterior dislocation, the deltoid contour is lost due to the absence of the humeral head lateral to the glenoid. The acromion appears prominent and the anterior axillary fold is lower on the affected side.

Axillary nerve neurapraxia occurs in up to one-third of patients. Circulation in the arm should be checked.

Imaging

Plain radiographs are performed to assess for associated injuries: fracture of the neck of humerus, greater tuberosity or glenoid rim. Fractures of the greater tuberosity are found in up to 30% of anterior dislocations. Glenoid rim fractures are found in up to 5% of anteroinferior shoulder dislocations.

The West Point axillary view is useful to detect for fractures of the glenoid rim. The Stryker notch view will show Hill–Sachs lesions (posterolateral humeral head defects). Most patients with suspected associated fractures should have a CT scan.

Management

Isolated dislocations of the humeral head are reduced by closed means under sedation and analgesia. The techniques described for reduction are -

- Hippocratic method—the foot is placed against the proximal end of the humerus and longitudinal traction is applied to the upper extremity. This is of historical interest only.
- Kocher's manoeuvre—comprises traction and external rotation of the arm, followed by adduction and internal rotation (Fig. 1.11). Although highly successful, this technique is associated with neurovascular complications and humeral head fractures, and is currently not favoured. TEAM is a pneumonic used to remember the sequence. (Traction and external rotation followed by adduction and medial or internal rotation).
- Milch method—This technique is first done by abducting the arm then applying external rotation. Fingers are kept in the axilla directly over the humeral head. Shoulder is reduced by a combination of gentle axial traction and direct pressure over the humeral head via the axilla (Milch, 1938).

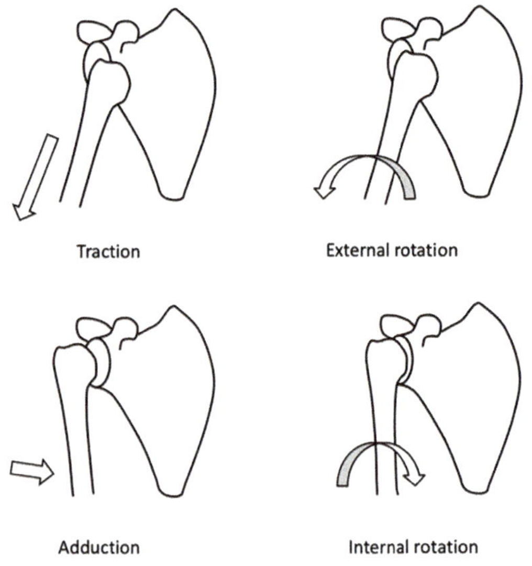

Fig. 1.11 Kocher manoeuvre for shoulder relocation

- Rockwood's method—the patient is supine with a sheet placed around the chest to apply countertraction. The arm is carefully pulled in the direction of the deformity and gentle rotational movements help disengage the humeral head.
- Spaso technique—With the patient supine, the affected arm is grasped around the wrist or distal forearm and gently lifted vertically. While maintaining vertical traction, the shoulder is slightly externally rotated. A clunk is heard or felt while reduction is done. Recent RCT comparing Spaso and Kocher's technique showed that both techniques had low complications however, Spaso technique was more effective, faster and easier to apply.

Rezende B da RM, de Almeida JI Sr, de Sousa UJ, Bomfim L de S, Ferreira MS Jr. Glenoumeral dislocation: a prospective randomized study comparing Spazo and Kocher maneuvers. Acta Ortop Bras. 2015;23(4):192–6.

Once reduction is achieved, radiographs will confirm the congruence as well as any associated fractures of the proximal humerus or scapula.

The arm is immobilised in adduction and internal rotation in a broad arm sling (e.g. Polysling). The duration of immobilisation after reduction, or the presence of a Hill–Sachs lesion, is not related to the risk of recurrence. A sling is advised for comfort and pendulum exercises are started early to minimise stiffness.

Hovelius L, Augustini BG, Fredin H, Johansson O, Norlin R, Thorling J. Primary anterior dislocation of the shoulder in young patients. A ten year prospective study. J Bone Joint Surg Br 1996;78(11):1677–84. This 10-year prospective study from Sweden reported on 245 patients aged 12–40 years. In 52% there was no further dislocation. With two recurrences within 1 year, 25% of patients were stable in long-term. A quarter of all patients needed stabilisation. The initial management had no effect on recurrence.

Bracing in external rotation (the gunslinger position) was proposed to reduce the risk of recurrence, but further studies have shown that this is no more effective than using the traditional sling in internal rotation.

Itoi E, Hatakeyama Y, Kido T, et al. A new method of immobilization after traumatic anterior dislocation of the shoulder: a preliminary study. J Shoulder Elbow Surg 2003;12:413–5. This study proposed bracing in external rotation.

Finestone A, Milgrom C, Radeva-Petrova DR, et al. Bracing in external rotation for traumatic anterior dislocation of the shoulder. J Bone Joint Surg Br 2009;91:918–21. This was a prospective randomised study in 51 patients. No advantage to bracing in external rotation was found.

Recent studies show that approximately half of the patients have recurrence within 2 years following traumatic anterior dislocation. There is moderate evidence suggesting that acute labral repair following first time traumatic dislocation helps to reduce the recurrence rates.

te Slaa RL, Wijffels MP, Brand R, Marti RK. The prognosis following acute primary glenohumeral dislocation. J Bone Joint Surg Br 2004;86(1):58–64. 105 patients with 4 year follow-up, overall recurrence was 26%. The recurrence rate was 64% in those aged less than 20 years compared with 6% in those aged more than 40 years.

Kavaja L, Lähdeoja T, Malmivaara A, Paavola M. Treatment after traumatic shoulder dislocation: a systematic review with a network meta-analysis. Br J Sports Med. 2018;52(23):1498–506.

Posterior Dislocation

Posterior dislocations represent approximately 4% of all shoulder dislocations. These dislocations are often missed at the initial evaluation, leading to permanent disability. Anterior trauma to an abducted and externally rotated shoulder is the most common mechanism of posterior dislocations. Additionally violent muscle contraction during seizures and electrocutions are associated with posterior dislocations.

Physical finding of locked internal rotation of shoulder provides a valuable clue on diagnosis. Standard AP radiographs are often inadequate for diagnosis. A recent review has shown that up to 70% of posterior shoulder dislocations were missed at initial evaluation. The 'light bulb sign' represents a symmetric proximal humerus on the AP view due to fixed internal rotation. The tuberosities are not visualised due to internal rotation. Additionally, there is no overlap of the humeral head and glenoid due to lateral displacement of the humeral head. Loss of a smooth scapulohumeral arch (Moloney line) is also evident.

Additional axially views and CT scan has shown to increase the diagnostic potential to up to 100%. Missed posterior dislocation leads to permanent reduction in ROM and loss of function (Fig. 1.12).

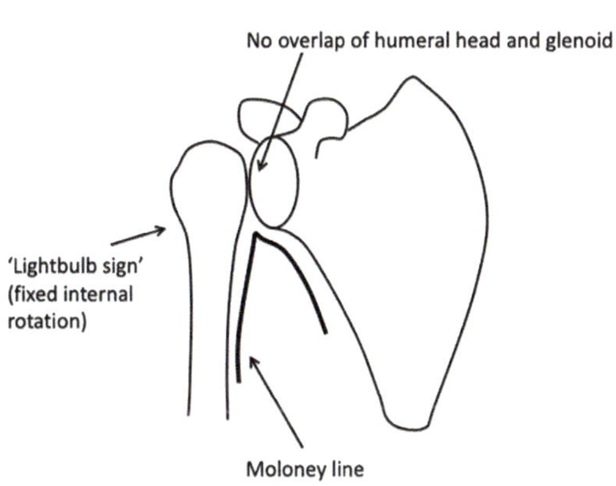

Fig. 1.12 Radiological signs of posterior glenohumeral dislocation

Closed reduction is successful under suitable anaesthesia. The arm is immobilised in external rotation and extension. Open reduction is usually performed through an anterior approach. If the impression fracture (reverse Hill–Sachs) is more than 25% of the humeral head, either subscapularis tendon (McLaughlin method) or the lesser tuberosity (Hughes and Neers procedure) is transferred into the defect.

Aydin N, Enes Kayaalp M, Asansu M, Karaismailoglu B. Treatment options for locked posterior shoulder dislocations and clinical outcomes. EFORT Open Rev. 2019 May 11;4(5):194–200.

Fracture of the Proximal Humerus

Fractures of the proximal humerus are common injuries and often caused by relatively low energy trauma in elderly osteopenic individuals. Four parts of the proximal humerus fracture were first described by Codman and later included in the classification by Neer (Fig. 1.13).

The humeral head is covered by the articular cartilage and hence has a poor blood supply. The lesser tuberosity has the attachment of the subscapularis and the greater tuberosity provides attachment to the remaining three rotator cuff muscles. The humeral shaft is separated from the proximal humerus by fracture of the surgical neck.

Neer CS 2nd. Displaced proximal humeral fractures. Part I. Classification and evaluation. Clin Orthop 1987;223:3–10.

The main blood supply of the humeral head is derived from the anterior circumflex humeral

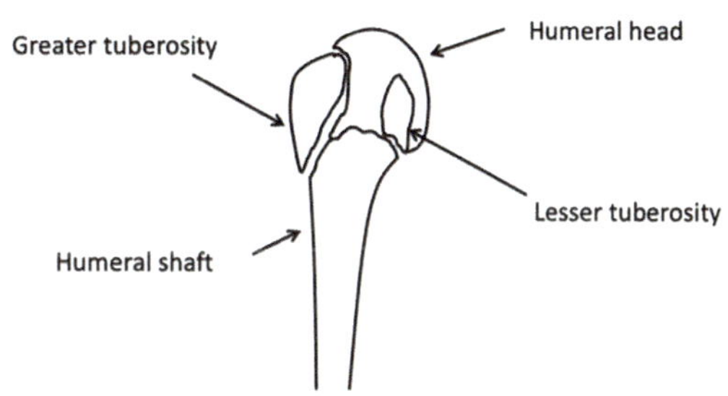

Fig. 1.13 Four parts of the proximal humerus

artery, a branch of the third part of axillary artery (Fig. 1.14). The arcuate artery arises from the anterior circumflex, runs proximally in the bicipital groove, and enters the head from the metaphysis. The posterior circumflex artery provides a small contribution and is, in itself, unable to maintain vascularity. Fracture of the lesser tuberosity implies a significant risk of loss of blood supply to the humeral head.

Classification

The Neer classification for displaced fractures is based on displacement of segments instead of actual fracture lines (see above). A segment is considered displaced if it is more than 45° angulated or more than 1 cm translated. Based on the number of displaced segments as described above, a fracture may be 2-part, 3-part or 4-part. This classification has poor interobserver reliability.

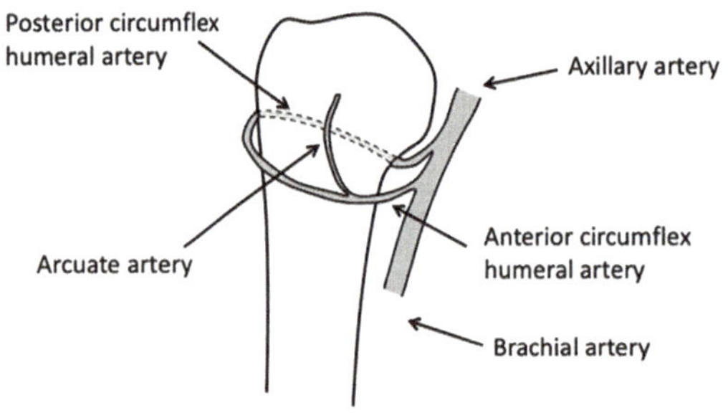

Fig. 1.14 Vascular supply to proximal humerus

Fragment stability is an important consideration. A compression fracture will heal faster than a shear fracture.

Hertel Criteria for Humeral Head Perfusion

It is important to determine if the blood supply and bone quality are adequate. The Hertel criteria for perfusion of the humeral head can be used to predict ischemia (Fig. 1.15). A metaphyseal extension of the humeral head of less than 8 mm and medial hinge disruption of more than 2 mm suggest poor humeral head blood supply. A combination of metaphyseal extension of the humeral head <8 mm, medial hinge disruption of more than 2 mm, and an anatomic neck fracture pattern has a 97% positive predictive value for humeral head ischemia. Such fractures may be best managed by arthroplasty.

Management

Impacted/Undisplaced Fractures

These fractures can be managed in a collar and cuff sling for 2 weeks, with pendulum exercises starting as soon as pain allows. These are followed by active range of motion exercises—usually within three weeks of injury.

Impacted fractures with unacceptable displacement in active patients require operative correction and stabilisation.

Fig. 1.15 Hertel criteria for poor prognosis in proximal humeral fractures

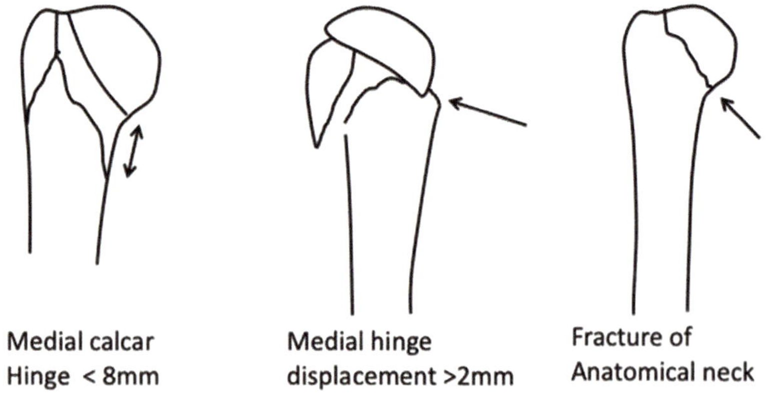

Displaced Two-Part Fractures

Displaced shear fractures in young patients are best managed by internal fixation.

For operative treatment, the choices are reduction and stabilisation with a proximal humeral locking plate, intramedullary nail, or percutaneous pins. The locking plate provides rigid fixation and is stable enough to allow early mobilisation, with consequent early rehabilitation.

Greater tuberosity fractures should be reduced and fixed if displaced more than 5 mm. The displaced fracture may block abduction or external rotation, and hence operative stabilisation is indicated. A tension-band wire or heavy suture or screw fixation can be used to achieve stability. These fractures are sometimes associated with anterior dislocation.

Lesser tuberosity fractures may be associated with posterior dislocation of the humeral head. Displaced fractures require rotator cuff repair and stabilisation.

Displaced anatomical neck fractures in young patients are managed by fixation with screws. Fixation will not prevent avascular necrosis (AVN), but the head may revascularise before collapse, if the fracture heals. In the elderly and low-demand patients, hemiarthroplasty is the treatment of choice.

Displaced Three-Part Fractures

Fixation of surgical neck fracture and stabilisation of the greater tuberosity is performed with a locking proximal humeral plate. The deltopectoral approach is commonly used. A delay of over two weeks before surgery makes reduction and fixation difficult. Almost one in four patients develop avascular necrosis, but this is frequently asymptomatic as it involves only a part of the head.

Displaced Four-Part Fracture

In valgus impacted fractures, minimal lateral displacement of the humeral head is associated with intact medial epiphyseal arteries and a viable head. The tuberosities maintain some blood supply to the humeral head. If head is not mechanically blocking abduction, these patients can be managed non-operatively.

The results of early arthroplasty are better than the results of arthroplasty after failed internal fixation. Neer reported 100% poor results with fixation and recommended hemiarthroplasty for all patients.

Neer CS 2nd. Four segment classification of proximal humeral fractures: purpose and reliable use. J Shoulder Elbow Surg 2002;11(4):389–400.

Fixation of Three- and Four-Part Proximal Humerus Fractures

The PROFHER trial (Proximal Fracture of the Humerus Evaluation by Randomisation) has provided new evidence towards optimum management of these injuries. No benefit was found through operative treatment of these injuries in this trial.

Rangan A, Handoll H, Brearley S. Surgical versus non surgical treatment of adults with displaced fractures of the proximal humerus. The PROFHER randomized clinical trial. JAMA 2015;313:1037–47. Multicentre trial with 231 patients with displaced proximal humerus fractures. Randomised to operative vs. nonoperative treatment. Choice of operative stabilisation was left to treating surgeon. No difference in the two groups over 2 years in Oxford shoulder score and SF-12 score.

Patients treated with internal fixation have a significant risk of complications.

Südkamp N, Bayer J, Hepp P, et al. Open reduction and internal fixation of proximal humeral fractures with use of the locking proximal humerus plate. Results of a prospective, multicenter, observational study. J Bone Joint Surg Am 2009;91:1320–8. From 187 patients 34% experienced a complication, of which 40% were related to the incorrect surgical technique. The reoperation rate was 19% within 1 year.

The oblique screw in the locking plate provides medial support and is the most important screw when fixing these fractures with a locking plate.

Reverse Total Shoulder Arthroplasty (RTSA) for Osteoporotic Three- and Four-Part Fractures

Traditionally hemiarthroplasty was considered as a treatment for unreconstructible 3 and 4 part fractures with moderate outcomes. The current trend seems to be shifted towards RTSA for such fractures. Healing of tuberosities is associated with improved functional outcomes.

Stone MA, Namdari S. Surgical considerations in the treatment of osteoporotic proximal humerus fractures. Orthop Clin North Am. 2019 Apr;50(2):223–31.

A recent meta-analysis comparing the reverse shoulder with hemiarthroplasty showed better clinical outcome with reverse shoulder replacement.

Gallinet D, Ohl X, Decroocq L, Dib C, Valenti P, Boileau P; French Society for Orthopaedic Surgery (SOFCOT). Is reverse total shoulder arthroplasty more effective than hemiarthroplasty for treating displaced proximal humerus fractures in older adults? A systematic review and meta-analysis. Orthop Traumatol Surg Res. 2018; 104(6):759–66.

See Chap. 2 for details on reverse shoulder replacement.

Fracture Dislocations of the Shoulder

Closed or open reduction of the humeral head may be used. ORIF is indicated in three-part fracture dislocations. In four-part dislocations, an effort should be made to preserve the humeral head in young patients. In older patients, reverse total shoulder may be the best option.

Articular surface impression defects are generally associated with dislocations of the glenohumeral joint with the glenoid making the impression on the head. Treatment options are

- For anterior defects—transfer of the subscapularis with or without the lesser tuberosity into the defect.
- For posterior defects—Remplissage or proximal humeral retroversion osteotomy.
- For large defects (>40%)—prosthetic replacement or autografting.

With humeral head splitting fractures, there is a high risk of AVN in fragments. Prosthetic replacement is often needed.

Surgical Approach

The deltopectoral approach provides extensile exposure. The deltoid can be reflected from the clavicle as an osteoperiosteal flap. This can be combined with an acromion osteotomy for further exposure of the proximal fragments. The acromion osteotomy is fixed back with screws.

For limited access, a deltoid splitting approach is an option.

Humeral Shaft Fracture

Humeral shaft fractures are commonly low-energy injuries. Humeral shaft fractures account for 3% of all fractures.

Ekholm R, Adami J, Tidermark J, et al. Fractures of the shaft of humerus. An epidemiological study of 401 fractures. J Bone Joint Surg Br 2006;88:1469–73. The incidence was 14.5 per 100,000 per year and increased with age. Radial nerve palsy was seen in 8% of 401 fractures. Two percent of fractures were open and 8% were pathological.

Classification

The AO classification for diaphyseal fractures is commonly used for humeral shaft fractures (Fig. 1.16)

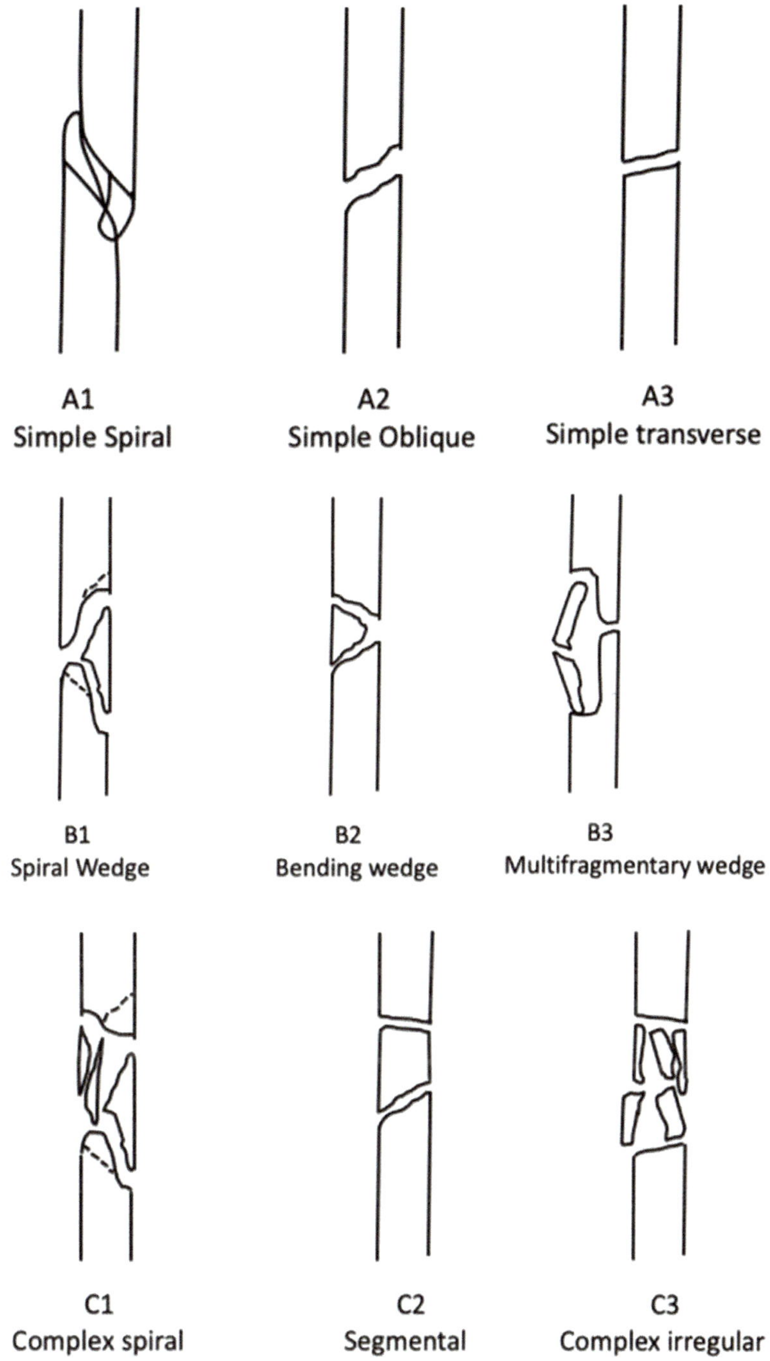

Fig. 1.16 AO diaphyseal fracture classification

Management

Most humeral shaft fractures are managed non-operatively. Bracing achieves healing in more than 90% of cases and can be preceded by a period of 1–2 weeks in a cast splint. However it often takes up to 12 weeks of immobilisation to achieve solid bony union. It can also be difficult to control fracture alignment in some patients. The current trend is towards an aggressive approach with a low threshold for internal fixation, particularly in young, active patients.

Klenerman L. Fractures of the shaft of the humerus. J Bone Joint Surg Br 1966; 48: 105–11. Twenty-degree anterior angulation, 30° varus angulation and up to 3 cm of shortening is well tolerated with little functional deficit.

The indications for surgery are as follows:

- Open fractures.
- Vascular injury.
- Pathologic fractures.
- Polytrauma.
- Segmental fractures.
- Irreducible fracture or unacceptable alignment with non-operative treatment (includes the long spiral fractures, which often have soft tissue interposition).
- Spiral fracture of the distal third (Holstein Lewis) with radial nerve palsy.
- Floating elbow.
- Patient unable to tolerate or adhere to non-operative treatment.
- Associated chest-wall trauma or bilateral fractures.
- Radial nerve palsy developing secondary to manipulation of the fracture.

The posterior approach allows exposure of 15 cm of the humerus above the lateral epicondyle (20 cm above the medial epicondyle) before the radial nerve is encountered. The recommended approach is to identify the nerve between the long and lateral head of the triceps (approximately 9 cm from the tip of the acromion) and identify it along its course.

Indications for exploring the radial nerve are

- Open fractures.
- Nerve palsy occurring after closed reduction.
- Holstein and Lewis fracture—closed spiral fracture at the distal third of the humerus where the radial nerve is at high risk of being trapped between the two fragments. If nerve palsy develops after closed reduction, exploration and internal fixation is indicated.

Ekholm R, Ponzer S, Törnkvist H, et al. The Holstein–Lewis humeral shaft fracture: aspects of radial nerve injury, primary treatment, and outcome. J Orthop Trauma 2008;22:693–7. This retrospective multicentre study looked at 27 patients with a Holstein–Lewis fracture. The risk of radial nerve injury was 22% compared with 8% for humeral fractures in general. Seven patients were managed operatively. Six patients had radial nerve injury (two managed non-operatively and four operatively). There was no relationship between radial nerve recovery and operative management.

In other situations, it may be advisable to wait for up to 3 months and observe the recovery of nerve function. In most instances the nerve will recover. If there is no recovery then nerve conduction studies are undertaken, followed by nerve repair/graft or tendon transfer.

Plating

Locking plates or dynamic compression plates are used. Fixation extending to eight cortices on either side of fracture is desirable. A 96% union rate with 2% incidence of radial nerve palsy has been reported. A broad plate with staggered holes is preferable to avoid the possibility of fissuring (longitudinal splitting) of the shaft.

In the upper two-thirds, plates are applied on the anterior or anterolateral surface to avoid injury to the radial nerve. The humeral shaft is exposed after splitting the brachialis, which carries a dual nerve supply. In the distal third, plates are easier to apply on the flat posterior surface.

The relationship of the radial nerve and plate should be recorded in the notes.

McCormack RG, Brien D, Buckley RE, et al. Fixation of fractures of the shaft of the humerus by dynamic compression plate or intramedullary nail. A prospective, randomised trial. J Bone Joint Surg Br 2000;82:336–9. This study randomised 44 patients with a 6 month follow-up. Six patients with fixation by an intramedullary nail experienced shoulder impingement, seven needed secondary surgery and 13 had a complication. Only three patients with a plate experienced a complication.

Intramedullary Nail

In antegrade humeral nailing, the rotator cuff should be repaired at the entry site and the proximal end of the nail should be under the surface of the bone. The intramedullary canal ends 2–3 cm above the olecranon fossa. The nail should be statically locked. Distal locking carries a risk of injury to the nerves around the elbow, but improves stability.

In retrograde nailing, the entry point is located posteriorly, 2.5 cm above the olecranon fossa. A triceps splitting approach is used. There is a risk of iatrogenic fracture and myositis ossificans in the triceps, leading to elbow stiffness.

Nailing is preferable for segmental fractures and pathologic fractures.

Crates J, Whittle AP. Antegrade interlocking nailing of acute humeral shaft fractures. Clin Orthop Relat Res 1998;350:40–50. From 73 acute fractures, the authors recorded non-union in 6%, transient radial nerve palsies in 3% and infection in 2%. Ninety percent of patients regained normal shoulder function and 96% regained normal elbow function.

External Fixation

Uniplanar lateral fixators are generally used. The radial nerve is at risk of injury during pin insertion. The usual indications are temporary stabilisation in polytrauma victims and for patients with open fractures.

Periprosthetic Humeral Fractures

Periprosthetic humeral fractures involve fracture of the humerus in the presence of a shoulder or elbow replacement prosthesis.

In well-fixed components, the aim is to achieve healing of the fracture with fixation rather than revision of the humeral stem. A shaft fracture can be stabilised with a compression plate supplemented with cable, strut graft or bone grafting. Revision of the prosthesis is considered if the components are loose.

Removal of plates from the humerus runs the risk of radial nerve injury. Adequate healing of the fracture should be confirmed before plate removal. Patients should abstain from heavy lifting for 6–8 weeks following plate removal to reduce the risk of fracture through the screw holes.

Fracture of the Distal Humerus

The distal humeral articular surface comprises the trochlea and the capitellum. The trochlea is shaped like an hourglass while the capitellum is spherical. The articular surface is angled anteriorly, in the sagittal plane, by 30° in relation to the shaft. Additionally, the articular surface is tilted laterally (valgus) in the coronal plane, giving the 'carrying angle' of the elbow (Fig. 1.17). The normal angle is 10–15° in males and 12–16° in females.

The medial collateral ligament extends between the medial epicondyle of humerus and the sublime tubercle of ulna and is tight in pronation. The lateral collateral ligament extends from the lateral epicondyle of humerus to the crista supinatorus of ulna and is tight in supination.

Anatomical Types

Supracondylar Fracture in Adults

These can be managed non-operatively with a hanging cast. Alternatively, ORIF can be used with crossed compression screws in the medial and lateral pillars. Contoured plates can be applied for comminuted fractures.

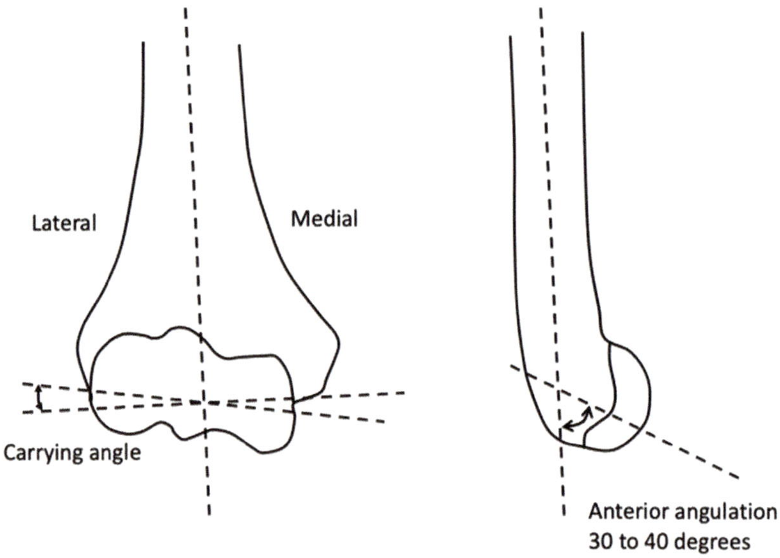

Fig. 1.17 Alignment of the distal humeral articular surface

Transcondylar Fractures

The fracture line in transcondylar fractures is intra-articular and runs across the condyles. These are unstable injuries and the callus itself may restrict motion. Percutaneous cannulated screws through both columns can enable early motion and restoration of function.

Intercondylar Fractures

A commonly used classification was given by Riseborough and Radin (Fig. 1.18).

Riseborough EJ, Radin EL. Intercondylar T fractures of the humerus in the adult. A comparison of operative and nonoperative treatment in 29 cases. J Bone Joint Surg Am 1969;51(1):130–41.

Jupiter and Mehne classified them as High T, Low T, Y, H, medial lambda and lateral lambda pattern based on fracture configuration. This system is purely descriptive.

The AO group has proposed a classification for distal humeral fractures (Fig. 1.19). This is useful in planning surgical approach and fixation.

Planning should be conducted preoperatively on radiographs. CT scans are also useful in planning. Intra-operative traction radiographs can be helpful in defining various fragments.

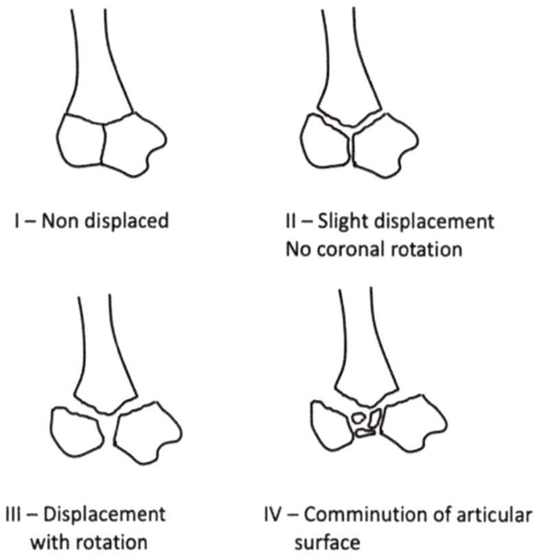

Fig. 1.18 Classification of intercondylar fractures

Doornberg J, Lindenhoivius A, Kloen P, van Dijk CN, Zurakowski D, Ring D. Two and three-dimensional computed tomography for the classification and management of distal humeral fractures. Evaluation of reliability and diagnostic accuracy. J Bone Joint Surg Am 2006;88:1795–801. CT scanning helps in classification but may not necessarily lead to better treatment decision making.

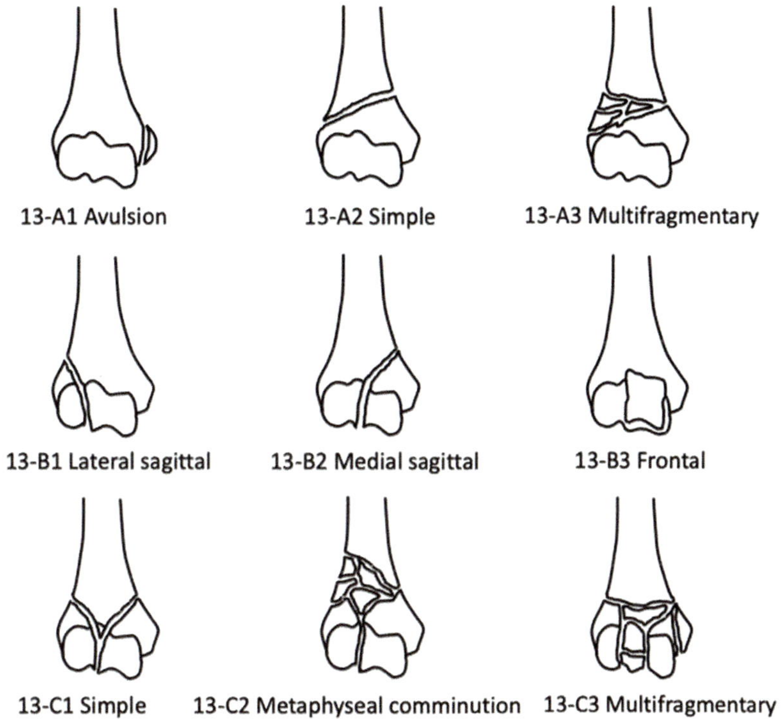

Fig. 1.19 AO classification of intercondylar fractures

Fracture of Medial or Lateral Humeral Condyle in Adults

Displaced fractures are fixed by a medial or a lateral incision. These are intra-articular injuries and require stable anatomic fixation and early mobilisation.

Fracture of the Lateral Epicondyle

These are generally associated with elbow dislocations. The fragment usually reduces once the elbow is reduced. If satisfactory alignment is achieved, the injury can be managed non-operatively. If rotated, internal fixation is advisable.

Fracture of the Medial Epicondyle

This is rare in adults and is usually the result of a direct injury or an avulsion fracture. Small, undisplaced fractures do not need surgery.

Indications for surgery include a fragment displaced into the elbow joint and displaced fractures in high-demand patients. Fixation is achieved with a screw and the ulnar nerve should be protected from iatrogenic injury.

Management

The choice of treatment depends on the patient's age, functional demand, degree of osteoporosis, type of fracture, degree of displacement, extent of joint involvement and the presence of compression fractures of joint surfaces.

Undisplaced fractures can be managed non-operatively. An initial cast is followed by gradual mobilisation. The elbow should not be immobilised for longer than three weeks to reduce risk of permanent stiffness.

Displaced fractures require internal fixation. Surgery is preferably performed within 48 h. An open fracture, associated vascular injury and other associated injuries are indications for urgent surgery. Open fractures should be debrided and internally fixed to reduce the risk of sepsis. In the presence of gross contamination and delayed presentation, spanning fixators can be used for temporary stabilisation.

As a treatment, traction imposes a long period of hospitalisation, results in stiffness and does not restore anatomical alignment. It is only for the rare situation where internal fixation is not possible.

Surgical Approach

Intra-articular fractures of the distal humerus are ideally treated with anatomic reduction, rigid internal fixation and early active mobilisation.

A variety of surgical approaches have been described including triceps splitting, triceps reflecting, TRAP (triceps reflecting anconeus pedicle), para tricipital or transolecranon (olecranon osteotomy). The paratricipital approach allows exposure along medial and lateral borders of the mobilised triceps and does not weaken the muscle. It can be extended through an olecranon osteotomy if further exposure is required of the articular surface.

The incision is posterior in the midline of the arm and ends distal to the olecranon, curving medially around the point of the elbow. Curving the incision medially is cosmetically more acceptable and gives easy access to the ulnar nerve. The ulnar nerve should always be identified and protected. Most fractures with intra-articular displacement or comminution are best visualised with a transolecranon approach.

Campbell's posterior approach involves elevation of a distally based U-flap of the triceps aponeurosis to expose the distal humerus.

An alternative approach of TRAP (triceps reflecting anconeus pedicle) with patient in supine position has also been descried. This approach provides adequate exposure of the distal humerus without complications associated with olecranon osteotomy.

O'Driscoll SW. The triceps-reflecting anconeus pedicle (TRAP) approach for distal humeral fractures and nonunions. Orthop Clin North Am. 2000;31(1):91–101.

In olecranon osteotomy (Fig. 1.20), extra-articular osteotomy provides unrestricted exposure. The technique is described in Chap. 18—Surgical approaches.

Olecranon osteotomy is relatively contraindicated if a total elbow replacement is being considered

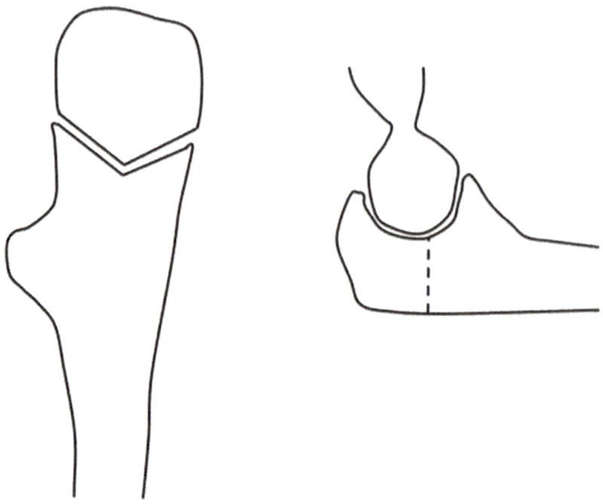

Fig. 1.20 Olecranon osteotomy

Principles of Surgery

Careful preoperative planning is essential to decide the fixation method and approach. Lateral positioning gives access to the posterior aspect of the arm and elbow. The draping should allow free movement of the extremity. Reconstruction of the articular fragments is performed first, and then the articular block is fixed to the diaphysis. Provisional stabilisation can be gained by K-wires or the guide wire of a cannulated screw system. Soft tissue attachments of the fragments should be protected to preserve vascularity.

The metalwork is placed on the medial and lateral columns and should not encroach on the olecranon fossa, coronoid fossa or radial fossa. Traditionally, two plates placed at 90° to each other were used. One plate was applied to the medial border and the other posterolaterally.

More recent biomechanical research has highlighted parallel plating provides greater stability. Precontoured plates are applied to the medial and lateral border of distal humerus. The screws interdigitate and provide better stability.

Stoffel K, Cunneen S, Morgan R, Nicholls R, Stachowiak G. Comparative stability of perpendicular versus parallel double-locking plating systems in osteoporotic comminuted distal humerus fractures. J Orthop Res 2008;26(6):778–784.

O'Driscoll SW. Optimizing stability in distal humeral fracture fixation. J Shoulder Elbow Surg. 2005;14(1 Suppl S):186S–194S.

However, expert opinion and biomechanical studies indicate that 90-90 plating (perpendicular plating or orthogonal plating) provides adequate stability to allow early functional movement of the reconstructed elbow. The parallel plating is perceived as technically more challenging and involves extensive soft tissue dissection.

Guitton TG, Juiter JB. 90-90 vs parallel plating of distal humeral fractures. Aofoundation.org. Expert zone. Chapter 28.

Precontoured plates with locking screws individually designed for the medial and lateral column provide stable fixation and multiple screw options (Fig. 1.21). These are preferable to intraoperatively contoured small fragment plates. Postoperatively, supervised active motion can be started after 48–72 h if stable fixation has been achieved. Immobilisation for 3 weeks in a cast leads to stiffness and early mobilisation is always preferable.

Complications

Complications include infection, nonunion, malunion, heterotopic ossification, nerve injury and failure of fixation.

Doornberg JN, van Duijn PJ, Linzel D, et al. Surgical treatment of intra-articular fractures of the distal part of the humerus. Functional outcome after twelve to thirty years. J Bone Joint Surg Am 2007;89(7):1524–32. This study conducted a long-term follow-up of 30 patients with an AO type C fracture. The average flexion arc was 106° and the average pronation–supination arc 165° at final follow up. Overall, 26 patients had a good or excellent result, and the rest had a fair or poor result.

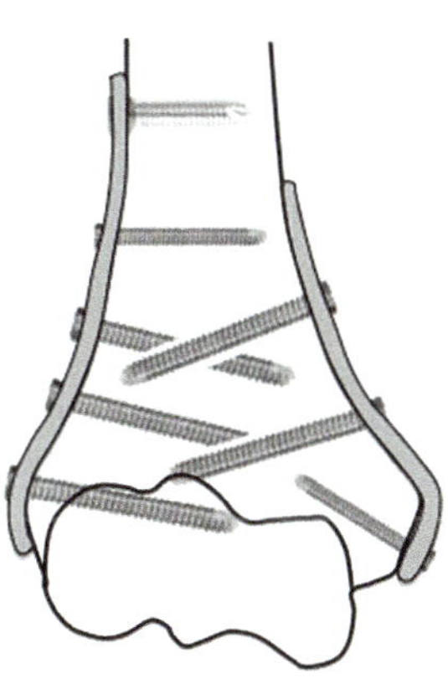

Fig. 1.21 Precontoured plates for medial and lateral column

ORIF is not contraindicated in elderly patients. Selective use of total elbow arthroplasty to treat fractures of the distal part of the humerus for infirm, less active older patients and patients with inflammatory arthritis has acceptable longevity in surviving patients, but at the cost of a number of major complications.

Barco R, Streubel PN, Morrey BF, Sanchez-Sotelo J. Total Elbow Arthroplasty for Distal Humeral Fractures: A Ten-Year-Minimum Follow-up Study. J Bone Joint Surg Am. 2017 Sep 20;99(18):1524–31.

Capitellum Fracture

The mechanism of a capitellum fracture is a shearing injury, because the centre of the capitellum is 12–15 mm anterior to the humeral shaft axis.

Classification

Classification is illustrated in Fig. 1.22.

Type I has a large fragment of bone and cartilage while type II is a superficial fracture of the subchondral bone and articular cartilage. Type IV is coronal shear of the capitellum and part of the trochlear ridge (described by McKee et al).

A double-arc sign on lateral X-ray indicates coronal shear fracture of the capitellum.

McKee MD, Jupiter JB, Bamburger HB. Coronal shear fractures of the distal end of humerus. J Bone Joint Surg Am 1996;78(1):49–54.

More complex articular fractures involving the lateral condyle and extending to the trochlea have been described by Ring.

Ring D, Jupiter JB, Gulotta L. Articular fractures of the distal part of the humerus. J Bone Joint Surg Am 2003;85(2):232–8.

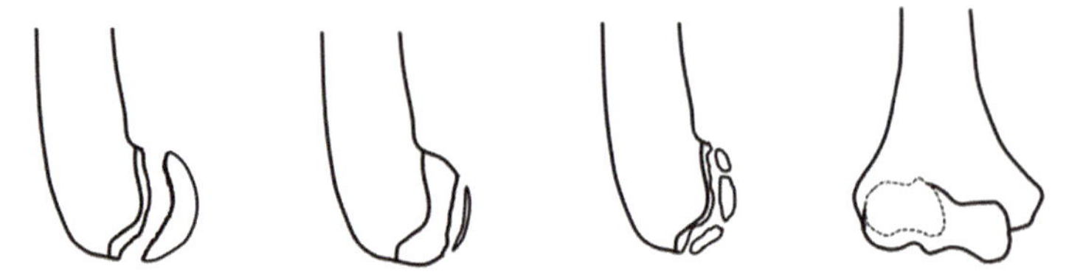

Fig. 1.22 Classification of capitellar fractures

Management

The anterior aspect of capitellum articulates with the radial head in the flexed elbow. The posterior surface of the capitellum is non-articular. The osteochondral fragment often displaces superiorly into the radial fossa of the distal humerus.

Type I fractures are managed with closed or open reduction and internal fixation. A lateral approach is taken between the anconeus and the extensor carpi ulnaris. Fixation is performed with headless screws (Herbert screw) or a posteroanterior lag screw. The screw is countersunk.

Type II and III fractures are managed with early excision. Small fragments are difficult to fix due to high shear forces and excision may provide the best chance for minimising disability.

Type IV fractures and other complex fractures with trochlear extension are best treated with internal fixation. These injuries can be clearly defined with preoperative CT scans. Most type IV fractures can be stabilised through a lateral approach, but some with medial extension warrant a posterior approach and lateral columnar plate fixation.

Complications

Complications include avascular necrosis, non-union, malunion and elbow stiffness.

Elbow Dislocations

The elbow centre of rotation is 12–15 mm anterior to the humeral shaft axis. The articular surface on the radial head covers an arc of 240°. There is a bare area on the lateral side of radial head of 110°, which is a safe area for fixation devices. The proximal ulna forms an arc of 60–80°, which articulates with the radius.

Elbow dislocation can be posterior, anterior, medial, lateral or divergent, based on the position of the forearm in relation to the distal humerus (Fig. 1.23). Combinations are possible and common. In divergent dislocation there is disruption of the radioulnar joint with separation of the radius and ulna.

Clinical Assessment

The direction of dislocation is assessed. Posterior or posterolateral dislocations are most common. Anterior dislocation is often associated with fracture of proximal ulna.

Injury to the median, ulnar or anterior interosseous nerve is evaluated. Most nerve injuries are neurapraxia due to stretch and resolve spontaneously.

Injury to brachial artery is also assessed. Intimal damage is due to stretching. This may cause acute vascular occlusion or delayed occlusion as a result of thrombosis. A vein graft may be needed if vascularity is not restored after reduction.

Management

Simple elbow dislocations without associated fractures are managed with prompt relocation and early active mobilisation. Close follow-up with X-rays is required to detect dislocation recurrence.

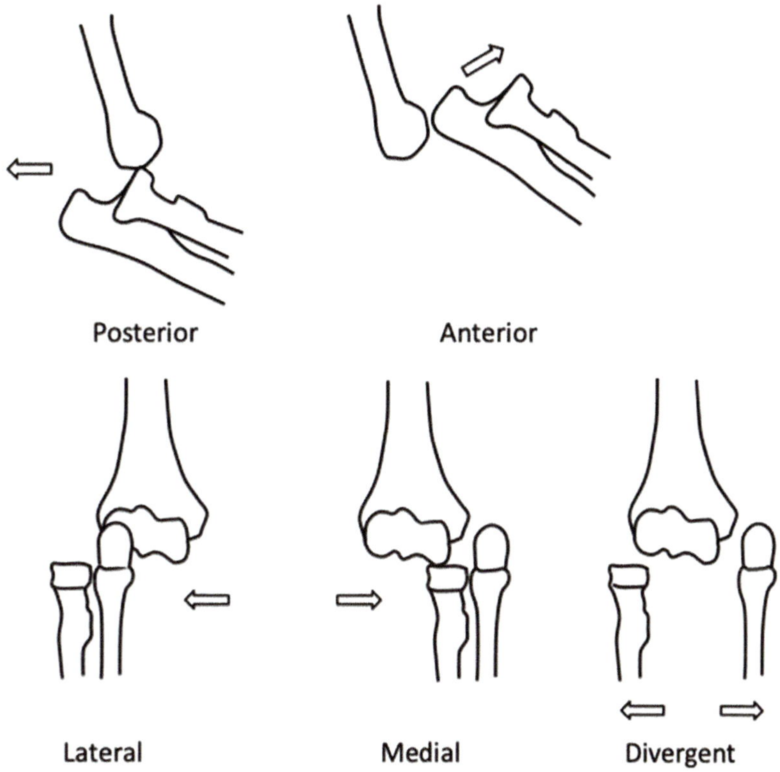

Fig. 1.23 Types of elbow dislocation

Open reduction is required if closed reduction is unsuccessful. A posterior approach gives access to both medial and lateral structures. The lateral approach may be useful if the dislocation is associated with a radial head fracture and ligament injury.

Traditionally, the elbow was kept immobilized for 3 weeks following dislocation. However, recent studies have shown that early active mobilization gives better short term clinical outcome and early return to work.

Fracture dislocations are screened for instability under anaesthesia. If unstable at or beyond 30° of extension, fixation of coronoid and radial head fractures, along with reconstruction of lateral ligament complex may be required.

Iordens GI et al; FuncSiE Trial Investigators. Early mobilisation versus plaster immobilisation of simple elbow dislocations: results of the FuncSiE multicentre randomised clinical trial. Br J Sports Med. 2017 Mar;51(6):531–538. 100 patients, prospective RCT. Early mobilisation resulted in faster return to work and no increase in complications.

Indications for Nerve Exploration

Exploration is considered if there is no recovery from nerve injury 3 months after dislocation. Onset of nerve palsy signs after reduction is a further indication for exploration.

Complications

Stiffness is common and most patients experience loss of 5–10° of terminal extension in the early rehabilitation period.

Posttraumatic arthritis may result from elbow fracture dislocations.

Heterotopic ossification can cause significant stiffness. It may appear radiologically within 4 weeks. It is related to soft tissue damage and possibly passive elbow mobilisation. Preventative measures include local radiation therapy, which is often impractical considering the presence of a fracture or surgical incision. Indomethacin can be given orally.

Ectopic calcification in the collateral ligaments and capsule is common and does not require treatment.

Terrible Triad

The 'terrible triad' describes dislocation of the elbow, coronoid fracture and radial head fracture (Fig. 1.24). The lateral ulnar collateral ligament is often torn in this pattern. This may lead to recurrent posterior subluxation or dislocation with a poor outcome.

Most series report uniformly poor result in patients with the terrible triad. Radial head excision in this situation is contraindicated as it often leads to redislocation and instability. Radial head fixation versus arthroplasty has been long debated. The choice of fixation versus replacement is dictated by fracture pattern. In general, fixation of radial head fractures with more than 3 parts is prone to early failure and arthroplasty may be preferred in such cases.

Overstuffing of the radiocapitellar joint is a major issue with radial head arthroplasty and should be avoided. Routine fixation of coronoid fractures is debated. However, if coronoid fixation is planned then the repair sequence should be from inside out: coronoid, radial head, and LCL complex. A hinged elbow external fixator can be applied to provide stability while the soft tissues heal. The hinge allows flexion and extension and the axis of the hinge is aligned with the axis of rotation of the elbow joint.

Chen NC, Ring D. Terrible Triad Injuries of the Elbow. J Hand Surg Am. 2015; 40(11):2297–303.

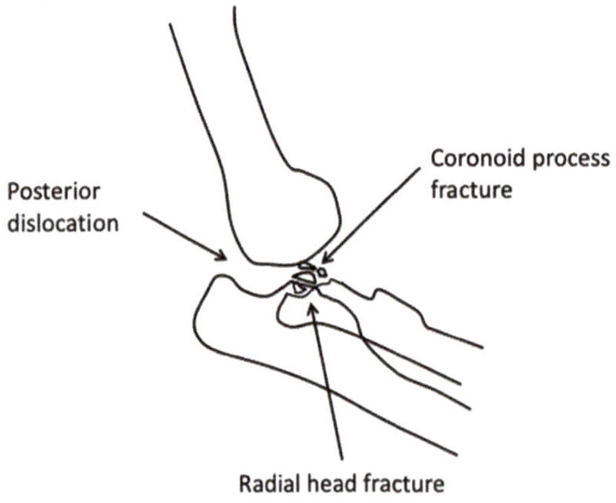

Fig. 1.24 Terrible triad of elbow dislocation

Recurrent Elbow Dislocation

Injury to the lateral collateral ligament leads to chronic posterolateral instability of the elbow. Clinically this causes pain, swelling, instability and clicking. A pivot shift test of the elbow is positive. Management is based on reconstructing the ligament using tendon grafts.

Coronoid Fracture

Classification

The classification was proposed by Regan and Morrey (Fig. 1.25). The tip of coronoid provides attachment to the brachialis and the capsule of the elbow joint. Fractures of the coronoid involving less than 50% of coronoid may not lead to instability. This system did not account for injuries to the anteromedial facet.

Regan W, Morrey B. Fractures of the coronoid process of the ulna. J Bone Joint Surg Am 1989;71(9):1348–54.

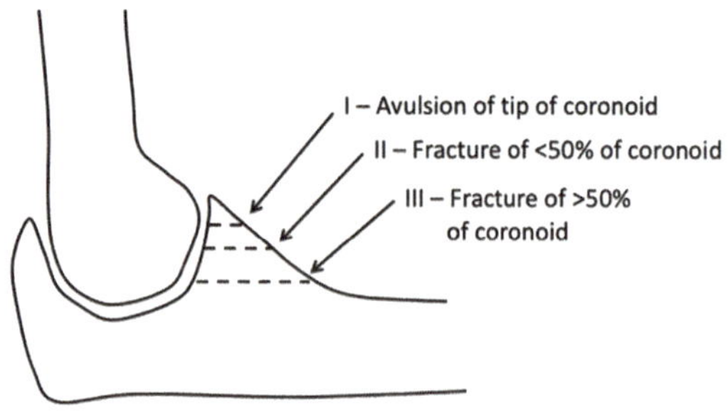

Fig. 1.25 Fractures of the coronoid

Management

Types I and II are managed with conservative treatment with early mobilisation. If the injury is associated with elbow dislocation, the brachialis is reattached with non-absorbable sutures passed through drill holes in the proximal ulna.

Type III fracture is managed with reduction and fixation with early mobilisation. These fractures are often associated with elbow dislocations. An interfragmentary screw is used to fix the fracture.

Anteromedial Facet Fracture of Coronoid

The anteromedial aspect of the coronoid is the part of coronoid which projects medially and is relatively unsupported (Fig. 1.26). Over 70% of the coronoid lies medial to the longitudinal axis of ulna. A compression fracture of the anteromedial facet of the coronoid has been described. The mechanism is predominantly varus force with concomitant injury to the lateral collateral ligament. This leads to posteromedial rotatory instability (PMRI) of the elbow.

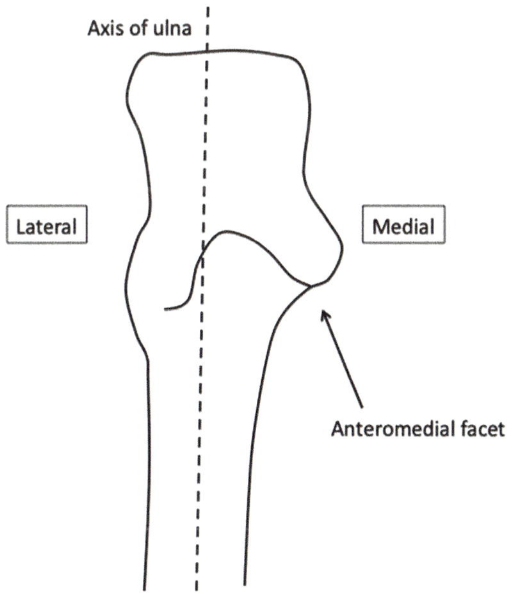

Fig. 1.26 The anteromedial facet of coronoid

Table 1.7 O'Driscoll classification of coronoid fractures

Type I	Fracture of tip of coronoid
Type II	Fracture of anteromedial facet of coronoid Subtype 1—Fracture of the rim Subtype 2—Fracture of rim and tip Subtype 3—Fracture of rim and sublime tubercle
Type III	Fracture of base and body of coronoid

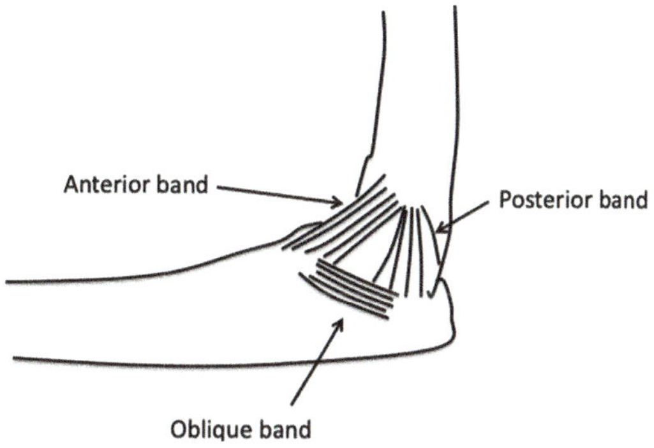

Fig. 1.27 Parts of the medial collateral ligament of elbow

The importance of the anteromedial facet of coronoid has been emphasised by O'Driscoll and a new classification system has been proposed for coronoid fractures (Table 1.7).

The medial ligament complex of the elbow has three bands (Fig. 1.27). The anterior band is the important stabilizer against posteromedial rotatory instability. It originates from the medial epicondyle and inserts on the sublime tubercle on the anteromedial aspect of base of coronoid.

CT scans are useful to determine the size of the fragment.

These fractures are fixed with an anteromedial buttress plate along with lateral ligament repair.

The lateral collateral ligament complex of elbow comprises the lateral ulnar collateral ligament (LUCL), radial collateral ligament (RCL) and the annular ligament (Fig. 1.28). The lateral ligaments prevent varus angulation and provide posterolateral stability.

Olecranon Fracture

The usual mechanism is a fall on the point of the elbow or a fall on an outstretched hand with the elbow in flexion.

Classification

The fracture can be undisplaced, displaced or associated with elbow instability based on the Mayo classification (Fig. 1.29).

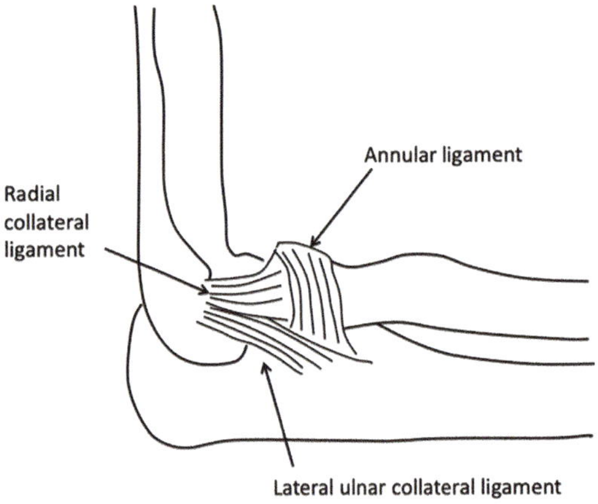

Fig. 1.28 The lateral stabilisers of the elbow

Management

The aim of treatment is to restore the articular surface, preserve the extensor mechanism and maintain elbow stability.

Type 1 fractures are managed with splinting with the elbow flexed to 90°.

Type 2A fractures are managed with tension-band wiring (TBW) with two knots. The superficial surface of the olecranon is the tension surface and placing the figure of eight on this surface provides compression across the fracture site as the elbow flexes.

The position of the patient is either supine with the arm in a trough across the chest or lateral position. Two parallel 1.6-mm Kirschner wires (K-wires) are placed antegrade across the fracture site, which should penetrate the anterior cortex in the distal fragment. The K-wires must not penetrate more than 10 mm through the anterior cortex of the distal fragment and lie no closer than 15 mm to the coronoid to avoid anterior neurovascular injury. The anterior interosseous nerve is most at risk. Wires should not be placed in the intramedullary canal due to the significant risk of backing out proximally. A 1 mm stainless steel wire is used in a figure of "8" fashion to complete the tension band wiring construct.

Fig. 1.29 Classification of olecranon fractures

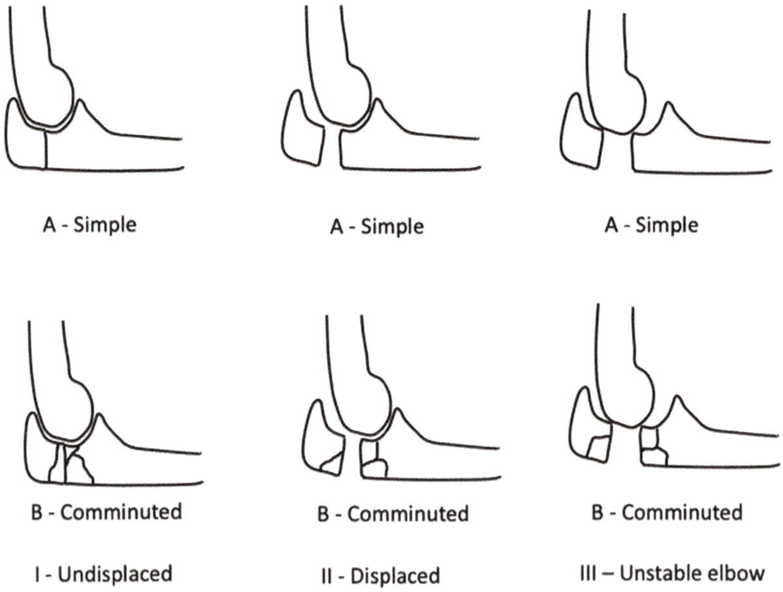

Displaced fractures that are comminuted, or show evidence of ulnohumeral incongruence (Mayo 2b, 3) and those of a simple two-part configuration with an oblique fracture line that extends distal to the midpoint of the sigmoid notch are regarded as unstable and unsuitable for wire fixation. Precontoured fixed angle locking plates are currently the preferred implant of choice for fixation.

Active range of motion exercises can be started after 7 days and splinting is discontinued within 3 weeks.

If associated with a coronoid fracture, open reduction and stabilisation by plating helps to fix the coronoid fracture as well as the olecranon. Olecranon fractures associated with radial head fractures indicate ligament injury. The radial head fracture should be reduced and fixed or the radial head replaced to restore stability.

There is no difference in clinical outcome or complications in TBW versus plating. However the need for hardware removal is more in the TBW group.

Radial Head Fracture

Fractures of the radial head are a common injury and about 10% of elbow dislocations are associated with radial head fracture. The mechanism of injury is a fall on the hand with a pronated forearm.

Thirty percent of radial head fractures are associated with coronoid fractures, medial collateral injury (ulnar collateral ligament) or ulnar nerve neurapraxia. A wrist examination is done to check for Essex Lopresti fracture (described later). Bruising on the medial aspect of the elbow may indicate a medial collateral ligament injury.

The radial head resists valgus stress along with the medial collateral ligament. Fracture of radial head, or injury to the medial collateral ligament, individually, does not result in valgus instability. However, the combination of these 2 injuries will lead to valgus instability.

A CT scan is helpful to look for injuries to coronoid process, if suspected.

Classification

Three types were proposed by Mason and a fourth type was added by Broberg-Morrey (Fig. 1.30).

Mason ML. Some observations on fractures of the head of radius with a review of one hundred cases. Br J Surg 1954;42(172):123–32.

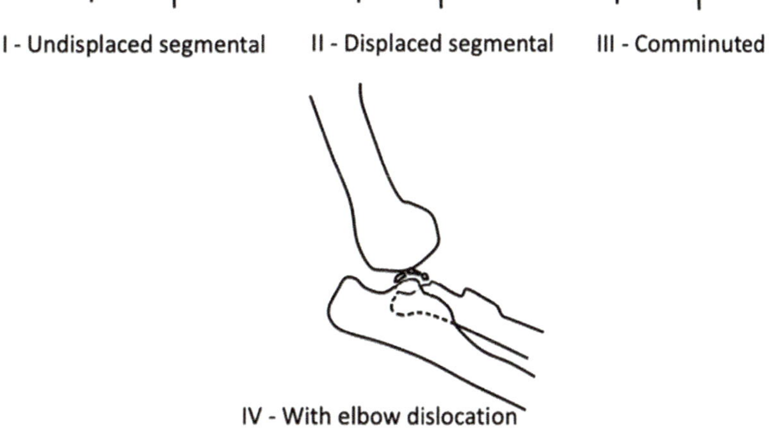

Fig. 1.30 Classification of radial head fractures

Broberg MA, Morrey BF. Results of treatment of fracture dislocations of the elbow. Clin Orthop 1987;216:109–19.

Management

Management is based on the classification:

Type I are managed nonoperatively with early active motion. One-third of patients are likely to experience restriction of full extension. The risk of non-union is 5%. Symptomatic non-union is managed with excision of the fragment.

For Type II injuries, if the radial head fragment is displaced less than 2 mm and the patient has normal pronation and supination then non-operative treatment is preferred. If there is a block to motion or displacement is more than 2 mm, internal fixation with screws and plate is considered. The block to motion is assessed in clinic after infiltration of local anaesthetic in the elbow.

For Type III injuries, nonoperative treatment yields unsatisfactory results. If there is no forearm pain (indicates absence of significant interosseous membrane injury), the coronoid is intact and the elbow is stable in valgus strain in 30° flexion, the radial head should be excised. If not, replacement of the radial head in needed to provide stability.

Type IV injuries are unstable. These are managed by repair of ligaments and replacement of radial head.

Indications for Surgery

- Loose intra-articular fragments.
- Associated olecranon fracture or medial collateral ligament injury.
- Block to motion from a displaced fragment.
- Axially unstable radius because of injury to the interosseous membrane or the distal radio-ulnar joint.

The radial head has a bare area of approximately 110° opposite to the articulation with the sigmoid notch. This is a non-articular part of the radial head and is suitable for the placement of metalwork for fixation.

In radial head fractures with associated medial collateral ligament injury, the radial head should be preserved if possible by internal fixation. If the fracture is not fixable, a radial head replacement is the option. Late excision is acceptable, but early (within 3 weeks) excision will impair the healing of the medial ligament.

Radial head excision/fixation can be performed through a posterolateral approach between the anconeus and extensor carpi ulnaris. The annular ligament is incised and all fragments are excised. The forearm must be kept pronated to protect the posterior interosseous nerve. Care must be taken to protect the lateral ulnar collateral ligament (LUCL). The Kaplan direct lateral approach, employing the interval between extensor digitorum communis (EDC) and extensor carpi radialis brevis may also be used. This approach will not disrupt the LUCL as it is more anterior.

Early motion reduces pericapsular scarring and increases range of motion. Excision of the radial head may lead to proximal migration of the ulna and posterolateral instability of the elbow.

Swenson SJ, Tyagi V, Uquillas C, Shakked RJ, Yoon RS, Liporace FA. Maximizing outcomes in the treatment of radial head fractures. J Orthop Traumatol. 2019;20(1):15.

Ikeda M, Sugiyama K, Kang C, et al. Comminuted fractures of the radial head. Comparison of resection and internal fixation. J Bone Joint Surg Am 2005;87:76–84. This study found no difference in range of motion between fixation and excision groups. The fixation group had significantly higher strength and functional scores.

Radial Head Replacement

The radial head can be replaced with silicone or metal implants. Swanson popularized silicone implants in 1970s. These have a high incidence of synovitis and are no longer used.

Metal implants provide more stability. Modular implants allow matching different size radial heads to different stem sizes. The stems can be cemented, cementless or free floating in the canal. Cementless stems are associated with a risk of microfractures during insertion and impaction. Stems which are loose in the canal allow self-alignment and radiolucencies around the stem do not appear to cause clinical problems.

Kocher's approach is used, with the plane between anconeus and extensor carpi ulnaris. The annular ligament is preserved and repaired at the end. The radial collateral ligament is preserved. Pronation helps protect the interosseous nerve. Lateral epicondyle osteotomy may be needed to insert the implant.

Replication of the diameter and thickness of the radial head, along with the supero-inferior positioning is important to improve outcome. An excessive superior placement will increase joint force and lead to degeneration. An inferior placement will not provide adequate stability.

Trial implants are used and checked in image intensifier.

The radial collateral ligament is usually avulsed from its proximal attachment and should be reattached. Muscles on the lateral epicondyle are reattached using suture anchors. A medial approach to repair the medial collateral ligament may be needed.

Frank SG, Grewal R, Johnson J, et al. Determination of correct implant size in radial head arthroplasty to avoid overlengthening. J Bone Joint Surg Am 2009;91:1738–46. The authors determined that incongruity of the lateral ulnohumeral joint is a reliable indicator of over-lengthening of the radius.

Burkhart KJ, Mattyasovszky SG, Runkel M, Schwarz C, Küchle R, Hessmann MH et al. Mid- to long-term results after bipolar radial head arthroplasty. J Shoulder Elbow Surg 2010;19:965–972. 60 to 80% have good results at 8 years despite development of humeroulnar osteoarthritis.

Radial Neck Fracture

Classification

Classification is similar to that of radial head fractures. Type I are undisplaced, type II have a displaced radial head with one large fragment and type III is comminuted radial head fracture.

Management

Undisplaced fractures are managed by early mobilization. Management options for displaced fractures are internal fixation by T-plate, interfragmentary screws and excision of the radial head.

Essex–Lopresti Fracture Dislocation

Essex–Lopresti fracture dislocation is fracture of the radial head or neck with disruption of the distal radioulnar joint. It is a rare injury and was described by Peter Essex-Lopresti in 1951.

The mechanism of injury is a fall on an outstretched hand. The distal radioulnar joint is disrupted, along with tearing of the interosseous membrane and fracture of the radial head or neck. The membrane normally stabilises the radius and prevents its proximal migration. If the radial head is excised in this injury, the radius will migrate proximally due to an incompetent interosseous membrane (Fig. 1.31). This will lead to

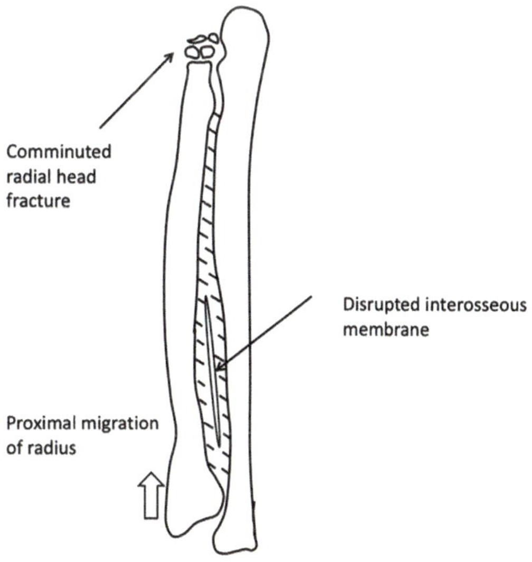

Fig. 1.31 Essex-Lopresti injury

radiocapitellar impingement at the elbow and ulnar carpal impingement at the wrist.

The diagnosis is indicated by radial head fracture along with pain along the forearm and at the distal radioulnar joint.

Plain x rays of the wrist, and possibly comparison x rays of the contralateral wrist are useful. An ultrasound of the forearm can reveal herniation of the forearm muscles into the interosseous space.

Management

Radial head excision is contraindicated in Essex–Lopresti fracture dislocation.

If the radial head is fixable, internal fixation is performed along with stabilisation of the distal radioulnar joint with a K-wire across the distal radius and ulna. The K-wire is removed after 6 weeks.

In comminuted fractures, the radial head is replaced and the distal joint stabilised with a K-wire.

Monteggia Lesions

Monteggia injury is fracture of the proximal ulna with dislocation of the radial head. This injury is named after the Italian surgeon Giovanni Monteggia. Typically, this results from a hyperpronation, hyperextension injury.

Classification

Classification was proposed by Bado from Uruguay (Fig. 1.32).

Imaging

A high index of suspicion is required for radial head dislocation in proximal ulna fractures, or in elbow injuries in general.

The long axis of the radius is drawn along the shaft of radius. This is the radiocapitellar line and should always pass through the capitellum in all radiographic views (Fig. 1.33). If the radial shaft does not line up with the capitellum, it indicates subluxation or dislocation of the radial head.

Management

An algorithm for the management of Monteggia lesions is shown in Fig. 1.34.

Reconstruction of the annular ligament can be performed using a strip from the forearm fascia or triceps aponeurosis. This is used to make a loop around the radial head.

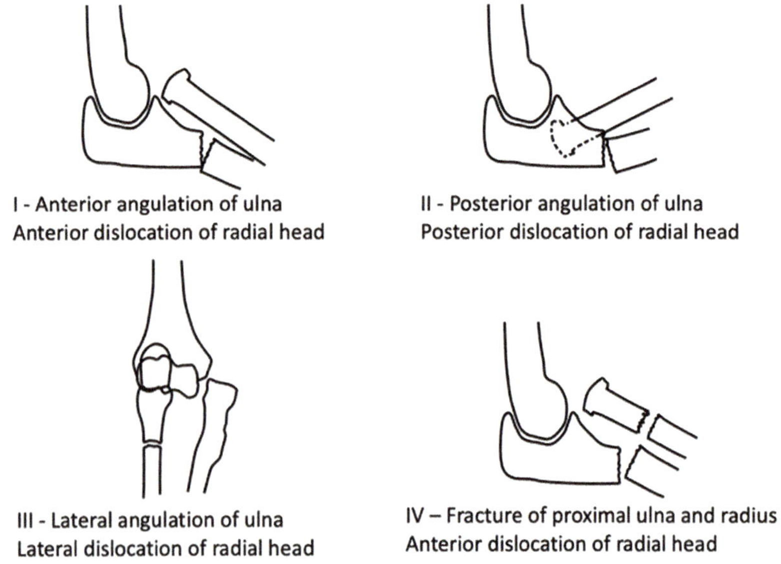

Fig. 1.32 Bado classification of Monteggia injuries

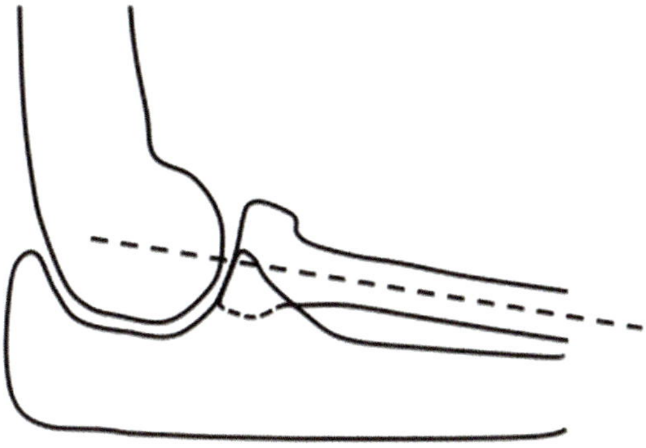

Fig. 1.33 Radiocapitellar line

If the ulnar fracture is associated with a fracture of the radial head, the radial head should either be fixed or replaced with radial head implant to restore stability at the time of ulnar fixation.

Pronation and supination exercises can be started under supervision at 4 weeks. Close follow-up with radiographs is advisable to ensure the radial head does not sublux or dislocate postoperatively.

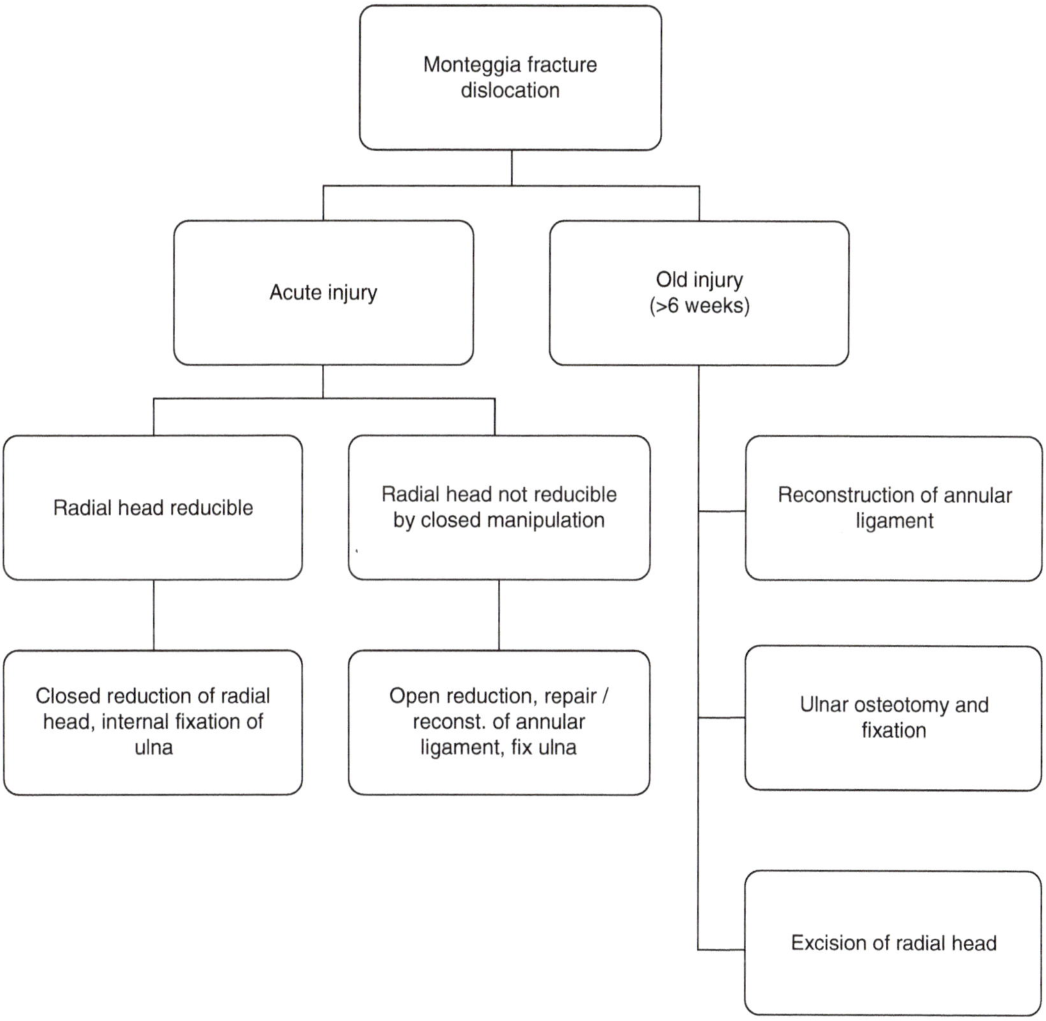

Fig. 1.34 Management of Monteggia injuries

Galeazzi Lesion

A Galeazzi lesion is a fracture anywhere in the radial shaft, with or without fracture of the ulna, with distal radioulnar joint injury.

Imaging

X ray shows signs of distal radioulnar joint injury. Widening of joint space on the anteroposterior view and dislocation of the radius on the lateral view may be evident. Radial shortening of more than 5 mm implies disruption of the distal radio-ulnar joint.

There may be an associated ulnar styloid fracture.

Management

Anatomic reduction is achieved by internal fixation using a compression plate. The distal radio-ulnar joint often reduces in supination when the radial fracture is reduced. Stability of the DRUJ should be assessed in supination. If the joint is unstable, it can be stabilised with a temporary K-wire.

Fracture of the Radius and Ulna Midshaft

Angulation of more than 10° in either bone restricts forearm function. Internal fixation is indicated with angulation of more 10° or displacement of more than 50% at the fracture site.

Management

In adults, this injury is best managed with anatomic reduction, rigid internal fixation and early mobilisation. Fixation may be achieved with intramedullary rods or dynamic compression plates.

Closed treatment is indicated with undisplaced fractures and with less than 10° angulation in an isolated distal ulna fracture. External fixation is an alternative to internal fixation in severe soft tissue injury.

Complications with intramedullary implants include poor rotational control, loss of radial bow, shortening and non-union.

Plate fixation achieves union in 96–98% of cases. The radial bow should be restored. Fixation is recommended in six cortices in each fragment. Plate fixation allows early mobilisation and no postoperative cast is required.

The dorsal approach (Thompson) carries a risk of injury to the posterior interosseous nerve. Henry's approach carries a risk of damage to the superficial branch of the radial nerve. The ulna is approached from the subcutaneous border.

Complications

Complications include malunion, synostosis and stress fracture. Osteotomies performed within 12 months regain better rotation.

Cross-union between the radius and ulna occurs in up to 5% of patients. Factors that predispose to increased incidence of synostosis are delayed ORIF, severely comminuted fractures and placement of a bone graft near the interosseous membrane.

The Vince and Miller classification is used, which is based on the site of synostosis (Table 1.8).

Resection and interposition of a silicon sheet or fat is successful in 50% of cases. This should be performed 1–3 years after injury.

Stress fracture can occur at the end of the plate, which is the junction of bone supported by the plate with the unsupported bone. Plate

Table 1.8 Classification of radioulnar synostosis

Type	Level of syndesmosis	Prognosis
Type I	Distal intra-articular part of the radius and ulna	Worst
Type II	Non-articular distal and middle third of the radius and ulna	Best
Type III	Proximal third of the radius and ulna	Intermediate

removal can be performed after 2 years but is not routinely advised. Indications for plate removal include irritation from a subcutaneous location of the plate. In addition, plate removal may be advised for athletes participating in contact sports. Following plate removal, the forearm should be protected in a splint for 6–8 weeks.

Fracture of the Distal Radius

The incidence of this injury is 1 in 500 persons per year. It follows a bimodal distribution—one peak in the second decade of life and a second in the seventh decade.

Abraham Colles was a professor of surgery in Ireland and described the distal radius fracture in 1814, before the development of x rays. Colles fracture is a simple transverse extraarticular fracture of the distal radius due to fall on the outstretched hand resulting in a dinner fork deformity.

Smith fracture is the reverse of Colles fracture and is caused by an impact on the dorsum of the wrist. This is characterised by volar displacement of the distal fragment.

A Barton's fracture is a fracture of the dorsal or volar margin of radius with dislocation of the radiocarpal joint. The volar Barton is commoner than dorsal Barton fracture.

Anatomy

The normal inclination of the distal radial articular surface is 23° in the AP view. The normal volar inclination of the distal radial articular surface (lunate fossa) is 11° in the lateral view (Fig. 1.35).

Radial height is measured as the distance between a line drawn through the tip of the radial styloid perpendicular to the long axis of radius and another line drawn through the distal articular surface of the ulna. Typically this distance is 12 mm. The distal radial articular surface is generally 1 mm distal to the distal ulnar articular surface. Ulna variance or Hulten variance is the relative position of the distal articular surface of radius and ulna (Fig. 1.36). In positive ulna variance, the ulna projects more than 2.5 mm distal compared to radius. In negative ulna variance, the ulna is more than 2.5 mm proximal to radius.

Classification

The AO group define periarticular fractures as type A (extra-articular), type B (partial articular) and type C (complete articular).

Other classification systems have been proposed by Frykman and Malone.

The universal classification is simple and descriptive and is commonly used (Fig. 1.37).

Evaluation

Standard wrist radiographs are used to assess the lunate fossa, scaphoid fossa and sigmoid notch. If there is suspicion of scaphoid fracture, further scaphoid views are obtained.

CT scans are very helpful to assess the joint surface irregularity or metaphyseal comminu-

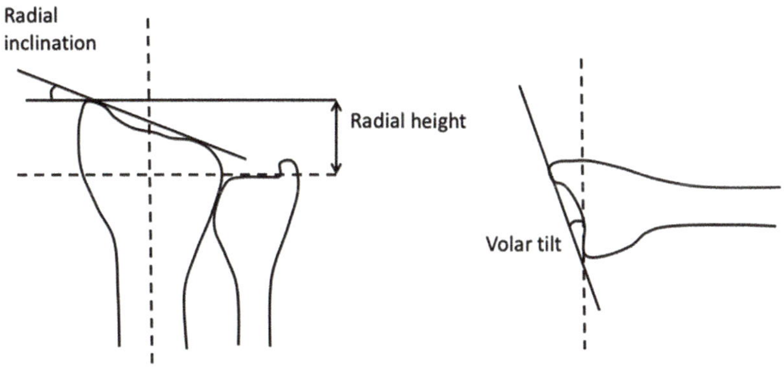

Fig. 1.35 Anatomical parameters of the distal radial articulation

tion. Magnetic resonance imaging (MRI) will demonstrate the soft tissue injuries.

Radial shortening (3–6 mm) may lead to a poor clinical result with symptoms of ulnar-sided pain, decreased forearm rotation, diminished grip and ulnar carpal impaction.

Barton T, Chambers C, Bannister G. A comparison between subjective outcome score and moderate radial shortening following a fractured distal radius in patients of mean age 69 years. J Hand Surg Eur Vol 2007;32:165–9. In this study, 60 patients were managed with K-wiring. Shortening of 8 mm did not correlate with poor outcome. The Frykman classification correlated with outcome.

Dorsal tilt leads to increased load transmission through the ulna. This can cause dorsal intercalated segment instability and extrinsic midcarpal instability.

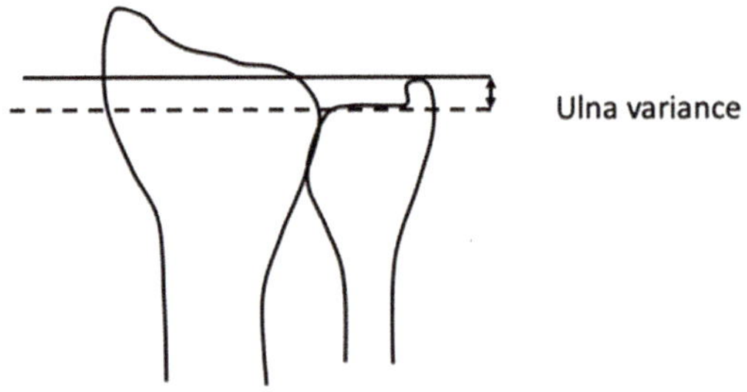

Fig. 1.36 An example of negative ulna variance

Loss of radial inclination leads to increased load transmission onto the lunate fossa.

An intra-articular step greater than the thickness of the articular cartilage leads to poor remodelling and increased contact stresses. The intra-articular step-off should be less than 2 mm.

Knirk JL, Jupiter JB. Intraarticular fractures of the distal end of radius in young adults. J Bone Joint Surg Am 1986;68(5):647–59. Retrospective study showed higher incidence of wrist arthritis in patients where accurate reduction was not achieved. 43 fractures with 6.7 year follow up.

Management

The aim of treatment is to restore the alignment of the distal radial articular surface and congruence of the radiocarpal and distal radioulnar joints. The acceptability criteria are summarised in Table 1.9.

The DRAFFT Trial was a pragmatic randomized controlled trial that compared functional outcome following acute fixation of distal radius fracture. This trial found no difference in functional outcome in patients with dorsally displaced fractures of the distal radius treated with Kirschner wires or volar locking plates.

Costa ML, Achten J, Parsons NR, Rangan A, Griffin D, Tubeuf S, Lamb SE; DRAFFT Study Group. Percutaneous fixation with Kirschner

Fig. 1.37 Universal classification for distal radius fractures

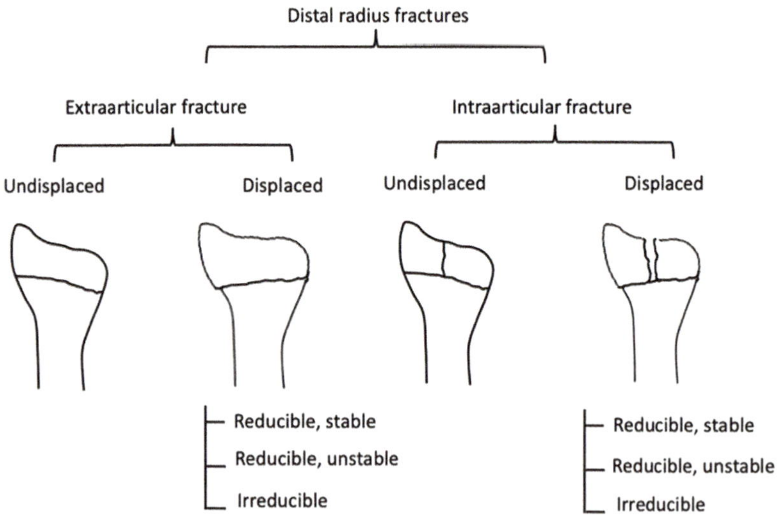

Table 1.9 Acceptability criteria for reduction of distal radius fracture

No	Criteria	Normal	Acceptable
1	Ulnar Variance	2 mm comparing level of lunate facet to ulnar head	No more than 2 mm shortening compared to ulnar head
2	Radial Height	11–12 mm (Range: 8–18 mm)	Not defined
3	Palmar Tilt	11 degrees (Range 0–28 degree)	Neutral
4	Radial Inclination	22–23 degrees (Range: 12–30 degree)	Up to 10 degree
5	Intra-articular Step	None	≤2 mm

Table 1.10 Summary of management options for fracture of the distal radius based on the universal classification

Type	Management
I	Cast
II	Manipulation under local/regional anaesthetic and cast If unstable, K-wires can be used If an irreducible or complex fracture, use ORIF and a volar plate
III	Cast If there is displacement on follow up, use K-wires or volar locking plate
IV	Reducible, stable: K-wire, interfragmentary screws, plates or external fixator Reducible, unstable: if >2 mm step or >5 mm shortening, use a K-wire, bone graft or external fixator with a limited open approach.

wires versus volar locking plate fixation in adults with dorsally displaced fracture of distal radius: Randomised controlled trial. BMJ. 2014 Aug 5;349:g4807

Management options are summarised in Table 1.10.

For fractures that cannot be reduced by closed methods, open reduction and internal fixation with or without bone grafting is required.

If an external fixator is used, a maximum of 1 mm distraction of the radiocarpal joint is permissible to prevent overdistraction and stiffness.

Cast

There is no demonstrable advantage of a long-arm cast over short-arm cast. Furthermore, there is no benefit in remanipulation in patients older than 60 years.

Mcqueen, MM, Hajducka C, Court-brown CM. Redisplaced unstable fractures of the distal radius. A prospective randomised comparison of four methods of treatment

J Bone Joint Surg Br 1996;78(3):404–9. No benefit of remanipulation in patients over 60 years of age.

The predictors of instability are degree of initial displacement, age (osteopenia), amount of dorsal comminution and intra-articular fractures.

Manipulation and K-Wire Stabilisation

Wiring is acceptable for stable fractures without significant comminution. A cross K-wire technique has been described, in which one 1.6 mm K-wire is inserted through the radial styloid and another from the dorsal metaphysis, or through the dorsal fracture site. Wires are removed 5–6 weeks after injury.

A limited open reduction to reduce the dorsal fragment is a useful adjunct to percutaneous pinning. The fragment is reduced under image-intensifier control by levering and a 1.6 mm K-wire is passed adjacent to the subchondral bone to support the fragment.

Metaphyseal bone defects may be managed with bone grafting: autograft, allograft or bone substitutes.

Kapandji A. Intrafocal pinning of fractures of the distal end of radius; 10 years later. Ann Chir Main 1987;6(1):57–63. Kapandji suggested using three separate pins to lever the fragment and then driving the pins through the volar cortex to allow early motion. This is known as intrafocal pinning, where the K-wires act as a buttress.

External Fixation

Reduction is achieved by ligamentotaxis.

Limited open exposure is performed to place the pins, avoiding injury to the cutaneous branches of the radial nerve. Drilling is performed before pin insertion. Two pins are placed in the radius and two in the dorsoradial aspect of the index finger metacarpal. The radiocarpal joint should not be more than 1 mm wider than the midcarpal joint. This is an indicator of overdistraction and may lead to stiffness. Ligamentotaxis does not reduce dorsal fragments, as volar ligaments tighten first. For these, limited open reduction can be used. The fixator can be retained for 6–8 weeks. The benefit of early dynamisation is debatable.

A non-bridging external fixator has been described by McQueen, in which the distal pins are placed into the distal fragment instead of the metacarpal. This is very effective for extra-articular fractures and fractures with simple intra-articular extension. Comminution and osteopenia may compromise fixation in the distal fragment.

Hayes AJ, Duffy PJ, McQueen MM. Bridging and nonbridging external fixation in the treatment of unstable fractures of the distal radius. A retrospective study of 588 patients. Acta Orthop 2008;79(4):540–7. Nonbridging external fixator is preferable, if possible to insert pins in the distal fragment.

Dynamic mobile fixators have been proposed. These allow movement at the wrist while maintaining tension across the fracture site, but their benefit is debatable.

Open Reduction and Internal Fixation

Open reduction and plate *Open reduction* osteosynthesis are indicated for intra-articular shearing-type injuries. These include volar and dorsal Barton injuries.

Complications

Potential complications include a stiff wrist, pin-site infection, extensor pollicis longus tendon rupture, median nerve compression, stiffness, posttraumatic arthritis, neuropathy, complex regional pain syndrome, malunion and non-union.

Prophylactic release of the carpal tunnel is not required at the time of plating.

Odumala O, Ayekoloye C, Packer G. Prophylactic carpal tunnel decompression during buttress plating of the distal radius—is it justified? Injury 2001;32:577–9. There was no benefit in prophylactic carpal tunnel decompression at the time of plating of distal radius.

Ng CY, McQueen MM. What are the radiological predictors of functional outcome following fractures of the distal radius? J Bone Joint Surg Br 2011;93(2):145–50. Predictors of good outcome are less than 2 mm of step or gap in the articular surface, less than 2 mm of shortening and restoration of normal carpal alignment.

Dorsal plates on the distal radius (also known at Pi plates because of their shape) have been used for comminuted fractures of the distal radius that require either a dorsal approach or a combined volar and dorsal approach. Concerns have been raised about the high complication rate with these plates. Potential complications include tendon adherence, wrist stiffness, tendon irritation and rupture.

Grewal R, Perey B, Wilmink M, Stothers K. A randomized prospective study on the treatment of intra-articular distal radius fractures: open reduction and internal fixation with dorsal plating versus mini open reduction, percutaneous fixation, and external fixation. J Hand Surg Am 2005;30:764–72. This study compared dorsal plates with percutaneous fixation and external fixation in patients with AO type C intra-articular fractures. Plate fixation resulted in higher levels of pain and reduced grip strength.

Volar Barton Fracture

Volar Barton fracture is a marginal fracture of the anterior margin of the distal radial articular surface with anterior dislocation of the carpus. It is best managed with ORIF with a volar buttress plate.

Ulnar Styloid Fractures

Ulnar styloid fractures are commonly associated with distal radius fractures. In most cases, the ulnar styloid does not require fixation once the distal radius fracture has been reduced and stabilised.

Kim JK, Koh YD, Do NH. Should an ulnar styloid fracture be fixed following volar plate fixation of a distal radial fracture? J Bone Joint Surg Am 2010;92:1–6. This study included 138 patients, of which 55% had an ulnar styloid fracture. There was no difference in outcomes for these patients compared with those without fracture.

In patients with instability of the distal radioulnar joint, the ulnar styloid may be fixed with a single K-wire supplemented with figure-of-eight tension-band wiring. The forearm should be immobilised for 6 weeks after fixation.

Fractures of the Scaphoid

Scaphoid fractures are the result of a fall on the outstretched hand or sudden dorsiflexion of the wrist.

Displacement is present in 20% of fractures of the waist of scaphoid and CT scans have better sensitivity to detect displacement.

Classification

Herbert classification system is summarised in Fig. 1.38.

Treatment

Undisplaced fractures have 90% healing rate in plaster cast. Displaced fractures have 80–85% healing in plaster cast. The cast is applied for 2 months and does not need to include the thumb CMC joint.

Complications

Nonunion is commoner in displaced fractures.

Pain can be present in up to 20% patients on long term follow up, even though strength and movements may be fully restored.

Malunited fractures can lead to posttraumatic arthritis affecting the radioscaphoid and scaphotrapezial joints. The risk of arthritis is 2–5% and operative fixation of displaced fractures has not shown to reduce the risk of development of arthritis.

Avascular non-union of the scaphoid can be treated by free vascularised iliac bone graft.

Arora R, Lutz M, Zimmermann R, Krappinger D, Niederwanger C, Gabl M. Free vascularised iliac bone graft for recalcitrant avascular nonunion of the scaphoid. J Bone Joint Surg Br 2010;92(2):224–9. 21 patients, mean age 32 years. Time between injury and surgery was 39 months. Mean follow up 5.6 years, union obtained in 16 patients. In the successful group, the procedure prevented progressive carpal collapse and gave good pain relief.

DISI Dorsal Intercalated Segment Instability can be present in 10% of patients, but the development of DISI does not correlate with functional outcome.

Hip Dislocation

Dislocations of the hip are the result of a severe force. The hip is inherently stable with strong ligaments and congruent articulation. Posterior hip dislocation is commoner than anterior.

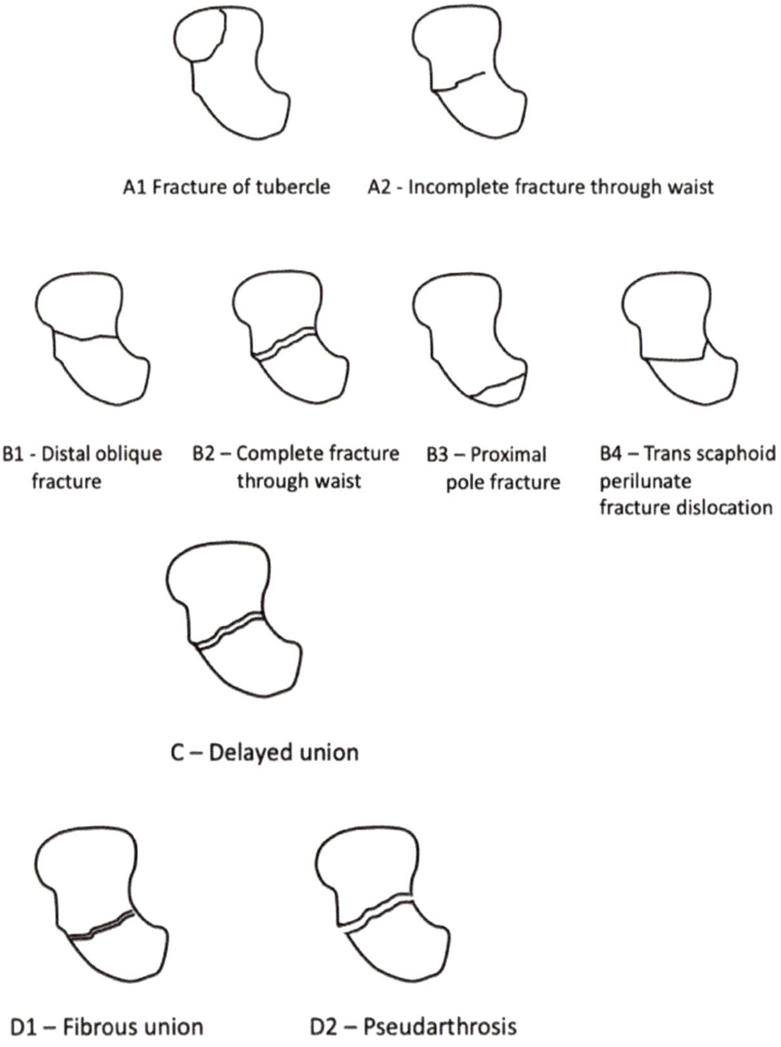

Fig. 1.38 Herbert classification for scaphoid fractures

Associated injuries should be checked. Impact from the dashboard in motor vehicle accidents exerts an axial force, which can lead to posterior dislocation. The classic position of the limb at the time of impact is flexion and adduction. Cruciate ligament injuries are frequent associated, as well as sciatic nerve injury.

Excess abduction and external rotation leads to anterior dislocation of the hip.

Posterior dislocation results in a flexed, adducted and internally rotated position of the hip. Anterior dislocation shows an abducted, externally rotated position.

Classification

Thompson and Epstein classified anterior hip dislocations into superior and inferior types (Fig. 1.39). Each of these has further subtypes of (a) no associated fractures; (b) associated fracture or impaction of the femoral head; and (c) with associated fracture of the acetabulum.

Thompson and Epstein also classified posterior hip dislocation, of which there are five types (Fig. 1.40).

Management of hip dislocation is an emergency. Current evidence promotes early reduction of hip dislocation to reduce the risk of avascular necrosis. In patients with dislocation without associated injury, the risk of avascular necrosis is less than 3% if the hip is reduced within 12 h. A delay in reduction of dislocation beyond 12 h leads to a 5.6 fold increase in the risk of developing AVN.

Kellam P, Ostrum RF. Systematic Review and Meta-Analysis of Avascular Necrosis and Posttraumatic Arthritis After Traumatic Hip Dislocation. J Orthop Trauma. 2016;30(1):10–6.

The risk of developing arthritis after isolated hip dislocation is approximately 18%. As a comparison, the risk of developing hip arthritis in the general population is around 3.5%.

Dislocations with an associated large posterior wall fragment are often unstable after reduction. Open reduction and internal fixation of the fragment is needed through a posterior approach. Associated femoral head fractures are fixed.

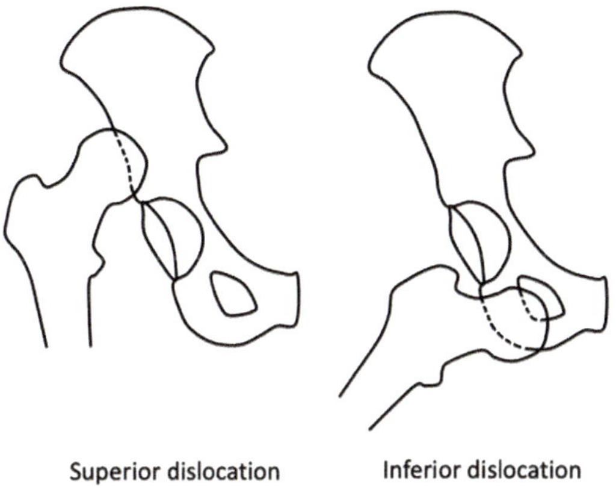

Fig. 1.39 Types of anterior hip dislocation

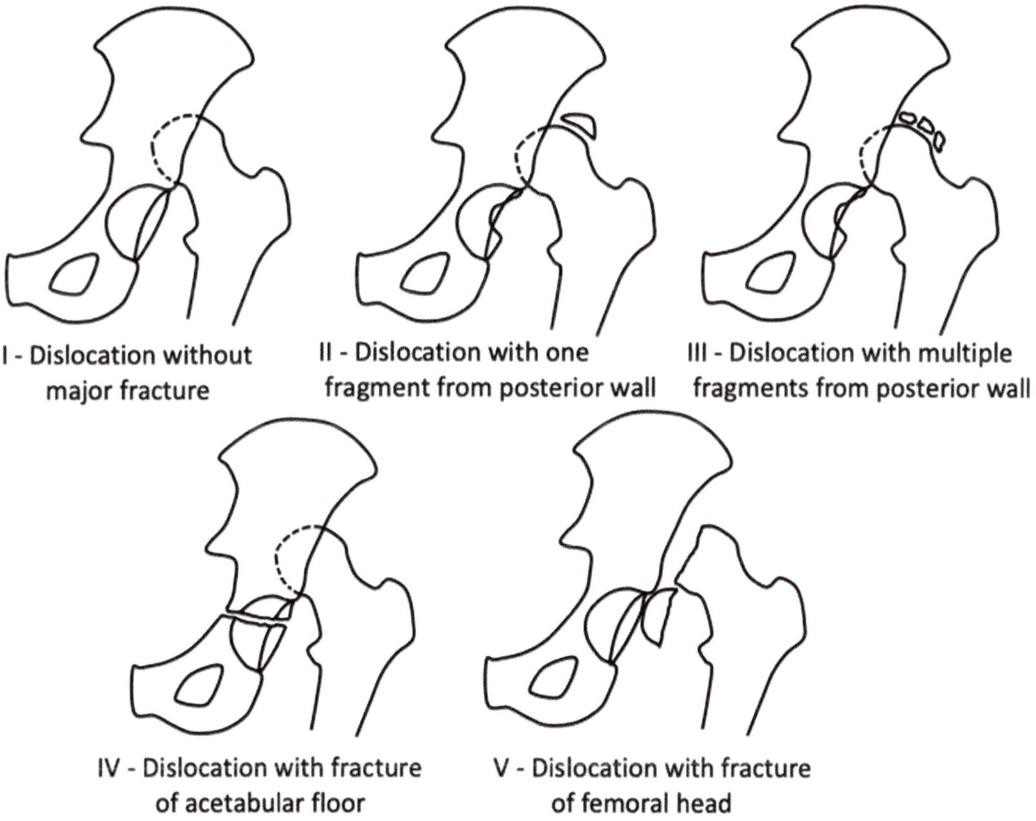

Fig. 1.40 Types of posterior hip dislocation

Femoral Head Fractures

Femoral head fractures are usually found in association with hip dislocations.

The classification of these injuries was proposed by Pipkin in 1957 (Fig. 1.41).

A closed reduction of the dislocated hip can be attempted in the emergency department. A post reduction CT scan is mandatory to look for congruency of the hip joint, and any remaining intra-articular fragments. Any residual incongruity of hip or retained intraarticular fracture fragments necessitates open reduction and internal fixation. Fragments that are too small to fix are excised.

An anterior approach (Smith Peterson) or a trochanteric flip approach for fixation of the femoral head fracture reduces the risk of avascular necrosis. Visualisation of the fragment is often better from the anterior approach. CT scans help in determining the optimal approach. Small fragments in the joint can be excised arthroscopically if there is no articular incongruence.

Beebe MJ, Bauer JM, Mir HR. Treatment of Hip Dislocations and Associated Injuries: Current State of Care. Orthop Clin North Am. 2016;47(3):527–49. Review article.

Femoral Neck Fracture

Femoral neck fractures predominantly occur in the elderly population and are more common in women. Only 3–5% of femoral neck fractures occur in people younger than 50 years and these are usually due to high-energy trauma.

Anatomy

Normal femoral anteversion is 10 ± 7°, while the neck shaft angle is 130 ± 7°. The tip of the greater

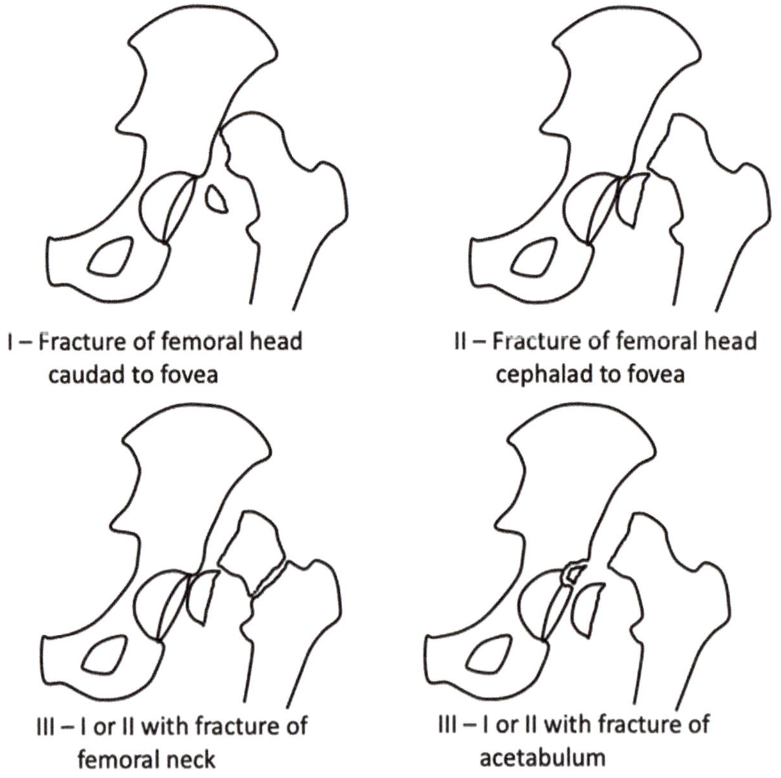

Fig. 1.41 Classification of femoral head fractures

trochanter is level with the centre of rotation of the femoral head in the axial plane. In a varus hip, the centre of the femoral head is lower, while in a valgus hip the centre of the femoral head is higher than the tip of trochanter. The lesser trochanter is posteromedial on the femoral shaft. The greater trochanter flares posteriorly in the proximal part.

The femoral neck lacks the cambium layer in the periosteum. This reduces the periosteal callus formation and is a possible contributor to the high risk of nonunion in these injuries. Additionally, the presence of synovial fluid at the fracture site may inhibit fracture healing.

Diagnosis

The clinical presentation is often typical, with a fall followed by pain in the hip. The leg may be shortened and externally rotated, but this sign is absent in impacted or undisplaced fractures. A full examination is essential to check for other injuries.

Plain radiographs in two planes are the mainstay of diagnosis. Further investigations can be used for fractures not evident on plain radiographs:

- T1-weighted MRI will demonstrate fracture in all cases.
- Fractures can be demonstrated on a bone scan within 72 h (or sometimes as early as 24 h).
- A CT scan may show the fracture line. The presence of lipohaemarthrosis on a CT scan is suggestive of fracture.
- Enhanced MRI is very effective for showing AVN at an early stage. A Tc99 bone scan within 72 h can predict AVN.

Hakkarinen DK, Banh KV, Hendey GW. Magnetic resonance imaging identifies occult hip fractures missed by 64-slice computed tomography. J Emerg Med 2012;43(2):303–7. CT scan missed 2% of femoral neck fractures compared to MR scan. CT does not completely exclude occult femoral neck fracture.

Classification

Garden (1964) classified femoral neck fractures into four types (Fig. 1.42).

Partially displaced fractures have loss of alignment of the trabeculae in the head and acetabulum. In completely displaced fractures, alignment of the trabeculae in the femoral head and acetabulum is restored as there is minimal contact across the fracture site.

The outcomes in type 1 and 2 are similar; and those in 3 and 4 are similar. Hence, the classification can be simplified into undisplaced (type I and II) and displaced fractures (type III and IV).

Pauwel's classification (1965) is based on the angle between the fracture surface on the femoral shaft fragment and a line perpendicular to the longitudinal axis of the femur (Fig. 1.43). In type I the angle of fracture line from the horizontal plane is 30° to 49°; in type II it is 50° to 69° and in type III it is more than 70°.

The importance of this classification lies in the emphasis on biomechanical forces in this area. A fracture with an angle of 30° is subject to predominantly compressive force and is more likely

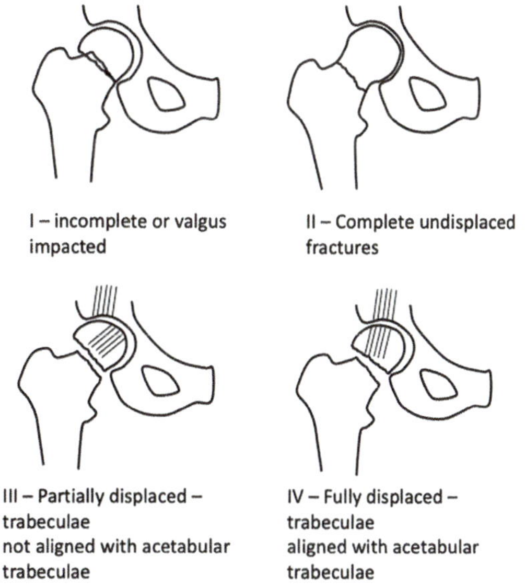

Fig. 1.42 Garden classification of femoral neck fractures

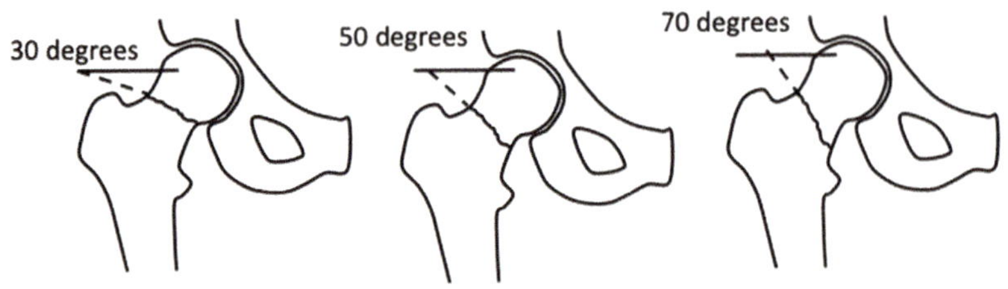

Fig. 1.43 Pauwel's angle for femoral neck fractures

to unite than a fracture with an angle of 70°, which is largely under shear stress.

Imaging

Standard plain radiographs in two planes are adequate in the vast majority of individuals. Occult fractures can be demonstrated on CT scan or MR scan. Imaging should not delay definitive management. CT scan is easily available and nearly as sensitive as MR scan, which is the gold standard.

Management

Femoral neck fracture is an absolute indication for surgical intervention: internal fixation or replacement. Non-operative management in indicated only when the patient is unfit for surgery. Every effort should be made to optimise the medical condition as soon as possible; a prolonged period of recumbency increases the risk of complications.

Ideally, joint medical and orthopaedic teams will assess and manage patients in the perioperative period. Postoperative care in a high-dependency unit helps reduce in-hospital mortality from femoral neck fractures.

Aspiration of the haemarthrosis was proposed to reduce the intraarticular pressure in the capsule. This was thought to improve circulation in the retinacular vessels. Studies have shown aspiration has no proven value in restoring vascularity.

Maruenda JI, Barrios C, Gomar-Sancho F. Intracapsular hip pressure after femoral neck fracture. Clin Orthop 1997;340:172–80. This prospective study with 34 patients found that patients with AVN after 7 years had intracapsular pressures that were lower than their diastolic pressures.

Timing of Surgery

NICE recommends (CG124—updated May 2017) surgery for femoral neck fracture on the day of admission, or the day after.

Many patients with a hip fracture requiring hemiarthroplasty have medical complications that must be optimised before surgery. Ideally these patients should be operated upon within 36 h. Delay after 48 h is associated with increased risk of hospital acquired pneumonia.

Sasabuchi Y, Matsui H, Lefor AK, Fushimi K, Yasunaga H. Timing of surgery for hip fractures in the elderly: A retrospective cohort study. Injury. 2018; 49(10):1848–54.

Moran CG, Wenn RT, Sikand M, Taylor AM. Early mortality after hip fracture: is delay before surgery important? J Bone Joint Surg Am 2005;87:483–9. In this prospective observational study of 2,660 patients, mortality was 9% at 30 days, 19% at 90 days and 30% at 12 months. Patients with medical conditions that delayed surgery had 2.5-times higher risk of mortality.

For patients with planned reduction and internal fixation, the literature is divided on the need for urgent surgery. Surgery is planned on the day of admission; or planned as the first operation on the following morning.

Papakostidis C, Panagiotopoulos A, Piccioli A, Giannoudis PV. Timing of internal fixation of femoral neck fractures. A systematic review and meta-analysis of the final outcome. Injury. 2015;46(3):459–66. Meta-analysis of 7 studies.

No demonstrable difference in rate of avascular necrosis based on timing of surgery.

Fracture Reduction

For displaced fractures where internal fixation is intended, a gentle closed reduction is the first step in managing the fracture. The femoral shaft fragment is displaced proximally and rotates externally as a result of the fracture. The reduction is achieved by traction in extension to correct the proximal displacement and internal rotation of the leg to correct the rotational alignment.

Different methods of closed reduction have been described. Reduction can be achieved either with traction in flexion or extension, followed by internal rotation.

Rarely, open reduction is needed. This can be performed with anterior capsulotomy and manipulating the femoral shaft fragment to the head fragment. The Smith Peterson approach is used. Anatomic reduction is desirable as inadequate reduction is a risk factor for failure of fixation. Varus positioning of femoral neck should be avoided at any cost.

Screw Fixation

Lag screw fixation is undertaken with three or four 6.5 mm cancellous screws or 7.3 mm cannulated cancellous screws.

The threads of the screws should cross the fracture site. Screws with 16 mm threads are preferred to those with 32 mm threads. In presence of postero-medial comminution, a fully threaded cancellous screw can be placed in the postero inferior sector to prevent the fracture from collapsing into varus and retroversion.

The screws are inserted in a triangular orientation parallel to each other. The apex of the triangle can be either superior or inferior, with the 'apex inferior' configuration being preferable. Finite element analysis supports 'apex inferior' placement to reduce screw cutout rate.

Oakey J, Stover M, Summers H, et al. Does screw configuration affect subtrochanteric fracture after femoral neck fixation? Clin Orthop Relat Res 2006;443:302–6. An inferior apex is preferable as a superior configuration is associated with a higher risk of subtrochanteric fracture.

The tips of the screws should be 5–10 mm from the subchondral bone ensuring the screws do not penetrate the femoral head cartilage. The entry point of screws on the lateral femoral cortex should be above the level of lesser trochanter. This reduces the risk of subtrochanteric fracture through the screw hole.

Parker MJ, Blundell C. Choice of implant for internal fixation of femoral neck fractures. Meta-analysis of 25 randomised trials including 4,925 patients. Acta Orthop Scand 1998;69:138–43. This meta-analysis included 4,925 patients in 25 series. There was no advantage to using side plates. Therefore, cannulated parallel screws are preferred.

Asnis SE, Wanek-Sgaglione L. Intracapsular fractures of the femoral neck. Results of cannulated screw fixation. J Bone Joint Surg Am 1994;76:1793–803. This 8-year follow-up of 141 patients reported that cannulated screws were associated with union in 96% of patients and with AVN in 22%.

The spread of screws in the lateral radiograph is related to failure. A wider spread reduces the failure rate.

Gursamy K, Parker MJ, Rowlands TK. The complications of displaced intracapsular fractures of the hip: the effect of screw positioning and angulation on fracture healing. J Bone Joint Surg Br 2005;87(5):632–5. Reduced spread of screws on the lateral view was associated with greater risk of nonunion.

Medical co-morbidities and delay in fixation of over 24 h correlate with higher risk of failure.

Duckworth AD, Bennet SJ, Aderinto J, Keating JF. Fixation of intracapsular fractures of the femoral neck in young patients: risk factors for failure. J Bone Joint Surg Br 2011;93(6):811–816. 122 patients, 58 month follow up, union in 68%, non-union 7.4% and avascular necrosis 11%. The risk factors for failure of fixation in young patients are considered to be delay in operation over 24 h, excess alcohol intake, existing renal, hepatic or respiratory disease.

Dynamic Hip Screw

Using a two-hole side plate with a dynamic hip screw is an option for femoral neck fractures. This provides secure fixation and may be advisable for basal neck fractures. It has a higher rate of AVN, but provides better fixation compared to cannulated screws. A dynamic hip screw is also advocated for Pauwel's type 3 fractures for its biomechanical advantage.

Liporace F, Gaines R, Collinge C, Haidukewych GJ. Results of internal fixation of Pauwels type-3 vertical femoral neck fractures. J Bone Joint Surg Am. 2008;90(8):1654–9.

There is a risk of rotational malalignment while inserting the hip screw and a guide wire inserted superior to the hip screw will prevent rotation. Subsequently, the guide wire can be removed or used to insert a lag screw parallel and superior to the dynamic hip screw.

In basicervical fractures, a dynamic hip screw with derotation screw should be used.

Deneka DA, Simonian PT, Stankewich CJ, Eckert D, Chapman JR, Tencer AF. Biomechanical comparison of internal fixation techniques for the treatment of unstable basicervical femoral neck fractures J Orthop Trauma 1997;11(5):337–43. Dynamic hip screw had a higher load to failure than cannulated screws.

Hemiarthroplasty

Displaced subcapital fractures in the elderly (over 80) with limited mobility requirements are managed with hemiarthroplasty.

Hoskins W, Webb D, Bingham R, Pirpiris M, Griffin XL. Evidence based management of intracapsular neck of femur fractures. Hip Int. 2017;27(5):415–24.

Leonardsson O, Sernbo I, Carlsson A, et al. Long-term follow-up of replacement compared with internal fixation for displaced femoral neck fractures: results at ten years in a randomised study of 450 patients. J Bone Joint Surg Br 2010;92:406–12. At 10 years, this randomised study reported a complication rate of 46% with screw fixation versus 9% with total or hemiarthroplasty. Mortality was 75% at 10 years in both groups. Better function was achieved in patients with replacement.

In patients with chronic renal failure and hyperparathyroidism, a cemented hemiarthroplasty is preferred.

Cemented hemiarthroplasty is preferred as it has 4 times less complication rate. Uncemented hemiarthroplasty can be done in low demand group but both types are associated with groin pain due to the articulation of the metal head against the acetabular cartilage. The Austin–Moore prosthesis was an uncemented design and is no longer in popular use. The fixation of Austin-Moore prosthesis in femur was poor as there was no coating on the metal surface for osseointegration. A loose femoral stem in the femur will lead to thigh pain.

Moerman S, Mathijssen NMC, Niesten DD, Riedijk R, Rijnberg WJ, Koëter S, Kremers van de Hei K, Tuinebreijer WE, Molenaar TL, Nelissen RGHH, Vochteloo AJH. More complications in uncemented compared to cemented hemiarthroplasty for displaced femoral neck fractures: a randomized controlled trial of 201 patients, with one year follow-up. BMC Musculoskelet Disord. 2017 Apr 21;18(1):169.

Song JSA, Dillman D, Wilson D, Dunbar M, Richardson G. Higher periprosthetic fracture rate associated with use of modern uncemented stems compared to cemented stems in femoral neck fractures. Hip Int. 2019;29(2):177–83. This study showed that the rate of periprosthetic fractures is more when uncemented stem is used for hemiarthroplasty.

Timperley AJ, Whitehouse SL. Mitigating surgical risk in patients undergoing hip arthroplasty for fractures of the proximal femur. J Bone Joint Surg Br 2009;91(7):851–4. This study found that cementation of hemiarthroplasty in fracture patients did not increase the risk of mortality. Patients with cemented implants had less pain and a lower revision rate, reoperation rate and risk of death.

Bipolar hemiarthroplasty designs have an additional articulation within the femoral head. This can theoretically reduce the movement at the metal—cartilage interface, reducing groin pain. Studies have shown better function with bipolar hemiarthroplasty.

Inngul C, Hedbeck CJ, Blomfeldt R, Lapidus G, Ponzer S, Enocson A. Unipolar hemiarthroplasty versus bipolar hemiarthroplasty in patients with displaced femoral neck fractures: a four-year follow-up of a randomised controlled trial. Int Orthop. 2013;37(12):2457–64. In patients over 80 years of age with displaced fractures, bipolar prosthesis was associated with better functional outcome. The rate of acetabular erosion was more at 12 months with unipolar hemiarthroplasty but the rates were similar at 24 and 48 months.

Figved W, Svenøy S, Röhrl SM, Dahl J, Nordsletten L, Frihagen F. Higher cartilage wear in unipolar than bipolar hemiarthroplasties of the hip at 2 years: A randomized controlled radiostereometric study in 19 fit elderly patients with femoral neck fractures. Acta Orthop. 2018;89(5):503–8. This showed higher acetabular cartilage wear in unipolar hemiarthroplasty when compared to bipolar hemiarthroplasty. Functional outcome was better in bipolar hemiarthroplasty. Bipolar hemiarthroplasty may be preferable in ambulatory elderly patients.

Total Hip Arthroplasty

Total hip arthroplasty is an option for patients with hip arthritis and femoral neck fracture. These patients are unlikely to do well with either fixation or hemiarthroplasty.

Total hip replacement is increasingly being used in patients with displaced fractures as a definitive treatment. The traditional concerns with hip arthroplasty in patients with femoral neck fractures have focused on a higher dislocation rate.

HEALTH Investigators, Bhandari, M., Einhorn, T. A., Guyatt, G., Schemitsch, E. H., Zura, R. D., Sprague, S., Frihagen, F., Guerra-Farfán, E., Kleinlugtenbelt, Y. V., Poolman, R. W., Rangan, A., Bzovsky, S., Heels-Ansdell, D., Thabane, L., Walter, S. D., & Devereaux, P. J. (2019). HEALTH investigators presented the short term results (24 months) of a multinational RCT (80 centres, 10 countries) comparing 1495 independently mobile patients who were >50 years old sustaining a displaced IC fracture treated by THA or HA. They found no statistically significant difference with respect to secondary hip procedure, dislocation rates (4.7% in THA, 2.4% in HA, HR=2.0), mortality, and serious adverse events between the two groups. Function and quality of life only modestly favoured THA over HA over 24 months. It must be noted that these are short term results only.

Wang F, Zhang H, Zhang Z, Ma C, Feng X. Comparison of bipolar hemiarthroplasty and total hip arthroplasty for displaced femoral neck fractures in the healthy elderly: a meta-analysis. BMC musculoskeletal disorders 2015; 16: 229. This meta-analysis included 8 RCTs from 1986 to 2013, which compared outcomes of bipolar HA versus THA in patient aged >65 with displaced IC fractures (1014 total patients with 523 HA and 491 THA) with follow up ranging from 12 months to 13 years. No significant difference was noted for HHS, infection rates, general complications, 1-year mortality, blood loss, and length of hospital stay between the two groups. Quality of life, mobility, and pain were better in THA, whereas surgical time was less in HA. Re-operation rates, acetabular wear were higher in the HA group after more than 4 years whereas dislocation rates were higher in THA within 4 years.

Management Planning

A simplified plan is presented in Fig. 1.44.

Patients with renal failure, neurologic deficit, Parkinsonism or hyperparathyroidism have a high failure rate with internal fixation and replacement options should be considered.

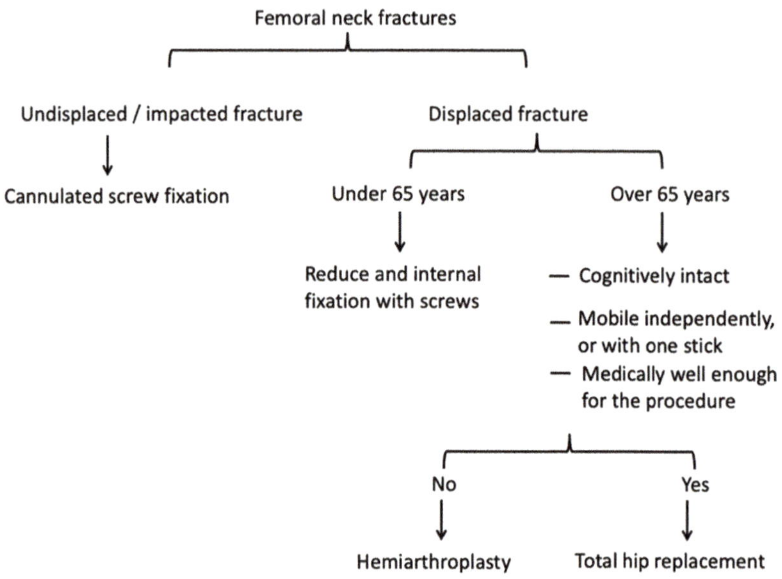

Fig. 1.44 Management plan for femoral neck fractures

Table 1.11 Management of anticoagulation

Aspirin alone	No need to delay surgery. No bridging therapy
Aspirin and Clopidogrel	Avoid neuraxial anesthesia. No need to delay surgery. No bridging therapy
DOACs	Delay surgery by 24 h. No bridging therapy
Warfarin	If INR is <1.5 then surgery can proceed without delay. If INR is more than 1.5 in low risk groups (AF with no previous TIA, DVT/PE>3 months) parenteral Vitamin K (3–5 mg) is given. INR is rechecked in 6 h and Vitamin K is repeated if required. In high risk group (VTE<3 months, recurrent VTEs, heart valve, AF with previous stroke) a multidisciplinary consultation is needed. Bridging therapy may be needed in the peri-operative period.

DOAC Direct Oral Anti Coagulants, *INR* International Normalised Ratio, *AF* Atrial fibrillation, *TIA* Transient ischemic attack, *DVT* Deep vein thrombosis, *PE* Pulmonary Embolism, *VTE* Venous thrombo embolism

Management of Anti-Coagulation

Most of the patients with neck of femur fractures are elderly with multiple co-morbidities. Many of these will be on anticoagulants on admission. Timing of surgery and need for reversal varies depending on the type of anticoagulant (Table 1.11).

Yassa R, Khalfaoui MY, Hujazi I, Sevenoaks H, Dunkow P. Management of anticoagulation in hip fractures: A pragmatic approach. EFORT Open Rev. 2017;2(9):394–402.

Complications

1. *Osteonecrosis*

The incidence of osteonecrosis is 10–45% after femoral neck fractures. The risk of osteonecrosis depends on the following:

- Initial displacement of the fracture.
- Time gap between injury and reduction.
- Adequacy of reduction (>20° varus/valgus leads to AVN).
- Associated dislocation of the hip.
- Comminution of the posterior part of the neck.

Treatment options include hemiarthroplasty, total hip replacement, arthrodesis of the hip, valgus osteotomy, core decompression and insufflation of the femoral head with methyl methacrylate. In view of good and reliable long-term results, total hip arthroplasty is often the preferred option for patients with osteonecrosis.

2. *Non-union*

The prevalence of non-union has been reported to be 10–30% after 12 months. If the head is viable on MRI scan then valgus osteotomy is an option in young patients. A free vascularised fibular graft can also be considered. If the head is not viable, and in relatively elderly patients, total hip arthroplasty is advisable.

3. *Failure of fixation*

This is best managed with total hip arthroplasty.

4. *Infection*

Urinary tract infection is present in up to one in four patients undergoing surgery for femoral neck fracture. Treatment is instituted as appropriate but surgery is not delayed unless there is systemic sepsis. Surgical site infection is rare after fixation.

5. *Transfusion requirement*

The requirement for transfusion varies with the procedure. The figures quoted are 45% after total hip replacement, 42% after cemented hemiarthroplasty, 29% after uncemented hemiarthroplasty, 19% after a dynamic hip screw and 0% after cannulated screws.

Swain DG, Nightingale PG, Patel JV. Blood transfusion requirements in femoral neck fracture. Injury. 2000;31(1):7–10.

There may be an increased risk of infection in patients receiving a blood transfusion.

6. *Mortality*

After femoral neck fracture, the 30-day mortality is 10% and 1-year mortality is 30%.

After cemented hemiarthroplasty, mortality is 20% at 6 months and 28% at 1 year.

Eiskjaer S. Risk factors influencing mortality after bipolar hemiarthroplasty in the treatment of fracture of the femoral neck. Clin Orthop 1991;270:295–300. Risk factors for high mortality include cardiac conditions, pulmonary disease, nursing home patients, high serum creatinine and pneumonia.

The preoperative albumin level has been shown to be an indicator of mortality.

Foster MR, Heppenstall RB, Friedenberg ZB, Hozack WJ. A prospective assessment of nutritional status and complications in patients with fractures of the hip. J Orthop Trauma 1990;4:49–57. A preoperative albumin level below 3.0 correlated with 70% mortality at 11 months, while levels over 3.0 corresponded to 18% mortality at 11 months.

Intertrochanteric Fracture

Intertrochanteric fractures involve the region of the greater and lesser trochanter of the femur (Fig. 1.45). These are different from femoral neck fractures as the extensive muscle attachments in this area provide good vascularity and hence good healing potential of the fracture, making non-union quite rare. AVN of the femoral head is also rare, with a reported incidence of 1%.

Diagnosis

Clinical features are similar to those of intracapsular fractures of the femoral neck. Patients are usually elderly and this fracture is more common in women. Young patients with this injury have high-energy impacts, in contrast to simple falls in

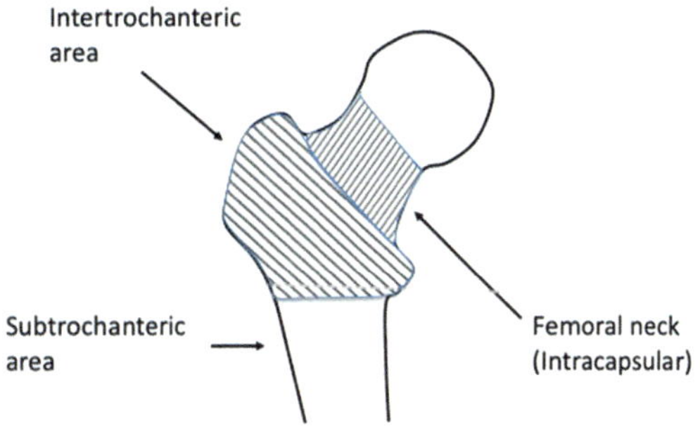

Fig. 1.45 The intertrochanteric area of femur

the older age group. The shortening and external rotation may be more marked in patients with intertrochanteric compared with femoral neck fractures.

The bone density bears a relationship to the risk of intertrochanteric fractures. Bone density of less than 0.6 g/cm^3 indicates an increased risk of fracture.

The family history is significant, as there is a two-fold increased risk of fracture in women whose mothers sustained a similar injury.

Imaging studies show similar patterns to those for femoral neck fracture. An X-ray in internal rotation may reveal an undisplaced fracture, which may not be obvious on standard images. A Tc-99 bone scan will be positive after 72 h. An MRI scan is the most sensitive modality to detect undisplaced fractures.

Classification

The difference between stable and unstable fractures is based on the ability to resist a medial compressive load on physiological loading. Medial comminution or reverse obliquity of the fracture line indicate instability.

Boyd Griffin classification is shown in Fig. 1.46.

Evans classified these based on the direction of the fracture line (Fig. 1.47). In type I, the main fracture line is along the intertrochanteric line. Type I fractures are further classified into those in which stability can be restored by anatomical reduction and those in which it cannot. In type II, the main fracture line extends downwards and laterally from the lesser trochanter (also known as reverse oblique fractures).

Other systems of classification include the Jensen–Michaelsen classification and the OTA classification.

Surgical Planning

Surgical stabilisation is the standard treatment for intertrochanteric fractures. Non-operative treatment can be considered only for patients who are medically unwell and unlikely to survive the anaesthetic/surgical procedure. Non-operative treatment carries risk of shortening, external rotation deformity and mortality.

Only the primary compressive trabeculae can provide sufficient hold for implant. Anatomic reduction is not always achievable, but stable reduction is mandatory. Mild valgus may be desirable. The Dimon–Hughston osteotomy was based on the principle of impaction of the neck into the medullary canal, hence medialising the shaft of the femur to improve stability. The

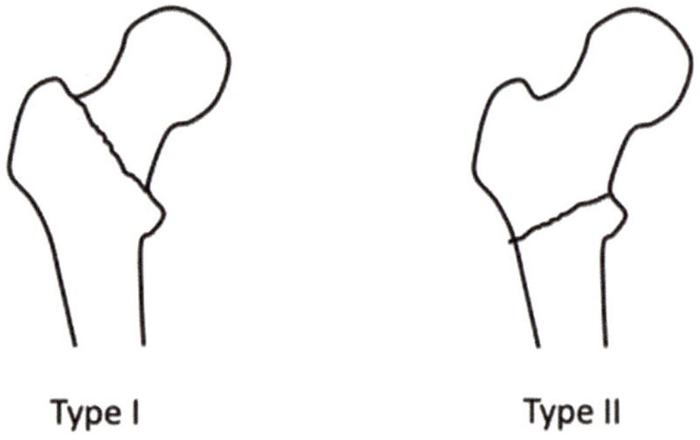

Fig. 1.47 Evans classification

Fig. 1.46 Boyd and Griffin classification

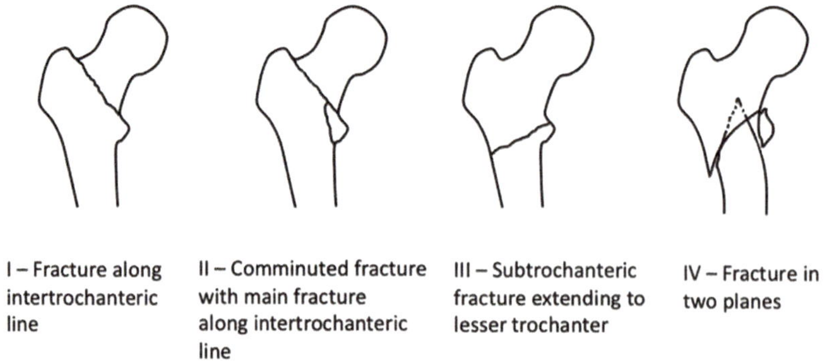

Sarmiento osteotomy describes resection of a lateral wedge so as to reduce the fracture to a more stable valgus position. These osteotomies are now largely historical and offer no definite benefit overstandard treatment for intertrochanteric fractu modern intramedullary fixation devices.

Choice of Implant

Historical implants used for fixation of these fractures include the Jewett nail plate, which was a fixed-angle, fixed-length device. The development of the sliding screw led to better outcomes as it allowed impaction of the fragments to a stable position with loading; and reduced the rate of implant cutout from the femoral head.

Currently, the most commonly used implant for stabilising these fractures is the dynamic hip screw (DHS). Intramedullary (IM) implants which allow fixation in the femoral head are used in unstable fracture patterns, reverse oblique fractures and fractures with subtrochanteric extension.

A recent randomized control trial showed that there is no significant difference in outcome following fixation of intertrochanteric fractures with DHS or IM nail but regaining mobility is better with IM nail.

Parker MJ. Sliding hip screw versus intramedullary nail for trochanteric hip fractures; a randomised trial of 1000 patients with presentation of results related to fracture stability. Injury 2017;48(12):2762–7. Regaining mobility better with IM implants. No difference in mortality, fracture healing complications, reoperations, hospital stay, length of surgery, medical complications, residual pain.

Implant Position

Screw placement in the femoral head should not be in the anterior or superior part of the head. Central, or slightly posterior and inferior, is acceptable.

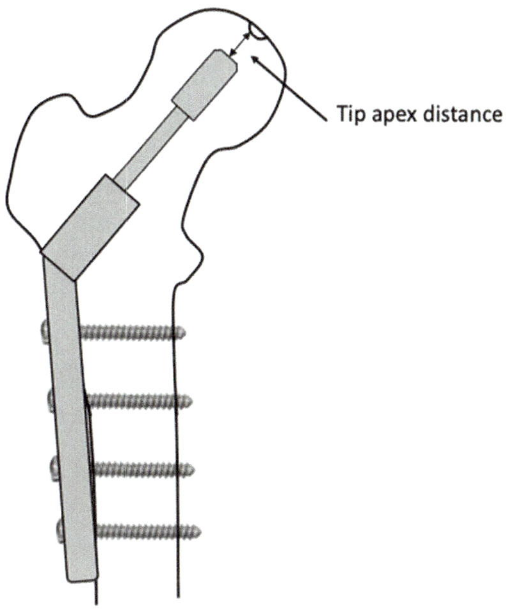

Fig. 1.48 The tip apex distance on AP view

The tip–apex distance predicts the risk of cut-out of the screw. This distance is the sum of distance from the tip of the screw to the fovea on the femoral head measured on AP and lateral radiographs (Fig. 1.48). The total distance should be less than 25 mm.

Baumgaertner MR Curtin SL, Lindskog DM, Keggi JM. The value of tip apex distance in predicting failure of fixation of peritrochateric fractures of the hip. J Bone Joint Surg Am 1995; 77(7): 1058–64. 198 fractures studied and tip apex distance described. 16 out of 19 failures were due to screw cutout from femoral head.

Baumgaertner MR, Solberg BD. Awareness of tip apex distance reduces failure of fixation of trochanteric fractures of the hip. J Bone Joint Surg Am 1997; 79(6): 969–71. Awareness of the tip–apex distance of 25 mm reduced the cutout rate from 8% to 0%.

The sliding hip screw acts as lateral tension band. A loss of sliding leads to a rigid construct and high failure rate.

Jacobs RR, McClain O, Armstrong HJ. Internal fixation of intertrochanteric hip fractures: a clinical and biomechanical study. Clin Orthop Relat Res 1980;146:62–70.

Telescoping of the screw within the barrel by 10 mm improves strength by 28%, and telescoping by 20 mm improves strength by 80%. The average settling of the screw is 5 mm in stable fractures and 15 mm in unstable fractures.

Posterior sag does not compromise fixation strength.

Factors which determine failure of sliding of DHS include

1. The ratio of length of screw beyond the barrel and the length of screw within the barrel. A longer contact area within the barrel allows better sliding. Short barrels can lead to jamming of the screw within the barrel.
2. DHS implants made of 316 stainless steel are more likely to jam compared to those made with Chromium—cobalt—molybdenum.
3. A higher angle allows sliding of the screw. A 150 degree screw will be more likely to slide compared to a 127 degree screw.

Kyle RF, Wright TM, Burstein AH. Biomechanical analysis of the sliding characteristics of compression hip screws. J Bone Joint Surg Am 1980;62(8):1308–14. Short contact within the barrel and stainless steel screws have higher risk of failure to slide.

The lateral wall thickness is a prognostic factor for failure of fixation following DHS (Fig. 1.49). The lateral wall thickness is measured along the axis of the neck of femur from a point 3 cm distal to innominate tubercle of trochanter to the fracture site.

Hsu C-E, Shih C-M, Wang C-C, Huang K-C. Lateral femoral wall thickness. A reliable predictor of postoperative lateral wall fracture in intertrochanteric fractures. Bone and Joint Journal 2013;95(8);1134–8. A lateral wall thickness less than 20.5 mm correlates with a higher rate of secondary lateral wall fracture if a Dynamic Hip Screw is used for fixation.

Seventy percent of patients need walking stick for 6 months postoperatively compared with 36% preoperatively. First-generation intramedullary nails have a 10° offset at the proximal end. The cutout rate is 3% and the incidence of thigh pain is 17%.

Second-generation nails have 4° angulation of the proximal end and a similar cutout rate to first-generation nails. In shorter nails, where the tip is in the diaphysis, a stress riser may be present, leading to cortical hypertrophy. These nails provide secure fixation and less shortening than a dynamic hip screw.

Intramedullary implants buttresses against collapse and shaft medialisation, thereby reducing shortening (Fig. 1.50). There is better calcar load sharing.

Intramedullary devices that end in the proximal half of femur are associated with a 3–6%

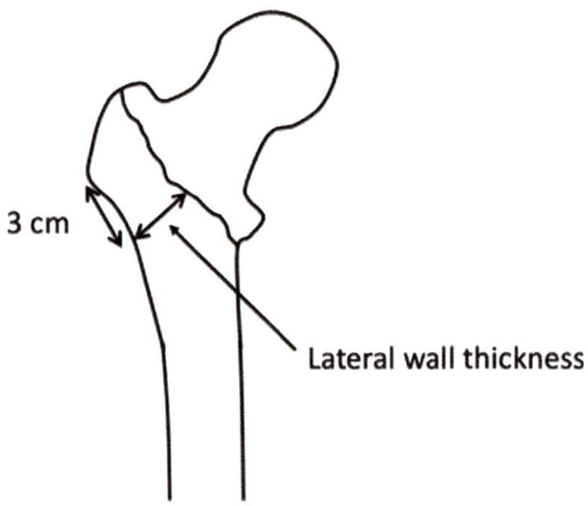

Fig. 1.49 Lateral wall thickness

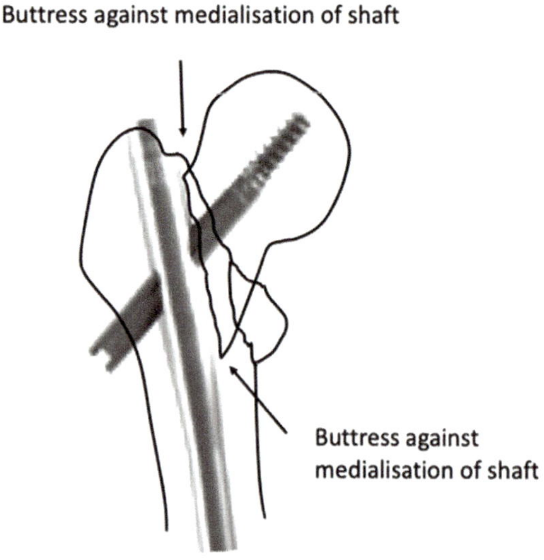

Fig. 1.50 Buttressing effect of intramedullary implants

incidence of secondary fracture at the tip of the stem. The advantage is easier distal locking using the jig. To reduce the risk of fracture, the locking screw is placed such that there is some length of nail beyond the screw.

Long intramedullary implants that are locked in the distal femur circumvent the problem of stress riser in the mid femur.

A 95° blade plate or screw device may be used for reverse obliquity fractures. Surgeon familiarity and ease of use of intramedullary implants has reduced the use of blade plates.

In recent years, there has been a surge in consideration of hemiarthroplasty/total hip replacement as a primary treatment for intertrochanteric fractures. However, a recent meta-analysis showed that there is no concrete evidence to support use of arthroplasty as the first line of surgical treatment in intertrochanteric fractures.

Arthroplasty in this situation is more complex. Calcar-substituting hemiarthroplasty or total replacement arthroplasty are useful for failed fixations. Bone pastes such as calcium phosphate cement can be used to augment fixation.

Nie B, Wu D, Yang Z, Liu Q. Comparison of intramedullary fixation and arthroplasty for the treatment of intertrochanteric hip fractures in the elderly: A meta-analysis. Medicine (Baltimore). 2017;96(27):e7446.

Patients should be allowed weight bearing to tolerance following surgery.

Ottesen TD, McLynn RP, Galivanche AR, Bagi PS, Zogg CK, Rubin LE, Grauer JN. Increased complications in geriatric patients with a fracture of the hip whose postoperative weight--bearing is restricted: an analysis of 4918 patients. Bone Joint J. 2018;100-B(10):1377–84. Immediate weight bearing as tolerated has less complications compared to restricted weight bearing.

Comparison of Different Implants

Schipper IB, Steyerberg EW, Castelein RM, et al. Treatment of unstable trochanteric fractures. Randomised comparison of the gamma nail and the proximal femoral nail. J Bone Joint Surg Br 2004;86(1):86–94. In this multicentre prospective trial, there was more lateral protrusion of the hip screw with the proximal femoral nail compared with the gamma nail. Both nails had similar complication and union rates, and the cutout rate was 7% cutout rate with both. A second screw in the proximal femoral nail had no benefit. There was no 'knife effect' of two screws in the proximal femoral nail leading to cutout.

Sadowski C, Lübbeke A, Saudan M, Riand N, Stern R, Hoffmeyer P. Treatment of reverse oblique and transverse intertrochanteric fractures with use of an intramedullary nail or a 95 degree screw plate. A prospective randomised study. J Bone Joint Surg Am 2002:84(3):372–81. In patients with a reverse oblique fracture, an intramedullary nail was found to be better than a 95° hip screw. The failure and non-union rate was 36% compared with 5%, respectively.

The sliding hip screw has been shown to be an effective implant for intertrochanteric fractures involving the lesser trochanter. Fractures of the lesser trochanter disrupt the medial weight-bearing axis and can lead to instability. However, a prospective randomised study has shown no difference in the failure rate of the sliding hip screw and nails.

Barton TM, Gleeson R, Topliss C, et al. A comparison of the long gamma nail with the sliding hip screw for the treatment of AO/OTA 31-A2 fractures of the proximal part of the femur: a prospective randomized trial. J Bone Joint Surg Am 2010;92(4):792–8. The reoperation rate was the same in 210 patients randomised to a long gamma nail or sliding hip screw.

Subtrochanteric Fractures

The subtrochanteric area is the segment of the femur at the level of the lesser trochanter and extending 5 cm distal to the lesser trochanter. Some fractures may extend proximally to involve the greater trochanter.

Muscle forces are considerable in the subtrochanteric region. The proximal fragment is abducted and externally rotated by the strong abductors. The femoral shaft provides attachment to the adductors, which pull the distal fragment away from the proximal fragment (Fig. 1.51). Shortening results from the combined action of the quadriceps, adductors and hamstring muscles.

The subtrochanteric area is a common site for metastasis. The possibility of pathologic fracture should be considered in all subtrochanteric fractures, particularly those with a transverse pattern of fractures.

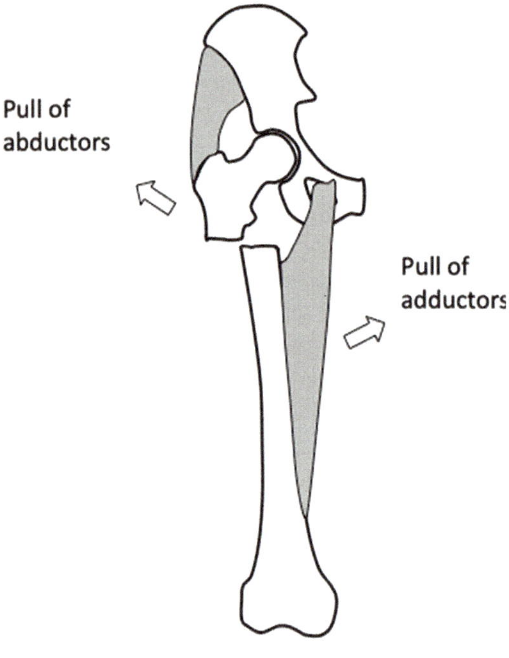

Fig. 1.51 Deforming forces in subtrochanteric fractures

Bisphosphonate related fractures are also common in the subtrochanteric area. Evidence of beaking of the cortex, prior pain in the local area and history of bisphosphonate use is relevant.

Classification

Classification was proposed by Russell Taylor (Fig. 1.52).

Management

Subtrochanteric fractures are best managed with internal fixation.

Second-generation nails are preferred for type I fractures. These provide secure fixation in the head of the femur and have good stability. The nails should not be locked in the diaphysis to avoid the risk of a stress fracture at the site of the screw hole. The nails should be long and locked in the distal metaphysis.

Type II fractures can be managed with the newer proximal femoral nails as these are inserted through the greater trochanter instead of the piriform fossa. Results of proximal femoral plates are encouraging in recent reports. Although IM devices have inherent biomechanical advantages, an extramedullary implant has shown to produce

Fig. 1.52 Classification of subtrochanteric fractures

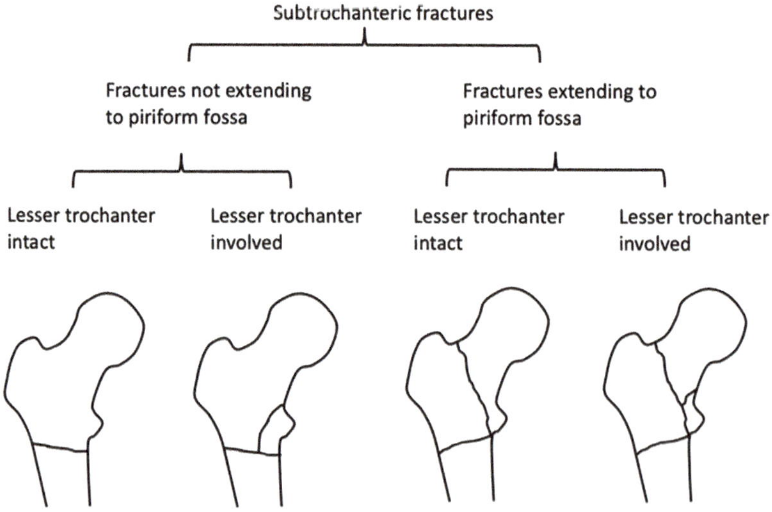

comparable outcome as long as varus malreduction is avoided.

Varus malreduction is a cause of failure and has to be avoided fastidiously. A low threshold is maintained for open reduction as opposed to accepting a malreduced fracture. A cerclage wire can be used to hold the reduction and this helps achieve anatomic reduction without an adverse impact.

Hoskins W, Bingham R, Joseph S, Liew D, Love D, Bucknill A, Oppy A, Griffin X. Subtrochanteric fracture: the effect of cerclage wire on fracture reduction and outcome. Injury. 2015;46(10):1992–5. 134 cases, 9.7% major complication rate. Cerclage wire used in 14.8%. No link of wire to complications. Complication rate was 11.4% if wire was not used.

Complications

Implant failure is relatively common because of high biomechanical forces in the subtrochanteric area. Varus positioning contributes to high risk of implant failure.

Non-union if there is no evidence of progression of healing after 6 months, a reamed statically locked intramedullary nail can be inserted.

Malunion is commonly due to varus malpositioning.

Femoral Shaft Fracture

Historically, femoral shaft fractures were treated by traction in a Thomas splint followed by hip spica. The Thomas splint, designed by Hugh Owen Thomas from Liverpool, was first used in 1865 and was used extensively in the First World War. Although a revolutionary treatment at the time, this often resulted in decubitus ulcers, deep vein thrombosis, osteoporosis, muscle wasting, knee stiffness, respiratory complication, shortening and malalignment.

The development of the Küntscher nail (K Nail) was a landmark in the management of these injuries. It was introduced in 1939 and was used by the German military in the Second World War. The nail had a clover leaf cross section which allowed firm fixation and quick return to mobility in the days when internal fixation of bones was in its infancy. Gerhard Küntscher also introduced the concept of reaming to allow a larger-diameter nail insertion and improve the contact area between the nail and the bone.

Clinical Evaluation

The diagnosis of femoral shaft fracture is usually obvious on clinical examination. Normal advanced trauma life support (ATLS) protocols should be followed as these are high-energy injuries and associated injuries may be present. Femoral neck fracture may be associated with a femoral shaft fracture and this should be checked before, during and after fracture fixation.

Classification

Classification is by Winquist and Hansen and the AO group. The Winquist classification is based on degree of comminution (Fig. 1.53).

In AO classification, femoral shaft is given the number 32. 32A is a simple fracture, 32B is a wedge fracture and 32C is a complex fracture.

Management

Non-operative treatment in the form of splinting or traction can be used as a temporary measure until internal fixation is performed. The definitive treatment of femoral shaft fractures in adults is by internal fixation. This should be undertaken as soon as the patient's physiologic condition has been stabilised.

Bone LB, Johnson KD, Weigelt J, Scheinberg R. Early versus late stabilization of femoral fractures. A prospective randomised study. J Bone Joint Surg 1989;71(3):336–40. Delays in internal stabilisation of femoral shaft fractures are associated with increased respiratory complications and acute respiratory distress syndrome.

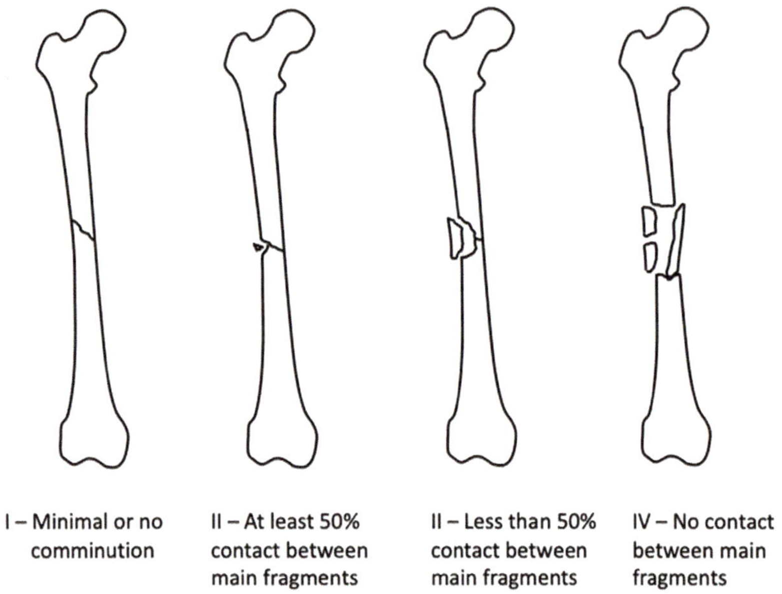

Fig. 1.53 Winquist classification of femoral shaft fractures

External Fixation

External fixation is an option for patients with severe open fractures or vascular injuries, or for initial stabilisation in haemodynamically unstable patients as part of damage control protocol. Once the vascular repair has been undertaken, physiology has been optimized, or soft tissue cover achieved, external fixation can be converted to an intramedullary nail within 3 weeks without an increased risk of infection.

Ipsilateral Femoral Neck and Shaft Fractures

Ipsilateral femoral shaft and neck fractures have an incidence of 5–10%. Traditionally, a cephalomedullary device, which enabled fixation of both fractures simultaneously using one implant, was used to manage these injuries. However due to high failure rates, the current trend is to treat both injuries as separate injuries.

Anatomic reduction of the neck fracture and the preservation of blood supply of the femoral head cannot be compromised. One strategy is to fix the femoral neck with multiple screws first. The shaft fracture is then stabilised with an intramedullary or extra medullary device. Either retrograde or antegrade nail can be used. A plate fixation is less preferable but may be used in certain cases.

Intramedullary Nail

An intramedullary nail is the most common method used to stabilise femoral shaft fractures. The development of locking nail expanded the indications for nailing and more comminuted fractures can now be managed satisfactorily. Fractures from the trochanteric to the supracondylar region can be managed with intramedullary nailing.

The first-generation nails were locked proximally and distally, but did not provide fixation into the femoral head. The second-generation nails have a screw or an alternative fixation device inserted along the femoral neck into the femoral head. This helped to extend the indications to subtrochanteric and intertrochanteric fractures, and for ipsilateral femoral neck and femoral shaft fractures.

Winquist RA Hansen ST Jr, Clawson DK. Closed intramedullary nailing of femoral fractures. A report of five hundred and twenty

cases. J Bone Joint Surg Am 1984;66(4):529–39. 99% union reported with intramedullary nails.

If Injury Severity Score (ISS) is more than 18, early stabilisation is associated with a lower rate of acute respiratory distress syndrome and pulmonary complications.

Brumback RJ. Intramedullary nailing of femoral shaft fractures. Part I: Decision making errors with interlocking fixation. J Bone Joint Surg Am 1988;70(10):1441–52. Static locking was better as dynamic locking was believed to lead to rotational instability and shortening.

Intramedullary nailing can be performed on the fracture table using the traction mechanism or on an ordinary radiolucent table with the help of a femoral distractor to achieve reduction. Rare complications with using the fracture table include pudendal, femoral or sciatic nerve palsy, perineal skin damage and occasionally 'well-leg' compartment syndrome.

Retrograde Nails

Retrograde nailing is an option in certain situations. The nail is inserted from the intercondylar notch in the distal femur and locked proximally. Indications for retrograde nailing include

- A femur fracture below a total hip replacement.
- A distal femoral fracture above a total knee replacement.
- Obesity that obstructs access to the proximal femur.
- Avoidance of radiation to the proximal femur in pregnant patients.
- Ipsilateral femoral fracture and acetabular fractures so as not to compromise acetabular exposure.
- A contaminated wound around the entry point for antegrade nailing.
- A femur fracture with hip dislocation.
- A femoral fracture with displaced femoral neck fractures requiring closed reduction
- Floating knee.

Floating Knee

A floating knee is a femoral shaft fracture with an ipsilateral tibial fracture. It can be managed with retrograde femoral and antegrade tibial nailing. Both procedures are performed through a single incision at the knee.

Complications that may result from retrograde nailing include a spread of infection to the knee joint in open fractures, a stiff knee, a 52% decrease in the anterior cruciate ligament blood supply, a 49% decrease in the posterior cruciate ligament blood supply and risk of patellofemoral joint damage if nail is prominent.

Union rates of 85–95% have been reported.

Reamed Versus Unreamed

Increased pulmonary complications with reaming in the presence of a chest injury in patients with multiple injuries were reported by Pape in 1990s. However, Bosse detected no adverse effect of reaming.

Pape HC, Regel G, Dwenger A, Krumm K, Schweitzer G, Krettek C, Sturm JA, Tscherne H. Influences of different methods of intramedullary femoral nailing on lung function in patients with multiple trauma. J Trauma 1993;35(5):709–16. Reaming was considered to increase risk of pulmonary complications compared to unreamed nailing.

Bosse MJ, MacKenzie EJ, Riemer BL, Brumback RJ, McCarthy ML, Burgess AR, Gens DR, Yasui Y. Adult respiratory distress syndrome, pneumonia, and mortality following thoracic injury and a femoral fracture treated with either an intramedullary nail with reaming or with a plate. J Bone Joint Surg Am 1997;79(6):799–809. There was no increased risk of ARDS after reaming for femoral fractures in patients with thoracic injury.

A recent meta-analysis of prospective RCTs comparing reamed versus unreamed nailing showed that reamed intramedullary nailing led to shorter time to union and lower rates of delayed-union, nonunion, and reoperation. Reamed intramedullary nailing did not increase blood loss or ARDS, implant failure, and mortality compared to unreamed intramedullary nailing. Therefore, the treatment of femoral fractures using reamed intramedullary nailing is recommended.

Li AB, Zhang WJ, Guo WJ, Wang XH, Jin HM, Zhao YM. Reamed versus unreamed intramedullary nailing for the treatment of femoral fractures: A meta-analysis of prospective randomized controlled trials. Medicine (Baltimore). 2016 Jul;95(29):e4248

One distal locking bolt is generally sufficient and the proximal hole out of the two distal holes should be used. There should be at least 5 cm of intact bone between the fracture and the bolt. In comminuted fractures, two bolts are recommended and early weight bearing can be allowed.

Complications of Femoral Fractures

1. The risk of infection is reported to be approximately 1% following internal fixation.
2. For delayed union or non-union—options are to dynamise the nail, perform a bone graft or exchange the nail. Exchange nailing is successful in approximately 80% patients with aseptic nonunion. Over 50% patients with septic nonunion need further procedures to achieve union.

Tsang ST, Mills LA, Baren J, Frantzias J, Keating JF, Simpson AH. Exchange nailing for femoral diaphyseal fracture non-unions: Risk factors for failure. Injury. 2015;46(12):2404–9.

Brown KM. Effect of Cox-2 specific inhibition on fracture healing in the rat femur. J Bone Joint Surg Am 2004;86(11):116–23. Cox-2 inhibitors interfere with healing of femur fractures.

3. Malunion in the distal third—rotational malalignment is common and averages 16° in some studies.
4. Compartment syndrome—rare.
5. Neurologic injury—the pudendal and sciatic nerves are at risk due to traction at the time of internal fixation.
6. Heterotopic ossification—present in 25% of patients, but routine prophylaxis is not recommended. The extent will depend on muscle damage and reaming. Pulsatile lavage does not reduce the risk.

Distal Femoral Fracture

The supracondylar area extends from the femoral condyles to up to 5 cm above the metaphyseal flare.

Clinical Assessment

The clinical assessment follows general principles. The physical examination should assess open injuries, neurological or vascular compromise and other associated injuries.

Imaging

Standard imaging includes AP and lateral views of the knee and femur, along with oblique views to detect fracture extension and configuration. In the lateral view, the lateral condyle appears larger and has a notch in the anterior half, which helps to differentiate it from the medial condyle.

CT scanning, including three-dimensional reconstruction, is very useful for determining the orientation of fracture lines and preoperative planning.

Classification

The fractures are commonly classified based on the comprehensive classification Fig. 1.54.

Management

Non-operative management of these injuries carries a poor prognosis and operative stabilisation is recommended.

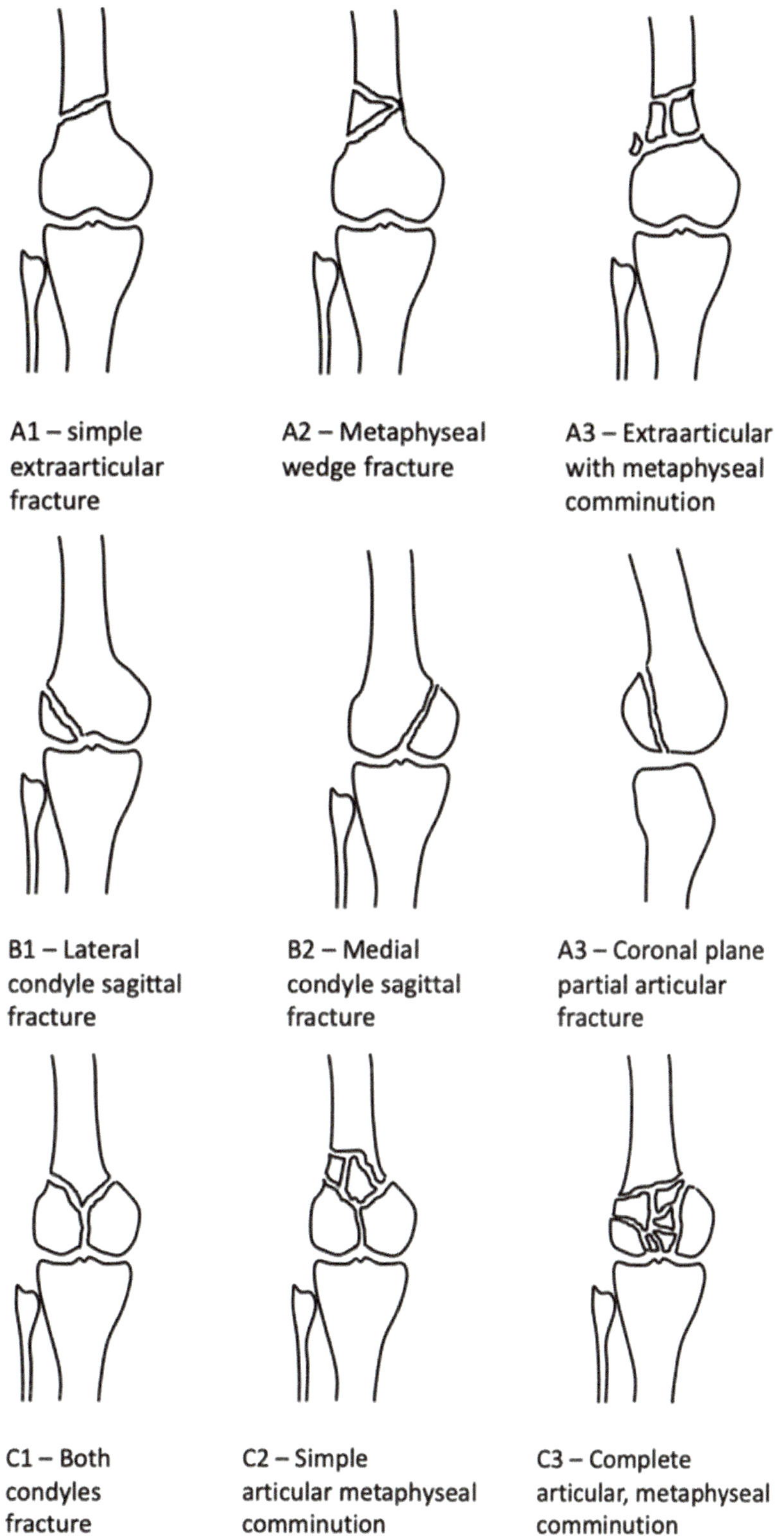

Fig. 1.54 Classification of distal femoral fractures

Fractures with intra-articular extension, fractures above total-knee replacement prosthesis, open injuries and fractures with vascular injury are absolute indications for operative stabilisation.

Treatment options are

- A 95° fixed-angle condylar screw.
- A 95° fixed-angle blade plate.
- Condylar buttress plate.
- Intramedullary nail—antegrade/retrograde.
- External fixation.
- Distal femoral locking plate.
- Distal femoral replacement.

In patients with metaphyseal comminution, the extramedullary fixation device is used as a bridging implant, without exposure of the metaphysis. This avoids devascularization of the fragments and stability is achieved by fixation in the distal and shaft fragments with near-far configuration.

Preoperative templating avoids surprises at the time of surgery. The blade or screws should be placed in the middle of the anterior half of the femoral condyle, which will coincide with the axis of the femoral shaft. The distal femur is trapezoid in cross-section, with the posterior aspect being the widest (Fig. 1.55). The blade or the screw will lie anterior to this and hence should be shorter than the widest diameter of the femur seen in the AP view of the image intensifier. A longer screw is likely to impinge on the medial collateral ligament and can be painful.

Locking plate functions as an internal fixator. It is inserted through a lateral incision and the plate is slid proximally from the femoral condyle to bridge the metaphysis. The screws are locking and proximal most screw can be unicortical to reduce stress concentration. Fixation into the femoral condyle is through multiple locking screws, which provide stable fixation. The ease of use and stability of fixation achieved with locking plates have made these the most commonly used implant for distal femoral fractures. Currently contoured distal femoral locking plates with options for bicortical fixation are the preferred choice and can be inserted through a MIPO (Minimally Invasive Plate Osteosynthesis) technique.

Distal femoral replacement is an option in the elderly with osteopenic bone. This allows immediate full weight bearing and is useful where restriction of weight bearing would not be possible or desirable.

Meluzio MC, Oliva MS, Minutillo F, Ziranu A, Saccomanno MF, Maccauro G. The use of knee mega-prosthesis for the management of distal femoral fractures: A systematic review. Injury. 2020:51 Suppl 3:S17–S22. This systematic review highlights the use of distal femoral replacement for acute distal femoral fractures,

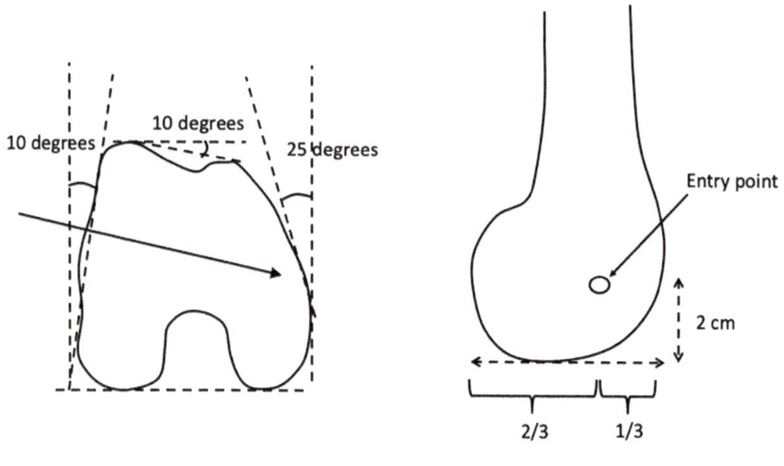

Fig. 1.55 Anatomical positioning of distal femoral compression screw or blade

periprosthetic fractures and distal femoral non unions. Distal femoral replacement allows immediate weight bearing, faster recovery of knee function and return to ADL.

Knee Dislocation

See Chap. 3—Knee.

Patellar Fracture

Patellar fractures are common. They can be the result of direct or indirect trauma.

Classification

Fractures of the patella can be of several types.

Osteochondral fractures are the result of patellar dislocation, whereby the injury causes a fracture of the medial facet of the patella. The fragment is largely cartilage and partly bone, and is sometimes difficult to visualise on plain radiographs.

The fragments can be replaced and fixed by arthroscopy or mini-arthrotomy. Bioabsorbable screws are useful in these cases. The tear in the medial extensor retinaculum can be repaired to restore stability to the patella.

Transverse fractures are generally the result of indirect trauma in which quadriceps pull results in fracture of the patella. Displaced fractures have an associated tear in the extensor expansion and, if present, will exhibit extensor lag. The gap in the patella is often palpable.

Vertical fractures are due to direct trauma and the extensor mechanism is not disrupted. As the fracture line is parallel to the pull of the quadriceps, the fracture is inherently stable. A step in the articular surface is an indication for open reduction and internal fixation.

Stellate fractures are comminuted fractures due to direct trauma, but the fragments are not displaced and the extensor retinaculum is intact. These can be managed non-operatively.

Comminuted fractures are caused by direct trauma and often need surgical stabilisation.

Management

Undisplaced fractures can be managed nonoperatively with an initial hinged brace or cylinder cast immobilisation followed by gradual supervised flexion. Full weight bearing in extension can be allowed from the outset.

Displaced fractures have tears in the extensor reticulum and should be managed surgically. Tension-band wiring of transverse fractures provides adequate fixation and early mobilisation. The presence of more than two fragments can often be dealt with using lag screws to reduce fragments to one another before fixing two main fragments with the tension band.

Weber MJ, Janecki CJ, McLeod P, et al. Efficacy of various forms of fixation of transverse fractures of the patella. J Bone Joint Surg Am 1980;62:215–20. Classic article describing the technique of tension-band wiring of the patella.

Cannulated screws can be used in place of K-wires and the wire loop can be passed through the screws. This is an alternative to tension-band wiring.

Postoperative early motion encourages compression at the fracture site. Weight bearing in extension is allowed as tolerated.

Patellar Tendon Rupture

Patellar tendon injuries are relatively rare and are usually the result of indirect trauma: flexion of the knee with an actively contracting extensor mechanism. Tendonitis of the patellar tendon or steroid injections in the local area predispose to rupture.

Patients exhibit reduced power of knee extension. A gap is usually palpable. Radiographs will reveal patella alta and an ultrasound scan will demonstrate the rupture.

Management

Rupture of the patellar tendon is managed with repair using a Kessler or Krackow suture.

The repair is protected with a cerclage wire passed along the superior pole of the patella and through the tibial tubercle. This can be a steel wire or non-absorbable suture, and is tightened with the knee flexed to 90° to maintain the length of the patellar tendon. The steel wire must be removed after 3 months, but cerclage sutures can be left *in situ*.

Proximal pole injuries are common and these can be repaired using locking sutures. The sutures are passed through three drill holes through the patella and tied at the proximal pole of patella (Fig. 1.56).

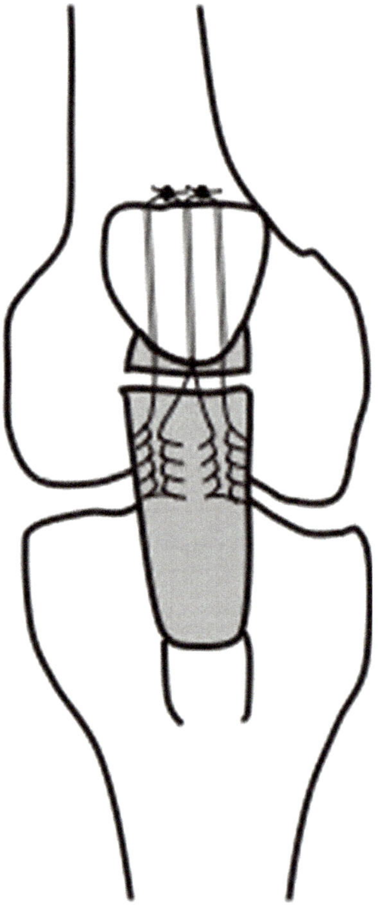

Fig. 1.56 Repair of proximal rupture of patellar tendon

Quadriceps Tendon Rupture

Quadriceps tendon rupture commonly occurs within 2 cm of the proximal pole of the patella. It is predisposed by steroid injections or diabetes.

Patients have a history of injury followed by pain and inability to actively extend the knee. In patients with an intact extensor mechanism, active extension may be possible but the power will be diminished.

A gap is often palpable and an ultrasound scan will demonstrate the tear.

Management

Direct repair of the tendon is performed. If there is inadequate tissue on the distal end, repair can be achieved by drill holes in the patella or through suture anchors in the patella. If using drill holes, the sutures is passed through the holes and tied at the distal pole of patella.

Postoperative knee flexion should start early if possible, starting from 0 to 30° flexion, and gradually increasing by 30 degrees every 2 weeks, so as to achieve unrestricted knee flexion by 6–8 weeks.

Tibial Spine Fracture

Tibial spine avulsion fractures are injuries of the tibial attachment of the anterior cruciate ligament. The injury to the knee can be hyperextension, twisting or excess varus or valgus strain. The knee is swollen and painful, with lipohaemarthrosis. Full extension may be blocked.

Classification

Classification was proposed by Meyers and McKeever (Table 1.12).

A further type IV was added by Zaricznyl, in which the tibial eminence is comminuted.

Meyers MH, McKeever FM. Fractures of the intercondylar eminence of the tibia. J Bone Joint

Surg Am 1970;52(8):1677–84. Classification of tibial spine fracture.

This system has poor interobserver reliability and predates MR scan. Consequently, it completely ignores the soft tissue injury associated with tibial spine avulsions. A more modern system was proposed by Green et al. for pediatric tibial spine avulsions (Fig. 1.57).

Green D, Tuca M, Luderowski E, Gausden E, Goodbody C, Konin G. A new, MRI-based classification system for tibial spine fractures changes clinical treatment recommendations when compared to Myers and Mckeever. Knee Surgery, Sports Traumatology, Arthroscopy 2019; 27:86–92.

Table 1.12 Myers and Mckeever classification

Type I	Anterior edge of the eminence is slightly elevated
Type II	Greater elevation of the anterior edge of the eminence
Type IIIA	Entire eminence is elevated and lies in its bed in the tibia
Type IIIB	Displaced eminence with loss of contact with the tibia

Imaging

Radiographs of the knee are obtained. A lipohaemarthrosis may be the only evidence of an undisplaced fracture. A CT scan will help to clearly define the fragment. MRI is helpful to identify concomitant injuries including osteochondral fractures, meniscal entrapment and cruciate ligament injury.

Management

The stability of the knee is checked, along with the ability to achieve passive full extension. If full extension is possible, a cast in full extension will reduce the fragment. Most type 1 and type 2 fractures can be managed nonoperatively.

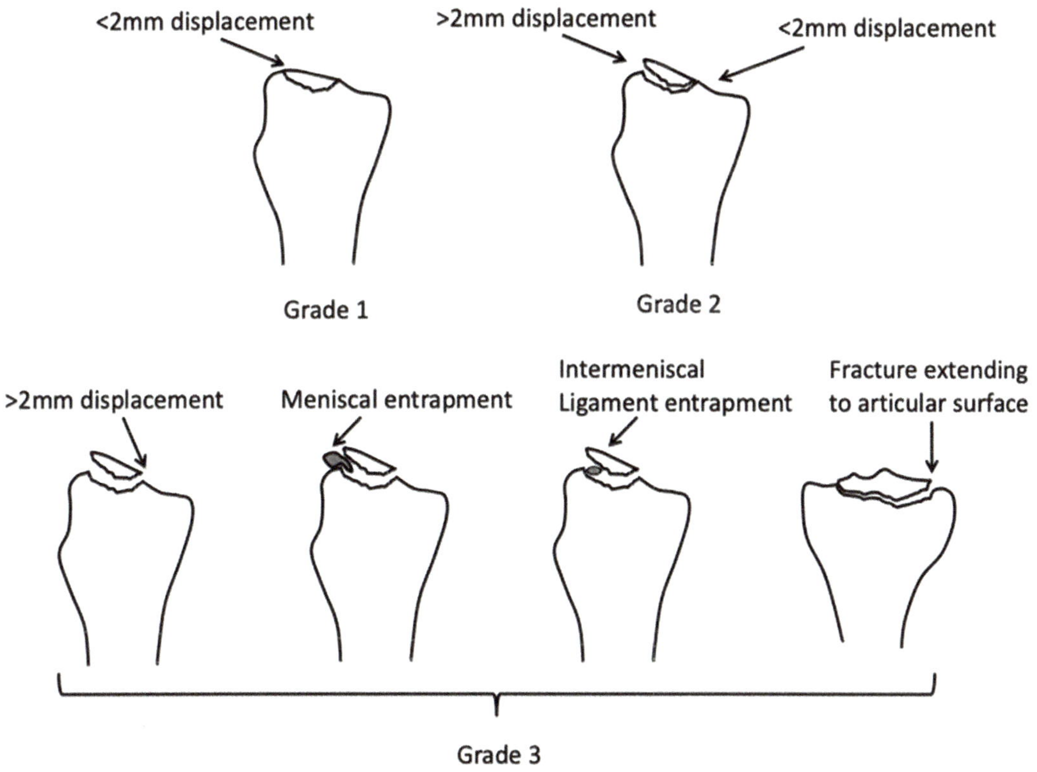

Fig. 1.57 Classification of tibial spine avulsions

Fixation of the fragment when there is a block to extension can be achieved by arthroscopic or mini open arthrotomy. The anterior horn of the medial or lateral meniscus can block full extension, in which case arthroscopic reduction will be needed. Displacement more than 5 mm can be considered as an indication for surgery. Fixation can be done using screws, wires or sutures. Residual cruciate laxity may be noticed postoperatively due to stretching of the ligament prior to bony avulsion at the time of bony injury. In the adult patient, arthroscopic tunnels can be made to pass sutures that reduce and stabilise the fragment.

Strauss EJ, Kaplan DJ, Weinberg ME, Egol J, Jazrawi LM. Arthroscopic Management of Tibial Spine Avulsion Fractures: Principles and Techniques. J Am Acad Orthop Surg. 2018;26(10):360–7. Description of surgical technique for arthroscopic fixation.

Tibial Plateau Fracture

Tibial plateau fractures are the result of varus, valgus or axial loading of the knee, which drives the femoral condyle into the proximal tibia. These are high-energy injuries in the young, but relatively low-energy injuries can cause tibial plateau fractures in osteopenic individuals.

Assessing the soft tissue component is an important aspect of management of tibial plateau fractures. This includes local soft tissue, skin cover, open injury and neurovascular assessment. A tilt of more than 5° or articular incongruity of more than 3 mm is an indication for surgery.

Imaging

Standard radiographic views, along with oblique films and, if necessary, radiographs of the uninjured contralateral side are obtained. CT scanning is useful for assessment and changes the classification in 10–15% of patients.

Approximately 50% of the patients have associated meniscal tears.

Classification

The Schatzker classification is most commonly used. It is based on the AP radiograph of the knee (Fig. 1.58).

The Schatzker classification, although useful, completely ignores posterior injury. More recently, the three column concept based on CT scans was proposed for tibial plateau fractures (Fig. 1.59). This recognizes three columns—anterolateral, anteromedial and posterior. Injury to any of these column requires appropriate approach for fixation. The posterior column is also subdivisible into a posterolateral and posteromedial fragment. In this system, a pure depression (Schatzker type 3) is classified as a zero column injury. Schatzker type 6 injuries could be three column injuries, which means each column is a separate articular fragment.

Luo CF, Sun H, Zhang B, Zeng BF. Three column fixation for complex tibial plateau fractures. J Orthop Trauma 2010;24(11):683–92. Prospective study of 29 patients classified on basis of three column concept and operated through a combined posterior and anterolateral approach.

The system helps guide treatment planning and surgical approach. The posterior slope of tibia is assessed and should be corrected at the time of surgery to prevent late instability.

Imaging

In addition to plain radiographs, CT scanning with reformats is useful in demonstrating the extent of the fracture and planning fixation. MRI can help to identify an associated torn or trapped meniscus.

Management

Non-operative treatment may be appropriate for minimally displaced fractures. A cast is initially required, followed by hinged bracing to allow knee flexion once the fracture is sufficiently

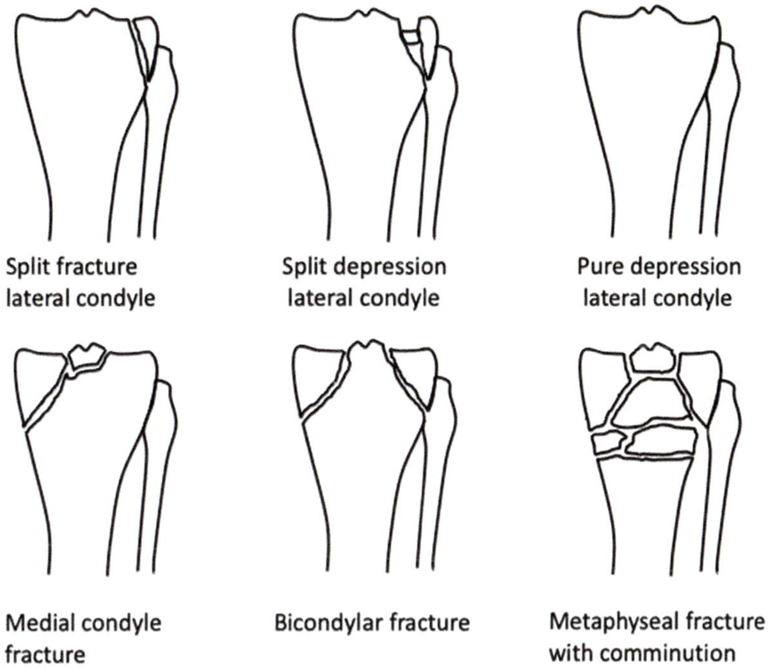

Fig. 1.58 Schatzker classification of tibial plateau fractures

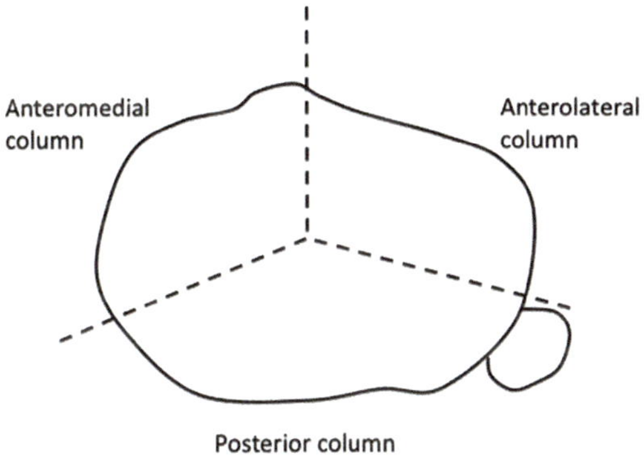

Fig. 1.59 Three column classification of tibial plateau fractures

healed. Weight bearing is restricted for 6–8 weeks.

Type I fractures are more common in young patients. If undisplaced, these fractures can be managed non-operatively with early mobilisation and avoiding weight bearing. Displaced fractures require reduction and internal fixation. The lateral meniscus is sometime trapped between the fragments; this can be resolved by arthroscopy. Percutaneous partially threaded screws are used for internal fixation.

Type II fractures are managed with open reduction, elevation of the depressed fragment, bone grafting and internal fixation. Early mobilisation limits knee stiffness. An anterolateral approach is used. If there is no anterior split, an option is opening a medial cortical window, elevating the fragment by a bone punch and bone grafting under the depressed fragments. Percutaneous screws can be used to buttress the elevated fragment.

Type III fractures are common in relatively older patients compared with type I fractures and are related to an osteoporotic proximal tibial bone. If the knee is unstable on examination under anaesthetic then open reduction, elevation of the condyle, bone grafting and internal fixation is performed. Stable fractures can be managed in a hinged brace without weight bearing.

Arthroscopic assisted internal fixation (ARIF) has been gaining popularity for management of Schatzker type I-III fractures. There are very few prospective trials comparing ARIF and ORIF.

Elabjer E, Benčić I, Ćuti T, Cerovečki T, Ćurić S, Vidović D. Tibial plateau fracture management: arthroscopically-assisted versus ORIF procedure—clinical and radiological compari-

son. Injury. 2017;48 Suppl 5:S61–S64. There was no significant difference in radiological or clinical outcome, however evaluation of intra-articular pathologies was better in the ORIF group.

Type IV fractures can be managed non-operatively if undisplaced. Close follow-up is needed to check for any late displacement. Displaced fractures need open reduction and internal fixation. These are often high energy injuries and are associated with ligament injuries.

Type V fractures are often unstable. Internal fixation offers the best chance of anatomic alignment.

Type VI fractures are difficult to manage. The principles of treatment are restoration of the articular surface anatomy and using a bridging implant to connect the epiphysis and diaphysis. Ring fixators have been used in these situations with good results. Locking plates to stabilise one or two pillars may be an option. Dual approach is often needed for these injuries.

Surgical Planning

The incisions used for fixation of the fracture are planned so as not to compromise any future reconstructive procedure. Protected weight bearing is instituted in the postoperative period and continues for 8–12 weeks. Early movement of the knee is encouraged. For bicondylar fractures, a double-incision technique can be employed: a posteromedial incision is made to manage the coronal split of the medial condyle, while a standard anterolateral approach is taken for the lateral condyle. Any extensile approach to both condyles through one incision, with or without tenotomy of the patellar tendon, is associated with a high rate of wound complications.

Wasserstein D, Henry P, Paterson JM, Kreder HJ, Jenkinson RR. Risk of total knee arthroplasty after operatively treated tibial plateau fracture. J Bone Joint Surg Am 2014,96(2):144–50. 8426 tibial plateau fractures. Knee replacement needed in 5.3% at 5 years and 7.3% at 10 years.

Tibial Shaft Fracture

Nicoll (1964) coined the term—'personality of fracture' to describe the differences in outcome based on degree of comminution, periosteal stripping and soft tissue injury.

Blood Supply of the Tibia

The vascular supply of tibia (or any long bone) comes from three sources:

- The nutrient vascular system.
- The periosteal vascular system.
- The epiphyseal metaphyseal system.

The nutrient artery arises from the posterior tibial artery and enters the posterior aspect of the tibia below the soleal line. It divides into an ascending and descending branch. The anterior tibial artery gives rise to most of the periosteal circulation. The nutrient vessels and the periosteal supply comprise the main vascular system involved in the healing of tibial shaft fractures.

Classification

The soft tissue injury component is crucial in tibial fractures. The classification of closed soft tissue injuries in tibial fractures was proposed by Oestern and Tscherne (Table 1.13).

The AO classification of long bone fractures is applicable to tibial shaft fractures.

Table 1.13 Classification of soft tissue injury in closed fractures

Grade 0	Indirect force, negligible soft tissue injury
Grade 1	Superficial contusion or abrasion, simple fracture
Grade 2	Deep abrasion, direct trauma and impending compartment syndrome
Grade 3	Extensive skin contusion, crushed skin, subcutaneous degloving and compartment syndrome

Clinical Assessment

The following factors influence the choice of treatment method

- Age of the patient.
- Presence of other injuries, polytrauma.
- Coexisting medical conditions.
- Open or closed fracture.
- Neurovascular conditions.
- Presence of or impending compartment syndrome.
- Fracture comminution.
- Presence or absence of fibular fracture and its level.
- Involvement of the ankle or knee joints.

Imaging

Plain radiographs are taken in two planes, including the knee and the ankle joint. Associated vascular injuries require angiography.

If there is any suspicion of compartment syndrome then compartment pressures should be measured and documented. Some centres recommend routine continuous compartment pressure monitoring.

Management

The treatment of tibial shaft fractures has changed with the evolution of orthopaedic practice. Non-operative methods—plaster casts, traction and functional bracing—were initially employed. The AO group proposed internal fixation to allow early mobilisation and minimise stiffness.

Non-operative treatment for selected tibial fractures continues to be used with good results. The ideal indication for non-operative treatment is a stable closed, isolated, minimally displaced fracture. A long leg cast is applied and weight bearing is limited in the initial stages of treatment, depending on the fracture configuration. Mobilisation is commenced with functional cast bracing after 2–3 weeks, when the fracture becomes 'sticky'.

The acceptable alignment is less than 5° of varus or valgus angulation and less than 10° angulation in the sagittal plane. There should be less than 10° external rotation, and less than 10 mm shortening. Any degree of internal rotation is not acceptable. Displacement of more than 50% of the shaft diameter is associated with delayed union.

Cast Treatment

Stable tibial fractures without significant comminution can be managed by cast immobilisation or intramedullary nailing. Some degree of stiffness of knee and ankle is seen after prolonged casting.

Bone LB, Sucato D, Stegemann PM, Rohrbacher BJ. Displaced isolated fractures of the tibial shaft treated with either a cast or intramedullary nailing. An outcome analysis of matched pairs of patients. J Bone Joint Surg Am 1997;79(9):1336–41. In this study of 97 closed fractures, the time to healing was 14 weeks with nailing compared with 22 weeks in cast. The rates of healing were 98% and 90%, respectively. Functional scores for the knee and ankle were better in the group managed with an intramedullary nail.

Potential complications with a cast include delayed union (19%), non-union (4%), malunion (13–20%) and ankle stiffness.

Indications for Surgery

- Comminuted fractures.
- Displaced intra-articular fractures.
- Open fractures or severe soft tissue injury.
- Unstable fractures.
- Segmental fractures.
- Bone loss.
- Coexistent injuries to the limb—'floating knee' fracture of the femur with tibia fracture.
- Polytrauma.
- Neurovascular injury.
- Compartment syndrome.

External Fixation

External fixators are reported to be associated with a 20% rate of malunion, 5% non-union and 50% pin-tract infection. External fixation can be used for temporary stabilisation prior to the insertion of a tibial nail in open fractures and polytrauma patients. The safe period for conversion without increasing the risk of infection is up to two weeks.

Bhandari M, Zlowodzki M, Tornetta P 3rd, et al. Intramedullary nailing following external fixation in femoral and tibial fractures. J Orthop Trauma 2005;19:140–4. In this meta-analysis, external fixation for more than 28 days was associated with a higher risk of infection compared to earlier conversion of external fixation to nail.

Ream Versus Unreamed Nails

Reaming the tibial canal is believed to disrupt the endosteal vasculature, but clinical studies comparing reamed and unreamed nails have shown quicker healing with reamed tibial nails.

Blachut PA, O'Brien PJ, Meek RN, Broekhuyse HM. Interlocking intramedullary nailing with and without reaming for the treatment of closed fractures of the tibial shaft. A prospective, randomized study. J Bone Joint Surg Am 1997;79:640–6. This RCT included 136 closed tibial fractures. The non-union rate was 4% in the reamed group and 11% in the unreamed group.

Court-Brown CM, Will E, Christie J, McQueen MM. Reamed or unreamed nailing for closed tibial shaft fractures. A prospective study in Tscherne C1 fractures. J Bone Joint Surg Br 1996;78:580–3. This study randomised 50 patients with closed tibial fractures. In the reamed group, the healing time was 15 weeks, screw breakage was 4% and union without further surgery was 100%. In the unreamed group, the average time to healing was 23 weeks, screw breakage was 52% and delayed union occurred in 20% of fractures. There was no difference between the groups in the incidence of compartment syndrome and knee pain.

Suprapatellar Versus Infrapatellar Nailing for Tibial Shaft Fractures

Tibial nails can be inserted using the suprapatellar approach where an incision is made proximal to the superior pole of the patella. A protective sleeve is inserted in the patellofemoral joint (PFJ) and standard nailing procedure is followed (Fig. 1.60).

The advantages are:

- Ability to do the procedure in semi-extended position hence obtaining intra-operative imaging is easier.
- More accurate entry point.
- Better alignment in proximal third fractures as hyperflexion required for standard nailing may cause excessive procurvatum at the fracture site.
- Less anterior knee pain. With traditional nailing technique using an infrapatellar incision, anterior knee pain is due to damage to patellar tendon and infra-patellar nerves. This is avoided by supra-patellar nailing.

The concern is potential damage to the patellofemoral joint.

MacDonald DRW, Caba-Doussoux P, Carnegie CA, Escriba I, Forward DP, Graf M, Johnstone AJ. Tibial nailing using a suprapatellar rather than an infrapatellar approach significantly reduces anterior knee pain postoperatively: a multicentre clinical trial. Bone Joint J. 2019;101(9):1138–43.

Xu H, Gu F, Xin J, Tian C, Chen F. A meta-analysis of suprapatellar versus infrapatellar intramedullary nailing for the treatment of tibial shaft fractures. Heliyon. 2019 Sep 6;5(9):e02199

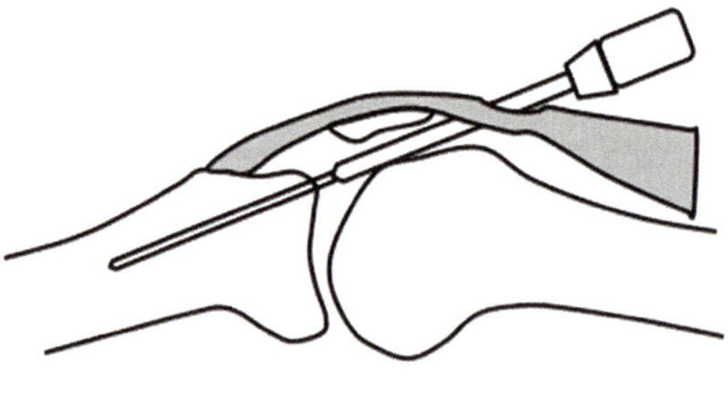

Fig. 1.60 Approach for suprapatellar nailing

Intramedullary nail fixation versus locking plate fixation for adults with a fracture of the (extra-articular) distal tibia: the UK FixDT RCT. The trial showed that the functional outcome, complications and need for removal of metal work was similar across both groups, however the IM nailing group had faster recovery and lesser cost.

Open Fractures

Open fractures are increasingly being managed with an intramedullary nail with soft tissue debridement and cover, and the use of external fixators has declined. The aim is to achieve definitive soft tissue cover within 72 h along with definitive skeletal stabilisation.

Henley MB, Chapman JR, Agel J, et al. Treatment of type II, IIIA, and IIIB open fractures of the tibial shaft: a prospective comparison of unreamed interlocking intramedullary nails and half-pin external fixators. J Orthop Trauma 1998;12:1–7. This RCT compared external fixation with an unreamed intramedullary nail in 174 type II and III open fractures. Malalignment was lower in the nail group at 8% versus 21%. Similar infection and healing rates were observed in the two groups.

Studies have shown no increase in infection rate when reamed nail was used compared to unreamed nails.

Keating JF, O'Brien PI, Blachut PA, Meek RN, Broekhuyse HM. Reamed interlocking intramedullary nailing of open fractures of the tibia. Clin Orthop 1997; 338: 182–91. 112 open fractures. Time to union was 29 weeks for Grade I open fractures, 32 weeks for grade II, 34 weeks for grade IIIA and 39 weeks for grade IIIB.

Court-Brown CM, Keating JF, McQueen MM, Infection after intramedullary nailing of the tibia. Incidence and protocol for management. J Bone Joint Surg Br 1992; 74(5): 770–4. Incidence of infection was 1.8% in closed and Type I fractures, 3.8% in type II, 5.5% in IIIA and 12.5% in IIIB open fractures.

In severe injuries, the decision to amputate is based on muscle damage, vascular damage and plantar sensation. These decisions should involve two consultants.

Intraarticular Fractures

Fractures that involve the proximal or distal articular surface of the tibia and extend into the metaphysis are managed with anatomic reduction of the articular surface, followed by stabilisation of the metaphysis. The metaphyseal comminution can be bridged with a locking plate or external ring fixator.

Minimally invasive plate osteosynthesis is achieved by the use of a locking plate to bridge the fracture site. The plate is inserted through a proximal incision and passed across the fracture without exposure of the fracture site. The screws are inserted with the help of a jig under image intensifier control. This technique causes minimal trauma to local tissues and provides a stable fixation, with each locking screw acting as a fixed-angle fixation device.

Complications

- Knee pain—occurs in 10–60% of patients and is more common with the patellar tendon splitting approach. Pain is greater on kneeling and is related to activity.
- Malalignment.
- Non-union—fracture non-union is declared after 9 months. If the fracture is axially stable, dynamisation of the nail can be considered. If not, exchange nailing is the preferred option.
- Compartment syndrome—the prevalence varies from 1% to 9% in tibial fractures. The diagnosis is based on the measurement of compartment pressures; a difference of 30 mmHg from the diastolic pressure is used as a cut-off for diagnosis.
- Reflex sympathetic dystrophy.
- Venous thromboembolism.

Keating JF, Orfaly R, O'Brien PJ. Knee pain after tibial nailing. J Orthop Trauma 1997;11(1):10–3. In 107 patients with 110 tibial fractures treated by interlocking tibial nailing, removal of the nail brought complete pain relief to 45% of patients, partial relief to 35% and no relief to 20%.

Connelly CL, Bucknall V, Jenkins PJ, Court-Brown CM, McQueen MM, Biant LC. Outcome at 12 to 22 years of 1502 tibial shaft fractures. Outcome data available for 568 patients including operated and non-operated patients, 11.5% had fasciotomies, 25% had ongoing knee pain, 10% had ongoing ankle pain and 17% had both.

Tibial Plafond (Pilon) Fracture

Pilon fractures are fractures of the distal tibial metaphysis with intra-articular extension. These comprise 5–10% of all tibial fractures. A fibular fracture in present in 75% of pilon fractures.

The main complications are fracture comminution, soft tissue injury and poor bone quality. The extent of soft tissue injury should be fully recognised even in closed injuries.

CT scans are routinely taken as plain radiographs often underestimate the injury.

Tornetta P 3rd, Gorup J. Axial computed tomography of pilon fractures. Clin Orthop Relat Res 1996;323:273–6. In this study, a CT scan led to change in the treatment plan in 64% of patients.

Classification

Several classifications systems are in use.

Ruedi and Allgower described three types (Table 1.14).

AO/ASIF (Association for Study of Internal Fixation) is illustrated in Fig. 1.61.

Severe fracture patterns are associated with more complications and poorer outcomes.

Table 1.14 Classification of pilon fractures

Type I	Undisplaced cleavage fractures involving the joint surface
Type II	Displaced cleavage fractures with minimal comminution
Type III	Metaphyseal and articular comminution

Surgical Approach

Multiple approaches have been defined for distal tibial fractures. Approach has to be tailor made to the type of injury in each patient. The cross sectional anatomy of lower end of tibia is illustrated in Fig. 1.62.

The approaches based on cross sectional anatomy are shown in Fig. 1.63.

Management

Initial management involves assessment of the patient, checking for neurovascular injury, soft tissue injury, swelling and checking for associated injuries. In presence of severe soft tissue injuries, a spanning external fixator may be considered to allow for soft tissue injuries to subside before considering ORIF.

A CT scan is obtained to determine fracture pattern in the axial plane and plan surgical management. A CT after spanning external fixator is preferable.

This is the "Span → Scan → Plan" principle.

Principles of management described in 1969 by Rüedi and Allgöwer are still undisputed and play an important role in ORIF:

- Reconstruction of fibular length
- Reconstruction of articular surface
- Stable internal fixation
- Filling of metaphyseal void with bone graft

In comminuted fractures, the surgical plan is to fix the fibula to restore length. Then the reconstruction of the articular surface is done with lag screws. Defects in the metaphysis from bone impaction are bone grafted. An antero-medial or anterolateral buttress plate, or a locking plate is applied as a neutralisation plate to maintain length.

Reudi in 1969 reported 74% good or excellent results at 4 and 9 years. Out of 75 fractures in this series, only three were open and almost half were low-energy injuries.

Temporary external fixation and delayed ORIF after 2 weeks had good results in 77% of cases. A useful plan is to stabilise the skeleton

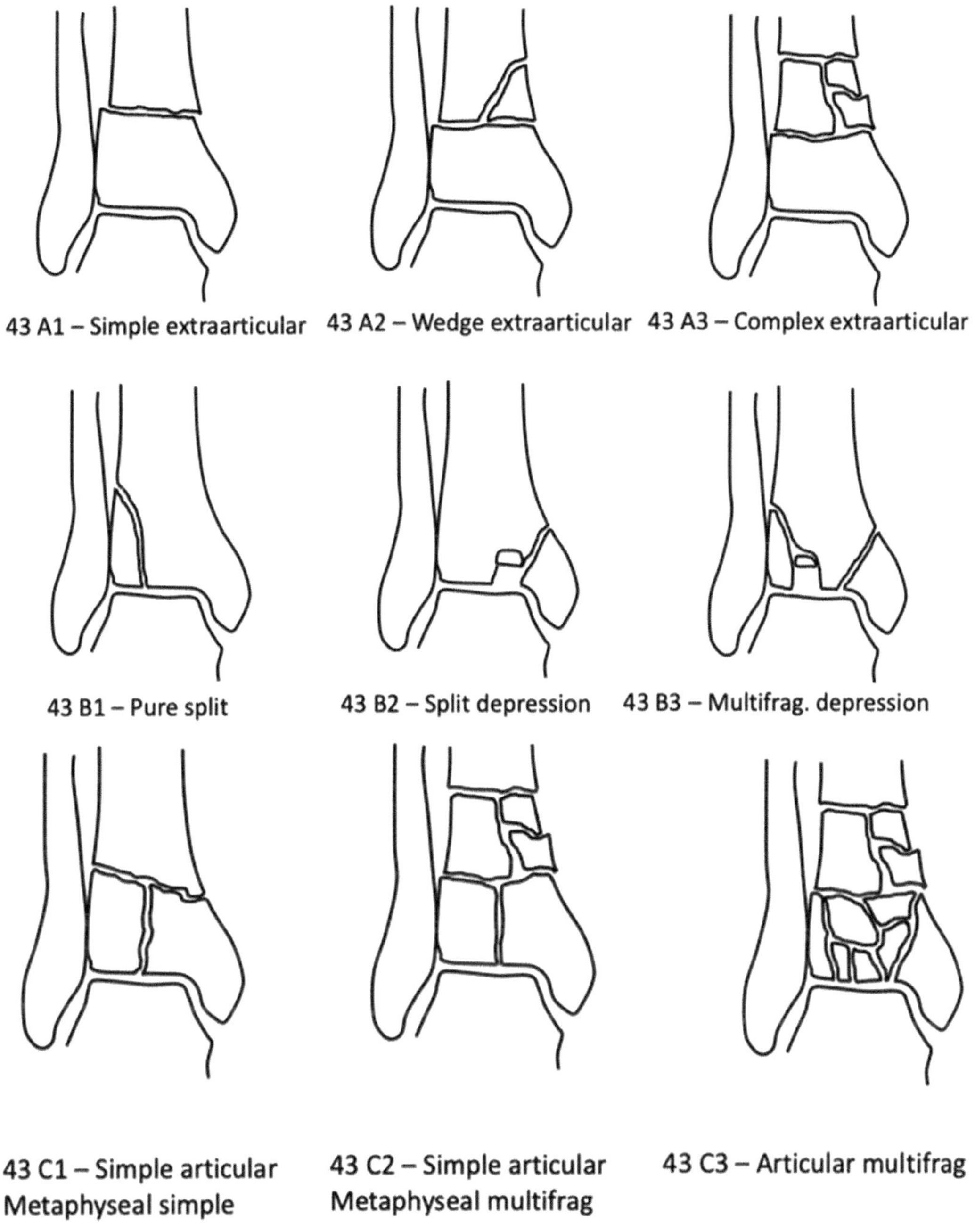

Fig. 1.61 AO classification of pilon fractures

and soft tissues with a spanning external fixator, with or without fixation of the fibular fracture (depending on the initial shortening). Delayed fixation with anatomical reduction of the articular surface and either bridge plating of the metaphysis or hybrid fixator application avoids soft tissue and wound complications.

Patterson MJ, Cole JD. Two stage delayed open reduction and internal fixation of severe pilon fractures. J Orthop Trauma 1999;13(2):85–91. 21 consecutive patients managed by fibular

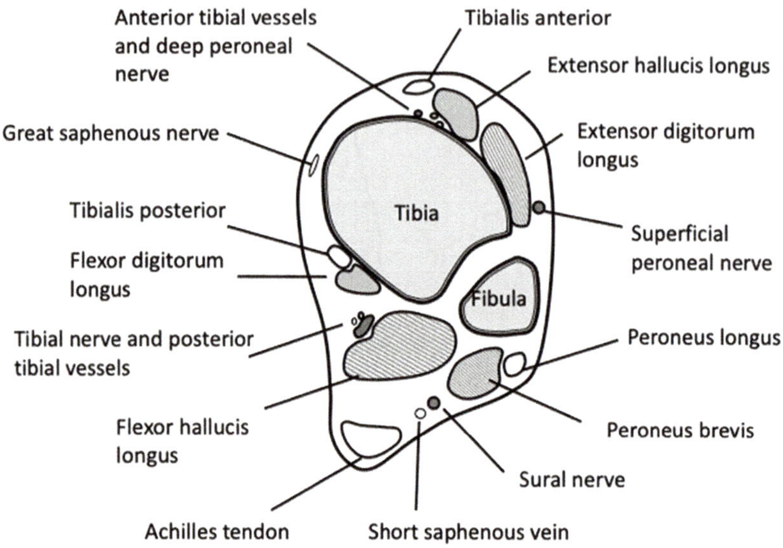

Fig. 1.62 Cross sectional anatomy of lower third of leg

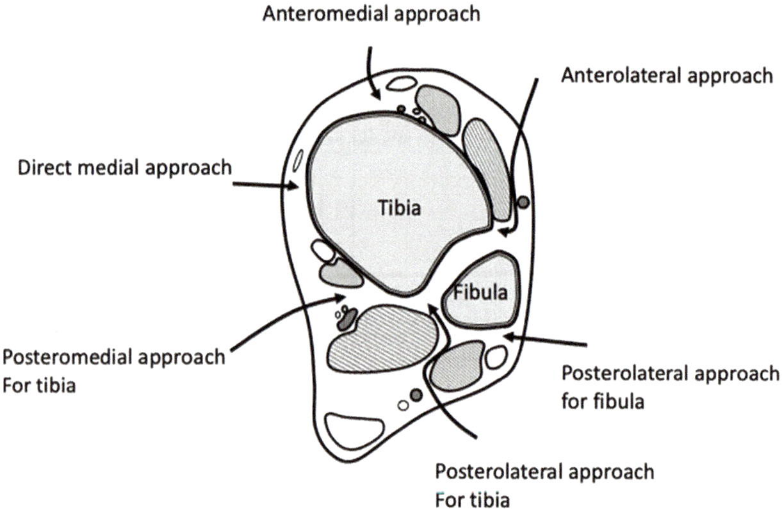

Fig. 1.63 Approaches to the lower third of tibia and fibula

fixation and medial spanning external fixator initially followed by removal of fixator and medial plate after an average of 24 days. No deep infections.

External fixators can be spanning, hybrid or articulated.

White TO, Guy P, Cooke CJ, Kennedy SA, Droll KP, Blachut PA, O'Brien PJ. The results of early primary open reduction and internal fixation for treatment of OTA 43.C type tibial pilon fractures: a cohort study. J Orthop Trauma 2010;24(12):757–63. 95 fractures treated with ORIF within 24 h in 70% and within 48 h in 88%. Risk of deep infection and wound dehiscence was 19% for open fractures and 2.7% for closed fractures.

Zelle BA, Dang KH, Ornell SS. High-energy tibial pilon fractures: an instructional review. International Orthopaedics 2019; 43(8):1939–1950. Article on strategies of management of pilon fractures. Description of approaches and principles of treatment.

Complications

- Malunion (varus) and non-union—the incidence is between 1% and 5%.
- Posttraumatic arthrosis—ankle fusion is an option for posttraumatic arthritis. Ankle fusion carries a risk of non-union, delayed union, leg-length discrepancy, arthritis in adjoining joints, chronic oedema and pain. Ankle replacement is increasingly being undertaken in posttraumatic arthritis.
- Wound breakdown—wound-healing problems are experienced by up to 10% of patients. Excess tension on the soft tissues and trauma to the tissues at the time of injury predispose to wound problems. Use of Allgower-Donati suture technique has been shown to improve oxygenation of the wound (Fig. 1.64).
- Infection—infection is reported in up to a third of patients. Removal of metalwork and extensive debridement may be needed for deep infection. Some patients may require amputation for persistent infection.

Stannard JP, Volgas DA, McGwin G 3rd, Stewart RL, Obremskey W, Moore T, Anglen JO. Incisional negative pressure wound therapy after high-risk lower extremity fractures. J Orthop Trauma 2012;26(1):37–42. In this prospective multicentre RCT, incidence of wound dehiscence and infections were lower when incisional negative pressure wound therapy was used on the surgical site immediately after wound closure.

Ankle Fractures

Ankle fractures are common and usually result from low energy injuries. Associated conditions like diabetes mellitus, peripheral neuropathy, peripheral vascular disease, osteoporosis, smoking, renal impairment and alcohol abuse should be assessed as these can affect the choice of treatment and outcome of these injuries.

Radiographs should be centred on the ankle and further images of the upper third of the leg may be required if a proximal fibular fracture is suspected. Careful assessment of skin condition, blisters, neurological integrity and circulatory function is essential.

Classification

Lauge and Hansen classified ankle fractures into five types based on the position of the foot at the time of injury and the direction of the deforming force; for example, 'supination adduction' implies an adduction force on the supinated foot.

The five types are supination adduction; supination external rotation; pronation abduction; pronation external rotation; and pronation dorsiflexion (Fig. 1.65).

Interobserver variability may be high, but the classification explains the injury mechanism. The grading is not a prognostic indicator.

Supination external rotation (SER) is the common injury pattern. The injury starts on the lateral aspect with a trans-syndesmotic fracture

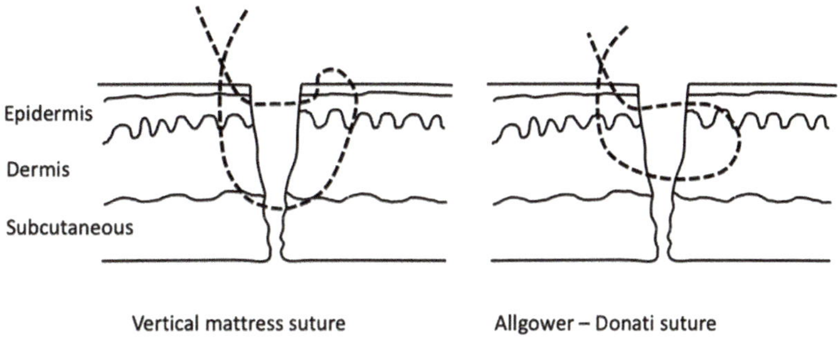

Fig. 1.64 Allgower—Donati suture to preserve viability of skin edges

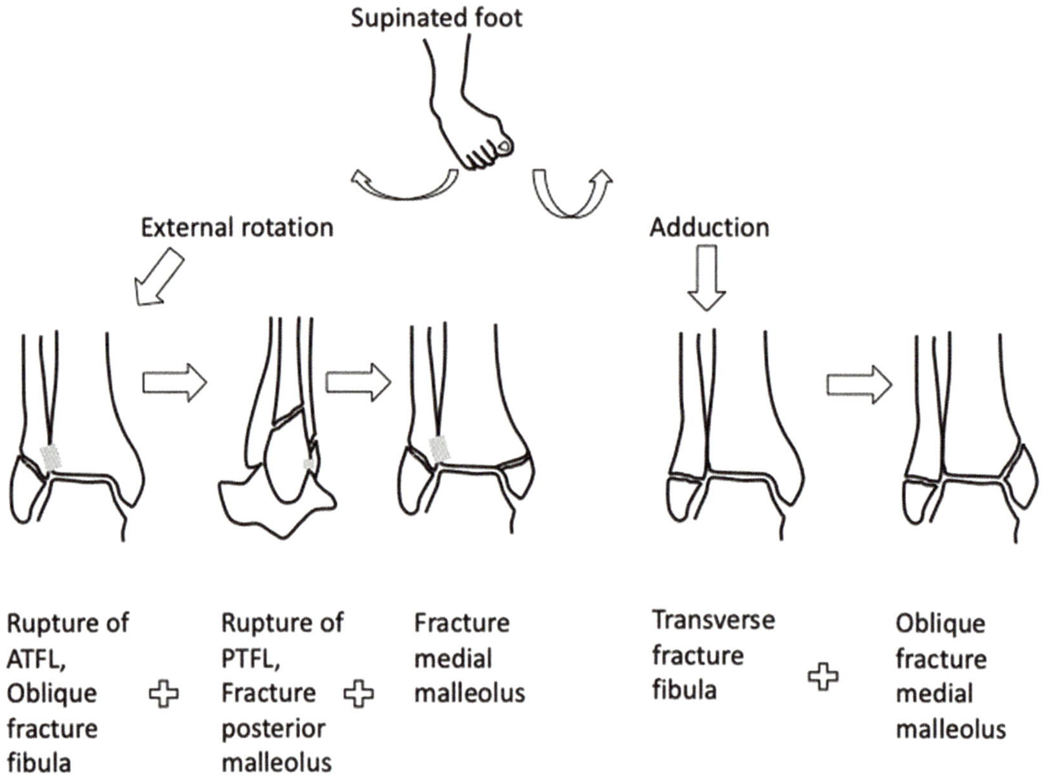

Fig. 1.65 Supination injuries of the ankle

of the fibula. Further force causes disruption of the syndesmosis (SER II injury). Progressive force can cause fracture of the posterior malleolus (SER III injury) or fracture of the medial malleolus or injury to deltoid ligament (SER IV injury). An SER IV injury will result in widening of the medial joint space, indicating an unstable injury.

The pronation external rotation (PER) injury starts on the medial side. This is followed by injury to the syndesmosis, a supra-syndesmotic fibular fracture and then posterior malleolus fracture (Fig. 1.66).

The Lauge Hansen classification is helpful in predicting ligamentous injury and determining the stability of the ankle joint.

The Danis–Weber classification is based on the level of the fibular fracture. Weber A fractures are generally stable and do not require surgical intervention. Weber B and C are potentially unstable and, if associated with talar shift, are managed by early internal fixation (Fig. 1.67).

Weber classification ignores the medial aspect of the ankle, and hence it is difficult to categorise fractures as stable or unstable purely on the basis of the Weber classification. The medial aspect of the ankle is an important contributor to stability of the ankle joint and has to be taken into consideration when deciding management options.

Determining Stability of the Ankle Joint

Bimalleolar and trimalleolar fractures are considered unstable. In isolated lateral malleolus fractures, determining the integrity of the deltoid ligament is essential. The deltoid ligament has a superficial and a deep component. The deep part has an anterior and a posterior band—anterior

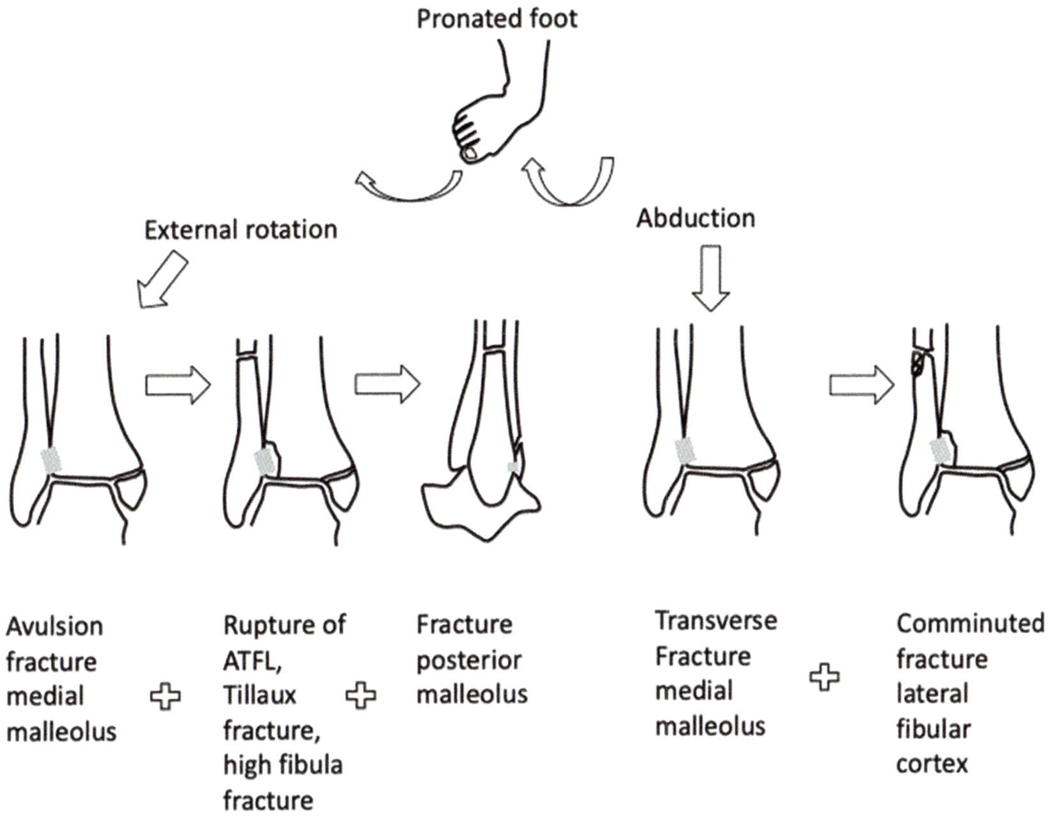

Fig. 1.66 Pronation injuries of the ankle

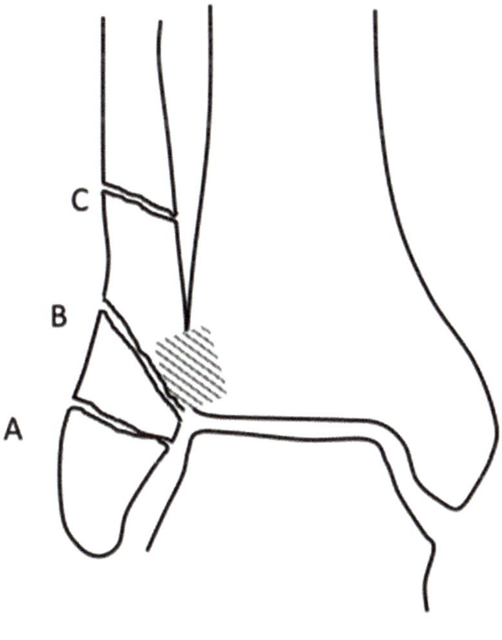

Fig. 1.67 Weber classification of ankle injuries

tibiotalar ligament and the posterior tibio talar ligament.

Determination of ankle stability is of paramount importance in determination of management. The methods which can be used to determine stability are

1. Evaluation of Medial Clear Space (MCS) on standard non weight bearing ankle mortice radiographs: This method is unreliable.
2. Presence of medial tenderness or bruising on examination. This method is also unreliable.
3. Manual external rotation stress radiographs: This is a reliable test, however, has poor reproducibility.
4. Gravity stress radiographs: These are as reliable as manual external rotation stress radio-

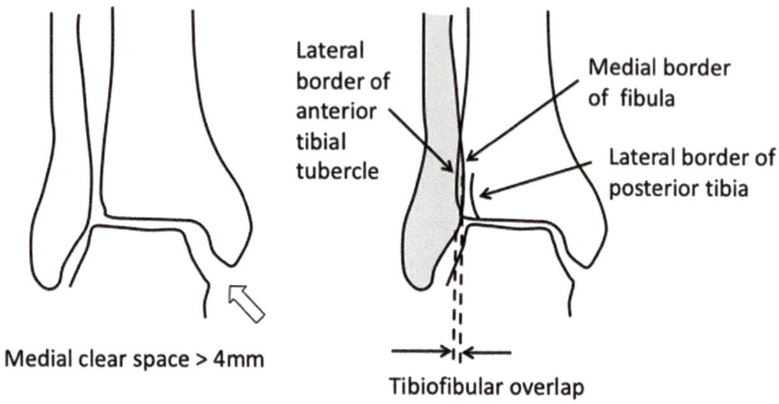

Fig. 1.68 Medial clear space and tibiofibular overlap

graphs but are less painful and avoid radiation exposure to the physician.

5. Weight bearing radiographs. This is the most useful method with good reproducibility and reliability. The radiographs are done 7 to 10 days after injury.

Dawe EJ, Shafafy R, Quayle J, et al. The effect of different methods of stability assessment on fixation rate and complications in supination external rotation (SER) 2/4 ankle fractures. Foot Ankle Surg 2015;21:86–90. Weight bearing radiographs reduced rate of unnecessary surgery in stable ankle injuries.

Gougoulias N, Sakellariou A. When Is a Simple Fracture of the Lateral Malleolus Not So Simple? How to Assess Stability, Which Ones to Fix and the Role of the Deltoid Ligament. Bone Joint J 2017;99(7):851–5.

Aiyer A, Zachwieja EC, Lawrie CM, Kaplan JRM. Management of isolated lateral malleolus fracture. J Am Acad Orthop Surg 2019;27(2):50–59.

Normal Radiographic Parameters of Ankle

The overlap in the mortise view should be at least 1 mm and is measure 1 cm above the distal tibial articular margin (Fig. 1.68). In the AP view, the overlap should be at least 6 mm.

The talocrural angle (Fig. 1.69) is formed between the distal tibial articular surface and the intermalleolar line. Normal value is 8 to 15 degrees. A reduced angle indicates fibular shortening.

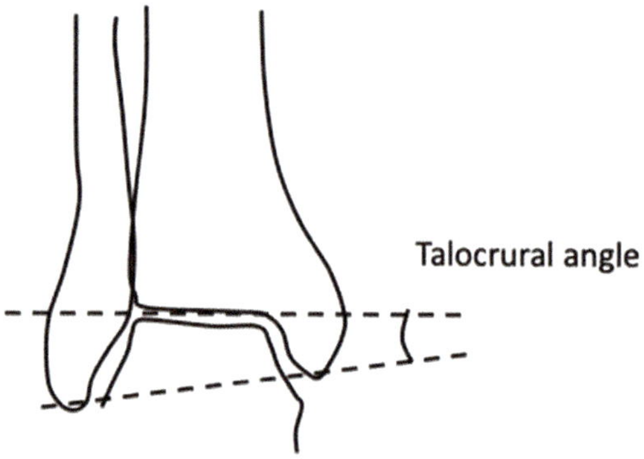

Fig. 1.69 The talocrural angle

Operative vs. Non-Operative Management of Unstable Ankle Fracture

There is agreement that most unstable ankle fractures in young individuals must be treated with ORIF. However, controversy exists amongst surgeons regarding optimal treatment of unstable ankle fracture in elderly patients due to increased risk of complications like local wound problems, infection etc. The AIM trail published in 2016 shows the efficacy of closed contact casting (CCC) done/supervised in theatre by a consultant trained in CCC. This trial showed that outcomes following CCC vs. ORIF were similar and the cost of treatment was less.

Keene DJ, Mistry D, Nam J, Tutton E, Handley R, Morgan L, Roberts E, Gray B, Briggs A, Lall R, Chesser TJ, Pallister I, Lamb SE, Willett K. The Ankle Injury Management (AIM) trial: a pragmatic, multicentre, equivalence randomised controlled trial and economic evaluation comparing close contact casting with open surgical reduction and internal fixation in the treatment of unstable ankle fractures in patients aged over 60 years. Health Technol Assess. 2016;20(75):1–158.

Isolated Medial Malleolus Fracture

Undisplaced fractures are usually treated non-operatively. Fixation may be required for high-demand individuals.

Displaced fractures are generally managed with internal fixation. Avulsion of the tip can be treated non-operatively, but fractures near the base of medial malleolus should be fixed. Tension-band wiring can be considered if the fragment is too small for two screws. There is a high rate of metalwork related problems with the use of tension band wiring.

Fixation is with two cannulated or partially threaded cancellous screws perpendicular to the fracture plane. In fractures oriented vertically, screws should be horizontal and an antiglide screw is used to prevent proximal displacement.

Bioabsorbable screws (polyglycolic acid or polylactic acid) have been used. These provide union rates similar to those with metal screws, but there have been reports of a higher local inflammatory response and sterile serous discharge with bioabsorbable screws.

Stress fracture of the medial malleolus may be seen in athletes and presents with tenderness over the medial malleolus. Diagnosis is by radiographs or bone scan and 4 to 5 months of restricted activity is necessary for healing. Displaced fractures can be treated with internal fixation.

Lateral Malleolus fractures

Reduction in the tibiotalar contact area increases the peak contact pressure. The deltoid ligament is a prime stabiliser against lateral displacement of the talus. Injury to deep deltoid ligament makes these injuries unstable, and is an indication for operative intervention.

Stable lateral malleolus fractures may be treated non operatively and allowed to weight bear as tolerated in a weight bearing cast or an air cast boot. Undisplaced fractures managed nonoperatively should have a weight bearing radiograph at 7–10 days. If stable, full weight bearing can be allowed.

In patients with an isolated lateral malleolus fracture with talar shift the medial ligament may get interposed in the joint, preventing accurate reduction. The medial aspect should be opened to retrieve the ligament, but primary repair does not appear to offer any significant advantage over simple retrieval of the ligament.

The CROSSBAT trial showed that fixation of isolated lateral malleolus fractures without talar shift led to higher complication rate without improvement in outcome.

Mittal R, Harris IA, Adie S, Naylor JM. CROSSBAT study group: Surgery for type B ankle fracture treatment. A combined randomized and observational study. BMJ Open 2017;7:013298.

Recent evidence has emerged in support of use of locked fibular nails for unstable lateral malleolus fracture (isolated or a part of bi-malleolar fractures). These are not indicated in young patients where anatomical reduction is required. Fibular nails may be used in elderly patients with co-morbidities like diabetes, peripheral neuropathy or vascular diseases. The advantage is avoidance of skin healing problems which often complicates plate fixation of lateral malleolus. It also has the advantage of allowing early weight bearing in a cast—as early as 24 h after surgery.

Tas DB, Smeeing DPJ, Emmink BL, Govaert GAM, Hietbrink F, Leenen LPH, Houwert RM. Intramedullary Fixation Versus Plate Fixation of Distal Fibular Fractures: A Systematic Review and Meta-Analysis of Randomized Controlled Trials and Observational Studies. J Foot Ankle Surg. 2019;58(1):119–26.

Bimalleolar Fractures

Most bimalleolar fractures are managed with fixation of both malleoli. A lateral plate on the fibula can lead to pain over the hardware and only half of patients experience relief with hardware removal.

Posterior plates avoid the problem of palpable hardware, but can cause peroneal tendonitis. A posterior antiglide plate is useful in osteopenic bone where bicortical screws distally achieve better fixation. Screws can be inserted through the plate to compress the fracture site.

Early surgery is recommended before the swelling increases. In the presence of fracture blisters or excess swelling, surgery may have to be delayed for 1–2 weeks. During this time, alignment of the ankle is maintained with a cast or external fixator.

An external fixator can be used for temporary stabilization if excess swelling precludes primary internal fixation.

Injury to the Syndesmosis

In syndesmotic injuries, the ankle pain is anterior, the squeeze test is positive and there is pain on external rotation of the ankle.

These injuries are caused by external rotation of the talus in the ankle mortise. They can be present in medial malleolus fractures without lateral malleolus fracture or with Weber type B or C fractures of the lateral malleolus.

Diagnosis is by demonstrating a widened gap between the distal tibia and fibula on radiographs or intraoperative stressing. Studies have shown that intra operative hook test is better at diagnosing syndesmotic injuries when compared to external rotation stress test.

A fibular fracture in the mid or distal third with a syndesmotic injury should be fixed along with stabilisation of the syndesmosis.

Fixation can be performed with 3.5 mm fully threaded cortical screws from the fibula to the tibia, engaging one or both tibial cortices. The screw should be 3 cm proximal and parallel to the tibial plafond. The direction of the screw is angled 30° anteriorly as the coronal plane of the fibula is posterior to the tibia. Two screws are used in large individuals. An alternative to screws is the tightrope suture. In recent years there has been a lot of debate on potential superiority of tightrope suture over screw fixation. However, a recent systemic review and meta-analysis failed to demonstrate a clear superiority of any implant.

McKenzie AC, Hesselholt KE, Larsen MS, Schmal H. A Systematic Review and Meta-Analysis on Treatment of Ankle Fractures With Syndesmotic Rupture: Suture-Button Fixation Versus Cortical Screw Fixation. J Foot Ankle Surg. 2019;58(5):946–53.

Routine removal of screws is controversial. Screws left *in situ* are liable to break, but removal before the syndesmosis is healed may cause diastasis. Currently there is no definitive evidence to support routine elective removal of syndesmotic screws. Screws should be left in situ for at least 4 months.

Dingemans SA, Rammelt S, White TO, Goslings JC, Schepers A. Should syndesmotic screws be removed after surgical fixation of unstable ankle fractures. Bone Joint J 2016; 98: 1497–1504. Systematic review of 9 studies. No difference in retaining versus removal of screw.

Bioabsorbable screws and tightropes have been used to avoid the issue of implant removal however both bioabsorbable and metallic screws yield similar clinical outcome. Moreover, a meta-analysis suggests that overall number of complications are more with bioabsorbable screws.

Van der Eng DM, Schep NW, Schepers T. Bioabsorbable Versus Metallic Screw Fixation for Tibiofibular Syndesmotic Ruptures: A Meta-Analysis. J Foot Ankle Surg. 2015;54(4):657–62.

Posterior Malleolus Fracture

The posterior malleolus fracture is increasingly of interest in ankle injuries. Accurate stabilisation of the posterior malleolus is important for restoring stability of the ankle. The posterior inferior tibiofibular ligament attaches to the posterior malleolus fragment. Non-anatomic healing of the posterior malleolus may lead to posterolateral talar instability.

All patients with a posterior malleolus fragment should have a preoperative CT scan. This aids in fracture classification and pre-op planning.

The Haraguchi classification is useful to assess the posterior malleolus fragment and determine the optimum approach for fixation (Fig. 1.70).

Haraguchi N, Haruyama H, Toga H, Kato F. Pathoanatomy of posterior malleolar fractures of the ankle. J Bone Joint Surg 2006; 88(5): 1085–1092.

In 2017, Mason et. al. published a modification of the Haraguchi classification. This classification helps the surgeon to decide on the approach required for fixation and the sequence of fixation (as in Type 2B #). This is shown in Fig. 1.71.

If a posterolateral approach is used, with the patient prone, the same approach can be used to place an antiglide plate on the posterior aspect of distal fibula instead of a lateral plate. This reduces hardware prominence problems.

Posteromedial approach is used for type II posterior malleolus fractures. The plane of approach is between the FDL tendon and the tibi-

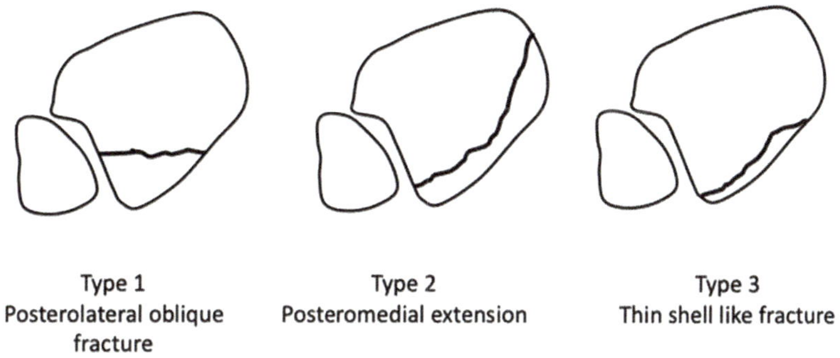

Fig. 1.70 Haraguchi classfication of posterior malleolus fractures

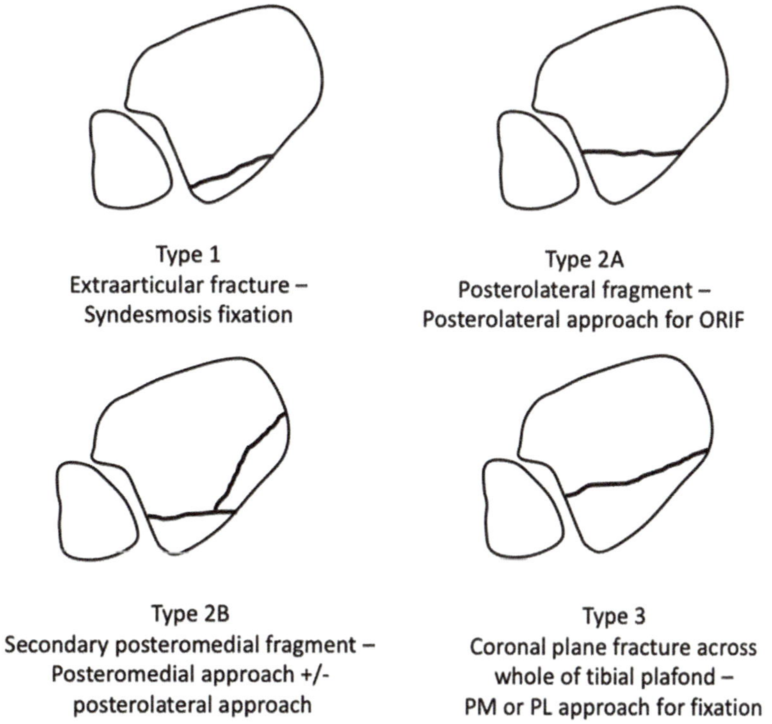

Fig. 1.71 Mason classification for posterior malleolus fractures

alis posterior. A plane can be developed between the neurovascular bundle and the FHL. A separate window can be created by retracting the neurovascular bundle posteriorly, to access the medial malleolus fracture for fixation.

Previous studies on fixation of posterior malleolus fractures did not show improvement in outcome following fixation of the posterior malleolus. However, with improvement in understanding of these fractures, better outcomes have been recently reported. Mason classification may also serve as a prognostic indicator as the severity of injury increases from Type 1 to Type 3 with outcomes being the best in Type 1.

Mason LW, Marlow WJ, Widnall J, Molloy AP. Pathoanatomy and Associated Injuries of Posterior Malleolus Fracture of the Ankle. Foot Ankle Int. 2017;38(11):1229–35.

Mason LW, Kaye A, Widnall J, Redfern J, Molloy A. Posterior Malleolar Ankle Fractures: An Effort at Improving Outcomes. JBJS Open Access. 2019 Jun 7;4(2):e0058

Complications of Ankle Fractures

Complications include infection, wound healing problems, malunion, non-union, posttraumatic arthritis, prominent metalwork and distal tibiofibular synostosis. Residual diastasis of the distal tibiofibular joint may require corrective surgery and is best diagnosed on axial CT scans and comparison with the contralateral side.

Fixation of ankle fractures is associated with a higher rate of non-union, infection and wound-healing problems in patients with diabetes. Prolonged immobilisation is required until fracture healing is satisfactory.

Ankle Sprain

The lateral ligament complex around the ankle includes the anterior and posterior talofibular ligaments and the calcaneofibular ligament. The lateral ligament complex provides stability against inversion stress.

Three grades of ankle sprain have been described—a stable ankle with ligament stretch, partial tear, or unstable ankle.

Management

Management is with proprioception training and acute repair. Acute repair has poor results compared with non-operative treatment.

Kaikkonen A, Kannus P, Järvinen M. Surgery versus functional treatment in ankle ligament tears. A prospective study. Clin Orthop Relat Res 1996;326:194–202. In this prospective study, 30 patients were treated with surgery and 30 were managed non-operatively. At 9 months, 60% of the surgically treated patients had excellent or good outcomes while 87% of the non-operatively managed patients had good or excellent outcomes.

Chronic Ankle Pain/Instability

Up to twenty percent of acute sprains develop chronic instability.

Clinically, the diagnosis is based on a positive anterior drawer test. Talar tilt and stress x-rays will demonstrate the instability.

Management

Management is with direct repair with suture anchors, with or without local tissue augmentation. A success rate of 85% is reported.

The peroneus brevis or plantaris tendon can be used for reconstruction of the lateral ligament complex.

Indications for ligament reconstruction are—old injury, failed anatomic repair, insufficient local tissue and osteoarthrosis of the ankle.

Achilles Tendon Rupture

The most common site for rupture of the Achilles tendon is 2–6 cm above insertion. Poor vascularity in this zone contributes to the high rupture rate. Risk factors are tendinopathy, local steroid injections, systemic steroids and quinolone antibiotics.

The injury follows an overload and presents with local pain and difficulty in walking. Patients may feel as if they have sustained a direct blow. There is weakness of plantar flexion with local swelling and bruising. A gap is often palpable on examination.

The Thompson test, first described by Simmonds in 1957, is conducted with the patient prone or kneeling on a chair. Squeezing the calf results in plantar flexion at the ankle if the Achilles in intact, and this is compared with the opposite side.

The Matles test is performed with the patient prone and the knees flexed to 90°. The ankle on the side of the rupture will have more dorsiflexion due to loss of the normal tone of the gastrosoleus complex.

In the O'Brien needle test, a needle is inserted into the muscle belly 10 cm proximal to musculotendinous junction. The ankle is plantarflexed and dorsiflexed. Lack of needle movement on movement of the ankle implies rupture of the tendon.

A sphygmomanometer cuff can be applied over the calf with the foot plantarflexed. Ankle dorsiflexion will elevate the pressure in the cuff if the Achilles tendon is intact. This test was described by Copeland.

Imaging

Distortion of the tendon outline may be evident on a lateral radiograph of the ankle. Kager's triangle is the fat pad bounded by the posterior aspect of the tibia, the anterior aspect of the Achilles tendon and the superior aspect of calcaneum, and can be disrupted in Achilles tendon ruptures.

Ultrasound of the tendon is helpful in diagnosis and for detecting partial ruptures. MRI scan is rarely needed, but is useful in chronic ruptures.

Management

It is debatable as to whether operative or non-operative treatment of acute rupture of the Achilles tendon is preferable. Surgery may allow earlier weight bearing with a reduced re-rupture rate, but wound-healing problems and superficial nerve injury are potential risks. Return to pre-injury activity level is possible even without surgery. Surgery is usually recommended for the active, young patient and nonoperative treatment is generally for relatively less active, lower demand patients. Supervised physiotherapy is needed for many months and return to sport takes 9 months.

Ochen Y, Beks RB, van Heijl M, Hietbrink F, Leenen LPH, van der Velde D, Heng M, van der Meijden O, Groenwold RHH, Houwert RM. Operative treatment versus nonoperative treatment of Achilles tendon ruptures: systematic review and meta-analysis. BMJ. 2019 Jan 7;364. A recent meta-analysis which included 10 RCTs and 19 observational studies. This study showed that the re-rupture rate is 2.3% following operative treatment vs 3.9% in non operative treatment. However, overall complications are significantly higher in operative group (4.9%) vs non-operative group (1.6%). 2.8% patients in the operative group had wound infections. There is no significant difference in functional outcome or return to sports/work in both groups.

Venous thromboembolism is a risk in patients treated in cast and consideration should be given for chemical thromboprophylaxis. Risk of VTE is approximately 1% in operative group vs. 1.2% in non-operative group.

Keene DJ, Alsousou J, Harrison P, Hulley P, Wagland S, Parsons SR, Thompson JY, O'Connor HM, Schlüssel MM, Dutton SJ, Lamb SE, Willett K; PATH-2 trial group. Platelet rich plasma injection for acute Achilles tendon rupture: PATH-2 randomised, placebo controlled, superiority trial. BMJ. 2019 Nov 20;367:l6132. This RCT showed that there is no objective improvement in muscle tendon function, functional outcome or quality of life with use of PRP. Hence, routine use of PRP is not advised.

Suchak AA, Bostick GP, Beaupré LA, Durand DC, Jomha NM. The influence of early weight-bearing compared with non-weight-bearing after surgical repair of the Achilles tendon. J Bone Joint Surg Am 2008;90:1876–83. This study randomised 110 patients to weight bearing 2 weeks after repair or non-weight bearing for 6 weeks. Early weight bearing had no detrimental effects and there was no difference between the two groups at 6 months.

Endoscopic methods have been employed for management and help in checking for adequate apposition of the tendon ends. There is risk of injury to the sural nerve.

Fortis AP, Dimas A, Lamprakis AA. Repair of Achilles tendon rupture under endoscopic control. Arthroscopy 2008;24:683–688.

Chronic ruptures of the Achilles tendon are those that remain 6 weeks following the injury. These are managed with open repair if the gap between the two ends is less than 2.5 cm. If there is wider separation between the two ends then management options include the following:

- V-Y-plasty of the proximal part of the tendon.
- Turndown flaps of the aponeurosis of the tendon.
- Use of the peroneus brevis, flexor hallucis longus, flexor digitorum longus, free tendon graft or fascia lata strip to bridge the defect.
- Fresh frozen Achilles allograft.

Talar Fracture

Two-thirds of the talus is covered by articular cartilage. The bone has no muscle or tendon attachments.

Blood Supply to the Talus

The blood supply to the talus is demonstrated in Fig. 1.72. The artery of the tarsal canal is one of the chief suppliers of blood (Fig. 1.73). It either arises from the posterior tibial artery 1 cm proximal to the origin of the medial plantar artery or occurs as a branch of the medial plantar artery.

The contribution from the anterior tibial artery is through the artery of the sinus tarsi. This anastomoses with the artery of the tarsal canal. There is also minimal contribution from peroneal artery through the perforating branch.

Talar Neck Fractures

Talar neck fractures commonly result from forced dorsiflexion of the ankle, with the anterior margin of the distal tibial articular surface striking the talar neck.

Classification

The Hawkins classification is commonly used (Fig. 1.74).

Disruption of joint implies subluxation or dislocation. Type IV was added later by Canale and Kelly.

Hawkins LG. Fractures of the neck of the talus. J Bone Joint Surg Am 1970;52(5):991–1002.

Canale ST, Kelly FB Jr. Fractures of the neck of the talus. Long term evaluation of seventy one cases. J Bone Joint Surg am 1978;60(2):143–56.

Management

Undisplaced fractures of the talar neck can be managed non-operatively in a below-knee non-weight-bearing cast, with close follow-up for late displacement.

Displaced fractures require urgent reduction to maintain the blood supply of the talus. A combined dorsomedial and posterolateral approach is used.

A posteroanterior direction of screws is preferred on the grounds of biomechanical stability. Two 4 mm screws are adequate. In the presence of gross comminution, compression by screws has to be avoided and plate fixation may be more appropriate. Specific plates for talus are available. Weight bearing is not permitted for 3 months, but ankle movements may be started.

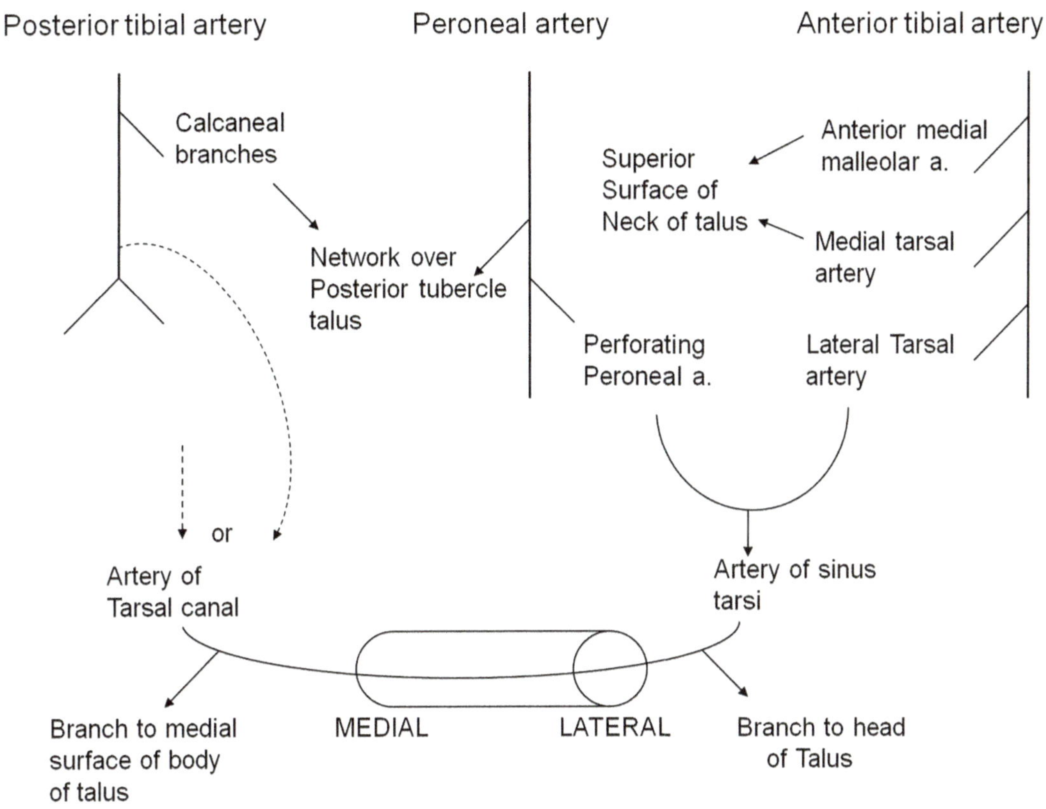

Fig. 1.72 Blood supply to talus

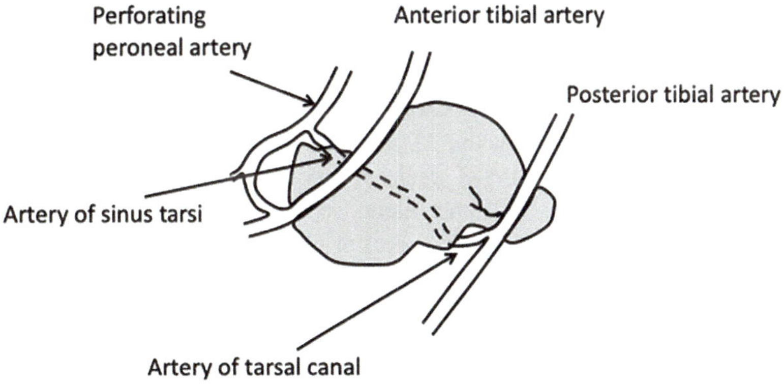

Fig. 1.73 Arterial anastomosis in the tarsal canal

Complications

- Delayed union or non-union—managed with bone grafting, with or without fixation.
- Malunion—commonly varus malunion of the fracture, which causes hindfoot varus and adduction of the forefoot. Triple arthrodesis is an option to relieve the pain and correct deformity.
- Posttraumatic arthritis of the subtalar and tibiotalar joints is common, occurring in up to 50% of patients.
- Avascular necrosis (AVN)—The risk of AVN correlates with the severity of injury

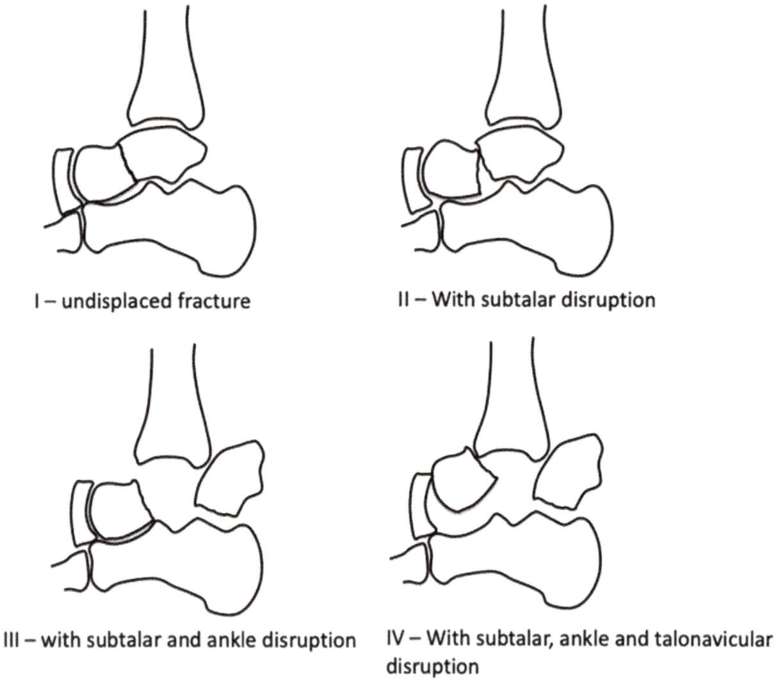

Fig. 1.74 Hawkins classification of talar neck fractures

Table 1.15 Risk of AVN with talar neck fractures

Classification	Risk of AVN
I	0–13%
II	20–50%
III	20–100%
IV	70–100%

(Table 1.15). Presence of subchondral lucency under the talar dome in the AP view of the ankle (Hawkins' sign) 6–8 weeks following the injury indicates an intact blood supply. AVN is managed with tibiocalcaneal or tibiotalar fusion (Blair fusion).

Calcaneal Fracture

The os calcis (calcaneum) is a weight-bearing bone. Fractures occur with a fall from a height or high-energy motor vehicle accidents resulting in an axial load. The talus is driven into the calcaneum and splits the bone into two or more parts.

The calcaneum has three facets on the superior surface. The posterior facet articulates with the talus and is separated from the middle and anterior facets by the tarsal canal and sinus tarsi.

The lateral process of the talus is driven into the 'angle of Gissane' on axial loading, resulting in a medial fragment that contains the sustentaculum tali and a lateral fragment.

Classification

The Essex—Lopresti classification is based on involvement of the subtalar joint and describes two types of intraarticular injuries (Fig. 1.75). In the 'tongue type' of fracture, the fracture line exits through the posterior aspect of the bone. The joint surface is therefore depressed but not directly involved in the fracture. In the 'joint depression type' of fracture, there are two primary fracture lines in the coronal plane. These result in the posterior facet being driven down into the cancellous bone. Both fracture lines extend to the superior surface of the calcaneum.

Sanders' classification of calcaneal fractures is based on CT scans—coronal Images

(Fig. 1.76). The posterior facet of the calcaneus is divided into three fracture lines (A, B, and C, corresponding to lateral, middle, and medial fracture lines, respectively). Thus, a total of four potential pieces can result: lateral, central, medial, and sustentaculum tali:

Type I is an undisplaced fractures regardless of the number of fracture lines. Type II is a two part fractures of the posterior facet. Subtypes IIA, IIB, IIC are based on the location of the primary fracture line. Type III is a three-part fracture with a centrally depressed fragment. Based on the

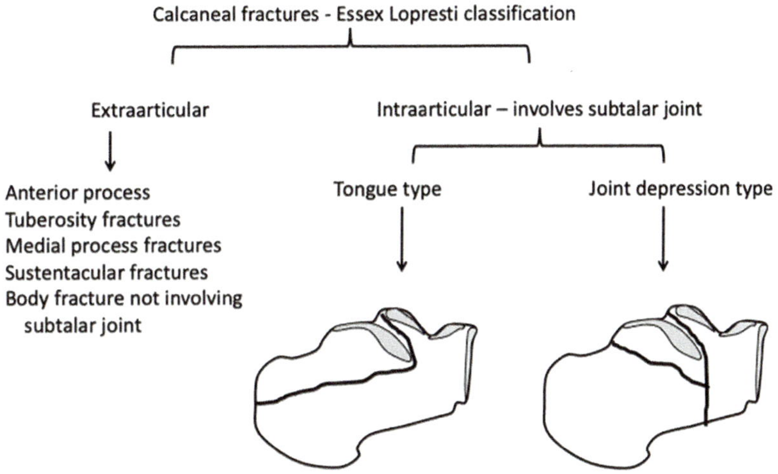

Fig. 1.75 The Essex-Lopresti classification

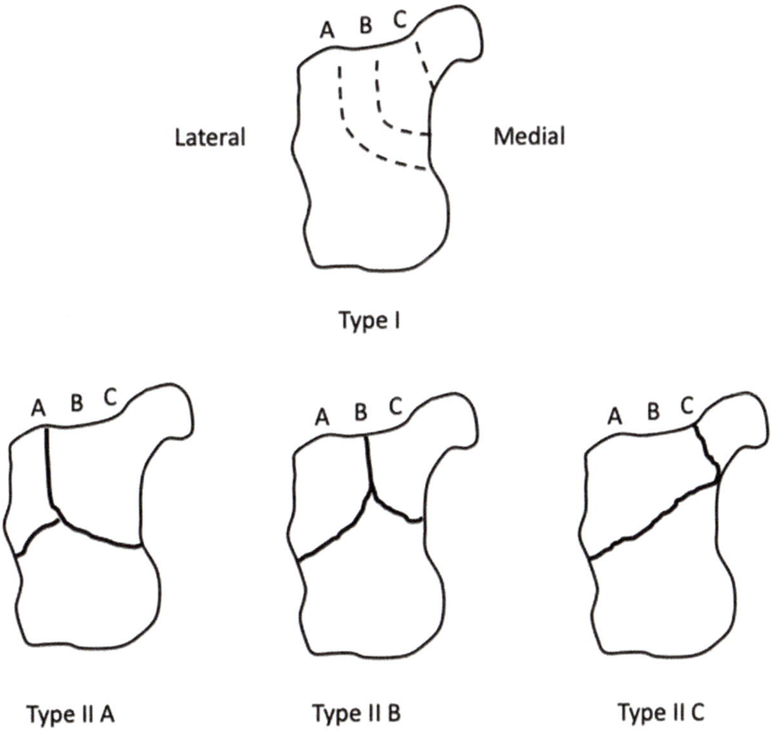

Fig. 1.76 Sanders classification for calcaneal fractures

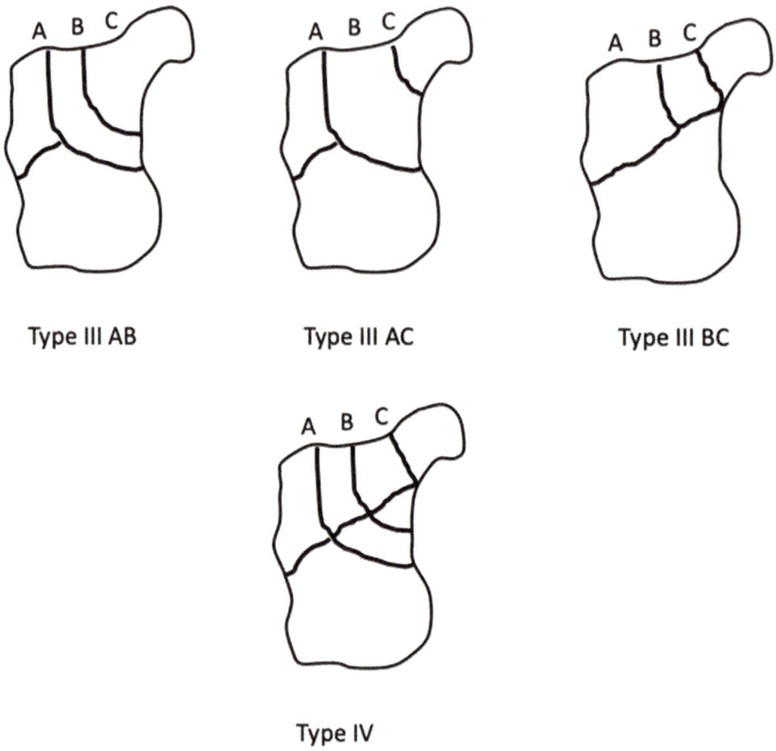

Fig. 1.76 (continued)

location of fracture lines for the depressed fragment, subtypes IIIAB, IIIAC, IIIBC have been described. Type IV is a comminuted articular fracture.

The Sanders classification considers only the posterior facet and not the relationship between the facets.

Clinical Features

The local soft tissues should be assessed carefully and a full examination conducted for associated injuries.

Management

Non-operative treatment is based on elevation, ice and early mobilisation, avoiding weight bearing for 8–12 weeks. Casts are unnecessary for calcaneal fractures.

Surgical treatment is undertaken to restore the alignment of the fragments and correct the widening of the heel. Surgery is delayed for 5–7 days after injury to allow soft tissue revascularisation and resolution of blisters.

In 2002, Buckley and colleagues published the largest RCT on operative versus non operative management of calcaneal fractures. This study of 471 patients suggested that functional outcome following both treatment options is similar.

Buckley R, Tough S, McCormack R, et al. Operative compared with nonoperative treatment of displaced intra-articular calcaneal fractures: a prospective, randomized, controlled multicenter trial. J bone Joint Surg Am 2002;84(10):1733–44.

However, most of the recent literature including meta-analysis suggest that anatomical reduction of posterior facet combined with restoration of calcaneal shape, alignment and height offers a better long term functional outcome and reduced risk of symptomatic sub-talar arthritis. Also, results of sub-talar fusion for sub-talar arthritis following ORIF are better than fusion following non operative management.

Gotha HE, Zide JR. Current Controversies in Management of Calcaneus Fractures. Orthop Clin North Am. 2017;48(1):91–103.

The lateral approach is the most common approach to the calcaneum. The fragments are reduced to the sustentaculum tali fragment and the lateral wall is plated. However, this approach is associated with 20–37% risk of wound complications. This is possibly due to extensive stripping of the fracture, larger surgical field, increased intra-operative time and disruption of the lateral calcaneal branch of the peroneal artery. Recently, sinus tarsi approach has been used as an alternative and most studies have shown a reduced risk of wound complications with this approach.

Xia S, Lu Y, Wang H, et al. Open reduction and internal fixation with conventional plate via L-shaped lateral approach versus internal fixation with percutaneous plate via a sinus tarsi approach for calcaneal fractures—a randomized controlled trial. Int J Surg 2014;12(5):475–80.

Primary subtalar arthrodesis is an option for the unreconstructable fracture. However, an RCT showed no difference in ORIF alone vs. ORIF with fusion at 2 years. Furthermore, simultaneous restoration of calcaneal anatomy and achieving fusion is technically challenging.

Buckley R, Leighton R, Sanders D, et al. Open reduction and internal fixation compared with ORIF and primary subtalar arthrodesis for the treatment of Sanders-Type IV calcaneal fractures: a randomized, multicenter trial. J Orthop Trauma 2014;28(10):577–83.

Malunited calcaneal fracture causes subtalar arthritis, loss of calcaneal height, tibiotalar impingement, increased calcaneal width causing fibulocalcaneal impingement and impingement of the peroneal tendons.

Lisfranc Injury

These injuries are named after a French surgeon—Jacques Lisfranc de Martin.

Lisfranc fracture dislocation involves the tarsometatarsal joint. The second metatarsal extends proximal to the other metatarsals and acts as a keystone to stabilise this joint. On average the base of second metatarsal is 8 mm proximal to the medial cuneiform and 4 mm proximal to the lateral cuneiform in the coronal plane. There are no interosseous ligaments between the first and second metatarsals. The base of second metatarsal is attached to the medial cuneiform via the dorsal, plantar and interosseous 'Lisfranc ligaments' (Figs. 1.77 and 1.78). Injuries to the Lisfranc joint can be bony, ligamentous or mixed and up to 20% can be missed on initial radiographs, leading to morbidity and poor outcome.

The Lisfranc joint is described in three columns. The medial column is composed of the medial cuneiform and the first metatarsal. The middle column comprises middle and lateral cuneiforms and second and third metatarsals. The lateral column is composed of the cuboid and the fourth and fifth metatarsals (Fig. 1.79).

Diagnosis

The mechanism of injury is axial loading of the foot and is often a high energy injury. It is usually seen in males in the third decade of life.

Local swelling and bruising will be seen in acute injury. Plantar ecchymosis is pathognomonic of this injury. Lateral compression test and axial stability test between the first and second metatarsal are indicative of Lisfranc ligament injury.

The oblique radiograph of the foot should normally show the medial border of the fourth metatarsal aligned with the medial border of the cuboid; the medial border of the second metatarsal aligned with the medial border of middle cuneiform; and the first metatarsal aligned with the medial cuneiform bone (Fig. 1.80). Any loss of alignment should raise the suspicion of a Lisfranc fracture dislocation.

The lateral radiograph should be assessed for any dorsal subluxation of the metatarsals in relation to the tarsal bones. A metatarsal lying superior or inferior to its respective tarsal bone on the

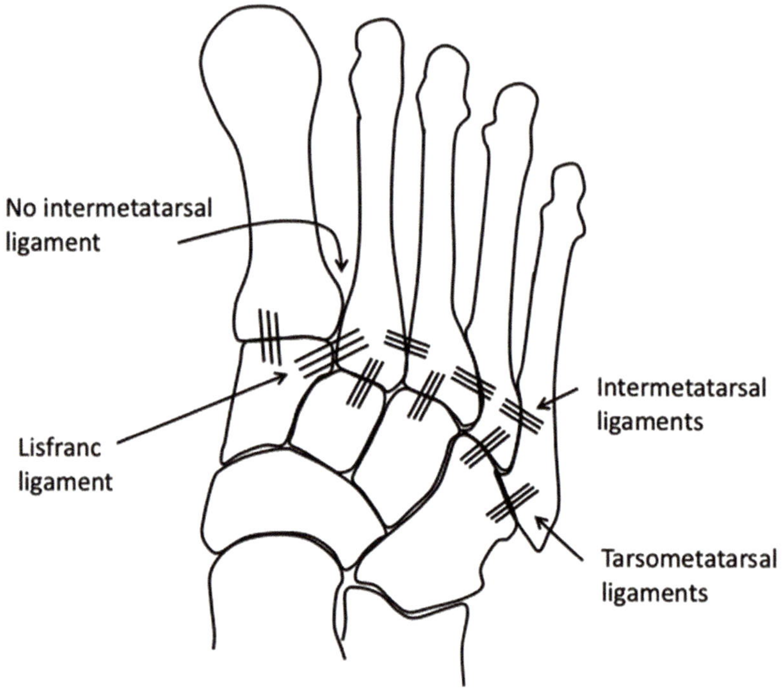

Fig. 1.77 Lisfranc ligament

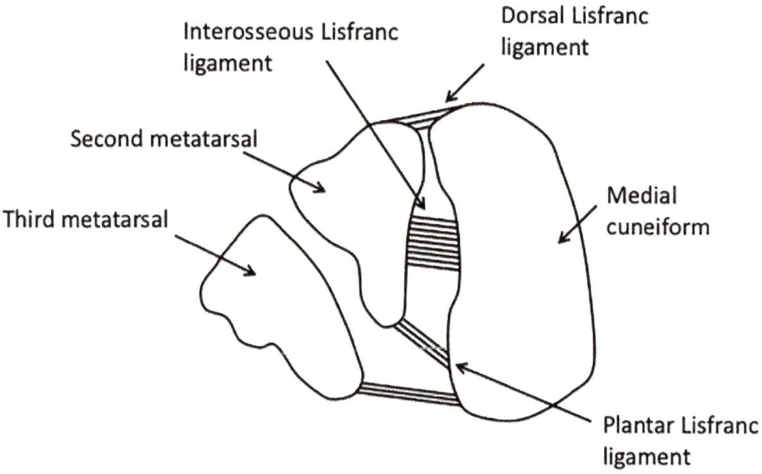

Fig. 1.78 The three components of the Lisfranc ligament

lateral view should raise suspicion of Lisfranc injury.

The "fleck" sign is avulsion of the Lisfranc ligament from the base of second metatarsal and is diagnostic of this injury.

A weight bearing radiograph (AP, lateral and oblique of both feet), if tolerated by the patient can reveal subtle instability. More than 2 mm diastasis between the base of second metatarsal and medial cuneiform indicates instability.

CT scans are helpful to detect occult fractures and confirm alignment of the tarsometatarsal joint. Rarely MR scans are done for ligamentous injuries.

Classification

Quenu and Kuss (1909) described three types of Lisfranc injury—Homolateral, Isolated and

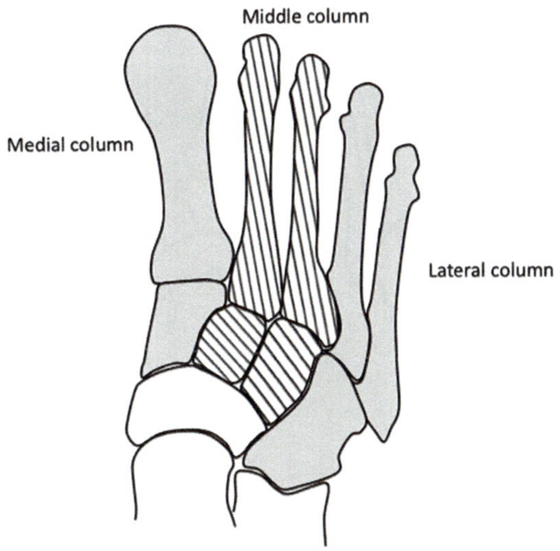

Fig. 1.79 Thee columns of Lisfranc articulation

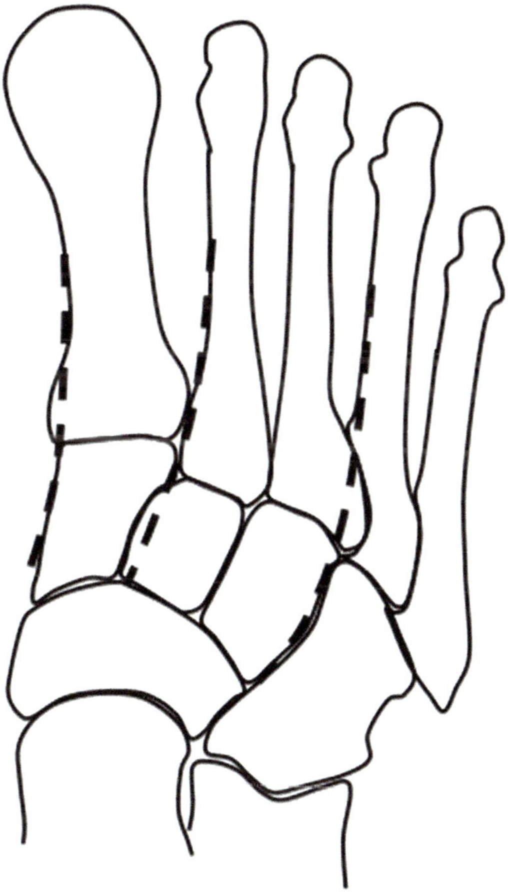

Fig. 1.80 Checking alignment of the metatarsals

Divergent (Fig. 1.81). Further classifications were proposed by Hardcastle and Myerson.

A more recent classification was proposed by Nunley and Vertullo (Table 1.16).

Nunley JA, Vertullo CJ. Classification, investigation and management of midfoot sprains; Lisfranc injuries in the athlete. Am J Sports Med 2002;30:871–8.

Management

Undisplaced injuries—where there is no displacement on proven stress radiographs or weight bearing films—can be managed non-operatively in a non weight bearing short-leg cast for 6–12 weeks. Restoration of alignment is the key to improving outcome.

Displaced fractures require accurate reduction and internal fixation. Open reduction is performed where soft tissue interposition impedes closed reduction. Fixation is achieved by stabilising the first ray to the medial cuneiform with screws, followed by stabilising the second and third metatarsals with screws to corresponding cuneiforms. The fourth and fifth metatarsals are fixed with K-wires to the cuboid for 6 weeks to maintain flexibility. Plate can be used to avoid damage to articular surface of the tarsometatarsal joints. Plates are also useful in cases of comminution of base of metatarsals or cuneiforms.

Moracia-Ochagavía I, Rodríguez-Merchán EC. Lisfranc fracture-dislocations: current management. EFORT Open Rev. 2019;4(7):430–44.

Weight bearing is not permitted for 6 weeks, and full weight bearing is not permitted for 3 months.

The chances of development of post traumatic arthritis depend on quality of reduction. Residual displacement of over 2 mm correlates with development of arthritis.

The role of primary arthrodesis is debatable at present.

Smith N, Stone C, Furey A. Does open reduction and internal fixation versus primary arthrodesis improve patient outcomes for Lisfranc trauma? A systematic review. Clin Orthop Relat

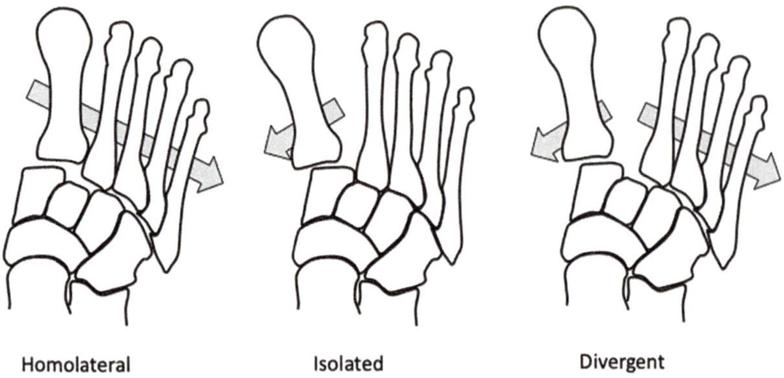

Fig. 1.81 Quenu and Kuss classification

Table 1.16 Classification of Lisfranc injuries

Stage	Injury	AP WB XRay	Lat. WB XRay	Bone scan
Stage 1	Lig. Sprain	Normal	Normal	+ve (100% sens.)
Stage 2	Lig. Rupture	2–5 mm diastasis	Normal	+ve
Stage 3	Lig. Rupture	2–5 mm diastasis	Loss of arch height	+ve

Res 2016;474(6):1445–52. This systematic review did not find any significant difference in functional outcome between ORIF and primary arthrodesis.

Coetzee JC, Ly TV. Treatment of primarily ligamentous Lisfranc joint injuries: primary arthrodesis compared with open reduction and internal fixation. Surgical technique. J Bone Joint Surg Am. 2007;89 Suppl 2 Pt1:122–7. Primary arthrodesis may have a role in pure ligamentous injuries. The above RCT of 41 patients showed that return to pre-injury level was 92% in primary arthrodesis group compared to 65% in ORIF group.

Hardware should be retained for 4 months. Return to full activity is expected after 6 to 9 months of injury.

Metatarsal Fractures

Most metatarsal fractures are managed nonoperatively with a good outcome. There is little evidence in support of operative intervention for metatarsal shaft fractures.

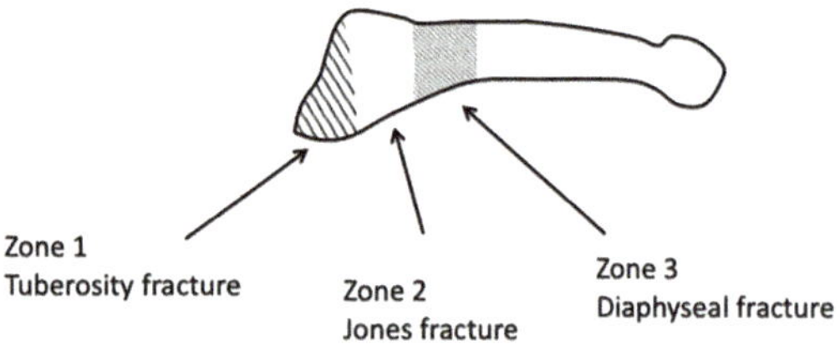

Fig. 1.82 Zones of fifth metatarsal fractures

Fracture of Base of Fifth Metatarsal

Fractures of the base of fifth metatarsal are common injuries resulting from an inversion force.

Three zones have been described for fractures of the fifth metatarsal (Fig. 1.82). The fracture at diaphyseo-metaphyseal junction carries a relatively unfavourable prognosis and this was first described by Sir Robert Jones in 1902, an injury he sustained himself while dancing.

Zone 1 fractures are avulsions and extend into the metatarsocuboid joint. Zone 2 fractures are typically Jones fractures, with the fracture line extending into the articulation between the fourth and fifth metatarsal. Zone 3 are diaphyseal fractures.

Metaphyseal fractures are generally managed nonoperatively.

Indications for surgery

1. Zone 1: More than 3 mm displacement or more than 30% involvement of metatarsocuboid joint
2. Zone 2:
   (a) Consider surgery for displacement >2 mm

   (b) Undisplaced fractures in athletes can be considered for early internal fixation as this results in early return to sport
   (c) Delayed/non union
3. Zone 3: Consider surgery for delayed or non union

Bowes J, Buckley R. Fifth metatarsal fractures and current treatment. World J Orthop. 2016;7(12):793–800.

Roche AJ, Calder JD. Treatment and return to sport following a Jones fracture of the fifth metatarsal: a systematic review. Knee Surg Sports Traumatol Arthrosc 2013;21:1307–15. 26 studies reviewed. Union rate for acute Jones fracture is 76% with non operative treatment and 96% with screw fixation. Nonunions treated with screw fixation healed in 97%. Acute fracture treated with screw fixation may have a slightly earlier return to sports.

Patients with undisplaced or minimally displaced (<3 mm) avulsion fractures can be allowed to bear weight as tolerated soon after the injury. Cast immobilisation is not superior to symptomatic treatment.

Akimau PI, Cawthron KL, Dakin WM, Chadwick C, Blundell CM, Davies MB. Symptomatic treatment or cast immobilisation for avulsion fractures of the base of the fifth metatarsal: a prospective, randomised, single-blinded non-inferiority controlled trial. Bone Joint J 2016;98(6):806–11.

Pelvic Ring Injuries

Pelvic ring fractures result from high-energy injuries such as motor vehicle accidents, falls and industrial crush injuries. Fractures in the elderly can result from simple falls, where osteoporosis is a contributory factor. High energy injuries can present as life threatening emergencies and need rapid and appropriate management.

Initial Evaluation

- ATLS protocol (Advanced Trauma Life Support)—Check Airway, Breathing, Circulation and Disability (ABCD) and manage as detailed in ATLS.
- Scrotal or labial swelling/bruising may be evident. Open fractures are rare.
- Compression and distraction of the pelvis should not be done. This has the potential of displacing clots and increasing the bleeding. Pelvic injury is diagnosed on radiographs/CT scans in the polytraumatised patients.
- Open laceration or skin degloving may be present. Extensive skin degloving is known as Morel–Lavallée lesion.
- Associated injuries such as urologic, neurologic and head injuries and limb trauma should be assessed.
- Rectal and vaginal examination is done to check for bone spike penetration into these cavities, if suspected on initial imaging.

During resuscitation, the following should be checked and corrected

- Hypotension—a systolic blood pressure below 90 mmHg is associated with a 38% mortality rate, compared with 3% in normotensive patients. Ninety percent of pelvic bleeding is venous and from fracture surfaces. Arterial bleeding arises from the internal pudendal, obturator or lateral sacral arteries.
- Hypothermia.
- Acidosis.
- Hypocalcaemia.

A CT scan of chest and abdomen is obtained to assess any associated injuries.

Imaging

For the polytraumatised patient, the current practice in trauma centres is to obtain a CT scan (trauma pan-scan) on presentation. This helps in diagnosing associated injuries as well as the pelvic injury.

For patients where a trauma scan is not done, a pelvis AP radiograph is obtained in the emergency department as part of the initial assessment. Approximately 90% of pelvic injuries are diagnosed on an AP view of the pelvis and resus-

Table 1.17 Signs of instability on plain radiographs

Signs of rotational instability	Signs of vertical instability
Widening of more than 2.5 cm of the pubic symphysis.	More than 1 cm cephalad migration of a hemipelvis
An avulsion fracture of the lateral sacrum or ischial spine	Sacral fractures with a gap (distraction).
Widening of the anterior sacroiliac (SI) joint	Avulsion of the tip of the L5 transverse process. This is the site of attachment of the iliolumbar ligament.

citation should commence based on this view. Inlet and outlet views are helpful to demonstrate AP and vertical displacement. The lateral lumbosacral view may sometimes be needed for suspected lower lumbar or sacral injuries.

Stability

Stability indicates the ability of the pelvis to withstand physiological loading without significant displacement. The signs of instability on plain radiographs are summarised in Table 1.17.

A CT scan is conducted to detect subtle associated fractures and injuries to the posterior part of the pelvic ring, retroperitoneal haematoma and other organ injuries. Definitive management of the pelvic ring is planned based on the CT scan.

Classification

Young and Burgess described four types of pelvic ring injuries—lateral compression, AP compression, vertical shear and combined mechanical (Fig. 1.83).

Lateral compression (LC) injuries are characterised by a horizontal fracture of pubic rami implying a lateral compressive force. Anteroposterior compression (APC) have a symphyseal diastasis and/or longitudinal rami fracture.

Crescent fracture is a type of lateral compression injury with dislocation of the SI joint and fracture of the posterior iliac wing. These fractures have been subdivided into three types (Table 1.18).

Day AC, Kinmont C, Bircher MD, Kumar S. Crescent fracture-dislocation of the sacroiliac joint: a functional classification. J Bone Joint Surg Br 2007;89:651–8.

Burgess AR et al. Pelvic ring disruptions: effective classification system and treatment protocols. J Trauma 1990:30(7);848–56. 210 consecutive patients. Classification system based protocols reduced mortality and morbidity.

The Tile classification proposed 3 types of injuries—Stable; rotationally unstable; and rotationally and vertically unstable (Fig. 1.84).

Classification of sacral fractures was proposed by Danis (Table 1.19).

Management

The initial management follows ATLS protocols.

Emergency Management

A Pelvic binder or a sheet is wrapped around the pelvic ring at the level of greater trochanters by paramedics/ambulance crew.

The lower limbs are internally rotated and tied together at the ankles and knees. Biomechanically, it has been shown to be comparable with anterior external fixation. It is currently the preferred method of initial stabilisation as it is simple, easy to apply and preserves the skin for future definitive surgery. Tranexamic acid is also administered at the scene in a bid to reduce hemorrhage.

Bonner TJ, Eardley WGP, Newell N, Masouros S, Matthews JJ, Gibb I, Clasper JC. Accurate placement of a pelvic binder improves reduction of unstable fractures of the pelvic ring. J Bone Joint Surg Br 2011;93(11):1524–8. The pelvic binder should be at the level of greater trochanters.

An anterior pelvic frame can be applied in the operating theatre with two or three pins in the anterior iliac crest. It is indicated in open-book injuries. If definitive fixation of pelvis cannot be carried out with in 48 h, pelvic binder is

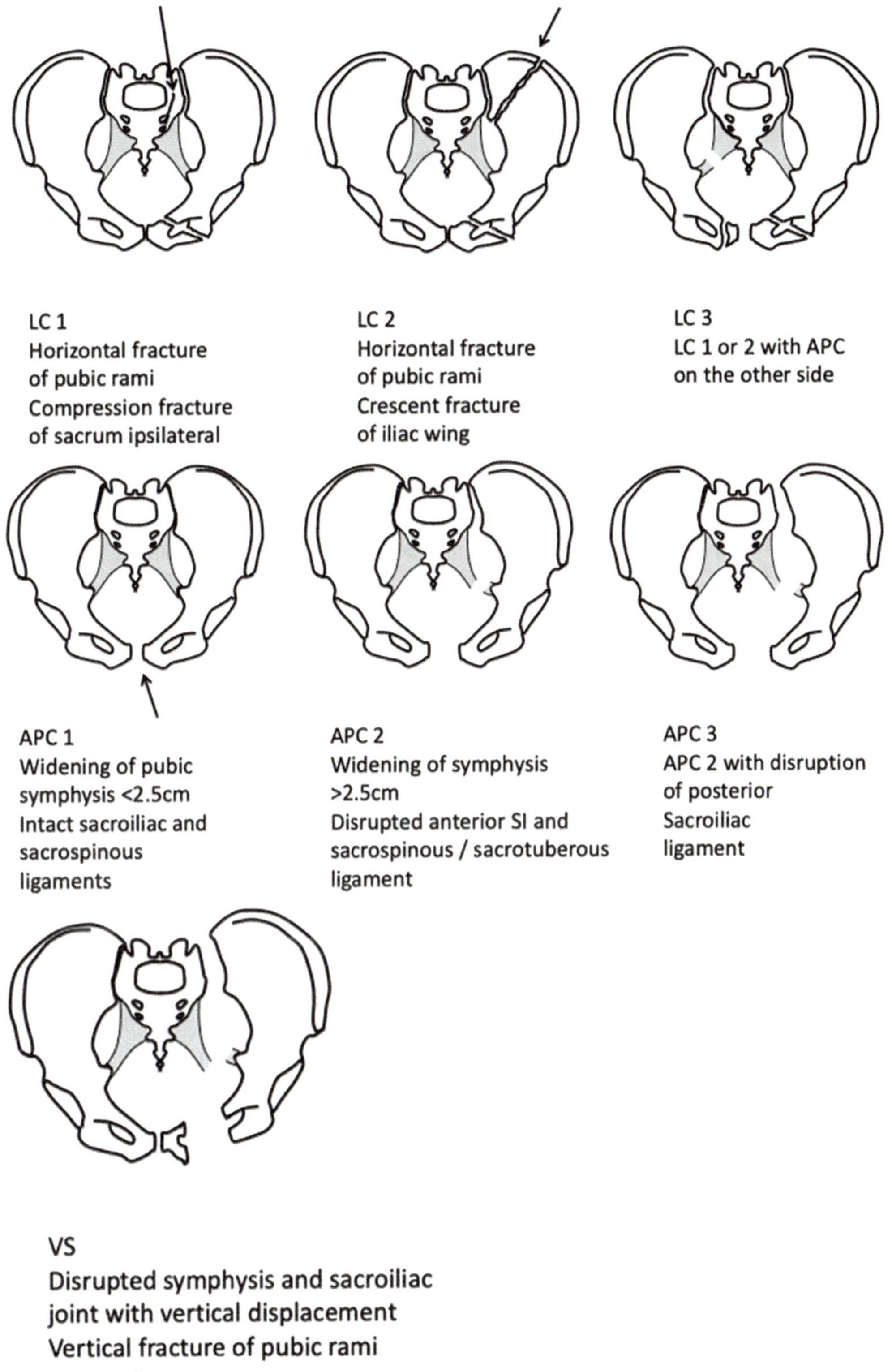

Fig. 1.83 Young and Burgess classification of pelvic ring injury

Table 1.18 Types of crescent fracture

Type I	A large crescent fragment with dislocation of less than one-third of the SI joint
Type II	An intermediate-size fragment with dislocation of a one- to two-third size fragment of the SI joint.
Type III	A small crescent fragment with dislocation of almost all the SI joint.

exchanged with an anterior external fixator. The C-clamp uses pins placed percutaneously over the region of the SI joints and helps to reduce posterior displacement. The C-clamp is solely an emergency device, while the anterior frame can be used as the definitive treatment in selected cases.

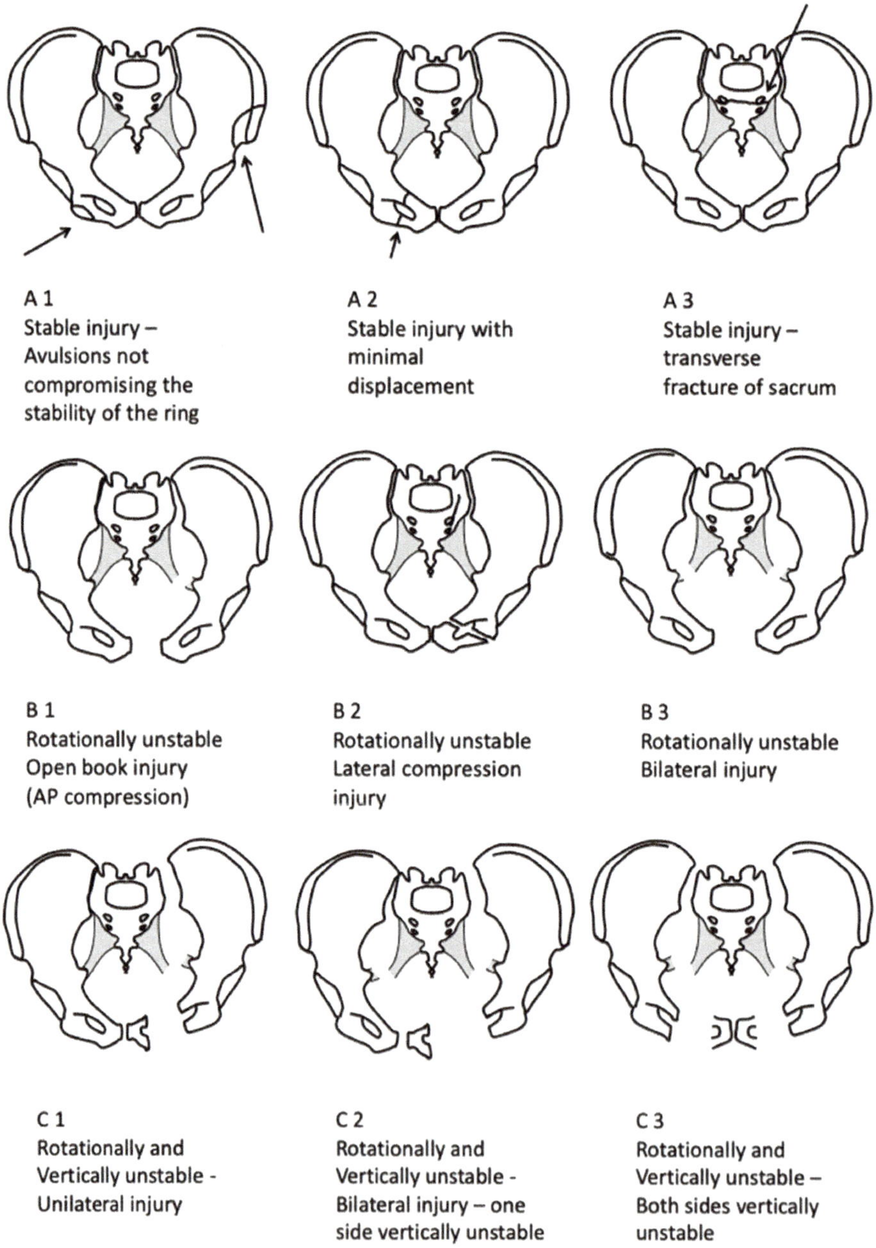

Fig. 1.84 Tile classification of pelvic ring injuries

Table 1.19 Classification of sacral fractures

Type I	The fracture line is lateral to the neural foramina
Type II	The fracture line is through the foramina
Type III	The fracture is medial to the neural foramina

Riemer BL, Butterfield SL, Diamond DL, et al. Acute mortality associated with injuries to the pelvic ring: the role of early patient mobilization and external fixation. J Trauma 1993;35:671–7. External fixation reduced the mortality rate of hypotensive patients from 41% to 21%. Historical study promoting the use of external fixation before the use of binders became common.

The use of CT scanning with contrast helps in the search for bleeding areas. Embolisation of the bleeding artery can be considered as long as bleeding is identified from the obturator artery, or superior gluteal artery or another branch of the internal iliac artery. Bleeding from the main trunk of internal iliac artery, venous bleeding and bleeding from bone surfaces cannot be controlled by embolisation.

Laparotomy and packing of true pelvis (below the pelvic brim) is also carried out in patients with uncontrolled hemorrhage who are *in extremis* and if angio-embolisation is not readily available.

Open pelvic fractures still carry a mortality rate of 40–50%. They are managed with aggressive debridement, surgical toilet, skeletal stabilisation and diversion of the bowel and bladder.

Management of Urological Injury Associated with Pelvic Fractures

All patients should have examination of the perineum and a digital rectal examination.

Bladder rupture, if intraperitoneal requires emergency laparotomy and repair. Extraperitoneal bladder rupture can be managed by catheter drainage alone.

A gentle attempt at catheterization can be undertaken for patients with suspected urethral injury. A retrograde urethrogram is done if passage is not possible and drainage is achieved with a suprapubic catheter. Suprapubic catheter, if needed should be inserted in the midline percutaneously, using a Seldinger technique under ultrasound control. The insertion should be at least 3 to 4 finger breadths above the pubic symphysis. An antegrade urethrogram is helpful to confirm/rule out urethral injury. Definitive treatment of urethral rupture is undertaken at 3 months post injury.

The BOA recommends (British Orthopaedic Association Audit Standards for Trauma—BOAST 14; August 2016) primary urethral repair (within 48 h) for patients with associated anorectal injury, perineal degloving, bladder neck injury, massive bladder displacement and penetrating injury to anterior urethra.

Definitive Treatment

Internal fixation of pelvic fractures can be delayed until the patient has been stabilised and other life-threatening associated injuries managed. This often translates to a delay of 5–7 days.

Stable injuries (Tile Type A) are managed with early mobilisation and analgesia. Type B and C injuries usually require operative stabilisation.

Rotationally unstable injuries can be managed with

- Anterior external fixator—acceptable as a definitive treatment as long as adequate reduction is achieved and maintained. For definitive management, supra-acetabular pins (low route) are preferred because the of the good fixation strength. However, hip joint penetration and injury to the lateral cutaneous nerve are notable complications with this procedure. Currently an 'Infix' where spinal pedicle screw systems are used to connect the supra-acetabular pins with a horizontal bar subcutaneously is gaining popularity. The infix has to be removed at 3 to 4 months post injury.
- Symphysis pubis plating—a single or double plate across the symphysis. With a Pfannenstiel

approach, the plate is placed on the superior and/or anterior aspect.

Vertically unstable injuries require posterior stabilisation in addition to anterior fixation. Posterior fixation can be achieved with the following:

- Iliosacral screws—for SI joint disruptions (percutaneous or open).
- Anterior plating of the SI joint with a retroperitoneal approach.
- Posterior fixation of sacral fractures and the SI joint through an open posterior approach.

For crescent fractures (fracture dislocation of the SI joint), open reduction and internal fixation is recommended.

Outcome

Patients with stable injuries generally do well and experience few long-term complications. Unstable injuries result in poorer outcomes with pain, non-union and malunion. The presence of urogenital and nerve injuries alongside pelvic fracture compromises the outcome.

Acetabular Fractures

The reduction achieved at surgery is the single most important factor affecting the outcome of the procedure and relates to the experience of the operating surgeon.

Radiographic evaluation is with an AP view of the pelvis and 45° oblique views (Judet views).

Medial roof arc should also be assessed. A vertical line is drawn through the centre of the acetabulum, with a second line drawn from the centre of the acetabulum to the fracture line crossing the dome of the acetabulum. If the angle between the lines is less than 45° in a displaced fracture then operative treatment should be considered (Matta). Similarly, anterior and posterior roof arcs can be measured on the Judet views.

On CT scans, the superior 10 mm of the acetabular roof corresponds to the 45° roof arc angle. Scans are taken with 3 mm intervals. Three-dimensional reconstructions are possible, but the best accuracy is achieved by correlating the plain radiographs with the two-dimensional CT images.

The acetabulum has a horseshoe-shaped articular surface surrounding a non-articular cotyloid fossa. The anterior column is composed of the anterior half of the acetabulum with the iliac crest, iliac spine and pubis, and is represented by the iliopectineal line. The posterior column comprises the posterior half of the acetabulum along with the ischium, ischial spine and posterior part of the ilium and is represented by the ilioischial line. The dome is the roof of the acetabulum. Restoration of the femoral head under the dome is the critical factor in determining the long-term outcome after an acetabular fracture. The neurovascular structures in the pelvis are at risk in acetabular injuries and should be checked.

Corona mortis is a large anastomosis between the external iliac, inferior epigastric and obturator arteries. It can lead to haemorrhage in the ilioinguinal approach.

Classification

There are 5 primary types (Fig. 1.85) and 5 complex types of fracture (Fig. 1.86).

Transverse fractures can be of three types (Table 1.20)

In associated both-column fractures, the articular fragments of the acetabulum do not maintain any continuity with the sacroiliac joint. The obturator oblique view demonstrates the spur sign, which is diagnostic of a both-column injury. This spur is the part of the ilium remaining attached to the SI joint and is seen lateral to the medially displaced acetabulum.

Initial Management

As these are often high energy injuries, initial management is based on the ATLS protocol. If

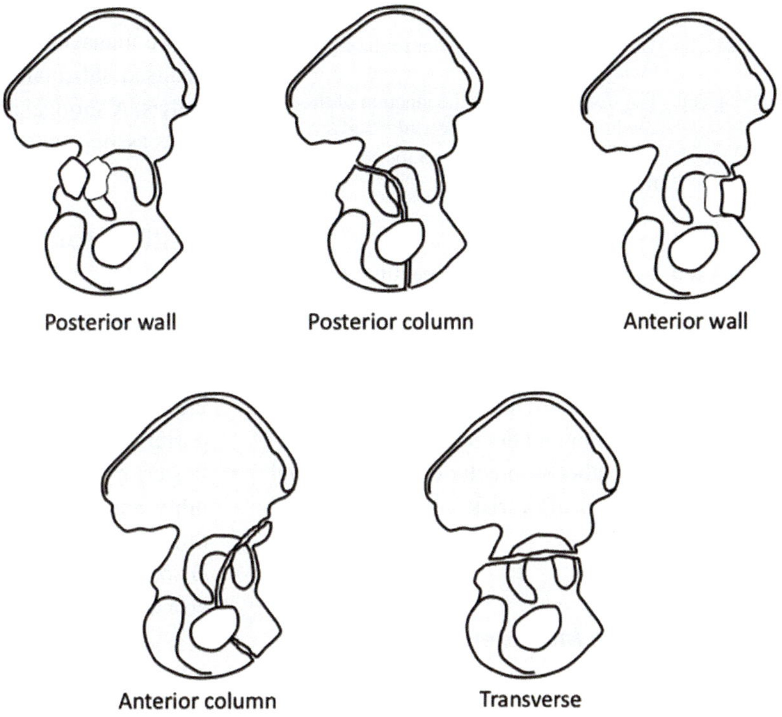

Fig. 1.85 Primary types of acetabular fractures

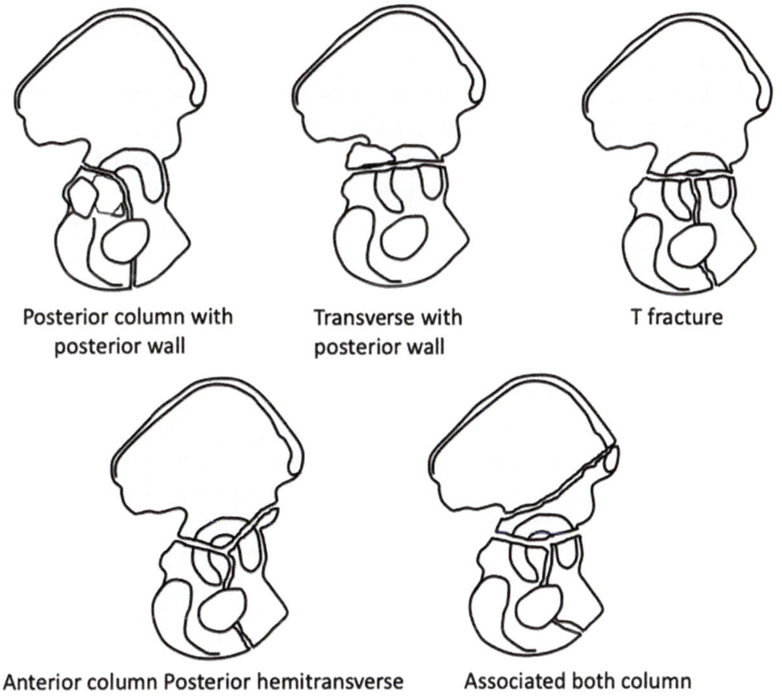

Fig. 1.86 Complex types of acetabular fractures

Table 1.20 Types of transverse fractures

Transtectal	The fracture line is superior to the cotyloid fossa
Juxtatectal	The fracture line is at the junction of the cotyloid fossa with the articular surface
Infratectal	The fracture line is through the cotyloid fossa

associated with dislocation of the hip, the hip should be reduced urgently in the emergency department or under image intensifier in the operating theatre. Posterior dislocation may be associated with injury to the sciatic nerve and this must be checked for and documented.

Suprapubic catheters preclude an ilioinguinal approach because of a risk of infection and should be avoided.

Non-Operative Management

Undisplaced fractures (<2 mm displacement) can be managed non-operatively. Traction or non-weight-bearing mobilisation is advised for 8 weeks, with regular radiographic monitoring.

Some comminuted both column fractures may have 'secondary congruence' in relation to the femoral head and can be managed non-operatively. The comminuted fragments are often displaced medially as a whole and may have gaps, but align themselves in the shape of an acetabulum.

Elderly osteoporotic and medically unfit patients can be considered for non-operative management. This carries problems of non weight bearing for a period of time, which is difficult in this group of patients. Fixation combined with total hip replacement as a single procedure within a few days of injury is an option to allow early mobilisation.

Local soft tissue infection indicates non-operative management. A Morel–Lavallée lesion is localised subcutaneous fat necrosis overlying the pelvis. A surgical approach made through this lesion is associated with a high infection rate.

Indications for Internal Fixation

- Displaced fractures (>2 mm displacement, based on the roof arc measurement). Roof arcs should be measured on the AP and Judet views, which will give the anterior, medial and posterior roof arcs.
- Posterior wall fractures can lead to hip instability and should be fixed if more than one-third of the posterior wall is fractured.
- Displaced fractures through the weight-bearing dome of the acetabulum should be fixed.
- Intra-articular fragments.

Relative Indications for Primary Total Hip Replacement

Primary total hip replacement is indicated in -

- Unreduced posterior fracture dislocation.
- Displaced acetabulum fracture with pre-existing arthritis or avascular necrosis of femoral head (AVN) in any age group
- Age >60 years with significant comminution of posterior wall & column/weight bearing dome
- Significant impaction of articular surfaces of femoral head and/or acetabulum/full thickness abrasive loss of articular cartilage
- Severe osteopenia & non-reconstructible acetabular comminution
- Associated femoral head or neck fractures

Surgical Approaches

Surgery should be performed within 5–7 days.

Standard approaches are summarised in Table 1.21.

Management of Different Fracture Patterns

The management is summarised in Table 1.22.

Surgical dislocation of the hip at the time of acetabular fracture fixation may help in reduction and improve outcome.

Tannast M, Krüger A, Mack PW, Powell JN, Hosalkar HS, Siebenrock KA. Surgical dislocation of the hip for the fixation of acetabular fractures. J Bone Joint Surg Br 2010;92(6):842–52. 54 patients followed for 4.4 years. Anatomical reduction achieved in 93% and four patients required total hip replacement within the follow up period.

Table 1.21 Surgical approaches for acetabular fractures

Standard approaches	Extensile approaches
Kocher–Langenbeck. Ilioinguinal. Modified Stoppa—a vertical/ transverse midline incision to expose the inner surface of the ilium	Extended ilioinguinal (Letournel and Judet). Triradiate approach (Mears and Rubash). T approach. KL approach with trochanteric flip (Ganz)

Postoperative Management

Prophylaxis should be provided against venous thrombosis, heterotopic ossification and infection. Toe-touch bearing is permitted 2 days after surgery and continues for 12 weeks.

Complications of acetabular fractures include

- Mortality (1–2.5%).
- Posttraumatic arthritis:
  - With anatomic reduction, 10% at 1 year.
  - Without anatomic reduction, 35% at 1 year.
- AVN (7.5% after posterior dislocation)
- Infection (up to 5%)—there is a higher risk of infection with a Morel–Lavallée lesion; if the posterior approach is used; and with a supra-

Table 1.22 Summary of treatment planning for acetabular fractures

Fracture pattern	Approach	Fixation	Comments
Posterior wall	Kocher–Langenbeck	Lag screw and reconstruction plate	Long-term results depend on marginal impaction, damage to femoral head and screw placement
Posterior column	Kocher–Langenbeck	Lag screw and reconstruction plate	Rotational malalignment must be corrected
Anterior wall	Ilioinguinal or iliofemoral	Buttress plate	May be associated with hip dislocation
Anterior column	Ilioinguinal or iliofemoral	Buttress plate	–
Transverse fractures	Posterior or ilioinguinal or both	Buttress plate on the exposed column and a lag screw in the other column	Juxta and transtectal fractures should be reduced anatomically
Posterior column and wall	Kocher–Langenbeck	Double plate posteriorly	–
Transverse and posterior wall	Extensile or combined	Based on the fracture pattern	Can be difficult to reduce an anterior fracture through a posterior approach
T fracture; and anterior column with posterior hemitransverse fracture	Ilioinguinal or combined	Plate along the pelvic brim	–
Both column	Iliinguinal or Combined approach	Based on the fracture pattern	–

pubic catheter if the ilioinguinal approach is used.

- Sciatic nerve injury—can be present in 10% of patients with acetabular fractures as part of the injury. The sciatic nerve is also at risk with the posterior approach (risk of injury is 2–6%).
- Heterotopic ossification—present in 50% of patients undergoing the posterior (Kocher–Langenbeck) or combined approach. The risk is lower with the ilioinguinal approach. Prophylaxis is with indomethacin (preferred; 25 mg three times a day for 6 weeks) or radiation.
- Thromboembolism—present in 50% of patients. If proximal deep vein thrombosis is detected then an inferior vena cava filter should be considered. Filters should also be used in high-risk patients. Preoperative prophylaxis is with low molecular-weight heparin, followed postoperatively by warfarin for 6 weeks.

Total Hip Replacement for Posttraumatic Arthritis Following Acetabular Fracture

The results of total hip replacement for posttraumatic arthritis are often not as good as primary total hip replacement for osteoarthritis. Complications include retained hardware, scarring, heterotopic ossification and early loosening.

Berry DJ, Halasy M. Uncemented acetabular components for arthritis after acetabular fracture. Clin Orthop Relat Res 2002;405:164–7. This study included 34 hips in 33 patients, with a 10-year follow-up. The mean patient age at surgery was 49 years. Nine patients underwent revision for osteolysis, loosening, poly wear or dislocation.

Acute Hip Replacement in Elderly Population for Acetabular Fracture

As mentioned above, there are some relative indications for primary THR following acetabular fractures.

Borg T, Hernefalk B, Hailer NP. Acute total hip arthroplasty combined with internal fixation for displaced acetabular fractures in the elderly: a short-term comparison with internal fixation alone after a minimum of two years. Bone Joint J. 2019;101(4):478–483. This is a prospective study of 27 patients with a minimum follow up of 2 years where 14 had ORIF and 13 had fracture fixation and acute THR. Survival for THR was 100% at 3 years as opposed to only 28.6% in ORIF group. THR group did not have any dislocation or deep infection. However, patient survival was lower in THR group at 3 years.

Hamlin K, Lazaraviciute G, Koullouros M, Chouari T, Stevenson IM, Hamilton S. Should total hip arthroplasty be performed acutely in the treatment of acetabular fractures in elderly or used as a salvage procedure only? Ind J Ortho 2017,51(4):421–33. Systematic review comparing results of primary and secondary THA for acetabulum fractures from 43 studies between 1976 to 2016. It included around 1,119 cases in total. Of note, rate of revisions due to any cause or due to aseptic loosening were higher for secondary THA compared to primary THA. Cemented arthroplasty had higher mortality rate in both primary and secondary THA groups compared to uncemented hip replacement.

Cervical Spine Injuries

Cervical spine injuries have a bimodal incidence. Up to 30% of such injuries occur in young men.

Mechanism

Cervical spine injuries are often the result of road traffic accidents or falls. Penetrating injuries and sports injuries also account for a small percentage. Cervical spine injury must be suspected in patients who cannot be adequately assessed because of head injury or impaired consciousness.

Vertebral artery injury occurs in about 20% of patients, with a higher risk in flexion distraction or flexion compression injuries. In 17% of patients there is reconstitution of the blood flow.

Table 1.23 Assessment of spinal injuries

General	Spine	Neurologic
Head injury Pupillary size Glasgow coma scale. Facial lacerations or fractures. Cerebrospinal fluid otorrhoea or rhinorrhoea. Urinary incontinence or retention.	Localised tenderness. Gaps in the spinous processes. Spinal shock—return of Bulbocavernosus reflex indicates end of spinal shock	*Sensory* Assess pin-prick sensation, light touch using a cotton ball and perianal sensation: 0 is absent, 1 is impaired, 2 is normal and NT is not testable. Proprioception is an important posterior column sensation. Babinski reflex Abdominal reflexes and Beevor's sign. *Motor* Assessed in 10 paired myotomes Tone.

Bilateral injuries can lead to delayed cortical blindness and quadriparesis. The assessment of spinal injuries is summarized in Table 1.23.

Bulbocavernosus reflex is contraction of anal sphincter in response to tugging on the indwelling urinary catheter or squeezing the glans penis.

Imaging

A CT scan of the entire spine (trauma pan scan) should be obtained in all patients with a suspected cervical spine injury. MRI scans are useful in patients with neurological deficit, although not needed urgently.

X-rays are notoriously difficult to interpret and miss a significant proportion of injuries. These are no longer part of initial imaging for cervical spine injuries.

The presence of a cervical spine injury should prompt a search for an associated second injury in the spine, the incidence of which is about 10%.

The five alignment lines should be identified on the lateral radiograph (Fig. 1.87).

1. Prevertebral line: Increase in the soft tissue outline by more than 7 mm anterior C2 or by more than 22 mm anterior to C6 is suggestive of cervical spine injury.
2. Anterior vertebral line: Along the anterior borders of the cervical vertebrae
3. Posterior vertebral line: Along the anterior extent of the spinal canal
4. Spino-laminar line: Along the posterior margin of the canal
5. Spinous process line: Connecting tips of spinous processes

Any step of more than 3 mm raises suspicion of a cervical spine injury. Unilateral facet dislocation produces a step in the vertebral alignment of less than 25% of the vertebral width. A step of 25–50% indicates bilateral facet dislocation.

Another indicator is the atlantodens interval, which is the space between the posterior border of the anterior arch of the atlas and the anterior margin of the odontoid process. The atlantodens interval should be less than 3 mm in adults and less than 5 mm in children.

On the open-mouth odontoid peg view, the distance between the odontoid and the lateral mass of the atlas should be equal on both sides, with the lateral margin of the mass in line with the lateral margin of the C2 body.

Management

The cervical spine is immobilised at the scene of accident.

The goals of treatment are stabilisation of spine, preventing progression of neurological deficit and allowing early rehabilitation.

The indications for surgical stabilisation are progressive neurological deficit, presence of associated injuries and spinal instability.

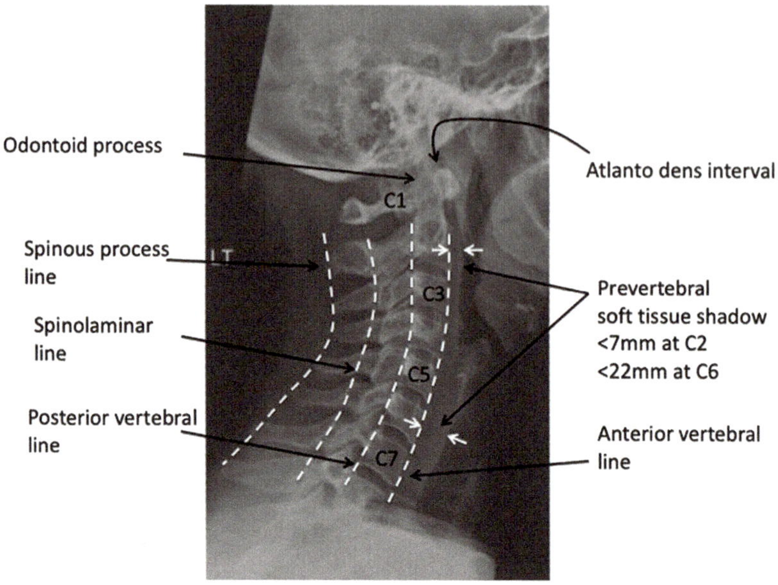

Fig. 1.87 Radiological parameters in lateral cervical spine radiograph

Thoracolumbar Spine Fracture

Holdsworth proposed the two-column concept of spinal stability. The posterior longitudinal ligament complex is the chief determinant of stability. If this is disrupted then the spine is unstable. Stable fractures include anterior wedge fractures, burst fractures and extension injuries. Unstable injuries are shear injuries and fracture dislocations. Denis proposed the three-column concept of spine stability. The anterior column includes the anterior half of vertebral body and the anterior longitudinal ligament. The middle column includes the posterior half of vertebral body and the posterior longitudinal ligament. The posterior column includes the posterior arch.

The transition zone is from T11 to L1. It is the junction of the immobile kyphotic thoracic spine and the mobile lordotic lumbar spine. Sixty percent of thoracolumbar spine fractures occur in this area.

Thoracolumbar spine fractures have been classified by Denis into four types—compression injuries, burst fractures, flexion distraction injuries and fracture dislocations.

Compression Fracture

In a compression fracture the anterior column fails under compression, the middle column remains intact and the posterior column remains intact or fails under tension (Fig. 1.88). These injuries commonly occur between T11 and L2. On plain X-rays, measure Cobb's angle and the percentage loss of vertebral height.

Kummell's disease is delayed progression of kyphotic deformity. It is characterised by worsening back pain and osteonecrosis of the vertebral body (posttraumatic). Patients may have neurological deficit.

Burst Fracture

Burst fractures involve failure of the anterior and middle column in axial load (Fig. 1.89). They commonly occur between T11 and L2. On X-rays, interpedicular widening is evident. The Cobb's angle and the percentage loss of vertebral height is measured.

Decision making in burst fractures is summarised in Table 1.24.

Fig. 1.88 Compression injuries

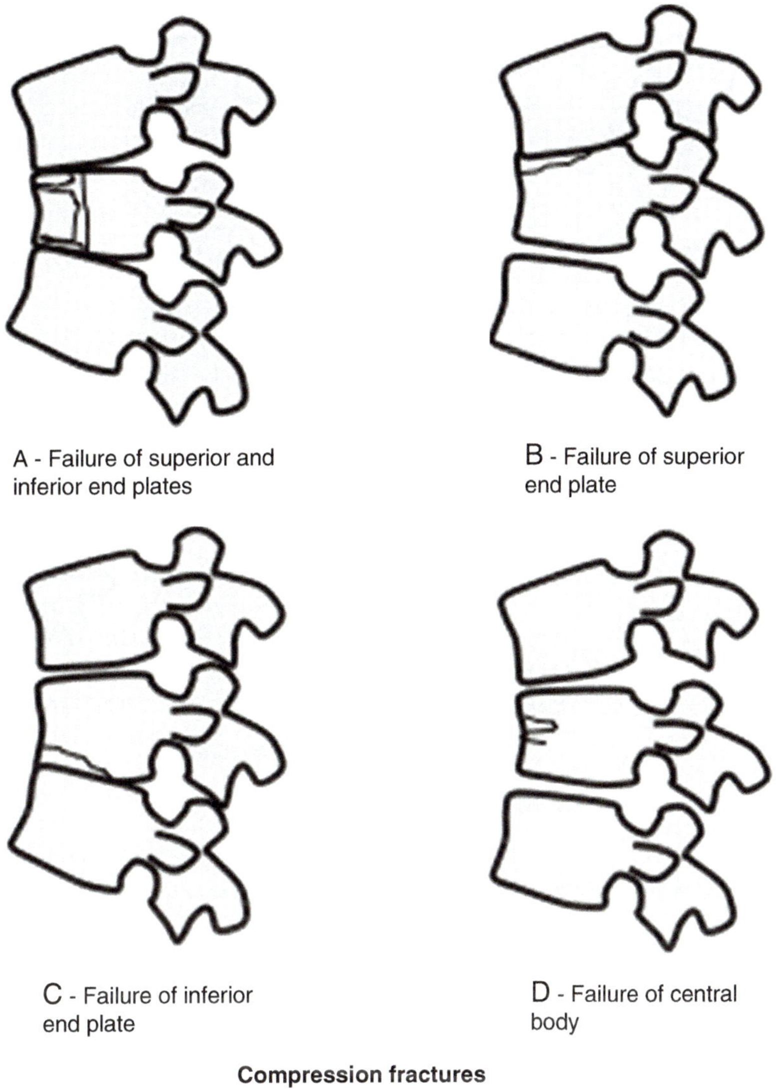

The TLICS (Thoraco Lumbar Injury Classification and Severity Scale is useful in determining the need for operative intervention (Table 1.25).

The TLICS was created by the Spine Trauma Study Group in 2005. The morphology is based on the pattern of injury rather than the mechanism of injury. The posterior ligamentous complex is assessed on MR scan. A score of less than 3 favours nonoperative treatment. A score of 4 needs individual decision making. Score more than 4 favours operative intervention.

Vaccaro AR, Lehman RA Jr, Hurlbert RJ, Anderson PA et al. A new classification of thoracolumbar injuries: the importance of injury morphology, the integrity of the posterior ligamentous complex, and neurologic status. Spine (Phila Pa 1976). 2005;30(20):2325–33.

Short-segment pedicle screws have a high failure rate if anterior stabilisation is not achieved and should be removed after 18 months.

An isolated anterior approach can be used if surgery is delayed for more than 2 weeks or if there is compression by the thecal sac.

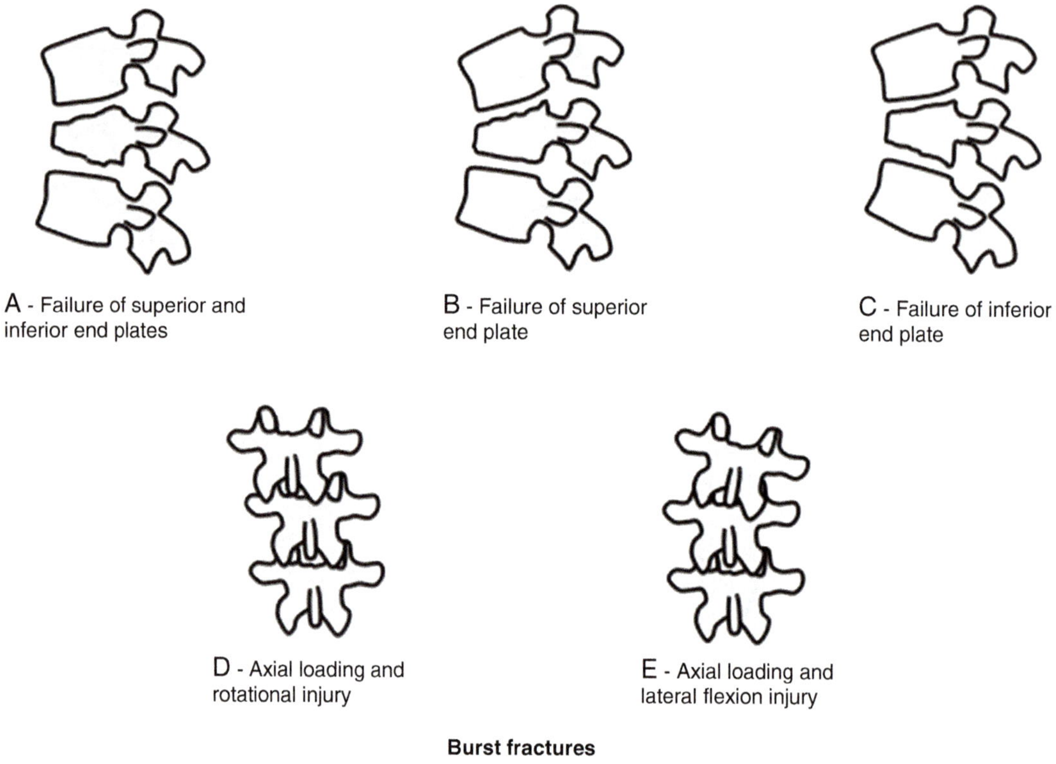

Fig. 1.89 Types of burst fractures

Table 1.24 Management planning in burst fractures

Signs of instability	Indications for surgery
• Progressive kyphosis. • Progressive neurologic deficit. • Substantial posterior column injury. • More than 50% loss of vertebral height with kyphosis.	• Kyphosis of more than 20–30°. • Subluxation of the posterior facets. • An increase in the interspinous process distance. • Loss of more than 50% of vertebral height.

Flexion Distraction Injury

The anterior column fails under tension or compression, the middle column fails under tension and the posterior column fails under tension (Fig. 1.90). MRI and CT with sagittal reconstructions should be obtained.

Associated intra-abdominal injuries occur in 45% of patients, and 10–15% experience neurologic deficit.

Table 1.25 The TLICS system for spinal injury

A. Morphology	
Compression	1 point
Burst	2 points
Translation/rotation	3 points
Distraction	4 points
B. Integrity of Posterior ligament complex	
Intact	0 points
Suspected/indeterminate	2 points
Injured	3 points
C. Neurological status	
Intact	0 points
Nerve root	2 points
Complete cord	2 points
Incomplete cord	3 points
Cauda Equina	3 points

In view of the good healing potential of bone, patients with no neurological deficit can be managed with a hyperextension cast or total-contact thoracolumbosacral orthosis for 3 months.

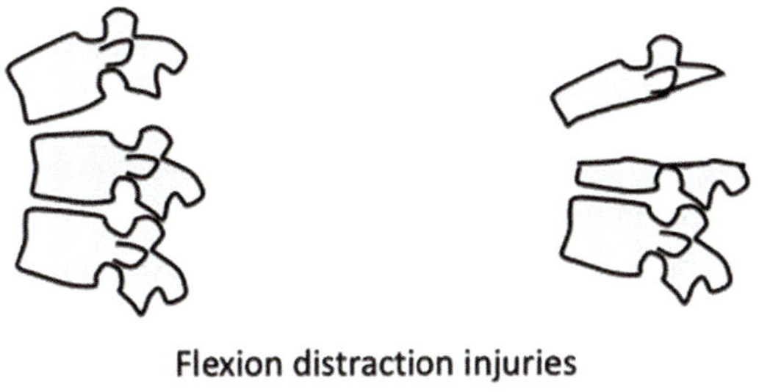

Fig. 1.90 Flexion distraction injuries

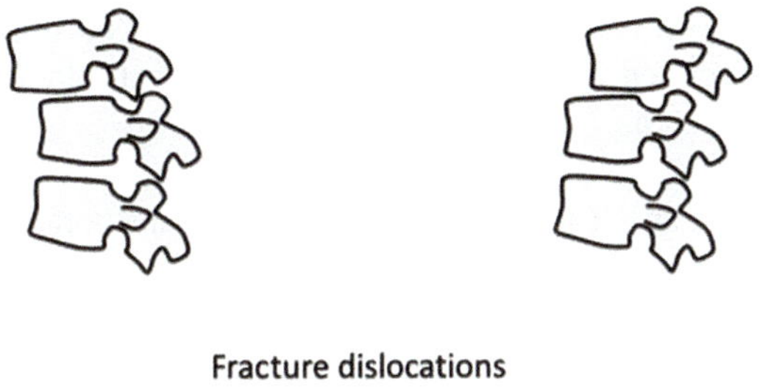

Fig. 1.91 Fracture dislocations

Fracture Dislocation

All three columns are disrupted. Horizontal translation or rotation will be evident on radiographs (Fig. 1.91).

Management is with multisegment posterior instrumentation. Stabilisation of two levels above and below the fracture is recommended.

Spinal Cord Injury

Two commonly used grading systems are those of Frankel (Table 1.26) and the American Spine Injury Association.

The American Spinal Injury Association (ASIA) charts are widely used. Motor function is documented from C5 to T1 and L2 to S1 and is graded from 0 to 5. Maximum motor score is 50 on either side.

Sensory function is graded from 0 to 2 for pin prick and light touch. Maximum score for each of these is 112 (56 on either side of the body).

Table 1.26 Frankel Spinal cord injury grading

Grade	Frankel
A	No motor or sensory function
B	Sensory function only, no motor function
C	Motor function is useless
D	Motor function is useful
E	Normal motor and sensory function

Emergency Treatment

A full neurological examination is carried out. It is important to rule out spinal shock by checking the bulbocavernosus reflex.

Sacral sparing may be the only indication that the injury is incomplete. In complete injuries, 80% of patients regain function in one root above the injury level while 20% regain two roots.

The National Acute Spinal Cord Injury Study determined a benefit of methylprednisolone infusion. A bolus of 30 mg/kg is administered followed by an infusion of 5.4 mg/kg/hr. The infusion is continued for 24 h if the bolus is given within 3 h of injury. If the bolus is given 3–8 h after injury, the infusion is carried on for 48 h.

There is, however, some controversy relating to the efficacy of steroids. Many centres do not use steroids as standard of care, but do include them as a treatment option. Currently, use of high dose methyl prednisolone is not recommended by NICE.

Bracken MB, Shepard MJ, Collins WF, et al. A randomized, controlled trial of methylprednisolone or naloxone in the treatment of acute spinal-cord injury. Results of the Second National Acute Spinal Cord Injury Study. N Engl J Med 1990;322:1405–11. In this study, 162 patients with an acute spinal-cord injury were given methylprednisolone, 154 were given naloxone and 171 were given placebo. A benefit was seen with methylprednisolone in patients with complete and incomplete lesions.

Hugenholtz H, Cass DE, Dvorak MF, et al. High-dose methylprednisolone for acute closed spinal cord injury—only a treatment option. Can J Neurol Sci 2002;29:227–35. This systematic review concluded that the evidence to support the use of methylprednisolone is weak (level I to II-1).

Evaniew N, Noonan VK, Fallah N, et al. Methylprednisolone for the treatment of patients with acute spinal cord injuries: a propensity score-matched cohort study from a Canadian Multi-Center Spinal Cord Injury Registry. J Neurotrauma. 2015;32:1674–1683. This study looked for neurological improvement in patients who received high dose steroid according to NASCIS II protocol. Patients who received high dose steroids did not show an improvement in motor function but had a significantly higher rate of complications.

Imaging

X-ray of the entire spine along with a CT scan is done. A wide transverse diameter indicates interpedicular widening. MRI is useful in patients with neurological deficit to assess cord damage and epidural haematoma.

Management

Stability is assessed on the basis of extent of damage to the posterior column, extent of collapse and extent of kyphosis.

The posterior column provides the greatest resistance to progressive kyphosis.

The neutral-zone theory of Panjabi describes a continuum between stability, hypermobility and frank instability.

Indications for surgery are

- Progressive neurologic deficit.
- Major neurological deficit with canal compromise.
- Progressive kyphosis.
- Substantial rotational or translational malalignment.
- Soft tissue chance fracture.

Approaches

The indications for an anterior approach are

- No injury to the posterior column.
- Incomplete neurologic deficit in flexion injury with canal compromise.
- Secondary decompression following posterior stabilisation.
- Significant anterior spinal instability.

An anterior approach provides direct decompression, but there is no difference in neurologic outcome.

- For T4–T9 injuries—right transthoracic approach.
- For T10–L1 injuries—thoracoabdominal approach with subphrenic extension.
- For T12–L5 injuries—subpleural retroperitoneal approach.
- For T2–T4 injuries—lateral extrapleural parascapular approach or extension of a cervical spine approach with partial manubriectomy and partial excision of the medial third of the clavicle. Sternal splitting may be needed.

In the posterior approach, instrumentation should be two or three levels above and two levels below. The distraction restores vertebral height and partial canal clearance is achieved by ligamentotaxis. Canal clearance of 40–75% is possible in acute injuries.

Posterior short-segment fusion (one level above and below) is associated with a high rate of proximal screw pullout if there is anterior column compromise. This technique is not commonly used.

In the 'rod long, fuse short' technique, rods are removed after 1 year. However, arthritis develops in unfused segments. Progressive kyphosis after rod removal and late back pain are other complications, and this technique is therefore not commonly used.

For fracture dislocations, fixation can be performed from the back initially with anterior reconstruction performed if needed. The fixation must extend three levels up and two or three levels below.

The extent of canal compromise has been correlated with neurological deficit in some studies, but this is not universally accepted. Any remaining canal compromise decreases by 50% with remodelling over the 12 months following the injury.

An anterior approach is used to reduce canal impingement; a posterior approach with ligamentotaxis may also reduce canal impingement. Sharpey's fibres help with reduction in the posterior approach. Indirect reduction should be performed within 3 days of injury. It is less effective in the presence of more than 67% canal compromise due to annular ligament disruption.

A 'flat back' after posterior instrumentation was a problem with the initial instrumentation systems, but square terminal-rod hook constructs allow sagittal contouring.

At the thoracolumbar junction, short-segment pedicle screw constructs have a high failure rate without anterior stabilisation.

Posterolateral Decompression

Posterolateral decompression allows access to the anterior thecal sac either through or lateral to the pedicle. Bone anterior to the retropulsed fragments is removed through curettes and pituitaries. This should only be performed in the lower lumbar spine below the conus.

Potential complications include neurologic damage, inadequate decompression and poor visualisation for grafting.

Complications of Surgery

- Neurologic deterioration (1%) caused by overdistraction, overcompression, malreduction or an instrument in the spinal canal.
- Instrumentation failure.
- Pseudarthrosis (2–8%).
- Delayed vascular erosion caused by metal–vessel contact in anterior instrumentation.
- Retrograde ejaculation caused by damage to autonomic nervous system (4%).
- Injury to the great vessels.
- Infection.

Surgery does not improve the chances of neurologic recovery. Animal studies, however, have shown better results with early decompression.

Kyphosis is not related to back pain and functional impairment. Damage to the discovertebral complex and posterior facet joints may be responsible for back pain.

Sacral Fractures

The S1 nerve root has the foraminal exit area, and the root occupies one-third of the area of the foramen. The S4 nerve root has the largest foraminal exit area, with the root occupying one-sixth of the area.

The anterior rami of S2–S5 conduct parasympathetic impulses for sexual, bladder and bowel function.

Evaluation

Bruising, tenderness, swelling and posterior sacral osseous prominence may be evident with sacral fracture, but 30% of cases are missed on the initial presentation.

A Morel–Lavallée lesion is indicated by degloving of the lumbosacral fascia and a subcutaneous fluid mass.

The examination should assess spontaneous and maximum anal sphincter contraction, light touch and pin-prick along the perianal S2–S5 dermatomes, and bulbocavernosus and cremasteric reflexes.

Imaging should include an X-ray of the pelvis: AP, inlet and outlet views.

X-ray signs include

- Fracture of the L5 transverse process—present in 51% of patients.
- A paradoxical inlet view of the sacrum seen on the AP view—92% of patients
- 'Stepladder sign'—anterior sacral foraminal disruption.

A CT, MRI, bone scan and single-photon emission CT can help to define the injury.

Perineal somatosensory evoked potentials and anal sphincter electromyography can assess neurological deficit from spinal injuries.

Classification

Denis proposed the three-zone classification (Fig. 1.92).

In zone 1, the fracture line is lateral to the neural foramen. In zone 2, the fracture involves the neural foramina and in zone 3, the fracture extends to the spinal canal.

Zone 3 is further subdivided based on the pattern of fracture lines into H type, U type, lambda fracture and the T fracture.

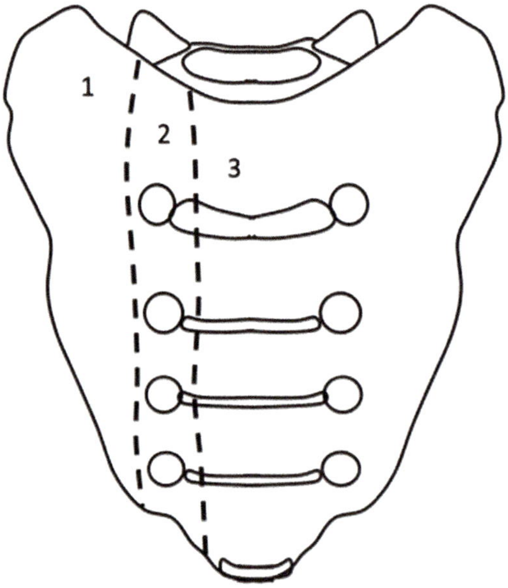

Fig. 1.92 Denis classification of sacral fractures

Management

Many sacral injuries are managed non-operatively, but the indications for surgery are being more clearly defined with an improved understanding of these injuries and their prognosis.

Indications for surgery include open injuries, fractures with neurological compromise and unstable fractures with progressive displacement.

Fixation of the sacrum can be achieved anteriorly or posteriorly. Percutaneously placed SI screws, plate fixation posteriorly, lumbar pedicle screws with iliac screw fixation and anterior plates are options for stabilising sacral injuries.

Fractures in Children

Hip Fracture

Hip fractures in children are a relatively rare compared with other childhood injuries.

Classification

The classification was proposed by Delbet (Fig. 1.93).

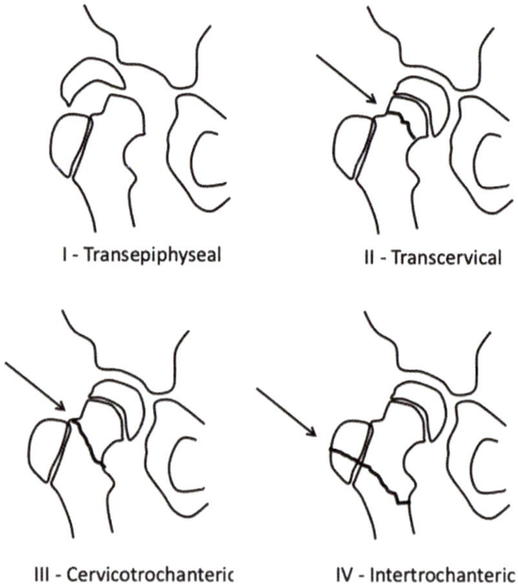

Fig. 1.93 Delbet classification of proximal femoral fractures in children

Blood Supply to the Femoral Head

From birth to the age of 4 years, the metaphyseal vessels arising from the medial and lateral circumflex femoral arteries are the major supply to the femoral head along with the artery along ligamentum teres. By the age of 4 years, the physis is more developed and the retinacular vessels become the major supply. These arise from the medial and lateral circumflex femoral artery.

Management

Type I fractures are treated with anatomic reduction (either closed or open) and stabilization with a pin or screws. These must cross the epiphyseal plate in order to stabilize the fracture and smooth pins should be used in children to minimise growth impairment at the physis. Type I injuries are associated with dislocation of the capital physis in 50% of children. This carries an almost 100% rate of AVN of the capital physis.

Type II and III fractures can be treated non-operatively with a cast in young children if they are undisplaced or if anatomic reduction can be achieved. ORIF may be needed for fracture which can not be reduced, but crossing the physis is avoided if possible. If the fracture is very proximal and the physis has to be crossed then it is advisable to cross the physis as close to the center as possible to avoid discrepancy in growth. Also, the physis must be crossed in a single attempt.

Type IV injuries have a low risk of AVN and are treated either in a spica or by internal fixation with a screw with a side plate (pediatric hip screws).

Complications

AVN is a complication related to initial displacement and a time lag between injury and reduction. The risk of AVN is highest with type I and lowest with type IV fractures.

Coxa vara can result from growth arrest at the physis, with relative overgrowth of the trochanteric physis. Malreduction or loss of alignment can also lead to coxa vara. Subtrochanteric valgus osteotomy is an option if the neck shaft angle is less than 110°.

Physeal growth arrest can be caused by damage at the time of injury or threaded pins crossing the physis.

Non-union is possible in patients where anatomic reduction is not achieved.

Chondrolysis is a rare complication.

Hip Dislocation

Hip dislocation is a rare injury in children. It is generally related to high-energy trauma. The diagnosis is evident on radiographs or cross-sectional imaging.

Treatment is directed towards concentric reduction, either with closed manipulation or open reduction.

Femoral Shaft Fracture

Femoral shaft fractures can occur from simple falls or high-energy injuries. Non-accidental injury (NAI) accounts for almost half of femoral shaft fractures in infants. There has to be high suspicion of NAI as 30% of femoral shaft fractures in infants (less than 1 year) and 12–14% in children <36 months are as a result of physical abuse. Also, femoral shaft fractures in non ambulatory children are commonly due to NAI.

Management

Femoral shaft fractures can be managed with various methods depending on the age of the child, and the treatment must be individualized according to the clinical situation. The options include spica application, traction followed by spica, external fixation, flexible intramedullary nails, rigid intramedullary nailing, minimally invasive sub-muscular plating and a dynamic compression plate. In general, children younger than 5 years can be managed in a spica cast. Beyond this age, flexible intramedullary nails are preferred. Antegrade femoral nailing is an option in skeletally mature patients.

Indications for surgery in young children include open fractures, multiple injuries, an associated head injury, neurovascular injury and floating knee (ipsilateral femoral and tibial fracture). Surgery is also indicated in situations where it is difficult to maintain reduction by closed methods.

Spica

The early application of spica is an option in children younger than 5 years. Children older than 5 years can be difficult to manage at home in a spica cast. It can be difficult to maintain reduction with spica and there is a possibility of shortening.

Traction

Traction used to be a common method of treatment, but the long period of hospitalization required has diminished its role in modern orthopaedics. Traction is usually applied for 2–4 weeks and is followed by spica cast application. It can be used on its own as a definitive treatment method.

External Fixation

External fixation is an effective method in children. It is easy to apply, minimally invasive and provides adequate stabilization. Conversely, external fixation is associated with pin-site infections, the inconvenience of a frame, knee stiffness and re-fractures after frame removal.

Flexible Intramedullary Nails

Flexible intramedullary nails are increasingly being used for femoral shaft fractures because of their minimally invasive nature and ability to maintain reduction effectively. They are generally inserted retrograde and the entry point is proximal to the distal femoral physis. The nails can be bent into a C- or S-shape to provide three-point fixation across the fracture.

Weight bearing is restricted until a callus is seen on the radiographs, but some stable fracture patterns can be progressed on weight bearing at an earlier point.

Dynamic Compression Plate

Plating of the femur provides a stable construct. Plating is associated with a relatively bigger scar and more blood loss. The risks are plate breakage and fracture through a screw hole after plate removal.

Submuscular bridge plating is a minimally invasive technique wherein a plate is inserted between the periosteum and vastus lateralis via small proximal and distal incisions.

Sutphen SA, Mendoza JD, Mundy AC, Yang JG, Beebe AC, Samora WP 3rd, Klingele KE. Pediatric Diaphyseal Femur Fractures: Submuscular Plating Compared With Intramedullary Nailing. Orthopedics. 2016;39(6):353–8.

Antegrade Femoral Nailing

Trochanteric entry femoral nails can be used in children older than 11 years or weighing >50 kg. These offer the advantage of early weight bearing. Piriformis entry nails are avoided due to risk of damage to blood supply of femoral head. Some children may develop narrowing of femoral neck or coxa valga due to early closure of trochanteric physis.

Complications

Leg-length discrepancy may occur due to malreduction and shortening of the injured limb. The shortening is compensated by overgrowth of the femur following fracture. This may be up to 1 cm.

Treatment Options For Various Age Groups are summarised in Table 1.27.

Table 1.27 Treatment option for femoral fractures in children

Age	Treatment
<6 months	Pavlik harness/early spica
6 months to 5 years	Early spica or traction followed by spica
5–11 years	• Flexible nailing • Submuscular plating
>11 years	• Submuscular plating • Lateral entry IM nailing • Flexible nailing

Supracondylar Femoral Fracture

These fractures are difficult to reduce and stabilize non-operatively because the pull of the gastrocnemius tends to flex the knee and produce angulation at the fracture site. Cross-pins or screws can be used.

Distal Femoral Physeal Fracture

These injuries can be seen in newborns, and are caused by pulling on the leg during delivery in a breech presentation. In older children, physeal separation is associated with high-energy trauma.

Undisplaced injuries can be managed with cast. Displaced fractures require reduction and can be stabilized with smooth pins crossing the physis or by screw fixation into the metaphyseal fragment.

Physeal injuries can lead to growth arrest with consequent angular deformity or limb-length discrepancy. The injury should be followed-up to skeletal maturity.

Patellar Fracture

Patellar fractures in children are managed in a similar manner to adult patellar fractures. A sleeve fracture of the patella is through non-ossified cartilage, and the radiographs may give a false appearance of a small fragment.

Patellar dislocations are common in children. Most dislocations or subluxations of the patella reduce spontaneously and present as a painful knee. Tenderness along the medial border of patella and apprehension on lateral subluxation indicate a possible patellar dislocation.

Acute patellar dislocations are managed with reduction and 1–2 weeks of immobilisation. Once the pain settles, quadriceps exercises can be started. Quadriceps setting exercises are started initially, followed by closed-chain exercises.

A significant number of patients with acute patellar dislocation have an osteochondral fracture involving the patellar surface or the lateral femoral condyle.

Tibial Tubercle Fracture

Avulsion injuries of the tibial tubercle can be classified into three types (Table 1.28).

Displaced fractures are managed with ORIF by screws. Interposition of periosteum makes closed reduction difficult. Arrest of physeal growth can lead to a recurvatum deformity in the growing child.

Tibial Fracture

Proximal tibial epiphyseal injuries can be Salter Harris type I or II. The close proximity of the arteries posteriorly means there is a risk of vascular injury.

Displaced fractures are managed with closed reduction and percutaneous pins. Open reduction is rarely needed. The physis should not be crossed with threaded pins. Growth arrest leading to deformity occurs in one in four patients and follow-up is advisable.

Fractures of the proximal tibial metaphysis are prone to late valgus deformity. These injuries should therefore be followed up. If a deformity

Table 1.28 Ogden classification of tibial tubercle avulsions in children

Type I	Avulsion of a small fragment of the tuberosity
Type II	Avulsion extending to the proximal tibial physis
Type III	Avulsion of the tuberosity extending to the proximal tibial articular surface

becomes evident, surgery to correct it should be delayed for 3 years as some deformities will spontaneously correct.

A toddler's fracture is an undisplaced oblique fracture of the distal tibia seen in infants and is the result of a low-energy trauma. A short-leg walking cast for 3 weeks is sufficient.

Tibial diaphyseal fractures in older children are managed with closed reduction and long-leg cast application. Surgical options for open fractures, irreducible fractures and unstable fractures are external fixation, flexible intramedullary nails and plate fixation.

Mashru et al defined acceptability criteria for tibial shaft fractures in children. Up to 10 degrees of coronal and sagittal angulation, 50% translation, and 10 mm of shortening is acceptable in children under the age of 8 years. Acceptable angulation decreases to 5 degrees in children over 8 years old.

Mashru RP, Herman MJ, Pizzutillo PD. Tibial shaft fractures in children and adolescents. J Am Acad Orthop Surg. 2005;13(5):345–52

Triplane Fracture

Triplane fractures are fractures of the distal tibia in the skeletally immature patient, involving the distal tibial growth plate. The fracture plane is sagittal in the epiphysis, horizontal through the growth plate and coronal through the posterior distal tibial metaphysis.

Triplane fractures are Salter Harris type IV injuries. They are often minimally displaced and can be managed in a cast with close monitoring for displacement. Displaced fractures require internal stabilization with one or two screws. A CT scan will show the displaced fragments.

There is a potential for growth arrest with these injuries.

Seymour Lesion

A Seymour lesion is an injury of the physis of the distal phalanx associated with injury to the skin and nail fold. The physeal plate is proximal in the phalanx, and is close to the nail fold. Displacement of this physis leads to an open injury. Operative intervention is required in Seymour lesion to ensure there is no soft tissue interposition in the fracture site. Missed injuries can lead to chronic osteomyelitis, physeal arrest and nail plate deformities.

Humeral Shaft Fracture

In neonates, fractures of the proximal end of humerus involving the growth plate are usually Salter Harris type I injuries. The growth plate is susceptible to injury. Older children have type II or III injuries. The vast majority are managed with non-operative methods due to good remodelling and quick healing.

Humeral shaft fractures are rare in children and non-operative measures such as a cast or brace with sling are adequate for immobilisation. Operative intervention is rarely needed.

Supracondylar Humerus Fracture

Supracondylar humerus fracture is a common elbow injury in children. It is sustained as a result of a fall on an outstretched hand. Rarely, it may be due to a direct fall onto the elbow.

Most common age of presentation is 4–7 years, as this a period of rapid metaphyseal remodelling. Most are hyperextension injuries. It is more common in boys.

Classification

Classification was proposed by Gartland (Fig. 1.94).

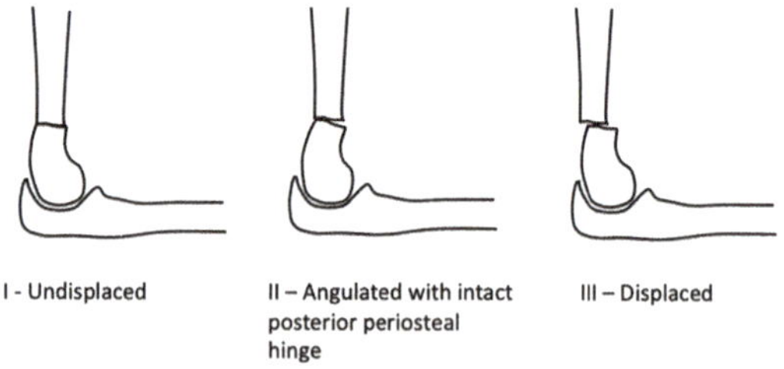

Fig. 1.94 Supracondylar fracture of distal humerus

Clinical Assessment

These fractures can be associated with neurovascular injury and a thorough assessment is vital.

There is often significant local swelling and tenderness. Open fractures require urgent debridement and K-wire stabilisation. In some closed fractures, the proximal fragment may be buttonholed through the brachialis and can pucker the skin on the anterior aspect of the elbow.

The nerves should be assessed and recorded. The anterior interosseous nerve is the most common nerve involved in this injury. The distal circulation is assessed, noting both the capillary refill time and the radial and ulnar pulses. Flexing the elbow can obstruct distal circulation; if this occurs, the arm should be splinted in a semi-flexed position until reduction and stabilisation can be performed.

Imaging

Baumann's angle is the angle between the longitudinal axis of the humerus and a line drawn along the axis of the capitellar physis. The normal angle is 10–25° (Fig. 1.95).

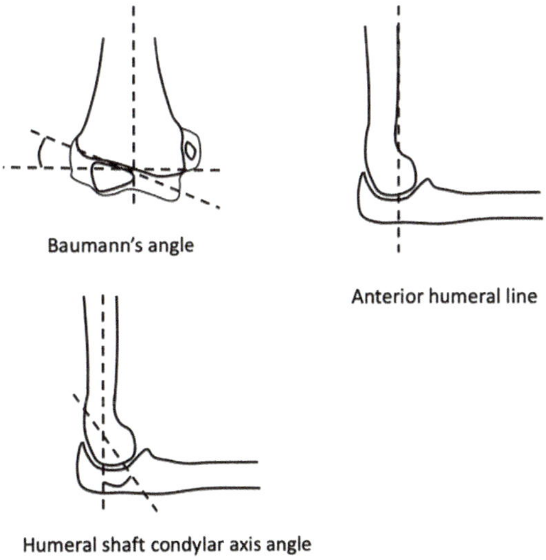

Fig. 1.95 Alignment parameters of the distal humerus

On the lateral view, a line drawn along the anterior cortex of the humerus should intersect the middle one-third of the capitellum. The angle between the humeral shaft axis on the lateral view and the axis of the condyles is 40 degrees.

Radiographs are helpful to classify the injury, assess displacement and look for associated injuries.

Management

In patients without vascular compromise, undisplaced (type I) injuries can be managed in a plaster splint.

Type II injuries require manipulation and splint application or K wire fixation to restore alignment. Moraleda et al studied the natural history of unreduced type II fractures and the arc of movement remained same as the opposite side but the affected elbow had significantly more hyper-extension (8 degree) and less flexion (7 degree). This suggested that not all type II fractures need surgery but due to change in arc of motion at elbow, a discussion should be done with the child and family while deciding treatment.

Moraleda L, Valencia M, Barco R, et al. Natural history of unreduced Gartland type-II supracondylar fractures of the humerus in children: a two to thirteen-year follow-up study. J Bone Joint Surg Am 2013;95(1):28–34.

Type III injuries are managed with closed reduction and percutaneous pin fixation. Open reduction is sometimes required if there is soft tissue interposition, or if the brachialis muscle is impaled by the fragment.

One pin is inserted from the medial epicondyle to engage the opposite cortex and the other is inserted from the lateral condyle. Crossed pinning is especially preferred in highly unstable fractures and fractures associated with medial comminution. Two diverging pins from the lateral side are acceptable, but will not be as mechanically stable as cross-pins. However, biomechanical stability of three well placed bicortical lateral entry pins with good spacing at the fracture site is similar to two crossed pins.

Larson L, Firoozbakhsh K, Passarelli R, et al. Biomechanical analysis of pinning techniques for pediatric supracondylar humerus fractures. J Pediatr Orthop 2006;26(5):573–8.

The timing of surgery has been a matter of some debate. It is advisable to undertake reduction before the local soft tissue swelling progresses to the extent of compromising circulation.

Sibinski M, Sharma H, Bennet GC. Early versus delayed treatment of extension type-3 supracondylar fractures of the humerus in children. J Bone Joint Surg Br 2006;88:380–1. In this study of 77 children, 43 children were pinned within 12 h and the rest were managed more than 12 h after the injury. There was no difference in outcome between the two groups.

Walmsley PJ, Kelly MB, Robb JE, et al. Delay increases the need for open reduction of type-III supracondylar fractures of the humerus. J Bone Joint Surg Br 2006;88:528–30. In this retrospective study of 171 children, 126 were managed within 8 h and 45 were managed after 8 h. Those in the delayed group were more likely to require open reduction.

Leet AI, Frisancho J, Ebramzadeh E. Delayed treatment of type 3 supracondylar humerus fractures in children. J Pediatr Orthop 2002;22:203–7. In this study of 158 patients, there was no increase in operative time, closed reduction and complications with delays in surgery of up to 21 h.

Olecranon pin insertion and traction is an option for the management of supracondylar fractures. It requires a hospital stay and is hence not a favoured method. Traction can be applied in a brace, which allows earlier discharge from hospital but has a relatively higher complication rate.

Matsuzaki K, Nakatani N, Harada M, Tamaki T. Treatment of supracondylar fracture of the humerus in children by skeletal traction in a brace. J Bone Joint Surg Br 2004;86:232–8. This study of 193 patients with supracondylar fracture, including 15 radial nerve injuries and 14 median nerve injuries, investigated bracing with skeletal traction using an olecranon pin. Four children (2%) developed cubitus varus and one child had restricted flexion. Lateral and posterior displacement was not significant.

Fractures with vascular compromise should be reduced as an emergency. In most cases, the distal circulation is impaired because of tenting of the artery over the fracture site and will be restored immediately or within few minutes of reduction.

'Cool pulseless hand' is a surgical emergency. Immediate closed/open reduction is done followed by stabilization. If the circulation is still impaired, exploration of the brachial artery is undertaken by a vascular surgeon. Intimal tears are managed with a vein graft and lacerations in the artery can be repaired directly or with a graft.

In many patients, the collateral circulation may be adequate to maintain perfusion. Management of the 'pink pulseless hand' following supracondylar fracture has been somewhat controversial. Close post operative neurovascular monitoring is required to ensure that the distal limb stays perfused. Vascular surgery opinion is essential, but surgery may not always be required.

Scannell BP, Jackson JB 3rd, Bray C, et al. The perfused, pulseless supracondylar humeral fracture: intermediate-term follow-up of vascular status and function. J Bone Joint Surg Am 2013; 95(21):1913–9. This study included 20 patients with pink pulseless hand and had a minimum of 6 months follow up. All patients had normal arm growth and good/excellent function. All children had palpable distal radial pulse at latest follow up even though 5 patients had brachial artery occlusion. These 5 children had excellent collateral circulation.

Nerve injuries in association with supracondylar fractures are usually neurapraxias and recover with time. If there is no recovery after 4–6 months then nerve conduction studies are undertaken and neurolysis considered. In presence of isolated nerve injury, urgent surgery is not always needed as timing of surgery does not necessarily result in faster nerve recovery.

Barrett KK, Skaggs DL, Sawyer JR, et al. Supracondylar humeral fractures with isolated anterior interosseous nerve injuries: is urgent treatment necessary? J Bone Joint Surg Am 2014;96(21):1793–7.

Complications of Supracondylar Fractures

- Nerve and vascular injury.
- Malunion.
- Elbow stiffness.
- Myositis ossificans.

The risk of malunion is minimised with pin fixation. Cubitus valgus is better tolerated, but can lead to stretching of the ulnar nerve. Cubitus varus is cosmetically disabling and a supracondylar dome or lateral closing wedge osteotomy is required for correction.

Separation of the Distal Humeral Physis

This injury is seen in neonates and young children. The cartilaginous capitellum is not visible on radiographs and the appearance may be of elbow dislocation. Elbow dislocations are extremely rare in neonates. Ultrasound is diagnostic and demonstrates the capitellum.

Treatment is with closed reduction and splintage in flexion.

Lateral Humeral Condyle Fracture

Lateral condyle fractures mainly involve the cartilaginous end of the distal humerus. There is little soft tissue cover to enable reduction and these fractures are likely to lose alignment if not internally stabilised.

Because these are intra-articular injuries there is a high rate of non-union. Fractures that are displaced more than 2 mm should be reduced and fixed.

Classification

Classification is by Milch (Fig. 1.96).

Type I are Salter Harris type IV injury involving the capitellum. The lateral part of the trochlear ridge remains attached to the humerus. Type II are Salter Harris type II injury involving the capitellum and the lateral part of the trochlear ridge.

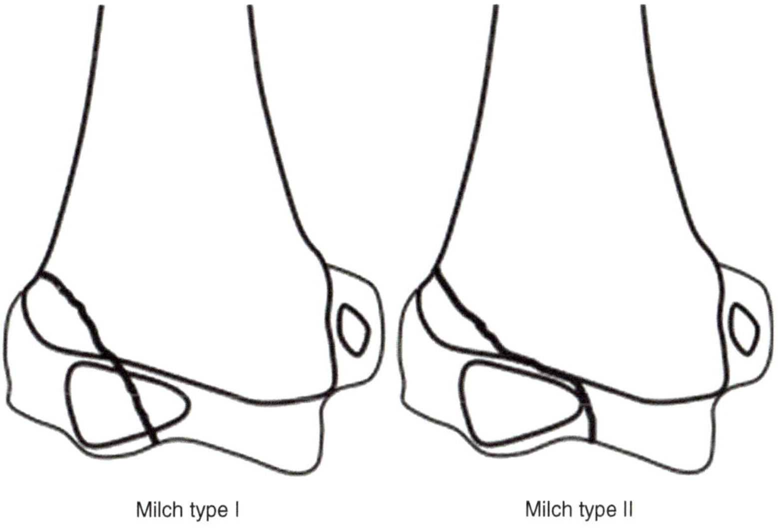

Fig. 1.96 Types of lateral condyle fracture

Management

Undisplaced fractures can be immobilised in a cast and followed-up closely to ensure there is no displacement.

Displaced fractures should be reduced (either closed or open) and stabilised with two smooth pins or 4 mm screws. Kocher's approach is used for exposure. The blood supply is from the posterior aspect and the soft tissues on this side should be protected. An anterior arthrotomy can be established to confirm the reduction.

The pins are removed at 4–6 weeks.

Complications

Complications include non-union, malunion and their consequences. Non-union is managed with bone grafting and fixation *in situ*. Cubitus valgus is possible in patients with malunion and can cause ulnar nerve palsy. Elbow stiffness may be encountered. Anterior transposition of the ulnar nerve will relieve stretch on the nerve.

Medial Epicondyle Fracture

These are avulsion injuries from a valgus force to the elbow. The fragment is separated and may become trapped within the elbow joint if the elbow was subluxed or dislocated at the time of injury.

In most patients, displaced fractures are managed by resting the arm in a sling. Fibrous union can be expected and functional limitation is minimal. Fixation of the fragment is indicated for open fractures and fractures with incarceration in the ulno-humeral joint. Surgery may be considered in high-demand patients as non union may lead to valgus instability or elbow and difficulty in throwing action. A single screw is adequate to achieve compression at the fracture site.

Radial Head Dislocation

Radial head dislocations in children may be congenital or traumatic.

Congenital dislocations have the appearance of a rounded radial head lacking concavity on the proximal aspect, relative overgrowth of the radius and a hypoplastic capitellum. Congenital dislocations have a poor outcome if reduction is attempted.

Traumatic dislocation can occur as an isolated injury or in association with ulnar fracture (known as the Monteggia injury).

Imaging

The longitudinal axis of the radius should be collinear with the capitellum in all views of the elbow (Fig. 1.97). Any loss of alignment indicates incongruence of the radiocapitellar joint.

Management

If diagnosed early, within 3–4 weeks, radial head dislocations can be reduced by closed manipulation.

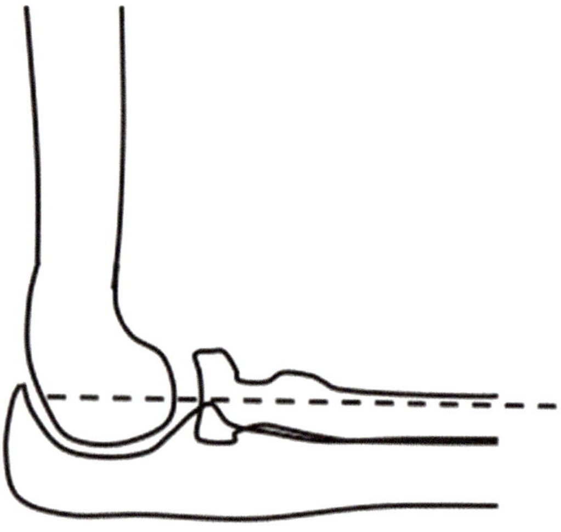

Fig. 1.97 Radial shaft and capitellum should be collinear in all views

If diagnosed late, open reduction is required. The annular ligament is reconstructed using strips of the triceps fascia passed through tunnels in the proximal ulna to maintain concentric reduction of the radial head. Many different techniques have been described. Bell Tawse used a strip from the central part of triceps fascia, while Lloyd-Roberts and Bucknill used the lateral part of the fascia. The harvested strip is left attached to the ulna at the distal end.

Lloyd-Roberts GC, Bucknill TM. Anterior dislocation of the radial head in children: aetiology, natural history and management. J Bone Joint Surg Br 1977;59-B:402–7.

Bell Tawse AJ. The treatment of malunited anterior Monteggia fractures in children. J Bone Joint Surg Br 1965;47:718–23.

Radial Neck Fractures

Radial neck fractures are the result of a valgus force on the elbow. There is good remodelling potential at this site in children and up to 30° of angulation can be accepted (Fig. 1.98).

Fractures angulated by more than 30° are managed with closed reduction and splintage/fixation.

Techniques of closed reduction:

1. Patterson technique: Traction and varus followed by direct pressure over radial head to reduce it
2. Israeli technique: Supination of flexed elbow to relax the capsule followed by direct pressure over radial head to reduce it
3. Esmarch bandage from distal forearm to elbow: Validation in literature is lacking.
4. Nehar and Torch: Elbow in traction and varus. Assistant pushes laterally on radial shaft to give counter-traction whilst surgeon pushes medially directly on radial head.

Techniques of percutaneous reduction:

Percutaneous reduction is done if closed reduction fails. Most fractures are stable after reduction and can be splinted for 2–3 weeks followed by immobilisation. A K-wire can be used across the fracture site to transfix the fragment, but a transcapitellar wire should be avoided because of risk of breakage.

1. A percutaneous pin can be used to physically push the fragment into alignment while applying a varus force to distract the joint. The

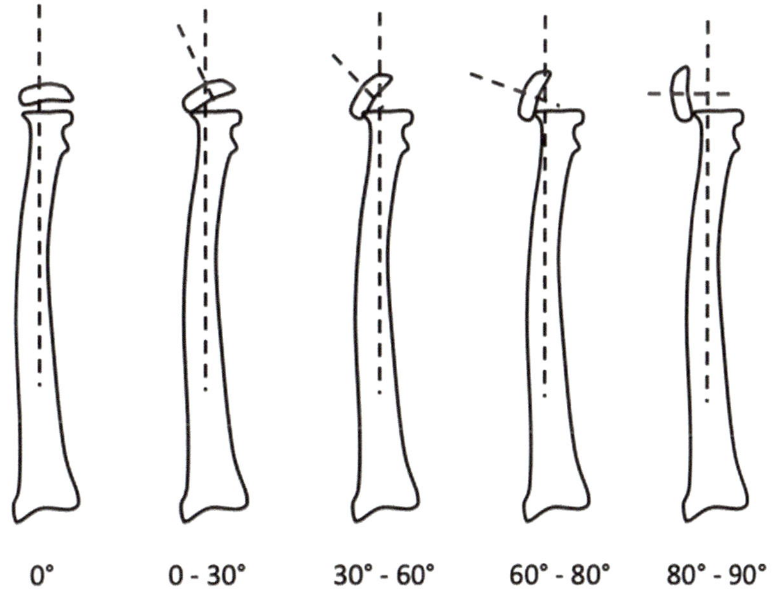

Fig. 1.98 Judet classification of proximal radial physeal disruptions

blunt end of a Steinmann pin or a 3.2 mm guide wire is useful for this purpose.
2. Metaizeau technique: A flexible nail is passed up the medullary canal of the radius with the tip bent. The wire is used to lever the fragment back into alignment with the tip of the nail (Fig. 1.99).

Open reduction is an option where closed reduction fails, but carries a high risk of damage to the growth plate.

Monteggia Fracture

A Monteggia fracture dislocation is a fracture of the ulna with dislocation of the radial head.

Acute injuries are managed with closed reduction of the radial head and immobilisation. Inability to achieve congruent reduction indicates an infolded annular ligament or button-holing of the radial head through the joint capsule; open reduction is needed. Ulnar fractures can be fixed internally for stability.

Injuries diagnosed late require either open reduction of the radial head or techniques to reconstruct the annular ligament. Ulnar corrective osteotomy can be combined with the procedure.

Radius and Ulna Diaphyseal Fracture

Fractures of the radius and ulna are the most common long-bone fractures in childhood. Accurate reduction is important to minimise loss of pronation and supination. The remodelling potential depends on the age of the patient, the extent of the deformity and the distance of the fracture from the physis.

Malrotation of the fragment translates into a similar loss of range of rotation. Rotational deformities do not remodel, but angulation in the plane of movement will improve with time in the growing child.

The proximal and distal radioulnar joints should be visualised on radiographs and checked for any dislocation or subluxation.

Management

Greenstick fractures are managed non-operatively with manipulation and a long-arm plaster cast.

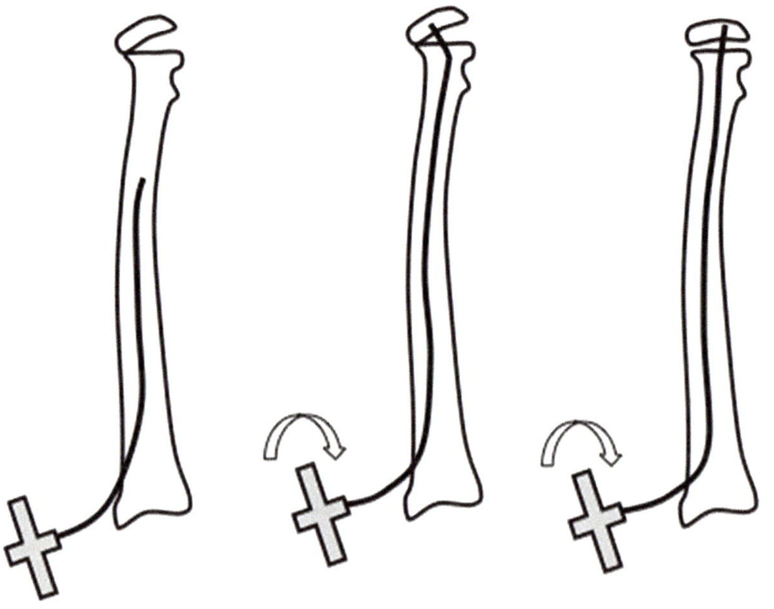

Fig. 1.99 Reduction of radial physis

Undisplaced fractures are also managed non-operatively. Acceptability criteria for pediatric forearm fractures are summarised in Table 1.29.

Displaced fractures of both the radius and ulna can be unstable and satisfactory reduction is important to restore function (Table 1.30).

Options for internal fixation are intramedullary titanium elastic nails or plate fixation.

Plate fixation provides anatomic rigid fixation with rotational control, but leaves longer scars. Plate fixation is preferred in adolescents nearing skeletal maturity.

Intramedullary nails can be inserted with minimal access and are effective in maintaining reduction but provide limited rotational control. Nails often require removal. These are currently the most preferred modality. If following fixation of single bone, the other one is well reduced then it is not necessary to fix the other one. External splintage with a cast is used in the early postoperative period.

Yong B, Yuan Z, Li J, Li Y, Southern EP, Canavese F, Xu H. Single Bone Fixation versus Both Bone Fixation for Pediatric Unstable Forearm Fractures: A Systematic Review and Metaanalysis. Indian J Orthop. 2018;52(5):529–535

Sinikumpu JJ, Serlo W. The shaft fractures of the radius and ulna in children: current concepts. J Pediatr Orthop B. 2015 May;24(3):200–206.

Table 1.29 Acceptability criteria for pediatric forearm fractures

Criteria	Age <8 years	Age >8 years
Angulation	10–15 degree	5–10 degree
Displacement	Up to 100% (bone diameter)	Up to 100% (bone diameter)
Rotation	Up to 45 degree	Up to 30 degree
Shortening	10 mm	10 mm

Table 1.30 Indications for surgery

Absolute	Relative
Open fractures	Oblique fracture of both bones
Segmental fractures	More than 10 mm displacement
Associated with dislocations	More than 45 degree angulation
Floating elbow	

Distal Radius Fractures

Fractures of the distal radial metaphysis not involving the growth plate are managed in a cast if minimally displaced. Fractures with an initial angulation of more than 30° and displacement of more than 50% are at high risk of malalignment. These fractures can be stabilised with one or two K-wires passed percutaneously to transfix the fracture.

Fractures of the distal radius at the level of the growth plate are very common. Most of these can be reduced by manipulation and maintained in a cast. There is some risk of growth arrest following these injuries. A single smooth pin inserted from the radial styloid crossing the physeal plate is used to stabilise unstable fractures.

Galeazzi fracture is a fracture of the distal third of the radius along with disruption of the distal radioulnar joint. It is managed with anatomic reduction and internal fixation of the radius. A Galeazzi equivalent is a distal radius fracture with separation of the distal ulnar physis.

Further Reading

Vallier HA, Wang X, Moore TA, Wilber JH, Como JJ. Timing of orthopaedic surgery in multiple trauma patients: development of a protocol for early appropriate care. J Orthop Trauma. 2013;27(10):543–51.

Gustilo RB, Anderson JT. Prevention of infection in the treatment of one thousand and twenty-five open fractures of the long bones: retrospective and prospective analyses. J Bone Joint Surg Am. 1976;58:453–8.

Gosselin RA, Roberts I, Gillespie WJ. Antibiotics for preventing infection in open limb fractures. Cochrane database Syst Rev. 2004;1:CD003764.

FLOW Investigators, Bhandari M, et al. A Trial of Wound Irrigation in the Initial Management of Open Fracture Wounds. N Engl J Med. 2015 Dec 31;373(27):2629–41.

Hassinger SM, Harding G, Wongworawat MD. High-pressure pulsatile lavage propagates bacteria into soft tissue. Clin Orthop Relat Res. 2005;439:27–31.

Ideberg R, Grevsten S, Larsson S. Epidemiology of scapular fractures. Incidence and classification of 338 fractures. Acta Orthop Scand. 1995;66(5):395–7.

Ogawa K, Yoshida A, Takahashi M, Ui M. Fractures of the coracoid process. J Bone Joint Surg Br. 1997;79(1):17–9.

Goss TP. Double disruptions of the superior shoulder suspensory complex. J Orthop Trauma. 1993;7(2):99–106.

Bartonicek J, Tucek M, Nanka O. Floating shoulder: myths and reality. J Bone Joint Surg Rev. 2018;6(10):e5.
Owens BD, Goss TP. The floating shoulder. J Bone Joint Surg Br. 2006;88(11):1419–24.
Nguyen V, Williams G, Rockwood C. Radiography of acromioclavicular dislocation and associated injuries. Crit Rev Diagn Imaging. 1991;32(3):191–228.
Phillips AM, Smart C, Groom AF. Acromioclavicular dislocation. Conservative or surgical therapy. Clin Orthop Relat Res. 1998;353:10–7.
Spencer EE Jr. Treatment of grade III acromioclavicular joint injuries. A systematic review. Clin Orthop Relat Res. 2007;455:38–44.
Weaver JK, Dunn HK. Management of acromioclavicular injuries, especially complete acromioclavicular separation. J Bone Joint Surg Am. 1972;54:1187–94.
Allman FL Jr. Fractures and ligamentous injuries of the clavicle and its articulation. J Bone Joint Surg Am. 1967;49(4):774–84.
Robinson CM, Court-Brown CM, McQueen MM, Wakefield AE. Estimating the risk of nonunion following nonoperative treatment of a clavicular fracture. J Bone Joint Surg Am. 2004;86:1359–65.
Canadian Orthopaedic Trauma Society. Nonoperative treatment compared with plate fixation of displaced midshaft clavicular fractures. J Bone Joint Surg Am. 2007;89:1–10.
Ahrens PM, Garlick NI, Barber J, Tims EM. Clavicle trial collaborative group. The clavicle trial: a multicentre, randomised controlled trial comparing operative with nonoperative treatment of displaced midshaft clavicle fractures. J Bone Joint Surg Am. 2017;99(16):1345–54.
Hill JM, McGuire MH, Crosby LA. Closed treatment of displaced middle-third fractures of the clavicle gives poor results. J Bone Joint Surg Br. 1997;79(4):537–8.
Neer CS 2nd. Fractures of the distal third of the clavicle. Clin Orthop. 1968;58:43–50.
Jackson WFM, Bayne G, Gregg-Smith SJ. Fractures of the lateral third of the clavicle: an Anatomic approach to treatment. J Trauma. 2006;61:222–5.
Morell DJ, Thyagarajan DS. Sternoclavicular joint dislocation and its management: a review of the literature. World J Orthop. 2016;7(4):244–50.
Rezende B da RM, de Almeida JI Sr, de Sousa UJ, Bomfim L de S, Ferreira MS Jr. Glenoumeral dislocation: a prospective randomized study comparing Spazo and Kocher maneuvers. Acta Ortop Bras. 2015;23(4):192-196.
Hovelius L, Augustini BG, Fredin H, Johansson O, Norlin R, Thorling J. Primary anterior dislocation of the shoulder in young patients. A ten year prospective study. J Bone Joint Surg Br. 1996;78(11):1677–84.
Itoi E, Hatakeyama Y, Kido T, et al. A new method of immobilization after traumatic anterior dislocation of the shoulder: a preliminary study. J Shoulder Elbow Surg. 2003;12:413–5.
Finestone A, Milgrom C, Radeva-Petrova DR, et al. Bracing in external rotation for traumatic anterior dislocation of the shoulder. J Bone Joint Surg Br. 2009;91:918–21.
te Slaa RL, Wijffels MP, Brand R, Marti RK. The prognosis following acute primary glenohumeral dislocation. J Bone Joint Surg Br. 2004;86(1):58–64.
Kavaja L, Lähdeoja T, Malmivaara A, Paavola M. Treatment after traumatic shoulder dislocation: a systematic review with a network meta-analysis. Br J Sports Med. 2018;52(23):1498–506.
Aydin N, Enes Kayaalp M, Asansu M, Karaismailoglu B. Treatment options for locked posterior shoulder dislocations and clinical outcomes. EFORT Open Rev. 2019 May 11;4(5):194–200.
Neer CS 2nd. Displaced proximal humeral fractures. Part I. Classification and evaluation. Clin Orthop. 1987;223:3–10.
Neer CS 2nd. Four segment classification of proximal humeral fractures: purpose and reliable use. J Shoulder Elbow Surg. 2002;11(4):389–400.
Rangan A, Handoll H, Brearley S. Surgical versus non surgical treatment of adults with displaced fractures of the proximal humerus. The PROFHER randomized clinical trial. JAMA. 2015;313:1037–47.
Südkamp N, Bayer J, Hepp P, et al. Open reduction and internal fixation of proximal humeral fractures with use of the locking proximal humerus plate. Results of a prospective, multicenter, observational study. J Bone Joint Surg Am. 2009;91:1320–8.
Stone MA, Namdari S. Surgical considerations in the treatment of osteoporotic proximal humerus fractures. Orthop Clin North Am. 2019 Apr;50(2):223–31.
Gallinet D, Ohl X, Decroocq L, Dib C, Valenti P. Boileau P; French Society for Orthopaedic Surgery (SOFCOT). Is reverse total shoulder arthroplasty more effective than hemiarthroplasty for treating displaced proximal humerus fractures in older adults? A systematic review and meta-analysis. Orthop Traumatol Surg Res. 2018;104(6):759–66.
Ekholm R, Adami J, Tidermark J, et al. Fractures of the shaft of humerus. An epidemiological study of 401 fractures. J Bone Joint Surg Br. 2006;88:1469–73.
Klenerman L. Fractures of the shaft of the humerus. J Bone Joint Surg Br. 1966;48:105–11.
Ekholm R, Ponzer S, Törnkvist H, et al. The Holstein–Lewis humeral shaft fracture: aspects of radial nerve injury, primary treatment, and outcome. J Orthop Trauma. 2008;22:693–7.
McCormack RG, Brien D, Buckley RE, et al. Fixation of fractures of the shaft of the humerus by dynamic compression plate or intramedullary nail. A prospective, randomised trial. J Bone Joint Surg Br. 2000;82:336–9.
Crates J, Whittle AP. Antegrade interlocking nailing of acute humeral shaft fractures. Clin Orthop Relat Res. 1998;350:40–50.
Riseborough EJ, Radin EL. Intercondylar T fractures of the humerus in the adult. A comparison of operative and nonoperative treatment in 29 cases. J Bone Joint Surg Am. 1969;51(1):130–41.

Doornberg J, Lindenhoivius A, Kloen P, van Dijk CN, Zurakowski D, Ring D. Two and three-dimensional computed tomography for the classification and management of distal humeral fractures. Evaluation of reliability and diagnostic accuracy. J Bone Joint Surg Am. 2006;88:1795–801.
O'Driscoll SW. The triceps-reflecting anconeus pedicle (TRAP) approach for distal humeral fractures and nonunions. Orthop Clin North Am. 2000;31(1):91–101.
Stoffel K, Cunneen S, Morgan R, Nicholls R, Stachowiak G. Comparative stability of perpendicular versus parallel double-locking plating systems in osteoporotic comminuted distal humerus fractures. J Orthop Res. 2008;26(6):778–84.
O'Driscoll SW. Optimizing stability in distal humeral fracture fixation. J Shoulder Elbow Surg. 2005;14(1 Suppl S):186S–94S.
Guitton TG, Juiter JB. 90-90 vs parallel plating of distal humeral fractures. Aofoundation.org. Expert zone. Chapter 28.
Doornberg JN, van Duijn PJ, Linzel D, et al. Surgical treatment of intra-articular fractures of the distal part of the humerus. Functional outcome after twelve to thirty years. J Bone Joint Surg Am. 2007;89(7):1524–32.
Barco R, Streubel PN, Morrey BF, Sanchez-Sotelo J. Total elbow arthroplasty for distal humeral fractures: a ten-year-minimum follow-up study. J Bone Joint Surg Am. 2017 Sep 20;99(18):1524–31.
McKee MD, Jupiter JB, Bamburger HB. Coronal shear fractures of the distal end of humerus. J Bone Joint Surg Am. 1996;78(1):49–54.
Ring D, Jupiter JB, Gulotta L. Articular fractures of the distal part of the humerus. J Bone Joint Surg Am. 2003;85(2):232–8.
Iordens GI, et al. FuncSiE trial investigators. Early mobilisation versus plaster immobilisation of simple elbow dislocations: results of the FuncSiE multicentre randomised clinical trial. Br J Sports Med. 2017 Mar;51(6):531–8.
Chen NC, Ring D. Terrible triad injuries of the elbow. J Hand Surg Am. 2015;40(11):2297–303.
Regan W, Morrey B. Fractures of the coronoid process of the ulna. J Bone Joint Surg Am. 1989;71(9):1348–54.
Mason ML. Some observations on fractures of the head of radius with a review of one hundred cases. Br J Surg. 1954;42(172):123–32.
Broberg MA, Morrey BF. Results of treatment of fracture dislocations of the elbow. Clin Orthop. 1987;216:109–19.
Swenson SJ, Tyagi V, Uquillas C, Shakked RJ, Yoon RS, Liporace FA. Maximizing outcomes in the treatment of radial head fractures. J Orthop Traumatol. 2019;20(1):15.
Ikeda M, Sugiyama K, Kang C, et al. Comminuted fractures of the radial head. Comparison of resection and internal fixation. J Bone Joint Surg Am. 2005;87:76–84.
Frank SG, Grewal R, Johnson J, et al. Determination of correct implant size in radial head arthroplasty to avoid overlengthening. J Bone Joint Surg Am. 2009;91:1738–46.
Burkhart KJ, Mattyasovszky SG, Runkel M, Schwarz C, Küchle R, Hessmann MH, et al. Mid- to long-term results after bipolar radial head arthroplasty. J Shoulder Elbow Surg. 2010;19:965–72.
Barton T, Chambers C, Bannister G. A comparison between subjective outcome score and moderate radial shortening following a fractured distal radius in patients of mean age 69 years. J Hand Surg Eur Vol. 2007;32:165–9.
Knirk JL, Jupiter JB. Intraarticular fractures of the distal end of radius in young adults. J Bone Joint Surg Am. 1986;68(5):647–59.
Costa ML, Achten J, Parsons NR, Rangan A, Griffin D, Tubeuf S, Lamb SE, DRAFFT Study Group. Percutaneous fixation with Kirschner wires versus volar locking plate fixation in adults with dorsally displaced fracture of distal radius: randomised controlled trial. BMJ. 2014 Aug 5;349:g4807.
Mcqueen MM, Hajducka C, Court-brown CM. Redisplaced unstable fractures of the distal radius. A prospective randomised comparison of four methods of treatment. J Bone Joint Surg Br. 1996;78(3):404–9.
Kapandji A. Intrafocal pinning of fractures of the distal end of radius; 10 years later. Ann Chir Main. 1987;6(1):57–63.
Hayes AJ, Duffy PJ, McQueen MM. Bridging and non-bridging external fixation in the treatment of unstable fractures of the distal radius. A retrospective study of 588 patients. Acta Orthop. 2008;79(4):540–7.
Odumala O, Ayekoloye C, Packer G. Prophylactic carpal tunnel decompression during buttress plating of the distal radius – is it justified? Injury. 2001;32:577–9.
Ng CY, McQueen MM. What are the radiological predictors of functional outcome following fractures of the distal radius? J Bone Joint Surg Br. 2011;93(2):145–50.
Grewal R, Perey B, Wilmink M, Stothers K. A randomized prospective study on the treatment of intra-articular distal radius fractures: open reduction and internal fixation with dorsal plating versus mini open reduction, percutaneous fixation, and external fixation. J Hand Surg Am. 2005;30:764–72.
Kim JK, Koh YD, Do NH. Should an ulnar styloid fracture be fixed following volar plate fixation of a distal radial fracture? J Bone Joint Surg Am. 2010;92:1–6.
Arora R, Lutz M, Zimmermann R, Krappinger D, Niederwanger C, Gabl M. Free vascularised iliac bone graft for recalcitrant avascular non-union of the scaphoid. J Bone Joint Surg Br. 2010;92(2):224–9.
Kellam P, Ostrum RF. Systematic review and meta-analysis of avascular necrosis and posttraumatic arthritis after traumatic hip dislocation. J Orthop Trauma. 2016;30(1):10–6.
Beebe MJ, Bauer JM, Mir HR. Treatment of hip dislocations and associated injuries: current state of care. Orthop Clin North Am. 2016;47(3):527–49.
Hakkarinen DK, Banh KV, Hendey GW. Magnetic resonance imaging identifies occult hip fractures missed

by 64-slice computed tomography. J Emerg Med. 2012;43(2):303–7.
Maruenda JI, Barrios C, Gomar-Sancho F. Intracapsular hip pressure after femoral neck fracture. Clin Orthop. 1997;340:172–80.
Sasabuchi Y, Matsui H, Lefor AK, Fushimi K, Yasunaga H. Timing of surgery for hip fractures in the elderly: A retrospective cohort study. Injury. 2018;49(10):1848–54.
Moran CG, Wenn RT, Sikand M, Taylor AM. Early mortality after hip fracture: is delay before surgery important? J Bone Joint Surg Am. 2005;87:483–9.
Papakostidis C, Panagiotopoulos A, Piccioli A, Giannoudis PV. Timing of internal fixation of femoral neck fractures. A systematic review and meta-analysis of the final outcome. Injury. 2015;46(3):459–66.
Oakey J, Stover M, Summers H, et al. Does screw configuration affect subtrochanteric fracture after femoral neck fixation? Clin Orthop Relat Res. 2006;443:302–6.
Parker MJ, Blundell C. Choice of implant for internal fixation of femoral neck fractures. Meta-analysis of 25 randomised trials including 4,925 patients. Acta Orthop Scand. 1998;69:138–43.
Asnis SE, Wanek-Sgaglione L. Intracapsular fractures of the femoral neck. Results of cannulated screw fixation. J Bone Joint Surg Am. 1994;76:1793–803.
Gursamy K, Parker MJ, Rowlands TK. The complications of displaced intracapsular fractures of the hip: the effect of screw positioning and angulation on fracture healing. J Bone Joint Surg Br. 2005;87(5):632–5.
Duckworth AD, Bennet SJ, Aderinto J, Keating JF. Fixation of intracapsular fractures of the femoral neck in young patients: risk factors for failure. J Bone Joint Surg Br. 2011;93(6):811–6.
Liporace F, Gaines R, Collinge C, Haidukewych GJ. Results of internal fixation of Pauwels type-3 vertical femoral neck fractures. J Bone Joint Surg Am. 2008;90(8):1654–9.
Deneka DA, Simonian PT, Stankewich CJ, Eckert D, Chapman JR, Tencer AF. Biomechanical comparison of internal fixation techniques for the treatment of unstable basicervical femoral neck fractures. J Orthop Trauma. 1997;11(5):337–43.
Hoskins W, Webb D, Bingham R, Pirpiris M, Griffin XL. Evidence based management of intracapsular neck of femur fractures. Hip Int. 2017;27(5):415–24.
Leonardsson O, Sernbo I, Carlsson A, et al. Long-term follow-up of replacement compared with internal fixation for displaced femoral neck fractures: results at ten years in a randomised study of 450 patients. J Bone Joint Surg Br. 2010;92:406–12.
Moerman S, Mathijssen NMC, Niesten DD, Riedijk R, Rijnberg WJ, Koëter S, Kremers van de Hei K, Tuinebreijer WE, Molenaar TL, RGHH N, AJH V. More complications in uncemented compared to cemented hemiarthroplasty for displaced femoral neck fractures: a randomized controlled trial of 201 patients, with one year follow-up. BMC Musculoskelet Disord. 2017 Apr 21;18(1):169.
Song JSA, Dillman D, Wilson D, Dunbar M, Richardson G. Higher periprosthetic fracture rate associated with use of modern uncemented stems compared to cemented stems in femoral neck fractures. Hip Int. 2019;29(2):177–83.
Timperley AJ, Whitehouse SL. Mitigating surgical risk in patients undergoing hip arthroplasty for fractures of the proximal femur. J Bone Joint Surg Br. 2009;91(7):851–4.
Inngul C, Hedbeck CJ, Blomfeldt R, Lapidus G, Ponzer S, Enocson A. Unipolar hemiarthroplasty versus bipolar hemiarthroplasty in patients with displaced femoral neck fractures: a four-year follow-up of a randomised controlled trial. Int Orthop. 2013;37(12):2457–64.
Figved W, Svenøy S, Röhrl SM, Dahl J, Nordsletten L, Frihagen F. Higher cartilage wear in unipolar than bipolar hemiarthroplasties of the hip at 2 years: A randomized controlled radiostereometric study in 19 fit elderly patients with femoral neck fractures. Acta Orthop. 2018;89(5):503–8.
Wang F, Zhang H, Zhang Z, Ma C, Feng X. Comparison of bipolar hemiarthroplasty and total hip arthroplasty for displaced femoral neck fractures in the healthy elderly: a meta-analysis. BMC Musculoskelet Disord. 2015;16:229.
Yassa R, Khalfaoui MY, Hujazi I, Sevenoaks H, Dunkow P. Management of anticoagulation in hip fractures: a pragmatic approach. EFORT Open Rev. 2017;2(9):394–402.
Swain DG, Nightingale PG, Patel JV. Blood transfusion requirements in femoral neck fracture. Injury. 2000;31(1):7–10.
Eiskjaer S. Risk factors influencing mortality after bipolar hemiarthroplasty in the treatment of fracture of the femoral neck. Clin Orthop. 1991;270:295–300.
Foster MR, Heppenstall RB, Friedenberg ZB, Hozack WJ. A prospective assessment of nutritional status and complications in patients with fractures of the hip. J Orthop Trauma. 1990;4:49–57.
Parker MJ. Sliding hip screw versus intramedullary nail for trochanteric hip fractures; a randomised trial of 1000 patients with presentation of results related to fracture stability. Injury. 2017;48(12):2762–7.
Baumgaertner MR, Curtin SL, Lindskog DM, Keggi JM. The value of tip apex distance in predicting failure of fixation of peritrochateric fractures of the hip. J Bone Joint Surg Am. 1995;77(7):1058–64.
Baumgaertner MR, Solberg BD. Awareness of tip apex distance reduces failure of fixation of trochanteric fractures of the hip. J Bone Joint Surg Am. 1997;79(6):969–71.
Jacobs RR, McClain O, Armstrong HJ. Internal fixation of intertrochanteric hip fractures: a clinical and biomechanical study. Clin Orthop Relat Res. 1980;146:62–70.
Kyle RF, Wright TM, Burstein AH. Biomechanical analysis of the sliding characteristics of compression hip screws. J Bone Joint Surg Am. 1980;62(8):1308–14.
Hsu C-E, Shih C-M, Wang C-C, Huang K-C. Lateral femoral wall thickness. A reliable predictor of postopera-

tive lateral wall fracture in intertrochanteric fractures. Bone and Joint Journal. 2013;95(8):1134–8.
Nie B, Wu D, Yang Z, Liu Q. Comparison of intramedullary fixation and arthroplasty for the treatment of intertrochanteric hip fractures in the elderly: a meta-analysis. Medicine (Baltimore). 2017;96(27):e7446.
Ottesen TD, McLynn RP, Galivanche AR, Bagi PS, Zogg CK, Rubin LE, Grauer JN. Increased complications in geriatric patients with a fracture of the hip whose postoperative weight-bearing is restricted: an analysis of 4918 patients. Bone Joint J. 2018;100-B(10):1377–84.
Schipper IB, Steyerberg EW, Castelein RM, et al. Treatment of unstable trochanteric fractures. Randomised comparison of the gamma nail and the proximal femoral nail. J Bone Joint Surg Br. 2004;86(1):86–94.
Sadowski C, Lübbeke A, Saudan M, Riand N, Stern R, Hoffmeyer P. Treatment of reverse oblique and transverse intertrochanteric fractures with use of an intramedullary nail or a 95 degree screw plate. A prospective randomised study. J Bone Joint Surg Am. 2002;84(3):372–81.
Barton TM, Gleeson R, Topliss C, et al. A comparison of the long gamma nail with the sliding hip screw for the treatment of AO/OTA 31-A2 fractures of the proximal part of the femur: a prospective randomized trial. J Bone Joint Surg Am. 2010;92(4):792–8.
Hoskins W, Bingham R, Joseph S, Liew D, Love D, Bucknill A, Oppy A, Griffin X. Subtrochanteric fracture: the effect of cerclage wire on fracture reduction and outcome. Injury. 2015;46(10):1992–5.
Bone LB, Johnson KD, Weigelt J, Scheinberg R. Early versus late stabilization of femoral fractures. A prospective randomised study. J Bone Joint Surg. 1989;71(3):336–40.
Winquist RA, Hansen ST Jr, Clawson DK. Closed intramedullary nailing of femoral fractures. A report of five hundred and twenty cases. J Bone Joint Surg Am. 1984;66(4):529–39.
Brumback RJ. Intramedullary nailing of femoral shaft fractures. Part I: decision making errors with interlocking fixation. J Bone Joint Surg Am. 1988;70(10):1441–52.
Pape HC, Regel G, Dwenger A, Krumm K, Schweitzer G, Krettek C, Sturm JA, Tscherne H. Influences of different methods of intramedullary femoral nailing on lung function in patients with multiple trauma. J Trauma. 1993;35(5):709–16.
Bosse MJ, MacKenzie EJ, Riemer BL, Brumback RJ, McCarthy ML, Burgess AR, Gens DR, Yasui Y. Adult respiratory distress syndrome, pneumonia, and mortality following thoracic injury and a femoral fracture treated with either an intramedullary nail with reaming or with a plate. J Bone Joint Surg Am. 1997;79(6):799–809.
Li AB, Zhang WJ, Guo WJ, Wang XH, Jin HM, Zhao YM. Reamed versus unreamed intramedullary nailing for the treatment of femoral fractures: a meta-analysis of prospective randomized controlled trials. Medicine (Baltimore). 2016 Jul;95(29):e4248.
Tsang ST, Mills LA, Baren J, Frantzias J, Keating JF, Simpson AH. Exchange nailing for femoral diaphyseal fracture non-unions: risk factors for failure. Injury. 2015;46(12):2404–9.
Brown KM. Effect of Cox-2 specific inhibition on fracture healing in the rat femur. J Bone Joint Surg Am. 2004;86(11):116–23.
Meluzio MC, Oliva MS, Minutillo F, Ziranu A, Saccomanno MF, Maccauro G. The use of knee mega-prosthesis for the management of distal femoral fractures: a systematic review. Injury. 2020;51(Suppl 3):S17–22.
Weber MJ, Janecki CJ, McLeod P, et al. Efficacy of various forms of fixation of transverse fractures of the patella. J Bone Joint Surg Am. 1980;62:215–20.
Meyers MH, McKeever FM. Fractures of the intercondylar eminence of the tibia. J Bone Joint Surg Am. 1970;52(8):1677–84.
Strauss EJ, Kaplan DJ, Weinberg ME, Egol J, Jazrawi LM. Arthroscopic management of tibial spine avulsion fractures: principles and techniques. J Am Acad Orthop Surg. 2018;26(10):360–7.
Luo CF, Sun H, Zhang B, Zeng BF. Three column fixation for complex tibial plateau fractures. J Orthop Trauma. 2010;24(11):683–92.
Elabjer E, Benčić I, Ćuti T, Cerovečki T, Ćurić S, Vidović D. Tibial plateau fracture management: arthroscopically-assisted versus ORIF procedure – clinical and radiological comparison. Injury. 2017;48(Suppl 5):S61–4.
Wasserstein D, Henry P, Paterson JM, Kreder HJ, Jenkinson RR. Risk of total knee arthroplasty after operatively treated tibial plateau fracture. J Bone Joint Surg Am. 2014;96(2):144–50.
Bone LB, Sucato D, Stegemann PM, Rohrbacher BJ. Displaced isolated fractures of the tibial shaft treated with either a cast or intramedullary nailing. An outcome analysis of matched pairs of patients. J Bone Joint Surg Am. 1997;79(9):1336–41.
Bhandari M, Zlowodzki M, Tornetta P 3rd, et al. Intramedullary nailing following external fixation in femoral and tibial fractures. J Orthop Trauma. 2005;19:140–4.
Blachut PA, O'Brien PJ, Meek RN, Broekhuyse HM. Interlocking intramedullary nailing with and without reaming for the treatment of closed fractures of the tibial shaft. A prospective, randomized study. J Bone Joint Surg Am. 1997;79:640–6.
Court-Brown CM, Will E, Christie J, McQueen MM. Reamed or unreamed nailing for closed tibial shaft fractures. A prospective study in Tscherne C1 fractures. J Bone Joint Surg Br. 1996;78:580–3.
MacDonald DRW, Caba-Doussoux P, Carnegie CA, Escriba I, Forward DP, Graf M, Johnstone AJ. Tibial nailing using a suprapatellar rather than an infrapatellar approach significantly reduces anterior knee pain postoperatively: a multicentre clinical trial. Bone Joint J. 2019;101(9):1138–43.
Xu H, Gu F, Xin J, Tian C, Chen F. A meta-analysis of suprapatellar versus infrapatellar intramedullary nail-

ing for the treatment of tibial shaft fractures. Heliyon. 2019 Sep 6;5(9):e02199.

Henley MB, Chapman JR, Agel J, et al. Treatment of type II, IIIA, and IIIB open fractures of the tibial shaft: a prospective comparison of unreamed interlocking intramedullary nails and half-pin external fixators. J Orthop Trauma. 1998;12:1–7.

Keating JF, O'Brien PI, Blachut PA, Meek RN, Broekhuyse HM. Reamed interlocking intramedullary nailing of open fractures of the tibia. Clin Orthop. 1997a;338:182–91.

Court-Brown CM, Keating JF, McQueen MM. Infection after intramedullary nailing of the tibia. Incidence and protocol for management. J Bone Joint Surg Br. 1992;74(5):770–4.

Keating JF, Orfaly R, O'Brien PJ. Knee pain after tibial nailing. J Orthop Trauma. 1997b;11(1):10–3.

Tornetta P 3rd, Gorup J. Axial computed tomography of pilon fractures. Clin Orthop Relat Res. 1996;323:273–6.

Patterson MJ, Cole JD. Two stage delayed open reduction and internal fixation of severe pilon fractures. J Orthop Trauma. 1999;13(2):85–91.

White TO, Guy P, Cooke CJ, Kennedy SA, Droll KP, Blachut PA, O'Brien PJ. The results of early primary open reduction and internal fixation for treatment of OTA 43.C type tibial pilon fractures: a cohort study. J Orthop Trauma. 2010;24(12):757–63.

Zelle BA, Dang KH, Ornell SS. High-energy tibial pilon fractures: an instructional review. International Orthopaedics. 2019;43(8):1939–50.

Stannard JP, Volgas DA, McGwin G 3rd, Stewart RL, Obremskey W, Moore T, Anglen JO. Incisional negative pressure wound therapy after high-risk lower extremity fractures. J Orthop Trauma. 2012;26(1):37–42.

Dawe EJ, Shafafy R, Quayle J, et al. The effect of different methods of stability assessment on fixation rate and complications in supination external rotation (SER) 2/4 ankle fractures. Foot Ankle Surg. 2015;21:86–90.

Gougoulias N, Sakellariou A. When is a simple fracture of the lateral malleolus not so simple? How to assess stability, which ones to fix and the role of the deltoid ligament. Bone Joint J. 2017;99(7):851–5.

Aiyer A, Zachwieja EC, Lawrie CM, Kaplan JRM. Management of isolated lateral malleolus fracture. J Am Acad Orthop Surg. 2019;27(2):50–9.

Keene DJ, Mistry D, Nam J, Tutton E, Handley R, Morgan L, Roberts E, Gray B, Briggs A, Lall R, Chesser TJ, Pallister I, Lamb SE, Willett K. The Ankle Injury Management (AIM) trial: a pragmatic, multicentre, equivalence randomised controlled trial and economic evaluation comparing close contact casting with open surgical reduction and internal fixation in the treatment of unstable ankle fractures in patients aged over 60 years. Health Technol Assess. 2016;20(75):1–158.

Mittal R, Harris IA, Adie S, Naylor JM. CROSSBAT study group: surgery for type B ankle fracture treatment. A combined randomized and observational study. BMJ Open. 2017;7:013298.

Tas DB, Smeeing DPJ, Emmink BL, Govaert GAM, Hietbrink F, Leenen LPH, Houwert RM. Intramedullary fixation versus plate fixation of distal fibular fractures: a systematic review and meta-analysis of randomized controlled trials and observational studies. J Foot Ankle Surg. 2019;58(1):119–26.

McKenzie AC, Hesselholt KE, Larsen MS, Schmal H. A systematic review and meta-analysis on treatment of ankle fractures with syndesmotic rupture: suture-button fixation versus cortical screw fixation. J Foot Ankle Surg. 2019;58(5):946–53.

Dingemans SA, Rammelt S, White TO, Goslings JC, Schepers A. Should syndesmotic screws be removed after surgical fixation of unstable ankle fractures. Bone Joint J. 2016;98:1497–504.

Van der Eng DM, Schep NW, Schepers T. Bioabsorbable versus metallic screw fixation for tibiofibular syndesmotic ruptures: a meta-analysis. J Foot Ankle Surg. 2015;54(4):657–62.

Haraguchi N, Haruyama H, Toga H, Kato F. Pathoanatomy of posterior malleolar fractures of the ankle. J Bone Joint Surg. 2006;88(5):1085–92.

Mason LW, Marlow WJ, Widnall J, Molloy AP. Pathoanatomy and associated injuries of posterior malleolus fracture of the ankle. Foot Ankle Int. 2017;38(11):1229–35.

Mason LW, Kaye A, Widnall J, Redfern J, Molloy A. Posterior malleolar ankle fractures: an effort at improving outcomes. JBJS Open Access. 2019 Jun 7;4(2):e0058.

Kaikkonen A, Kannus P, Järvinen M. Surgery versus functional treatment in ankle ligament tears. A prospective study. Clin Orthop Relat Res. 1996;326:194–202.

Ochen Y, Beks RB, van Heijl M, Hietbrink F, Leenen LPH, van der Velde D, Heng M, van der Meijden O, Groenwold RHH, Houwert RM. Operative treatment versus nonoperative treatment of Achilles tendon ruptures: systematic review and meta-analysis. BMJ. 2019 Jan 7;364:k5120.

Keene DJ, Alsousou J, Harrison P, Hulley P, Wagland S, Parsons SR, Thompson JY, O'Connor HM, Schlüssel MM, Dutton SJ, Lamb SE, Willett K. PATH-2 trial group. Platelet rich plasma injection for acute Achilles tendon rupture: PATH-2 randomised, placebo controlled, superiority trial. BMJ. 2019 Nov 20;367:16132.

Suchak AA, Bostick GP, Beaupré LA, Durand DC, Jomha NM. The influence of early weight-bearing compared with non-weight-bearing after surgical repair of the Achilles tendon. J Bone Joint Surg Am. 2008;90:1876–83.

Fortis AP, Dimas A, Lamprakis AA. Repair of Achilles tendon rupture under endoscopic control. Arthroscopy. 2008;24:683–8.

Hawkins LG. Fractures of the neck of the talus. J Bone Joint Surg Am. 1970;52(5):991–1002.

Canale ST, Kelly FB Jr. Fractures of the neck of the talus. Long term evaluation of seventy one cases. J Bone Joint Surg am. 1978;60(2):143–56.

Buckley R, Tough S, McCormack R, et al. Operative compared with nonoperative treatment of displaced intra-articular calcaneal fractures: a prospective, randomized, controlled multicenter trial. J bone Joint Surg Am. 2002;84(10):1733–44.

Gotha HE, Zide JR. Current controversies in management of calcaneus fractures. Orthop Clin North Am. 2017;48(1):91–103.

Xia S, Lu Y, Wang H, et al. Open reduction and internal fixation with conventional plate via L-shaped lateral approach versus internal fixation with percutaneous plate via a sinus tarsi approach for calcaneal fractures – a randomized controlled trial. Int J Surg. 2014;12(5):475–80.

Buckley R, Leighton R, Sanders D, et al. Open reduction and internal fixation compared with ORIF and primary subtalar arthrodesis for the treatment of Sanders-Type IV calcaneal fractures: a randomized, multicenter trial. J Orthop Trauma. 2014;28(10):577–83.

Nunley JA, Vertullo CJ. Claissfication, investigation and management of midfoot sprains; Lisfranc injuries in the athlete. Am J Sports Med. 2002;30:871–8.

Moracia-Ochagavía I, Rodríguez-Merchán EC. Lisfranc fracture-dislocations: current management. EFORT Open Rev. 2019;4(7):430–44.

Smith N, Stone C, Furey A. Does open reduction and internal fixation versus primary arthrodesis improve patient outcomes for Lisfranc trauma? A systematic review. Clin Orthop Relat Res. 2016;474(6):1445–52.

Coetzee JC, Ly TV. Treatment of primarily ligamentous Lisfranc joint injuries: primary arthrodesis compared with open reduction and internal fixation. Surgical technique. J Bone Joint Surg Am. 2007;89(Suppl 2 Pt1):122–7.

Bowes J, Buckley R. Fifth metatarsal fractures and current treatment. World J Orthop. 2016;7(12):793–800.

Roche AJ, Calder JD. Treatment and return to sport following a Jones fracture of the fifth metatarsal: a systematic review. Knee Surg Sports Traumatol Arthrosc. 2013;21:1307–15.

Akimau PI, Cawthron KL, Dakin WM, Chadwick C, Blundell CM, Davies MB. Symptomatic treatment or cast immobilisation for avulsion fractures of the base of the fifth metatarsal: a prospective, randomised, single-blinded non-inferiority controlled trial. Bone Joint J. 2016;98(6):806–11.

Day AC, Kinmont C, Bircher MD, Kumar S. Crescent fracture-dislocation of the sacroiliac joint: a functional classification. J Bone Joint Surg Br. 2007;89:651–8.

Burgess AR, et al. Pelvic ring disruptions: effective classification system and treatment protocols. J Trauma. 1990;30(7):848–56.

Bonner TJ, Eardley WGP, Newell N, Masouros S, Matthews JJ, Gibb I, Clasper JC. Accurate placement of a pelvic binder improves reduction of unstable fractures of the pelvic ring. J Bone Joint Surg Br. 2011;93(11):1524–8.

Riemer BL, Butterfield SL, Diamond DL, et al. Acute mortality associated with injuries to the pelvic ring: the role of early patient mobilization and external fixation. J Trauma. 1993;35:671–7.

Tannast M, Krüger A, Mack PW, Powell JN, Hosalkar HS, Siebenrock KA. Surgical dislocation of the hip for the fixation of acetabular fractures. J Bone Joint Surg Br. 2010;92(6):842–52.

Berry DJ, Halasy M. Uncemented acetabular components for arthritis after acetabular fracture. Clin Orthop Relat Res. 2002;405:164–7.

Borg T, Hernefalk B, Hailer NP. Acute total hip arthroplasty combined with internal fixation for displaced acetabular fractures in the elderly: a short-term comparison with internal fixation alone after a minimum of two years. Bone Joint J. 2019;101(4):478–83.

Hamlin K, Lazaraviciute G, Koullouros M, Chouari T, Stevenson IM, Hamilton S. Should total hip arthroplasty be performed acutely in the treatment of acetabular fractures in elderly or used as a salvage procedure only? Ind J Ortho. 2017;51(4):421–33.

Vaccaro AR, Lehman RA Jr, Hurlbert RJ, Anderson PA, et al. A new classification of thoracolumbar injuries: the importance of injury morphology, the integrity of the posterior ligamentous complex, and neurologic status. Spine (Phila Pa 1976). 2005;30(20):2325–33.

Bracken MB, Shepard MJ, Collins WF, et al. A randomized, controlled trial of methylprednisolone or naloxone in the treatment of acute spinal-cord injury. Results of the second national acute spinal cord injury study. N Engl J Med. 1990;322:1405–11.

Hugenholtz H, Cass DE, Dvorak MF, et al. High-dose methylprednisolone for acute closed spinal cord injury – only a treatment option. Can J Neurol Sci. 2002;29:227–35.

Evaniew N, Noonan VK, Fallah N, et al. Methylprednisolone for the treatment of patients with acute spinal cord injuries: a propensity score-matched cohort study from a Canadian multi-center spinal cord injury registry. J Neurotrauma. 2015;32:1674–83.

Sutphen SA, Mendoza JD, Mundy AC, Yang JG, Beebe AC, Samora WP 3rd, Klingele KE. Pediatric diaphyseal femur fractures: submuscular plating compared with intramedullary nailing. Orthopedics. 2016;39(6):353–8.

Mashru RP, Herman MJ, Pizzutillo PD. Tibial shaft fractures in children and adolescents. J Am Acad Orthop Surg. 2005;13(5):345–52.

Moraleda L, Valencia M, Barco R, et al. Natural history of unreduced Gartland type-II supracondylar fractures of the humerus in children: a two to thirteen-year follow-up study. J Bone Joint Surg Am. 2013;95(1):28–34.

Larson L, Firoozbakhsh K, Passarelli R, et al. Biomechanical analysis of pinning techniques for pediatric supracondylar humerus fractures. J Pediatr Orthop. 2006;26(5):573–8.

Sibinski M, Sharma H, Bennet GC. Early versus delayed treatment of extension type-3 supracondylar fractures of the humerus in children. J Bone Joint Surg Br. 2006;88:380–1.

Walmsley PJ, Kelly MB, Robb JE, et al. Delay increases the need for open reduction of type-III supracondylar fractures of the humerus. J Bone Joint Surg Br. 2006;88:528–30.

Leet AI, Frisancho J, Ebramzadeh E. Delayed treatment of type 3 supracondylar humerus fractures in children. J Pediatr Orthop. 2002;22:203–7.

Matsuzaki K, Nakatani N, Harada M, Tamaki T. Treatment of supracondylar fracture of the humerus in children by skeletal traction in a brace. J Bone Joint Surg Br. 2004;86:232–8.

Scannell BP, Jackson JB 3rd, Bray C, et al. The perfused, pulseless supracondylar humeral fracture: intermediate-term follow-up of vascular status and function. J Bone Joint Surg Am. 2013;95(21):1913–9.

Barrett KK, Skaggs DL, Sawyer JR, et al. Supracondylar humeral fractures with isolated anterior interosseous nerve injuries: is urgent treatment necessary? J Bone Joint Surg Am. 2014;96(21):1793–7.

Lloyd-Roberts GC, Bucknill TM. Anterior dislocation of the radial head in children: aetiology, natural history and management. J Bone Joint Surg Br. 1977;59-B:402–7.

Bell Tawse AJ. The treatment of malunited anterior Monteggia fractures in children. J Bone Joint Surg Br. 1965;47:718–23.

Yong B, Yuan Z, Li J, Li Y, Southern EP, Canavese F, Xu H. Single bone fixation versus both bone fixation for pediatric unstable forearm fractures: a systematic review and metaanalysis. Indian J Orthop. 2018;52(5):529–35.

Sinikumpu JJ, Serlo W. The shaft fractures of the radius and ulna in children: current concepts. J Pediatr Orthop B. 2015 May;24(3):200–6.

Shoulder Disorders

2

Oliver Donaldson and Alastair Jones

Osseous Anatomy

The glenohumeral joint is often referred to as the shoulder joint, but functional shoulder movement takes place through four separate articulations as shown in Fig. 2.1.

The glenohumeral joint is the most mobile joint in the body. To allow this, the glenoid is shallow and therefore does not offer stability. The glenoid is 1–9 degrees retroverted when compared to the scapula plane, but the scapula is 30 degrees anteverted as it lies on the posterior thorax, meaning that the glenoid is 21–29 degrees anteverted when viewed in the coronal plane. The humeral head, on average, is retroverted 26 degrees when compared to the transepicondylar axis (Fig. 2.2).

Matsumura N, Ogawa K, Kobayashi S, Oki S, Watanabe A, Ikegami H, Toyama Y. Morphologic features of humeral head and glenoid version in the normal glenohumeral joint. J Shoulder Elbow Surg 2014; 23(11): 1724–30

Welsch G, Mamisch TC, Kikinis R, Schmidt R, Lang P, Forst R, Fitz W. CT-Based Preoperative Analysis of Scapula Morphology and Glenohumeral Joint Geometry. Journal of computer aided surgery 2003;8:264–8.

The morphology of the acromion is variable, and this can be clinically relevant in impingement or os acromiale. The acromion develops from three secondary ossification centres, which normally fuse before the age of 25. The meta-acromion, meso-acromion and the pre-acromion (Fig. 2.3) are the origin sites for posterior, middle and anterior fibres of the deltoid respectively. Failure of fusion of one of the ossification centres is called an os acromiale. The commonest site for this to occur is between the meta-acromion and meso-acromion.

The acromion also has variations in its morphology in the sagittal plane as described by Bigliani. This can be clinically important in symptoms of impingement. Most individuals have a type B acromion. There is an increased incidence of impingement amongst individuals with a type C acromion (Fig. 2.4).

The acromioclavicular joint (ACJ) is ellipsoid and has a small surface area of contact. The orientation can be vertical, oblique or curved, and should be noted preoperatively when planning surgery in this area. The joint rotates during abduction and flexion. There is a small meniscus of cartilage in the joint, which can become degenerate.

The glenohumeral joint relies on soft tissue stabilisers to maintain congruity. These are static or dynamic.

O. Donaldson (✉)
Consultant Orthopaedic Surgeon, Yeovil District Hospital, Yeovil, UK
e-mail: oliver.donaldson@ydh.nhs.uk

A. Jones
Consultant Orthopaedic Surgeon, Taunton, UK
e-mail: alijones@doctors.net.uk

S. Agarwal (ed.), *Current Orthopaedic Practice*, https://doi.org/10.1007/978-3-030-78529-1_2

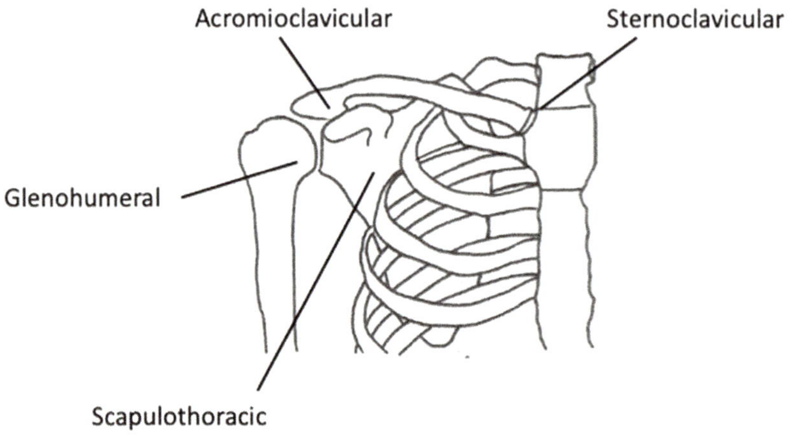

Fig. 2.1 The four articulations of the shoulder girdle

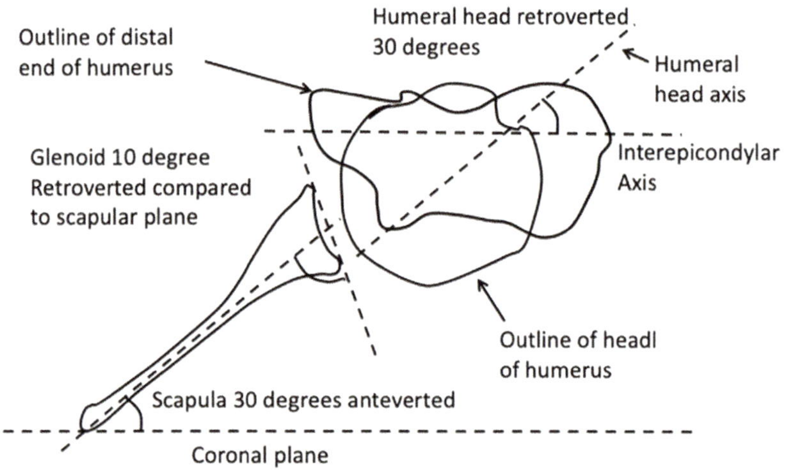

Fig. 2.2 Relative version of glenoid and humeral head. Approximate version drawn to indicate relative positioning

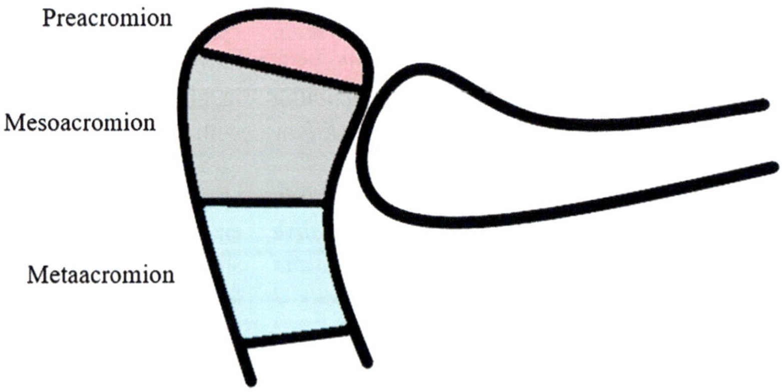

Fig. 2.3 The ossification centres of the acromion

Static Stabilisers

The static stabilisers are the glenoid labrum, osseous anatomy, capsuloligamentous complex and vacuum effect.

The labrum is cartilaginous and conforms to the shape of the humeral head. It deepens the glenoid by 50%. The strongest areas are posterosuperior and anteroinferior, which are the areas detached in SLAP tears (Superior Labrum Anterior and Posterior) and Bankart lesions respectively.

The capsule has condensations or glenohumeral ligaments in three distinct areas (Fig. 2.5).

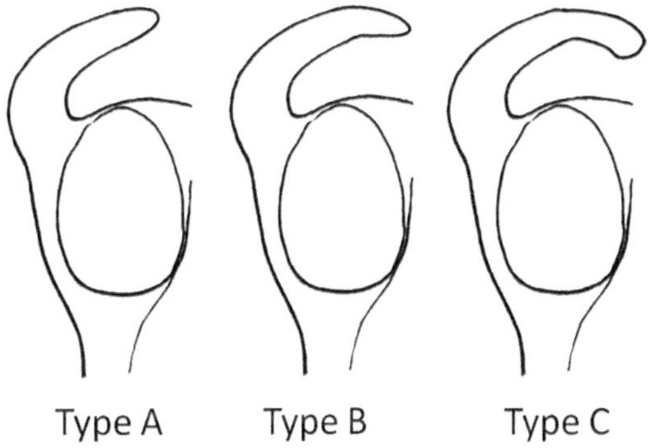

Fig. 2.4 Acromial morphology as described by Bigliani

These contain elastin and collagen and are biochemically distinct from other areas of capsule. The ligaments are under tension in differing positions of the glenohumeral joint and together resist translation of the humeral head throughout the arc of abduction (Table 2.1).

There is a negative pressure within the glenohumeral joint which resists translation of the humeral head and distraction forces. The force required to distract the glenohumeral joint surfaces is significantly reduced once an arthrotomy has been made.

Dynamic Stabilisers

Dynamic stabilisers include the 4 rotator cuff muscles, the long head of biceps and the scapular stabilisers.

The rotator cuff muscles create a net force that pulls in a medial direction, essentially hugging the head of the humerus into the glenoid, causing concavity compression. This allows the shoulder girdle muscles such as deltoid to act without causing glenohumeral translation. This action takes place throughout the range of movement of the glenohumeral joint.

Fig. 2.5 Glenohumeral ligaments

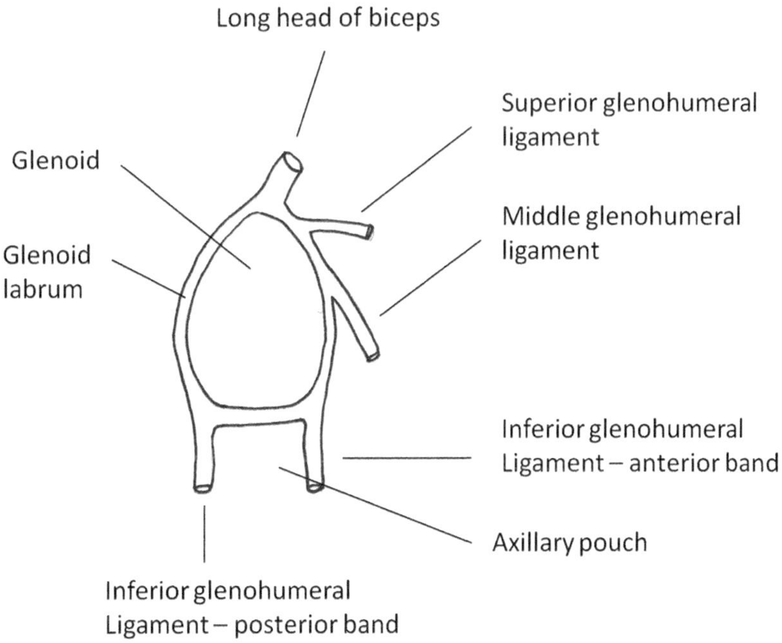

Table 2.1 Glenohumeral ligaments

Ligament	Function
Inferior Glenohumeral Ligament (IGHL)	Anterior band is primary restraint to anterior/inferior translation in 90 degrees abduction/external rotation Posterior band is primary restraint to posterior translation in 90 degrees flexion/adduction
Middle Glenohumeral Ligament (MGHL)	Resists anterior and posterior translation in mid-abduction
Superior Glenohumeral Ligament (SGHL)	Resists inferior translation with arm adducted to 0 degrees

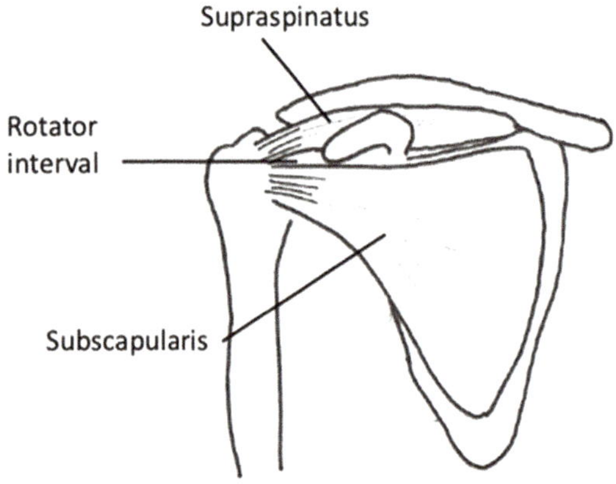

Fig. 2.6 The rotator interval

Each rotator cuff muscle contributes to planar shoulder movements. Supraspinatus initiates abduction, infraspinatus and teres minor externally rotate the arm and subscapularis internally rotates the arm. The key role they play together is to ensure the humeral head remains centred on the glenoid during shoulder movement. Consequently, in rotator cuff deficient shoulders the humeral head is seen to migrate proximally due to unrestrained superior pull of the deltoid.

The long head of biceps tendon arises from the superior glenoid fossa and crosses the superior humeral head acting as a restraint to superior migration. This is itself stabilised by the subscapularis tendon and superior glenohumeral ligament.

The rotator interval (Fig. 2.6) is a triangular space formed by the interposition of the coracoid between the inferior border of supraspinatus and the superior border of subscapularis. The interval contains the superior glenohumeral ligament, the coracohumeral ligament, long head of biceps and the rotator interval capsule. The rotator interval capsule is the anterosuperior part of the glenohumeral joint capsule which merges with the coracohumeral and SGHL.

Scapula

The scapula is a flat, triangular shaped bone that articulates with the posterior border of the rib cage. The only synovial joints involving the scapula are the acromioclavicular and glenohumeral joints. Thus the scapula is connected to the body via the acromioclavicular and sternoclavicular joints (SCJ). The scapulothoracic articulation though moves in multiple planes—rotation in the coronal plane, protraction/retraction (rotation in the axial plane) and superiorly and inferiorly (translation in the coronal plane). All movements cause a consequent movement of the AC or SC joint, explaining the increased incidence of ACJ arthritis with age.

The scapula has 16 muscles that either originate or attach to it. A further 2 muscles, pectoralis major and latissimus dorsi, act across the scapula. The latissimus dorsi has an attachment at the inferior angle of scapula. Table 2.2 gives a summary of the muscles around the scapula, excluding omohyoid as this is not relevant to shoulder movement.

The Axillary Spaces

There are 3 anatomical spaces in the axilla of the shoulder formed by bony and muscular boundaries (Fig. 2.7). These are relevant as neurovascular structures pass through them in order to pass from the anterior aspect of the shoulder to the posterior aspect, or vice versa.

Quadrangular Space

The quadrangular space, as its names suggests, has four borders and conveys 3 structures; the axillary nerve, posterior circumflex artery and posterior cir-

Table 2.2 The muscles around the shoulder

Muscle	Origin	Insertion	Innervation	Action
Subscapularis	Medial 2/3 of subscapular fossa	Lesser tuberosity	Upper subscapular, lower subscapular	Shoulder internal rotation
Supraspinatus	Medial 2/3 supraspinous fossa	Greater tuberosity	Suprascapular	Shoulder initiation of abduction
Infraspinatus	Medial 2/3 of infraspinous fossa	Greater tuberosity	Suprascapular	Shoulder external rotation
Teres Minor	Lateral border of scapula	Greater tuberosity	Axillary	Shoulder external rotation with arm in abduction
Deltoid	Acromion and scapula spine	Deltoid tuberosity of humerus	Axillary	Shoulder flexion, abduction
Coracobrachialis	Coracoid process	Anteromedial surface of humerus	Musculocutaneous	Shoulder flexion, adduction
Biceps	Supraglenoid tubercle (Long head) Coracoid process (short head)	Radial tuberosity	Musculocutaneous	Elbow flexion and supination Shoulder flexion (weak)
Triceps	Infraglenoid tubercle (Long head)	Olecranon process	Radial	Elbow extension
Levator Scapulae	C1-C4	Medial border of scapula	Dorsal scapular, C4/5	Scapula elevation, rotation
Rhomboid Major	T2-T5	Medial border of scapula	Dorsal scapular	Scapula retraction, rotation
Rhomboid Minor	C7-T1	Medial border of scapula	Dorsal scapular	Scapula retraction, rotation
Trapezius	Occiput, C1-T12	Scapula spine	Spinal accessory	Scapula elevation
Serratus Anterior	Ribs 1–9	Ventral border of scapula	Long thoracic	Scapula protraction
Teres Major	Lower border of scapula (dorsal)	Intertubercular groove of humerus	Thoracodorsal, lower subscapular	Shoulder adduction, internal rotation
Pectoralis Minor	2nd–4th Ribs	Medial border of coracoid	Medial pectoral	Scapula protraction
Latissimus Dorsi	Inferior angle of scapula, T7-L5	Intertubercular groove of humerus	Thoracodorsal	Shoulder extension, adduction
Pectoralis Major	Sternum and clavicle	Lateral aspect of bicipital groove	Lateral and medial pectoral	Shoulder flexion, adduction, internal rotation

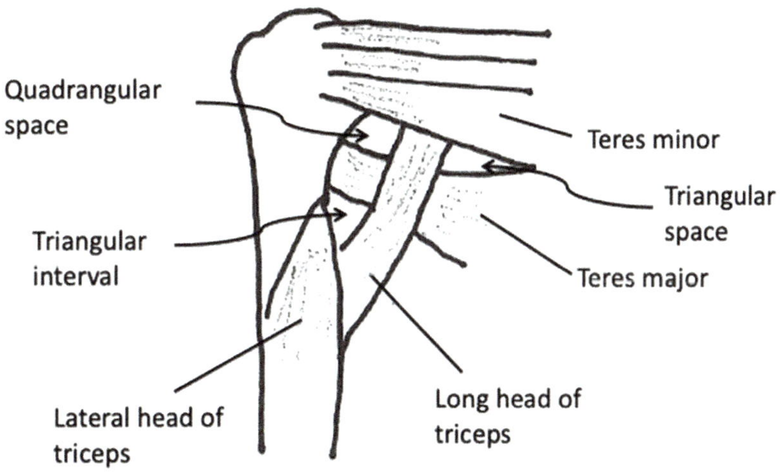

Fig. 2.7 The axillary spaces

cumflex vein. The boundaries are—teres minor—superiorly; teres major—inferiorly; long head of triceps—medially; and humerus—laterally.

Triangular Space

The triangular space sits inferomedial to the quadrangular space, separated by the long head of triceps. It has 3 borders and transmits the scapular circumflex vessels. The boundaries are—teres minor/subscapularis—superiorly; teres major—inferiorly; and long head of triceps—laterally.

Triangular Interval

The triangular interval sits inferolateral to the quadrangular space, separated by teres major. It conveys the radial nerve and profunda brachii artery. The boundaries are—teres major—superiorly; long head of triceps—medially; and lateral head of triceps/humerus—laterally.

Shoulder Pathology

Instability and pain are two commonest presenting complaints with regards to the shoulder. These are considered in the next two sections.

The Unstable Shoulder

The shoulder joint is the most unstable joint in the body due to the large humeral head and comparatively shallow glenoid. Over 90% of shoulder dislocations are attributed to trauma with the remainder, secondary to muscle patterning issues. Matsen proposed a widely used classification for instability, which is a useful reminder as to the pathogenesis and management of shoulder instability. It describes two types of shoulder instability. TUBS is **T**raumatic, **U**nidirectional, has a **B**ankart lesion, and responds to **S**urgery. AMBRI is **A**traumatic, **M**ultidirectional, **B**ilateral, **R**ehabilitation is the mainstay of treatment, and **I**nferior capsular shift may be rarely required.

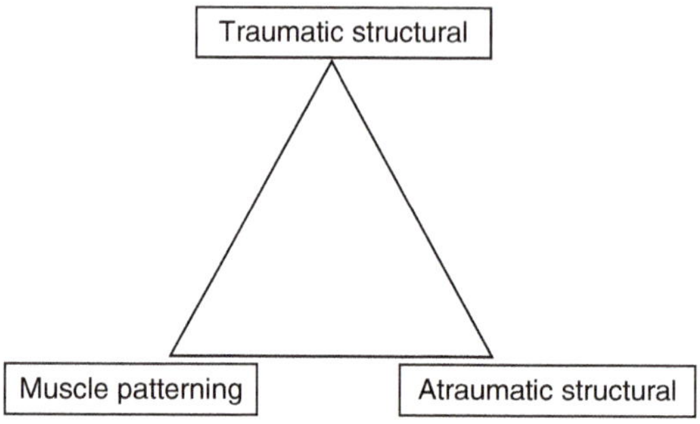

Fig. 2.8 Stanmore triangle for shoulder instability

This classification has now been superseded by the Stanmore triangle (Fig. 2.8). This recognises the group of patients that fall between the *polar type 1* traumatic instabilities with structural lesions and the *polar type 3* atraumatic instabilities with functional issues. This third group of patients are considered to have muscle patterning related shoulder instability. Muscles, apart from the rotator cuff, can help to stabilise the shoulder, as well as cause instability by abnormal activation. Further, patients can lie along the spectrum of these three patterns without conforming to one specific type.

Jaggi A, Lambert S. Rehabilitation for shoulder instability. Br J Sports Med 2010;44:333–40.

Anterior Traumatic Instability

The direction of dislocation is determined by the position of the arm when force is applied to it. 95% of traumatic instability is anterior with the remaining being either posterior or inferior (luxatio erecta).

Anterior traumatic shoulder dislocation is the most common presentation of shoulder instability. It is over twice as common in males compared to females. There is a bimodal distribution with 50% of dislocations occurring in patients between the ages of 15 and 29 and a second peak in elderly females.

Zacchilli MA, Owens BD. Epidemiology of shoulder dislocations presenting to the emergency departments in the United States. J Bone Joint Surg Am 2010;92:542–9. Incidence of shoulder dislocation is 23.9 per 100,000 person-years. Young men are more likely to sustain a shoulder dislocation.

The most common mode of injury is a fall onto an outstretched hand. This causes the shoulder to externally rotate in an abducted position forcing the humeral head anteriorly and inferiorly. The pathological lesions caused by the dislocation can be varied and are illustrated in Table 2.3.

Table 2.3 Lesions in anterior shoulder instability

Bankart lesion—avulsion of anterior labrum from 3'o clock to 6'o clock position	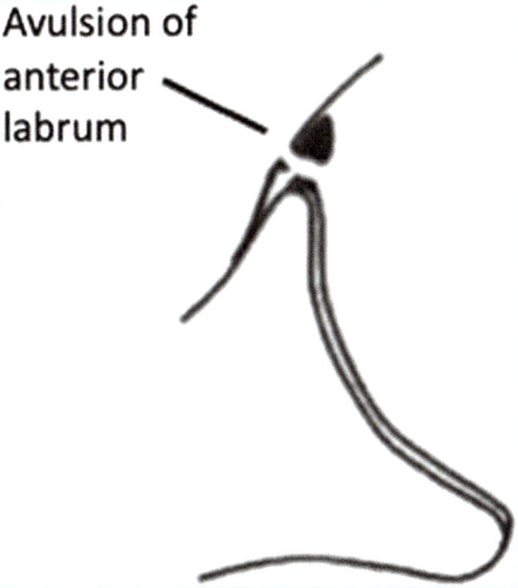
Bony Bankart lesion	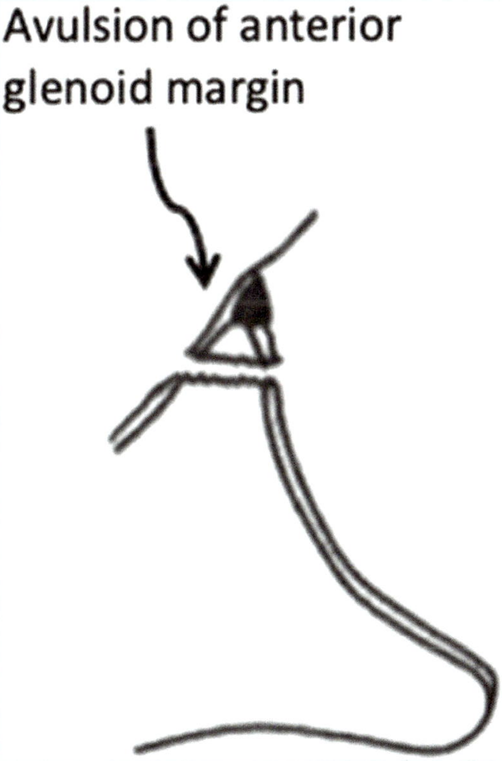

(continued)

Table 2.3 (continued)

Perthes lesion—Detachment of anteroinferior labrum (3–6'o clock) but intact periosteum	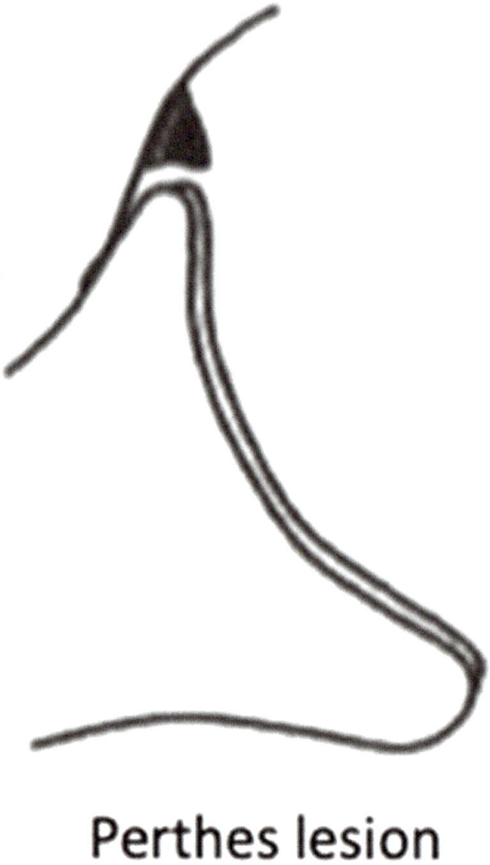
ALPSA (Anterior labral periosteal sleeve avulsion)—medial displacement of labrum—ligamentous complex	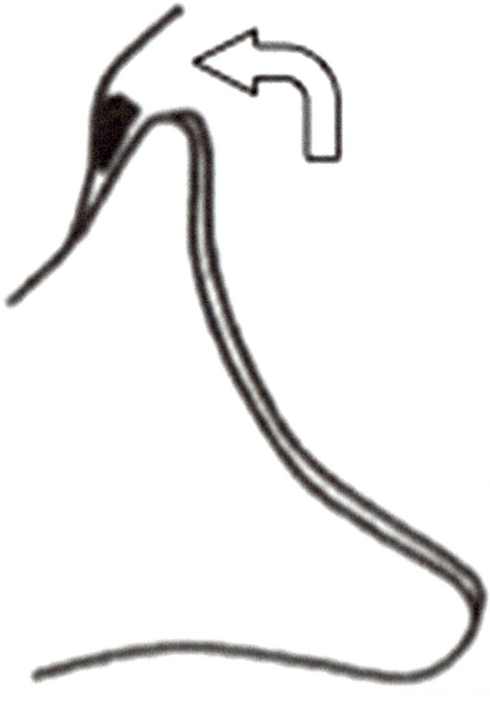

Table 2.3 (continued)

GLAD (Glenolabral articular disruption). Partial tear of labrum with adjacent cartilage damage.	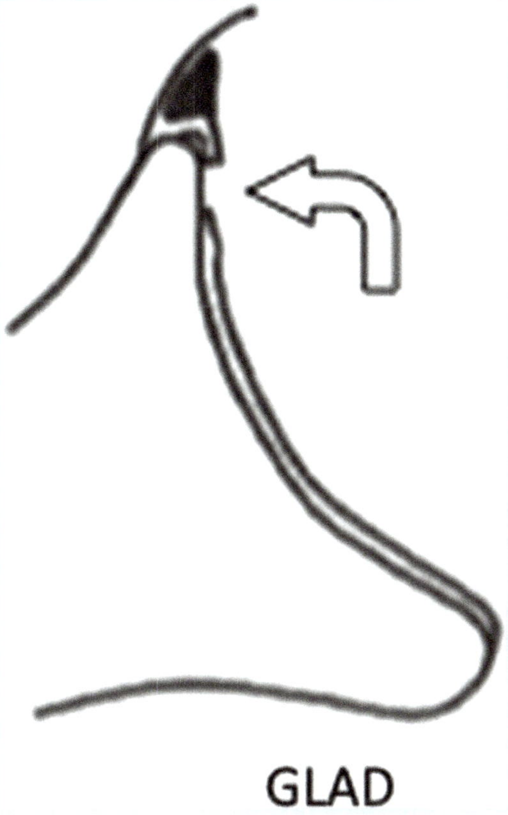
HAGL (Humeral avulsion of the inferior glenohumeral ligament)	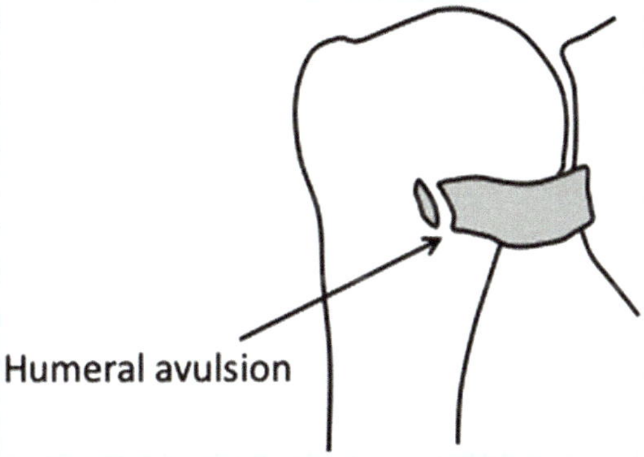
SLAP (Superior Labrum Anterior to Posterior) tear	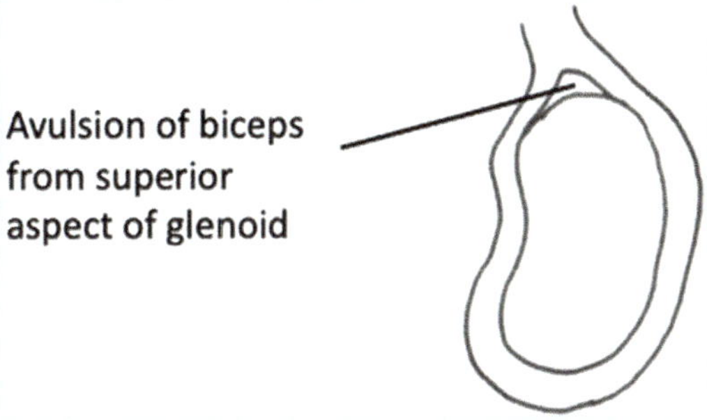

(continued)

Table 2.3 (continued)

Hill-Sachs lesion (compression fracture to posterior aspect of humeral head)	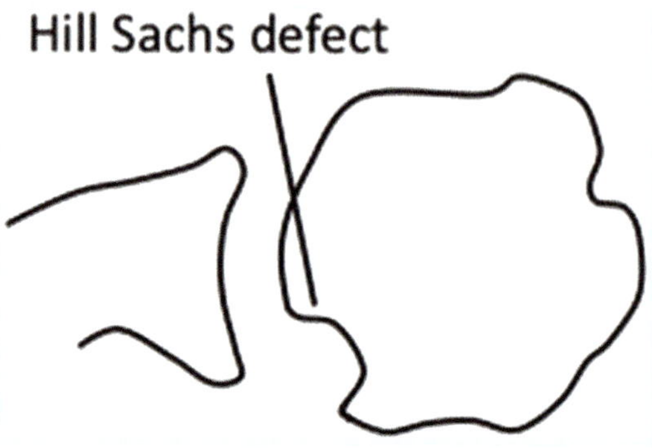
Rotator cuff tear/injury	
Neurological injury (Axillary nerve injury is most common)	

Natural History and Recurrent Instability

The likelihood of recurrent instability is related to the age and sex of the patient. 90% of recurrent dislocations will occur within 2 years of the primary incident. Young males have the highest redislocation rate with a 20 year old having a 72% risk of redislocation. A 20 year old female, however, has a 40% risk. By the age of 35, the risk of recurrent instability drops significantly to 29% and 13% respectively for male and female patients.

Robinson CM, Howes J, Murdoch H, Will E, Graham C. Functional outcome and risk of recurrent instability after primary anterior shoulder dislocation in young patients. J Bone Joint Surg Am 2006;88:2326–36. 86% of all young males who developed instability had this within the first 2 years.

Recurrent dislocations carry a risk of ongoing damage to the shoulder. The most important of these is the Bankart lesion (also known as Perthes–Bankart lesion), which is an anteroinferior labral tear that is found in nearly all young patients with first-time traumatic anterior dislocation. This was first described by Bankart in 1923, who identified the anteroinferior labral avulsion in 4 consecutive cases.

Bankart AS. Recurrent or habitual dislocation of the shoulder joint. BMJ 1923 15;2(3285): 1132–3

The Bankart lesion can be associated with a bony avulsion of the anterior rim of the glenoid, which in more severe cases can lead to glenoid deficiency. Glenoid bone loss of 20% or greater, especially on the antero-inferior rim, significantly increases the risk of recurrent instability. This was described as "the inverted-pear" glenoid by Burkhart depicting the change of the normal "pear-shaped" glenoid to an inverted pear with a wider glenoid superiorly compared to inferiorly.

Burkhart SS, De Beer JF. Traumatic glenohumeral bone defects and their relationship to failure of arthroscopic Bankart repairs: significance of the inverted-pear glenoid and the humeral engaging Hill-Sachs lesion. Arthroscopy 2000;16(7):677–94. Inverted pear glenoid and engaging Hill Sachs lesion were associated with higher failure rate after arthroscopic repair.

Some Bankart lesions (anterior labral periosteal sleeve avulsion; ALPSA) take a periosteal sleeve with them from the anterior glenoid margin. ALPSA predisposes to recurrent dislocation.

Neviaser TJ. The anterior labroligamentous periosteal sleeve avulsion lesion: a cause of anterior instability of the shoulder. Arthroscopy 1993;9(1):17–21.

Another consistent pathology is the Hill–Sachs lesion on the posterosuperior humeral head due to impaction of the humeral head on the anteroinferior glenoid. Large Hill–Sachs lesions can cause recurrent instability despite anterior repair (engaging Hill–Sachs) and will need intervention to prevent recurrence.

Hill-Sachs lesions were traditionally determined to be engaging or non-engaging based on an examination under anaesthesia. Itoi et al have devised a method for predicting which Hill-Sachs lesions will cause dislocation in abduction and external rotation. The 'track' that the glenoid makes as the posterolateral humeral head passes over it in abduction external rotation is mapped on to a 3D reconstruction of the humeral head.

Hill Sachs defects contained within this track ("on-track") are unlikely to become engaged and cause dislocation. Hill Sachs lesions that expand beyond the track margins ("off-track") are likely to engage and cause recurrent dislocation.

Radiologically, the 'glenoid track' is the contact area between glenoid and humeral head. It is considered to be approximately 83% of glenoid width. A Hill-Sachs lesion smaller than this measurement will have a lesser risk of engagement and instability. These are termed 'on track' Hill Sachs lesions. Larger defects will cause instability and are termed 'off track' (or engaging) Hill-Sachs lesions.

More severe and recurrent injuries leave an anteroinferior capsular redundancy, humeral avulsion of the glenohumeral ligament (HAGL) or SLAP lesions. Capsular deficiency is usually demonstrable in recurrent dislocations. The 'drive-through sign' on arthroscopy indicates laxity and may also be present in SLAP lesions due to anterior pseudolaxity.

Chronic anterior dislocation is sometimes seen in elderly patients, patients with multiple trauma and patients with impaired cognition.

Acute Management

The acute management of shoulder dislocations is usually performed by the emergency department. Clinical history should focus on the age, sex and hand dominance of the patient, the mechanism of injury and whether this was a primary or recurrent dislocation. Examination must include a detailed and documented neurological examination. While the axillary nerve is the most likely neurological injury any part of the brachial plexus can be injured. A documented sensory and motor evaluation of all the peripheral nerves is essential before and after shoulder reduction.

Orthogonal radiographs (AP and lateral scapular or modified axial view) should be performed prior to attempted shoulder reduction. A number of methods of shoulder reduction have been described. The principles of safe shoulder reduction include ensuring adequate analgesia, avoiding rotational forces and performing post-reduction radiographs and neurological examination.

Brownson P, Donaldson O, et al. BESS/BOA Patient care pathways. Traumatic anterior shoulder instability. Shoulder and Elbow 2015;7(3):214–26.

Investigations

Further investigations will depend on the age of the patient, number of dislocations, suspicion of associated rotator cuff tears and presence of associated fractures.

Cross sectional imaging should be performed in primary dislocations under the age of 25 or recurrent instability. MR arthrography has 90% sensitivity and specificity for identifying labral pathology and is the investigation of choice in this cohort. MR arthrography in the ABER (abducted, externally rotated) position improves accuracy but is impractical for all patients.

Smith TO, Drew BT, Toms AP. A meta-analysis of the diagnostic test accuracy of MRA and MRI for the detection of glenoid labral injury. Arch Orthop Trauma Surg 2012; 132:905–19. Meta-analysis of 60 studies. MR arthrography was more accurate for detection of labral pathology compared to MRI scan.

Associated Injuries

Clinically relevant rotator cuff tears (i.e. patients with new shoulder symptoms following dislocation) affect approximately 1 in 10 patients.

Robinson CM, Shur N, Sharpe T, Ray A, Murray IR. Injuries associated with traumatic anterior glenohumeral dislocations. J Bone Joint Surg Am 2012;94:18–26. Approximately 13.5% of dislocations sustain a neurological injury and 16% a greater tuberosity fracture.

The incidence of associated rotator cuff tears is significantly greater in patients over the age of 40. A careful assessment and a low threshold in diagnostic imaging of the rotator cuff are advisable in this cohort. US and MRI are both acceptable modalities to assess rotator cuff integrity. Early rotator cuff repair (within 3 months) is considered for patients with new symptoms (e.g. cuff weakness, pain) and a radiologically proven rotator cuff tear. New symptoms are important in this decision making process as a significant proportion of radiologically proven rotator cuff tears will be chronic.

Greater tuberosity fractures associated with dislocations can migrate in the first 3 weeks. Regular radiographs should be performed during this period to identify this. Operative fixation is considered for displacement of greater than 5 mm.

Platzer P, Thalhammer G, Oberleitner G, et al. Displaced fractures of the greater tuberosity: a comparison of operative and nonoperative treatment. J Trauma 2008;65:843–8. Retrospective review of 52 patients treated with internal fixation of displaced greater tuberosity fractures. Operative treatment resulted in better outcome.

Non-Surgical Management

Initial management, following a congruent reduction, is immobilisation in a sling with early mobilization as comfort dictates. Immobilisation in external rotation was proposed by Miller on the basis of a cadaveric study, which showed maximum contact between the labrum and glenoid in 45° external rotation.

Miller BS, Sonnabend DH, Hatrick C, O'leary S, Goldberg J, Harper W, Walsh WR. Should acute dislocations of the shoulder be immobilized in external rotation? A cadaveric study. J Shoulder Elbow Surg 2004;13(6):589–92.

Itoi conducted a prospective randomised controlled trial comparing external rotation orthosis with a simple sling. They demonstrated a reduction in recurrent instability from 42% to 26% with the use of external rotation orthosis. Further studies have not demonstrated similar results and long-term follow-up demonstrates no benefit, hence this is no longer routine practice.

Surgical Management

Surgical intervention depends on associated injuries (see above), the likelihood of recurrence and the demands the patient will place on their shoulder.

The risk of recurrent instability in young (<25 years) males is high and so labral (Bankart) repair should be considered even after the primary dislocation and certainly after recurrent dislocations. The principle of surgical management is to repair the labrum in its anatomical position and this can be performed through open or arthroscopic procedures. Historical procedures have included non-anatomic repair, such as the Putti-Platt procedure, where the subscapularis tendon and anterior capsule were surgically tightened. This resulted in early secondary osteoarthritis and consequently is not performed any longer.

Until recently, open Bankart repair was considered the gold standard for treating traumatic shoulder instability. However, the evolving techniques of shoulder arthroscopy have resulted in arthroscopic stabilization being as effective as open repair.

Harris JD, Gupta AK, Mann NA, et al. Long-term outcomes after Bankart shoulder stabilization. Arthroscopy 2013; 29:920–33.

Arthroscopic Bankart repair is now the preferred surgical procedure. Arthroscopy also has the advantage of less soft tissue damage, earlier rehabilitation and the ability to treat concomitant lesions such as cuff tears and especially SLAP and HAGL lesions.

Bankart repair is only appropriate when the patient has adequate bone stock. Bony surgical procedures should be considered in cases when glenoid bone stock is reduced by 20% or a patient has recurrent instability despite a previous Bankart repair.

An 'engaging' or 'off-track' Hill Sachs lesion (Fig. 2.9) can predispose to recurrent dislocation. The term engaging refers to when the anterior glenoid "falls" into the Hill-Sachs defect in abduction and external rotation due to the reduced excursion distance of the glenohumeral joint.

A Latarjet procedure can be used for large, engaging Hill-Sachs defects. In the Latarjet procedure, the coracoid process with the attached conjoint tendon is transferred to the face of the anteroinferior glenoid. Iliac crest graft can also be used.

The Latarjet procedure increases the excursion distance required to dislocate the humeral head (Fig. 2.10). Other techniques to manage an engaging Hill-Sachs lesion include 'Remplissage', in which the posterior capsule and infraspinatus are secured into the Hill-Sachs defect.

The Magnuson Stack procedure is advancement of subscapularis while the Putti Platt repair is imbrication and shortening of the subscapularis. These are rarely used anymore due to the risk of secondary osteoarthritis. Excess version of the humeral head may require derotation osteotomy.

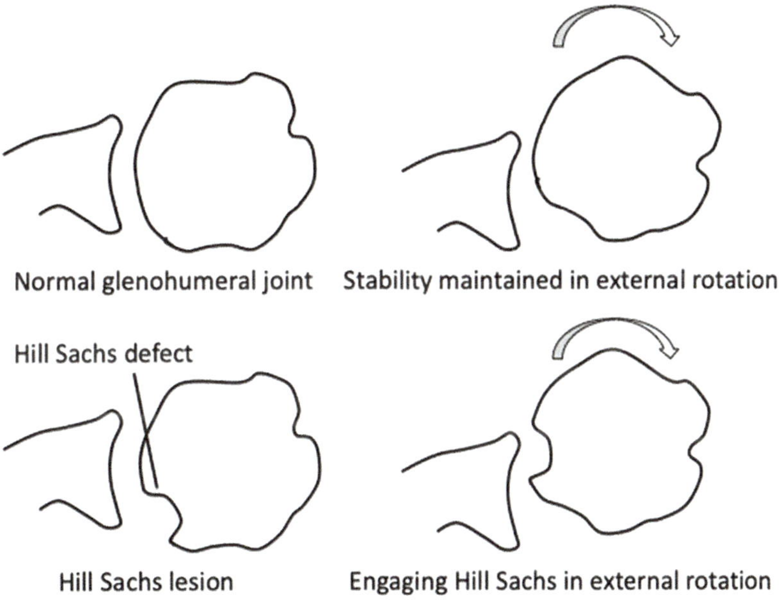

Fig. 2.9 Engaging Hill Sachs lesion

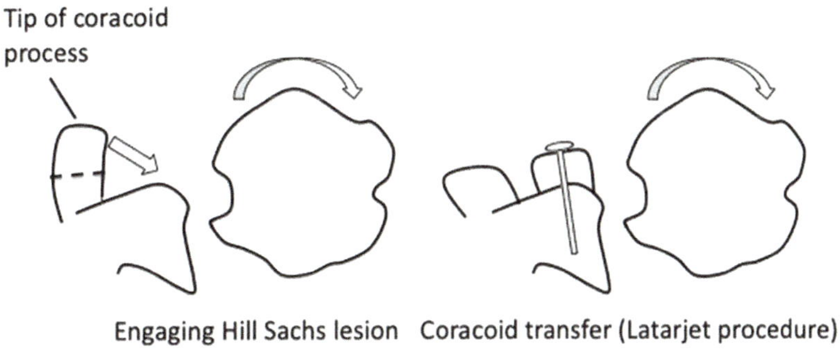

Fig. 2.10 Latarjet procedure

Posterior Shoulder Instability

Posterior dislocations account for approximately 5% of all shoulder dislocations. Almost 50% of these may be missed on initial presentation.

Recurrent posterior instability is significantly more common than an acute traumatic posterior dislocation. This is because it occurs as a result of repetitive micro trauma with the instability manifesting itself as pain, weakness or clunking. Predisposing conditions for acute posterior dislocation include seizures, alcoholism, electrocution or a direct blow on the anterior aspect of the shoulder.

The shoulder is usually held in an internally rotated and adducted position. Lack of active and passive external rotation should raise the suspicion of a posterior dislocation.

AP radiographs of the shoulder show the classic 'light-bulb sign', which means the humeral head appears symmetrical. This is because the greater tuberosity is not visible on the AP view due to internal rotation of the arm. It should be noted that most patients who have injured their shoulder naturally hold their arm in an internally rotated position as the position of comfort. Orthogonal radiographs in the form of a lateral scapular (Y) view or modified axillary with the AP radiograph are vital in the diagnosis. A CT scan is useful if doubt still remains following plain radiographs.

Injuries associated with an acute posterior dislocation include:

- Fracture of surgical neck of humerus
- Reverse Hill-Sachs lesion (compression fracture of the anterior aspect of the humeral head)
- Posterior labral tear
- Posterior glenoid rim fracture
- Rotator cuff tear (particularly subscapularis)
- Lesser tuberosity fracture/avulsion

It is important to carefully assess the radiographs to rule out an associated surgical neck of humerus fracture before considering closed reduction of the dislocation. Reduction is achieved by 'in-line traction' with avoidance of rotational forces and a sling is advised for 3–4 weeks. If unstable, an abduction/ER brace can be used for 6 weeks and a further clinical assessment is made.

Surgery is indicated for symptomatic instability. This usually occurs due to an engaging reverse Hill-Sachs defect. A modified McLaughlin procedure (the technique originally described by McLaughlin transferred only the subscapularis into the humeral head defect) in which the lesser tuberosity and attached subscapularis is transferred into the humeral head defect is an effective method of managing this.

McLaughlin HL. Posterior dislocation of the shoulder. J Bone Joint Surg Am 1952;24:584–90.

Recurrent posterior instability falls into the polar type 2 instability on the Stanmore triangle. The history of trauma is usually absent or subtle and there is usually no relocation history. Recurrent posterior instability usually occurs in a patient aged 20–30 years. The presentation is one of recurrent subluxation, usually with the individual perceiving pain or weakness at relocation. It is common that specific activities that put the shoulder in an "at risk" position (such as push-ups) precipitate symptoms.

Detailed clinical examination and comparison to the contralateral shoulder aid in diagnosis. Scapulothoracic dyskinesia during active movement (both concentric and eccentric) should be looked for. Specific tests, all performed with the patient in the sitting position, include:

- Posterior load and shift test—with the arm by the side, the scapula is stabilized with one hand and the other hand attempts to shift the humeral head off the glenoid in a posterior direction. A positive finding is greater than 50% excursion posteriorly
- Jerk test/Posterior apprehension test. The shoulder is held in a flexed and internally rotated position. Axial compression is applied to the shoulder while it is moved into adduction. A clunk/apprehension is suggestive of posterior instability
- Kim test. The arm is held in 90° abduction and an axial force is applied. The shoulder is then elevated diagonally in to a forward flexed and

adducted position, maintaining an axial force while the other hand applies a posteroinferior translation force on the humerus. A clunk or pain indicates a positive test.

A combination of a positive jerk and Kim test is highly sensitive for posteroinferior labral pathology.

Kim SH, Park JS, Jeong WK, Shin SK. The Kim test: a novel test for posteroinferior labral lesion of the shoulder—a comparison to the jerk test. Am J Sports Med 2005;33:1188–92.

Investigations

MR arthrography is the most accurate at identifying the underlying soft tissue pathology. CT can be useful if glenoid retroversion or bone loss is considered to be a significant contributing factor. It is common to see posterior capsule redundancy at arthroscopy in addition to posterior labral pathology. A Kim lesion (an incomplete and concealed avulsion of the posteroinferior aspect of the labrum) may be present and should not be mistaken for an intact posterior labrum. This is usually seen as a crack at the junction between the articular cartilage and posterior labrum. When this is surgically developed, an avulsion of the deep part of the posteroinferior labral complex becomes evident.

Kim SH, Ha KI, Yoo JC, Noh KC. Kim's lesion: an incomplete and concealed avulsion of the posteroinferior labrum in posterior or multidirectional posteroinferior instability of the shoulder. Arthroscopy. 2004;20:712–20.

Treatment

Initial treatment should involve physical therapy, posture and proprioceptive feedback exercises. Activity modification, seizure control, pain relief, cuff and scapulothoracic muscle rehabilitation should be the mainstay of therapy.

Surgery is increasingly being recognised as a way to address structural defects early in order to better rehabilitate the patient. This is especially true with an antecedent history of trauma. The most commonly performed procedure involves treatment of the posterior capsulolabral lesion through either open or arthroscopic surgery.

Arthroscopic labral repair using suture anchors is the preferred surgical treatment as it allows management of concomitant intra-articular pathology. This includes capsular plication to address the redundant posterior joint capsule.

Bony procedures are considered for patients with an engaging Hill Sachs defect in the form of a modified McLaughlin procedure. Rarely, posterior bone block augmentation for glenoid bone loss or glenoid osteotomy for glenoid retroversion associated with posterior instability is considered.

Non-Traumatic Instability (Polar Type 3)

Polar type 3 instability includes patients with structurally normal shoulders who have instability associated with muscle patterning problems, joint laxity or a combination of both. This is commonly associated with scapular dyskinesia during physiological shoulder movement with the shoulder subluxing or dislocating in the mid-range of movement or at rest. The direction of instability (or symptomatic instability) can be anterior, posterior or true multidirectional.

Clinical history rarely identifies a traumatic episode. It is significantly more common in adolescent female patients with a range of symptoms including subluxation, clunking, insecurity, pain and frank dislocation. Patients may have symptoms affecting multiple joints indicating a generalised joint laxity and so all patients should undergo a Beighton score (Table 2.4). Psychosocial factors can also influence symptoms and so should be considered.

Higher score indicates higher likelihood of hypermobility and joint laxity.

Examination should include an assessment of core stability and the kinetic chain. Patients should be asked to stand on each leg paying close attention to ankle stability, hip position (abductor

Table 2.4 The Beighton score

Hyperextension of little finger MCP joints	1 point for each side
Thumb can be passively extended to forearm in pronation	1 point for each side
Elbow hyperextension over 10 degrees	1 point for each side
Knee hyperextension on standing greater than 10 degrees	1 point for each side
Ability to touch palms to the floor while standing and keeping knees straight	1 point
Maximum score	9

strength), overall balance and shoulder position. Gagey (hyperabduction) test is performed to assess for inferior capsular laxity along with other instability tests described above. An assessment of scapular control through active shoulder range of movement should also be performed. Subtle scapular dyskinesia is more apparent during eccentric movement (i.e. lowering the arm from an elevated position).

An overactive pectoralis major or latissimus dorsi is a common feature of anterior instability. Overactive latissimus dorsi or infraspinatus contribute to posterior instability.

The mainstay of treating polar type 3 instability is a structured physiotherapy rehabilitation program. Treatment should include correcting abnormalities of the lower extremities and trunk. Correcting posture and strengthening the trunk are the first elements to be addressed in the kinetic chain, followed by the scapular and the shoulder musculature. Surgery is rarely indicated in these patients and is reserved for patients with evidence of capsular laxity who have exhausted physiotherapy treatment.

SLAP (Superior Labrum tears Anterior to Posterior) Lesions

SLAP lesions can be associated with shoulder instability or cuff tears. These are labral detachments in the region of attachment of the biceps tendon on the superior labrum (Fig. 2.11). The term SLAP lesion was first described and classified by Snyder.

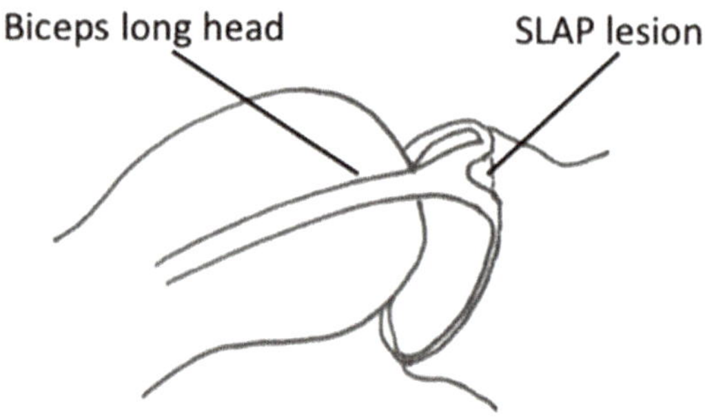

Fig. 2.11 The SLAP lesion

Table 2.5 Types of SLAP lesions

Type of lesion	Pathology
Type I	Fraying in the region of attachment of biceps tendon. Tendon intact
Type II	Detachment of biceps and superior labrum from the glenoid rim
Type III	Bucket handle tear of the labrum, intact biceps tendon
Type IV	Bucket handle tear of the labrum, intrasubstance tear of biceps tendon

Types of SLAP lesions are summarised in Table 2.5. Many further types have been described, which are variations/extensions of the original classification.

Type I and III are managed with arthroscopic debridement, while type II and IV require arthroscopic repair of the detached tendon.

The Painful Shoulder

Shoulder pain presents a diagnostic conundrum full of pitfalls. Pain can be broadly categorized according to location:

- Glenohumeral joint pain
- Subacromial pain
- Shoulder girdle pain
- Referred pain

Certain shoulder pathologies have a well-defined age distribution, and this can be used to further narrow the list of differential diagnoses. There is often overlap of symptoms and signs,

Table 2.6 Causes of shoulder pain

Location of pathology	Younger adults	Older adults (>30)
Glenohumeral joint	Labral tear SLAP tear Avascular necrosis Rheumatoid Arthritis Primary bone tumours	Osteoarthritis Rheumatoid arthritis Frozen shoulder Metastatic deposits
Subacromial	Rotator cuff tear ACJ trauma Internal Impingement Os acromiale	Rotator cuff degeneration Subacromial bursitis Rotator cuff tears Calcific tendinitis Bicipital tendinopathy ACJ arthritis
Shoulder Girdle	Scapulothoracic bursitis	
Referred	Suprascapular nerve entrapment Cervical radiculopathy Brachial Neuritis	Cervical radiculopathy

making shoulder pain often difficult to attribute to a single cause. A careful history, directed clinical examination and judicious use of different imaging modalities are essential. The causes of shoulder pain are listed in Table 2.6.

Glenohumeral Pain

Pain resulting from instability, such as labral tears is discussed in the instability section above.

Avascular Necrosis

The humeral head is the second most common site affected by avascular necrosis after the hip. The blood supply to the humeral head becomes interrupted resulting in osteonecrosis and subchondral collapse. Fracture of the humeral head and neck causes AVN in proportion to the severity of injury: 3-part and valgus impacted 4-part fractures have a risk of 10–15%. In displaced 4-part fractures the rate is 45%, and with an associated dislocation approaches 100%. The most common non-traumatic cause is steroid medication. Cruess has classified humeral head AVN in to five stages which determine the best treatment modality, as shown in Table 2.7.

Frozen Shoulder

This condition was first described by Codman in 1934. It is characterized by pain and limited movement at the glenohumeral joint. Frozen shoulder has been classified by Zuckerman as primary, where there is no identifiable cause; and secondary, where a cause or associated condition is present. Secondary frozen shoulder is further subdivided into intrinsic, extrinsic and systemic based on the location of the associated feature. The secondary causes are summarised in Table 2.8.

Table 2.7 The Cruess classification of humeral head avascular necrosis

Stage	Radiological appearances	Treatment
I	Normal. Can be detected on MRI	Core Decompression
II	Sclerosis. Mottled, Area of osteopenia. Sphericity maintained	Core Decompression
III	Crescent sign, subchondral fracture, minimal depression of articular surface	Resurfacing or hemiarthroplasty
IV	Flattening. Collapse. Loose bodies. Secondary arthritis	Resurfacing or hemiarthroplasty
V	Degenerative changes extend to include glenoid	Total Shoulder Arthroplasty

Table 2.8 Secondary causes of frozen shoulder

Intrinsic	Extrinsic	Systemic
Rotator cuff tear Calcific tendonitis Bicipital tendonitis	Clavicle fracture Proximal humeral fracture ACJ arthritis Chest wall tumours Ipsilateral breast surgery Cerebrovascular accident	Diabetes mellitus Thyroid disease Depuytren's disease Antiretroviral medication

Zuckerman JD, Rokito A. Frozen shoulder: a consensus definition. J Shoulder Elbow Surg. 2011;20(2):322–5.

Pathophysiology

The cause of frozen shoulder is unknown, although a number of theories have been proposed. Bunker and Anthony found consistent features were capsular thickening with increased vascularity, together with proliferation of fibroblasts, transformation to myofibroblasts and increased collagen deposition, similar to Dupuytren's disease. They found the synovium to be normal with no inflammatory changes.

Bunker TD, Anthony PP. The pathology of frozen shoulder. A Dupuytrens like disease. J Bone Joint Surg Br 1995;77:677–683.

Other studies indicate that the main pathology is an inflammatory contracture of the shoulder joint capsule. This is associated with an increased amount of collagen, fibrotic growth factors such as transforming growth factor-beta, and inflammatory cytokines such as tumour necrosis factor-alpha and interleukins. Capsular biopsies from patients with frozen shoulder have shown the presence of proliferating fibroblasts and chronic inflammatory cells. The infiltrate of chronic inflammatory cells is predominantly made up of mast cells, along with T cells, B cells and macrophages. These findings show a chronic inflammatory response with fibroblastic proliferation, which may be immunomodulated.

Hand GC, Athanasou NA, Matthews T, Carr AJ. The pathology of frozen shoulder. J Bone Joint Surg Br. 2007;89:928–32.

The clinical picture of initial pain followed by stiffness suggests an initial inflammatory phase followed by fibrosis. Fibrosis is characterised by excessive production of collagen types I and III. These form a matrix which then contracts. Matrix metalloproteinases and their inhibitors control matrix remodelling, and MMP inhibitors used in some forms of cancer chemotherapy have been shown to induce frozen shoulder.

Clinical Presentation

Frozen shoulder is a disease of the 5th and 6th decades, with a peak incidence in the mid-50s. Women are more often affected than men. There is an insidious onset of pain in the deltoid region with examination findings of a loss of passive external rotation (<50% of the contralateral limb) and pain at the extreme of external rotation. There is no crepitus on movement. Hannafin and Chiaia have described four stages of frozen shoulder (Table 2.9).

Hannafin JA, Chiaia TA. Adhesive capsulitis. A treatment approach. Clin Orthop Relat Res. 2000;372:95–109

Investigations

Diagnosis is clinical but radiographs are essential to rule out an arthritic glenohumeral joint.

Management

Management options include the following:

- Analgesia
- Physiotherapy
- Steroid injection
- Hydrodilatation/capsular distension
- Manipulation under anaesthesia
- Arthroscopic release

Table 2.9 Stages of frozen shoulder

Stage 1	Occurs during the first 3 months and is characterised by pain with little loss of motion.
Stage 2 (the freezing stage)	Occurs between 3 and 9 months and is characterized by pain with loss of active and passive motion.
Stage 3 (the frozen stage)	Occurs at 9–15 months and is characterized by little pain but with loss of motion.
Stage 4 (thawing phase)	Occurs after 15–24 month, with little pain and a progressive improvement in the range of motion.

The aim of treatment is to maintain a useful range of pain free movement of the shoulder. Management of frozen shoulder will differ according to the stage of disease. Analgesia is necessary in stage 1 and 2.

Physiotherapy is useful to maintain range of movement in the early stages and also to rehabilitate after hydrodilatation or release by manipulation or arthroscopy. A Cochrane review (2014) showed that a combination of manual therapy and exercise may not be as effective as glucocorticoid injection in the short-term. It is unclear whether a combination of manual therapy, exercise and electrotherapy is an effective adjunct to glucocorticoid injection or oral NSAID. Following arthrographic joint distension with glucocorticoid and saline, manual therapy and exercise may confer effects similar to those of sham ultrasound in terms of overall pain, function and quality of life, but may provide greater patient-reported treatment success and active range of motion.

Capsular distension involves an intra-articular injection of local anaesthetic (+/- corticosteroid) followed by an intra-articular injection under pressure of normal saline or air. The purpose of the injection is to stretch or rupture the joint capsule, and has been shown to significantly improve symptoms in patients with frozen shoulder with a low repeat intervention rate.

Nicholson JA, Slader B, Martindale A, Mckie S, Robinson M. Distension arthrogram in the treatment of adhesive capsulitis has a low rate of repeat intervention. Bone Joint J 2020;102(5):606–10.

Capsular distension, when compared to manipulation under anaesthetic, showed similar improvements in range of movement at 6 months but a higher satisfaction rate at final follow up (94% vs. 81%).

Quraishi NA, Johnston P, Bayer J, Crowe M, Chakrabarti AJ. Thawing the frozen shoulder. A randomised trial comparing manipulation under anaesthesia with hydrodilatation. J Bone Joint Surg Br. 2007;89(9):1197–200. This study compared manipulation under anaesthetic with hydrodilatation, and showed range of movement improved in all patients at six months, but was not significantly different between the groups. At the final follow-up, 94% of patients were satisfied or very satisfied after hydrodilatation compared with 81% of those receiving a manipulation.

Manipulation under anaesthetic with a concomitant steroid injection has long been the mainstay of treatment in the frozen phase. Thomas et al showed that manipulation confers a significant improvement in patient symptoms in the long term. Timing of intervention has no bearing on outcome.

Thomas WJ, Jenkins EF, Owen JM, Sangster MJ, Kirubanandan R, Beynon C, Woods DA. Treatment of frozen shoulder by manipulation under anaesthetic: does the timing of treatment affect the outcome? J Bone Joint Surg Br. 2011;93(10):1377–81.

Complications are rare but potentially serious, and include humeral and glenoid rim fractures. 18% of patients require a further MUA, and this increases to 38% in patients with diabetes mellitus. These patients can be offered a repeat MUA and expect a good outcome.

Woods DA, Loganathan K. Recurrence of frozen shoulder after manipulation under anaesthetic (MUA); the results of repeating the MUA. Bone Joint J. 2017;99(6):812–817

Arthroscopic release reduces the risk of fracture and so is preferred by some surgeons. The humerus is weakest in rotation and so releasing the rotator interval prior to manipulation reduces the rotational forces required during manipulation. Division of the anterior capsule is often sufficient, but posterior capsule can be released if required. Postoperative full range of movement has been reported as 90%, falling to 71% in diabetic patients.

Mehta SS, Singh HP, Pandey R. Comparative outcome of arthroscopic release for frozen shoulder in patients with and without diabetes. Bone Joint J. 2014;96(10):1355–8

Inflammatory Arthritis

Inflammatory arthropathies, including rheumatoid arthritis, psoriatic arthritis and juvenile chronic arthritis can affect the glenohumeral joint. Rheumatoid arthritis of the shoulder usually affects the glenohumeral joint, but cervical spine and acromioclavicular joint involvement can cause symptoms around the shoulder. For this reason imaging is a fundamental part of clinical assessment in these patients. Progression of disease involves the entire shoulder, with glenohumeral erosive arthritis, cuff tears and acromioclavicular joint involvement.

Operative treatment can range from synovectomy and glenohumeral debridement to arthroplasty depending on the severity of disease. Hemiarthroplasty has been shown to have inferior outcomes when compared to total shoulder replacement in patients with an intact rotator cuff and adequate glenoid bone stock (Collins et al.). In cuff deficient patients reverse shoulder arthroplasty can be used if there is adequate bone stock. In severe glenoid erosion where implantation of a glenosphere or glenoid resurfacing is not possible, hemiarthroplasty can offer some pain relief. However, the advances in prosthesis design have made glenoid reconstruction with bone graft or custom implants possible.

Collins DN, Harryman DT 2nd, Wirth MA. Shoulder arthroplasty for the treatment of inflammatory arthritis. J Bone Joint Surg Am. 2004;86:2489–96.

Osteoarthritis

The clinical presentation of osteoarthritis of the glenohumeral joint (GHJ) is progressive pain and stiffness. The radiological hallmarks of subchondral sclerosis, cysts, osteophytes and loss of joint space are present. In osteoarthritis of the glenohumeral joint, wear of posterior glenoid is a feature. This is the area of maximal joint reaction force. As the glenoid erodes posteriorly the humeral head can sublux posteriorly in advanced cases.

The rotator cuff tends to be intact in GHJ osteoarthritis, allowing anatomical TSR to be employed in cases where nonoperative measures have failed. Intraarticular steroid injections may give several months of pain relief, and can be used in younger patients, patients with less severe disease and those patients not fit enough to consider general anaesthetic. Total shoulder replacement (Fig. 2.12) has been shown to provide more pain relief and better function than humeral resurfacing alone.

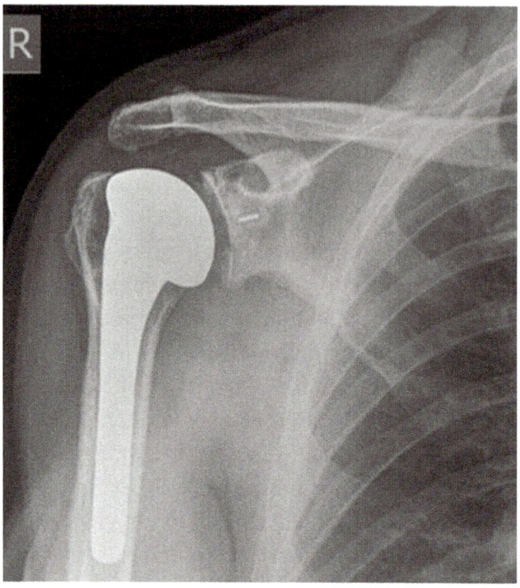

Fig. 2.12 Anatomic shoulder replacement

Bryant D, Litchfield R, Sandow M, et al. A comparison of pain, strength, range of motion, and functional outcomes after hemiarthroplasty and total shoulder arthroplasty in patients with osteoarthritis of the shoulder: a systematic review and meta-analysis. J Bone Joint Surg [Am] 2005;87-A:1947–56.

Humeral implants can be stemmed, stemless or resurfacing with the surgical intention of maintaining humeral bone stock while ensuring adequate glenoid exposure. Stemmed implants are often platform stems, which allow for retention of the stem and conversion of the modular components in revision situations, for example, conversion of anatomic total shoulder replacement to reverse total shoulder replacement for cuff failure.

Complications of anatomic shoulder replacement are similar to those of other joint replacements, and include infection, aseptic loosening (especially of the glenoid component), dislocation and periprosthetic fracture. Acute or chronic rotator cuff failure is a complication specific to anatomic shoulder replacement. While it is possible to perform a total shoulder replacement through a subscapularis sparing approach, this is surgically challenging and is not routinely used. Successful repair of subscapularis is essential in ensuring a good functional outcome. A lesser tuberosity osteotomy is used by some surgeons for access, and may provide more reliable healing potential.

The incidence of cuff deficiency increases with age and so careful assessment of cuff integrity and quality is vital. CT scans are useful at assessing glenoid morphology, degree of wear, and also give an indication of rotator cuff muscle quality. The Goutallier classification is used to assess rotator cuff muscle quality (see rotator cuff section) with a Goutallier grading of 3 and above a relative contraindication for anatomic total shoulder replacement.

MRI or US scan can be used if there is any ongoing concern. Anatomic total shoulder replacement in patients with evidence of cuff deficiency and osteoarthritis should be avoided. These patients should be managed in a similar way to patients with cuff tear arthropathy.

Rotator Cuff Arthropathy

Rotator cuff, or cuff tear arthropathy is characterised by the following:

- Rotator cuff insufficiency
- Proximal migration of the humeral head
- Glenohumeral cartilage destruction
- Subchondral disuse osteopenia

Pathogenesis

The normal rotator cuff provides concavity compression, forcing the humeral head into its relatively shallow socket. This function maintains joint congruity during glenohumeral movements. In patients with rotator cuff insufficiency this concavity compression is lost, allowing translation at the glenohumeral joint interface. In severe cases the proximal humeral migration causes articulation between the acromion and humeral head. Over time, wear of the superior glenoid and inferior acromion produces acetabularisation of the scapular components and femoralisation of the humeral head. Anterosuperior escape, where the coracoacromial ligament is deficient/absent allowing for the humeral head to "escape" on elevation, can be seen in extreme cases.

Clinical Presentation

Rotator cuff arthropathy classically affects older women. The symptoms may be bilateral and may have been present for several years with intermittent flares of pain and swelling. Examination findings will be positive for rotator cuff insufficiency and loss of muscle bulk in the supraspinatus and infraspinatus fossae. The humeral head may be palpable anteriorly and superiorly. There may be a subcutaneous effusion due to leakage of synovial fluid from the deficient capsule. Radiologically the unopposed deltoid will cause an anterosuperior displacement of the humeral head with humeral and glenoid bone loss, subchondral sclerosis and inferomedial subchondral disuse osteopenia. If operative intervention is to be considered a CT scan is useful to assess levels of glenoid bone stock.

Management

The aims of management are pain relief and maintenance of useful range of movement. In early disease or younger patients glenohumeral steroid injections may be of symptomatic benefit but will not slow progression of disease. Physiotherapy in the form of an anterior deltoid strengthening programme can assist in maintaining function, particularly in the early stages of the condition.

In cuff tear arthropathy the rotator cuff is either absent or non-functional, with the glenohumeral joint being moved by deltoid primarily. This gives the typical proximally migrated humeral head appearance on radiographs. Anatomical total shoulder arthroplasty may give some pain relief but excessive shear forces at the joint interface will cause excessive wear of polyethylene components and useful movements will be negligible. It is therefore contraindicated.

In the absence of a functional rotator cuff the deltoid can be recruited by using a reverse polarity total shoulder replacement (see later). This medialises the centre of rotation, lengthening the lever arm for deltoid and therefore increasing its efficiency.

Subacromial Pain

The rotator cuff is an important tendon complex that helps in the movements and stability of the shoulder joint. It is prone to degeneration and tendinosis, and can undergo attrition rupture. The muscle action is complex and the articular surface of the tendon is closely applied to the bone and cartilage of the humeral head. On its bursal surface it is separated from the acromion and the coracoacromial ligament by the subacromial bursa. The acromioclavicular joint is also applied closely to the supraspinatus tendon and osteophytes can impinge on the tendon. The bursa itself has a rich nerve supply and can be painful. Subacromial pain can be diagnosed by considering the potential underlying processes: inflammatory, structural or functional. Patients may have a mixture of these, with many having a functional problem with underlying inflammatory or structural problem (Fig. 2.13 and Table 2.10).

Calcific Tendinitis

The prevalence of calcium deposits within the supraspinatus tendon has been found to be between 2.4 and 7.8% in asymptomatic patients in recent studies. In patients with a subacromial pain syndrome this increases to 42.5%. Calcific deposits occur just medial to the insertion of the supraspinatus tendon, in the watershed area that displays poor vascularisation. There is an increased incidence in women and people with diabetes mellitus. Genetic links have also been suggested. During the calcific stage of tendinitis cells excrete calcium, which then coalesces into discrete deposits. After the resting phase the deposits start to be reabsorbed. This is usually the painful stage. The onset of pain can be acute or subacute and can be so severe that sufferers attend the emergency department. Treatment is non-operative with exercises, oral anti-inflammatory medications with or without a subacromial injection in 90% of cases. In cases where these measures fail, ultrasound guided barbotage is useful in the resorptive stage. Arthroscopic removal can also be performed in recalcitrant cases with good outcomes.

Louwerens JK et al. Prevalence of calcific deposits within the rotator cuff tendons in adults with and without subacromial pain syndrome: clinical and radiologic analysis of 1219 patients. J Shoulder Elbow Surg. 2015;24(10):1588–93.

Fig. 2.13 The causes of subacromial pain

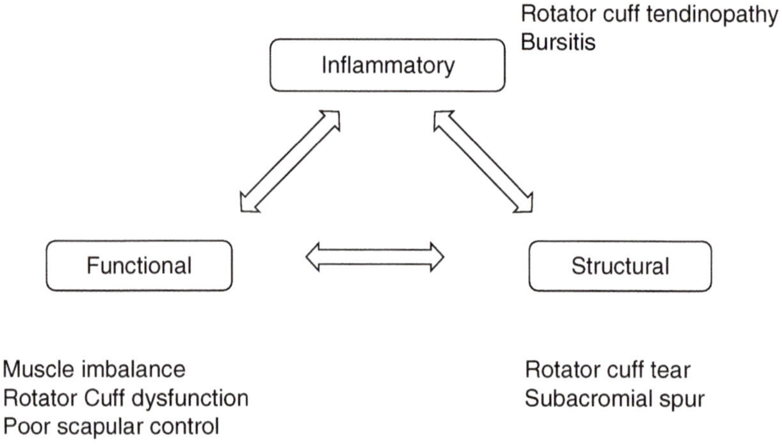

Table 2.10 Alternative causes of subacromial pain

Diagnosis	Presentation	Investigations	Treatment	Outcomes
Calcific tendonitis	Age 30–60 Male: Female 1:2 Diabetic association	Radiographs	NSAIDs, PT USS guided barbotage Arthroscopic removal	60–70% improved 6 months
ACJ osteoarthritis	Pain in ACJ. Repetitive overhead activities. Tender ACJ. Positive Scarf test	Radiographs Diagnostic LA injection	LA/steroid injection, excision of distal clavicle	Expect good/excellent outcomes
Os acromiale	Painful synchondrosis Posttraumatic pain Impingement pain	Axillary radiograph CT Diagnostic LA injection	Non operative in most cases Fusion+/- bone grafting Excision of pre-acromion fragment	Frequently need second stage fusion for metalwork removal/revision Deltoid dysfunction in large fragment excision.
Bicipital tendinopathy	Associated with impingement and bicipital groove stenosis. Pain anterior arm to elbow. Tender over bicipital groove. Positive Speed's test	Ultrasound shoulder MRI shoulder	NSAIDs and steroid injection around tendon. Tenodesis/ Tenotomy	Tenotomy for majority of patients—small risk of "Popeye" deformity. Tenodesis for younger patients—lower chance of being pain free
Internal impingement	Shoulder pain in throwing athletes. Posterior pain. Loss of internal rotation.	MR arthrogram as associated with SLAP tears/labral tears	Activity modification. Posterior stretching Rotator cuff debridement/ repair Labral repair	Worse outcomes if progresses to cuff tear.

Rotator Cuff Tendinosis

The basic pathology of tendinosis is degeneration within the tendon with age. Some studies have implicated genetic and mechanical factors. The role of the coracoacromial arch, especially the under surface of the acromion is known to perpetuate the pain.

Intrinsic factors:

- Muscle fatigue and overload in tension, especially in overhead activities
- Tendinosis
- Overuse of the shoulder

Extrinsic factors

- Malunion of greater tuberosity fractures
- Shoulder instability
- ACJ Osteophytes
- Hooked acromial spur

Charles Neer described three stages of impingement:

1. Reversible oedema and haemorrhage
2. Fibrosis and tendinitis
3. Tears and bone spurs on the acromion

He also divided impingement into outlet impingement due to the coracoacromial arch and non-outlet impingement due to an inflamed bursa or tendon, and advocated excising the anteroinferior acromion.

Clinical Presentation

The pain is usually felt in the upper lateral aspect of the arm and can radiate to the elbow. It is a dull ache associated with activity and can be sharp in certain positions of the arm such as abduction and internal rotation. Lying on the affected side is painful. Stiffness can develop in the posterior capsule and can manifest as reduced internal rotation.

There is a painful arc of abduction with pain between 70 and 90 degrees of elevation in the scapular plane (Neer's Sign). Several clinical tests are described for impingement and aim to elicit pain with narrowing of the subacromial space by the greater tuberosity. The Hawkins sign is a provocative test eliciting pain on passive internal rotation with the shoulder and elbow in 90° flexion. The Jobe "empty can test" attempts to provoke pain or weakness within the supraspinatus muscle. The patient resists downward pressure with their arm elevated in the scapular plane with the elbow extended and thumb pointing towards the floor (maximal internal rotation). The Neer's test is elimination of a positive Neer's sign after injection of local anaesthetic.

Rotator cuff tears, ACJ arthritis and long head of biceps tendinitis can commonly occur in association with subacromial pain and so routine examination to rule out these should be the norm. While clinical weakness in the rotator cuff is not particularly sensitive or specific in the diagnosis of rotator cuff tears, clinical examination is important in developing an overall clinical picture as to the diagnosis. Test both shoulders at the same time to allow direct comparison of strength.

Supraspinatus strength is best tested in the scapular plane using the "empty can test". Supraspinatus tears can be present without weakness due to deltoid compensation. Resisted external rotation with the arm by the patient's side can elicit infraspinatus weakness. Subscapularis is tested by Gerber's lift off test, in which the patient has their hand behind their back and are able to lift the dorsum of the hand away. Pain commonly prohibits this test and so assessment of internal rotation strength can also be performed with the arm in front of the body, e.g. Napoleon/belly press test.

Symptoms associated with ACJ arthritis is "high arc" pain when the arm is nearing maximum elevation. Examination reveals point tenderness over the ACJ. Scarf or cross body adduction test can also be performed but is less reliable than point tenderness over the ACJ. Speed's test is performed to assess for long head of biceps pathology. The hand is facing upwards (externally rotated) with shoulder flexed and elbow straight. A positive test is pain or weakness when a downward force is applied to the arm in this position.

Imaging

Radiographs may be normal or show greater tuberosity and/or acromion sclerosis and cysts. There may be ACJ osteoarthritis or an os acromiale. Ultrasound and MRI can show inflammation of the subacromial bursa, identify cuff tears and look for biceps pathology or fluid within the biceps tendon sheath.

Treatment

Nonoperative management should be the initial approach. A meta-analysis of 2300 patients demonstrated that steroid injection combined with physical therapy produces the best results. Injection alone gives a worse outcome.

Dong W, Goost H, Lin XB, Burger C, Paul C, Wang ZL, Zhang TY, Jiang ZC, Welle K, Kabir K. Treatment for shoulder impingement syndrome: a PRISMA systematic review and network meta-analysis. Medicine (Baltimore). 2015;94(10):e510

Surgical intervention is reserved for patients who have failed a prolonged course of conservative management. The intention of subacromial decompression is to increase the space under the acromion to allow the rotator cuff muscles to move freely. It involves releasing the coracoacromial ligament from the acromion and shaving away the undersurface of the acromion or acromial spur. All symptomatic pathology should be managed at surgery, including ACJ arthritis, biceps tendinitis and rotator cuff tears.

There is currently debate about the value of arthroscopic subacromial decompression in these patients. The CSAW Study compared outcomes at 6 months and 1 year after no treatment, diagnostic arthroscopy alone or arthroscopic subacromial decompression. The best results were in the surgical group, but there was no significant difference between diagnostic arthroscopy alone and ASAD. Surgery over no treatment was an average of 4.2 points better on the Oxford shoulder score, a difference which the authors do not see as clinically significant.

Beard DJ, et al. Arthroscopic subacromial decompression for subacromial shoulder pain (CSAW): a multicentre, pragmatic, parallel group, placebo-controlled, three-group, randomised surgical trial. The Lancet 2018;391(10118):329–38.

Rotator Cuff Tears

The rotator cuff maintains a balanced force couple that helps the shoulder move in space and keeps the fulcrum centred within the joint. The aim of repair surgery is to balance this force couple in all planes when it is disrupted as well as to relieve pain.

Rotator cuff tears can be asymptomatic or symptomatic and partial thickness or full thickness. Partial thickness tears are further classified into articular sided, mid-substance or bursal sided tears. Articular sided tears are common due to impaired blood supply in that area. The Ellman classification is based on depth of partial thickness tears—Grade I (less than 3 mm depth), Grade II (3–6 mm depth) and grade III (over 6 mm deep or more than half the thickness of the tendon).

The most common location is the supraspinatus tendon. Tears are commonly posterosuperior or less commonly anterosuperior.

The Cofield classification is based on size of tears—small (less than 1cm), medium (1–3 cm), large (3 5 cm) and massive (more than 5 cm). The anatomical classification describes the shape of tears—longitudinal, L shaped, U shaped or a crescent.

Pathology

Theories have described extrinsic and intrinsic influences in the development of rotator cuff tears. Traditional thinking has placed emphasis on extrinsic compression on the tendon from, for example, acromial spurs leading to degeneration and tears. However, basic science research has placed a greater importance on intrinsic factors including tendinosis and rotator cuff vascularity.

Reduced cellularity and metabolism have been shown at the edges of tears, especially in large tears, which may influence capacity to heal.

Matthews TJW et al. In-vivo measurement of tissue metabolism in rotator cuff tendons: implications for surgical management. J Bone Joint Surg Br 2007;89:633–8.

Tears usually occur following degeneration of the tendon. Eccentric load is an important factor in tear propagation. Traumatic tears occur in patients younger than 50 years. In the elderly, minimal trauma can cause a tear in a degenerate cuff.

Clinical Presentation

The incidence of asymptomatic rotator cuff tears in those over 60 is 30% and increases with age. It should be noted that rotator cuff tendinosis and consequently tears are part of a normal aging process. Most tendon tears will occur in the presence of pre-existing tendinosis. When a tear occurs the remaining rotator cuff will compensate for this, hence the possibility of having an asymptomatic tear. As the tear progresses the ability to compensate reduces, increasing the chance of symptoms. Symptoms generally mimic those of subacromial pain. Massive cuff tears present with clear weakness in the affected rotator cuff, scapular hitching or pseudo paralysis indicating a decompensated rotator cuff. A full rotator cuff muscle testing is done as described in the preceding section. Wasting might be evident in the supraspinous and infraspinous area.

Traumatic rotator cuff tears occur after an obvious injury, for example, glenohumeral dislocation or fall onto an outstretched hand. The tears can be sub classified into acute traumatic tears or acute-on-chronic, in which a pre-existing tear worsens following trauma. Traumatic tears are more likely to be symptomatic as the remaining rotator cuff has not had the ability to compensate.

Rotator cuff tears can be demonstrated with a rotator lag sign. This is where the arm is passively placed in maximal external rotation and the arm drops as the patient is unable to maintain the position with muscle contraction. External rotation lag is more easily demonstrable than abductor weakness due to deltoid compensation. An inability to externally rotate in abduction indicates an infraspinatus tear which can be technically more difficult to repair.

Other muscles can be tested with the lag test. Subscapularis tear occurs in around 5% of patients and is demonstrated with internal rotation weakness. Asking the patient to keep the hand lifted off the lumbar spine in full internal rotation is used to assess this. Full thickness subscapularis tears can also demonstrate increased passive external rotation. In supraspinatus tears, the patient is unable to sustain the empty can position. The 'hornblower sign' is used to test teres minor—the patient is unable to sustain a position of abduction, external rotation and forward elevation.

Investigation

In addition to size it is important to characterise the chronicity, traumatic or atraumatic tear, degree of retraction, quality of tissue, delamination, wasting of the muscles, fatty infiltration, and any associated stiffness.

Investigations should start with an AP and axillary radiograph. The gold standard investigation is MRI which has good specificity and can identify fatty infiltration as well as other shoulder pathology.

Ultrasound is cheaper and faster but is operator dependent. Sensitivity and specificity is very good for medium to large tears, but smaller or partial thickness tears can be difficult to diagnose. Ultrasound will not give an accurate assessment of the degree of muscle wasting and fatty infiltration.

Muscle Changes in Cuff Tears

The chronicity of a cuff tear can affect management decisions. Wasting is evident in the supraspinatus and infraspinatus fossa in longstanding tears, and there may be stiffness and radiographic changes

Goutallier classified the degree of muscle involvement on CT (Table 2.11).

In practice grade 3 and 4 indicate a poor prognosis, as even if the cuff is repairable, the muscle is unlikely to function.

Management

There is surprisingly poor quality evidence on the management of rotator cuff tears given the prevalence of the condition. With an increasing prevalence of rotator cuff tears with age they can be considered a normal aging process. Conservative and surgical management have been advocated with evidence to support both modalities. Interestingly, Khatri performed a meta-analysis looking at the natural history of rotator cuff tears in patients enrolled in randomised controlled trials. They demonstrated a consistent pattern of improvement in tears treated both conservatively and surgically. Therefore, patients with degenerate rotator cuff tears should undergo a period of conservative management before considering surgical intervention.

Khatri C, Ahmed I, Parsons H, Smith NA, Lawrence TM, Modi CS, Drews SJ, Bhabra G, Parsons NR, Underwood M, Metcalfe AJ. The natural history of full-thickness rotator cuff tears

Table 2.11 Goutallier classification

Grade 0	Normal muscle
Grade 1	Some fatty streaks
Grade 2	Less than 50% fatty muscle atrophy
Grade 3	50% fatty muscle atrophy
Grade 4	Greater than 50% fatty muscle atrophy

in randomized controlled trials: a systematic review and meta-analysis. Am J Sports Med. 2019;47(7):1734–43.

Surgical management depends on patient factors and tear characteristics. Patient characteristics include age, smoking status, co morbidities and occupation. Tear characteristics include size, location, chronicity, muscle involvement, mechanism and associated arthritis. A greater age of patient (>70) and size of tear confers a poorer outcome. Arthroscopic and open techniques for surgical repair using contemporary suture anchor techniques are comparable. Published rates of re-tear are as high as 45%, which does appear to have a small negative affect on outcome compared to healed rotator cuff repairs. However, a significant increase in Oxford shoulder score was seen for all surgery with outcome reducing by approximately 3 points for healed repairs, re-tears and irreparable tears respectively.

Carr A, Cooper C, Campbell MK, Rees J, Moser J, Beard DJ, Fitzpatrick R, Gray A, Dawson J, Murphy J, Bruhn H, Cooper D, Ramsay C. Effectiveness of open and arthroscopic rotator cuff repair (UKUFF): a randomised controlled trial. Bone Joint J. 2017;99(1):107–15.

Symptoms from traumatic cuff tears are more challenging to manage and surgical repair should be considered at an early stage. Repairable traumatic cuff tears in younger patients can become irreparable in time. 40–50% of patients with full thickness cuff tears treated non-operatively had a progression in size over 18–24 months.

Maman E, Harris C, White L, Tomlinson G, Shashank M, Boynton E. Outcome of nonoperative treatment of symptomatic rotator cuff tears monitored by magnetic resonance imaging. J. Bone Joint Surg Am 2009;91(8):1898–906.

Mall NA, Kim HM, Keener JD, Steger-May K, Teefey SA, Middleton WD, Stobbs G, Yamaguchi K. Symptomatic progression of asymptomatic rotator cuff tears: a prospective study of clinical and sonographic variables. J. Bone Joint Surg Am. 2010;92(16):2623–33.

Acromioclavicular Joint Osteoarthritis

The acromioclavicular joint (ACJ) is usually the first in the body to develop osteoarthritic changes. Its small surface area combined with a large load demand means that force per unit area is very high and resulting repetitive micro-trauma leads to cartilage loss. Degenerative changes can be seen as early as the second decade. The ACJ has a small meniscus that can become degenerate, similar to the menisci in the knee. Therefore, symptoms can be present without any radiological changes. Repetitive load bearing above shoulder height accelerates degeneration.

Osteolysis of the distal clavicle is a rare condition that can affect the young (<40) patient, often with a history of lifting heavy weights. The condition is poorly understood but most likely relates to overload of the ACJ.

If activity modification and NSAIDs are ineffective then steroid injection of the joint can be considered. This is more effective in younger than older patients, and benefit can be felt for up to five years. In cases resistant to non-operative measures ACJ excision can be performed arthroscopically or open. The distal 1 cm of the clavicle is removed. Arthroscopic surgery has the benefit of allowing other pathologies to be addressed during the same sitting. There is a very high proportion of good or excellent outcomes after ACJ excision in patients with confirmed osteoarthritis.

Hossain S, Jacobs LG, Hashmi R. The long-term effectiveness of steroid injections in primary acromioclavicular joint arthritis: a five-year prospective study. J Shoulder Elbow Surg. 2008;17(4):535–8.

Kay SP, Dragoo JL, Lee R. Long-term results of arthroscopic resection of the distal clavicle with concomitant subacromial decompression. Arthroscopy. 2003;19(8):805–9.

Os Acromiale

This results from an unfused secondary ossification centre and is present in 3% of the population. It is a normal finding up to the age of 25. Os acromiale most commonly occurs at the junction of the meso- and meta-acromion. It is rare for an os acromiale to cause symptoms in isolation. Imaging of the rotator cuff is important due to the increased incidence of rotator cuff tears. Clinical features include pain on palpation of the os acromiale. Ultrasound guided injections are useful to confirm the diagnosis.

Treatment is challenging but surgical options are excision or fusion. Excision is reserved for os acromiale between the pre and meso acromion. Fusion with bone grafting is challenging with unpredictable outcomes. Many fusion patients will require a second stage to remove metalwork or to perform an acromioplasty.

Biceps Tendinopathy

The long head of biceps passes through the glenohumeral joint and the bicipital groove. The overlying glenohumeral ligament can stretch and cause instability of the tendon and subluxation medially. Patients feel anterior pain radiating down towards the elbow. Yergason's test and Speed test are specific for biceps tendinopathy. Ultrasound or MRI can show tendinopathy, fluid within the biceps tendon sheath, subluxation or dislocation.

Management depends on the severity of the symptoms and the state of the biceps tendon. Spontaneous rupture can occur in severe cases of biceps tendinopathy causing a consequent "popeye" sign. Interestingly, this often resolves the patient's preceding symptoms and does not require further treatment unless associated with a symptomatic rotator cuff tear. Conservative management includes physiotherapy with or without an injection into the biceps tendon sheath. Subluxation or dislocation can put the subscapularis tendon at risk and so there should be a lower threshold for surgical intervention. Surgical options are long head of biceps tenotomy or tenodesis. There is no difference in function or pain between the two techniques. Tenotomy is simpler and cheaper so should be used in the majority of cases.

Gurnani N, van Deurzen DF, Janmaat VT, van den Bekerom MP. Tenotomy or tenodesis for pathology of the long head of the biceps brachii; a systematic review and meta-analysis. Knee Surg Sports Traumatol Arthrosc. 2016;24(12):3765–71.

Scapulothoracic Pain

Scapulothoracic pain is associated with muscle patterning abnormalities which are covered in the instability section of this chapter. Snapping scapula can be present in the normal shoulder, with overuse or with normal use in shoulders with a structural abnormality. The causes are illustrated in Fig. 2.14. The mainstay of treatment for functional and inflammatory causes is non-operative, with physical therapy and NSAIDs. Bursae can be injected with steroid and excised in recalcitrant cases. Surgical intervention is rare.

Total Shoulder Replacement

Charles Neer is credited with the development of modern techniques for shoulder replacement. Initially, humeral head replacement was designed for proximal humeral fractures; as good results were obtained, the scope was extended to arthritis of the shoulder.

The first replacement of the humeral head was performed by Neer using a Vitallium prosthesis in 1951. Glenoid components were developed in the early 1970s to improve shoulder biomechanics and function. Stability, restoration of version, balance of soft tissues and tension in the soft tissues are critical to good function.

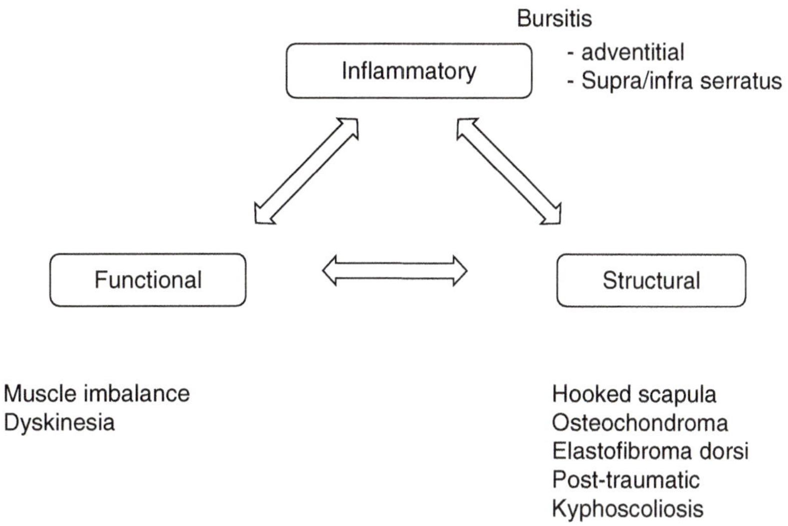

Fig. 2.14 Causes of scapulothoracic pain

Anatomical Relationships

Humeral Head

The average radius of curvature of the humeral head is 24 mm and the average thickness is 19 mm. The absolute values vary in different patients, but the inter-relationship of these two variables is relatively constant at a ratio of 0.7–0.9.

The humeral head is retroverted by 10–55°; compared to the transepicondylar axis; the average is approximately 30°.

The superior extent of the humeral head lies 8–10 mm superior to the highest point of the greater tuberosity. The centre of rotation of the humeral head is medial and posterior to the axis of the humeral shaft.

The neck shaft angle is described as the angle between the axis of the humeral shaft and the base of the articular fragment. The angle is 40–45° (Fig. 2.15).

Glenoid

The glenoid is pear-shaped (wider inferiorly). The articular cartilage is thin at the centre and thicker at the periphery. This makes the glenoid articular surface more concave to match the convexity of the humeral head. The bony glenoid is relatively flat. The radius of curvature of the humeral head is 2–3 mm less than the radius of curvature of the glenoid.

Glenoid offset is the perpendicular distance between the deepest part of the glenoid and the lateral aspect of base of coracoid. Lateral glenohumeral offset is the perpendicular distance between the lateral border of greater tuberosity and the lateral aspect of the base of the coracoid process. If this distance is reduced then the lever arm of the deltoid is also reduced, impairing abduction power. If the distance is increased following arthroplasty then the joint is overstuffed, resulting in loss of movement.

Glenoid depth is the percentage of the humeral head that is covered by the glenoid and labrum. It is approximately 28% on average.

Component Design in Total Shoulder Replacement

Humeral Component Design

Humeral component design can be split into resurfacing, stemless or stemmed. Hemiarthroplasty was traditionally the favoured

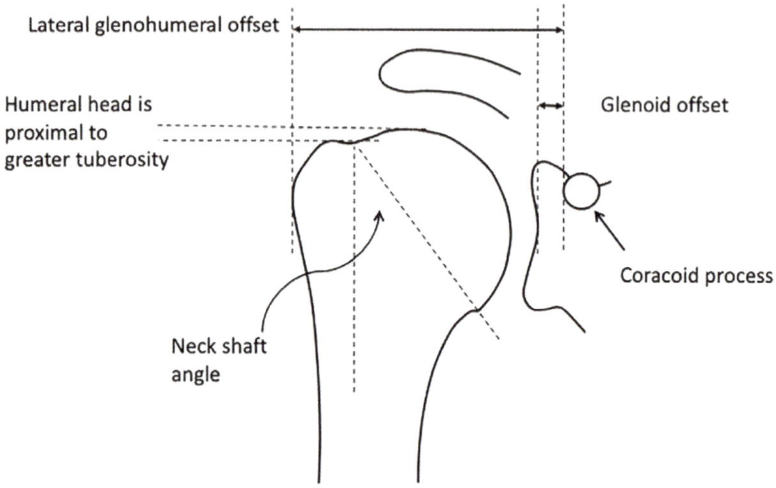

Fig. 2.15 The anatomical relationships of bony landmarks around the shoulder

operation for shoulder arthritis. Resurfacing hemiarthroplasty was, therefore, a common operation to ensure humerus bone stock was maintained. Total shoulder replacement has now superseded hemiarthoplasty due to its improved outcomes and consequently resurfacing has becoming less popular due to the challenges of getting good glenoid exposure.

Stemless humeral components were designed to overcome the challenge of glenoid exposure while maintaining humeral bone stock. It relies on metaphyseal fixation. Some stemmed designs have the additional advantage of being modular, thus allowing the stem to remain in situ during revision cases and exchange of the bearing surfaces, e.g. anatomic to reverse. These are commonly termed "platform" stems.

For all component design, the humeral head should be reconstructed close to its anatomical shape and size to restore lateral glenohumeral offset. The perpendicular distance between the lateral margin of the acromion and the lateral aspect of greater tuberosity is an indicator of restoration of offset.

Modular heads enable different head sizes to be matched to different stems to achieve the best fit. Any overhang of the humeral head either anteriorly or posteriorly should be avoided (Table 2.12).

An offset humeral head matches the normal anatomy more closely, as opposed to components where the centre of the humeral head is in line with the humeral shaft axis. This is because the anatomical humeral head centre is medial and posterior to the axis of the humeral shaft. Proximal cementation of the stem seems to work as well as full cementation.

Glenoid Component Design

The bony glenoid is pear-shaped and hence a prosthetic pear-shaped glenoid will achieve maximum bone cover and bone support. An oval glenoid will overhang anterosuperiorly and anteroinferiorly and pressure from the humeral head in these areas may lead to loosening. In addition, a pear-shaped glenoid allows greater ROM before internal impingement occurs compared with an oval glenoid.

Adequate bone support of the glenoid component is important for better survival. Concentric reaming is used to improve contact.

Non-contained defects in the glenoid rim require augmentation by bone graft or metal augments. Cement does not function well in non-contained defects.

Metal-backed glenoid components tend to increase the thickness of the component, which can lateralise the joint line and weaken the abductor lever arm. If a metal-backed component is chosen, more reaming of the glenoid may be required. There is a risk of dissociation of polyethylene from the metal backing.

Table 2.12 The result of humeral component malpositioning

Humeral component malpositioning	Effect on function
Anterior overhang of humeral head	Excess tension on the subscapularis Posterior impingement of uncovered metaphysis on the glenoid
Oversizing the humeral head	Increase in the lateral glenohumeral offset Tightening of the soft tissue envelope Reduction in the range of motion Rupture of the subscapularis
Undersizing the humeral head	Reduction of the lever arm of the deltoid Internal impingement of the humerus and cuff on the glenoid Instability
Inferior positioning of the humeral head	Prominence of greater tuberosity Impingement of greater tuberosity against the acromion
Varus stem alignment	Head will be medial and inferior Overstuffed joint Increased lateral glenohumeral offset Greater tuberosity may be prominent and impinge on the acromion
Valgus stem positioning	Head will be superior and laterally placed
Retroversion of the head	Posterior instability Rotator cuff rupture
Anteversion of the head	Loss of external rotation

Cemented all-poly glenoid components are the most commonly used. Multiple small pegs are preferred to counter the shear stress. Keeled components are an option in rheumatoid arthritis and these tend to compensate, to some extent, increased shear forces due to the absence of the rotator cuff. These have however fallen out of favour on account of loosening due to the 'windshield wiper' effect. Reverse shoulder replacements are commonly used in patients with deficient cuff.

Erosion of the posterior margin of the glenoid may occur in osteoarthritis causing either a biconcave glenoid (Walch B2) or retroverted glenoid. This produces a more surgically challenging glenoid reconstruction. Techniques to correct the retroversion include the use of augmented glenoids, bone grafting the defect or eccentric reaming of the anterior glenoid. Hemiarthroplasty should be avoided if possible in patients with posterior glenoid erosion due to less favourable outcomes.

Types of Shoulder Replacement Prostheses

There are several types of prostheses depending on the degree of constraint.

- Unconstrained—no constraint between the humeral head and the glenoid. This group includes Neer-type shoulder replacements and cup arthroplasty.
- Semiconstrained—this group includes hooded glenoid components, which provide some constraint to humeral head movement. Examples are the Neer hooded replacement and DANA (Designed after Natural Anatomy).
- Constrained ball and socket—the glenoid is specially designed to capture the humeral head and improve stability. Disadvantages include breakage and loosening.
- Constrained reverse ball and socket—the ball is mounted on the glenoid and the socket is placed on the humeral head.

Indications

The indications for shoulder arthroplasty are osteoarthritis, rheumatoid arthritis, traumatic arthritis, osteonecrosis and rotator cuff arthropathy.

Contraindications

Contraindications for shoulder arthroplasty are active infection, loss of both deltoid and rotator cuff function and gross instability. Massive rotator cuff tear is a contraindication for total shoulder replacement, although hemiarthroplasty with a cuff tear arthropathy head can be performed if a reverse total shoulder replacement is not feasible.

Surgical Considerations

Several surgical aspects should be considered prior to shoulder arthroplasty:

- Glenoid morphology—CT scans are helpful in determining the exact glenoid morphology. Retroversion should be corrected into normal parameters.
- Subscapularis management—Deltopectoral approach is the gold standard for anatomic total shoulder arthroplasty. A recognized complication is subscapularis failure. Therefore, careful consideration should be made as to how subscapularis is released and repaired. Options for subscapularis release are:
  - Subscapularis tenotomy
  - Subscapularis peel (the whole of the subscapularis insertion is peeled off)
  - Lesser tuberosity osteotomy
  - Subscapularis sparing approaches (in which the superior tendinous portion is kept attached and windows above and below are utilized—surgically challenging)
- Soft tissue balance—the soft tissues must be balanced to provide optimum function. Osteoarthritis commonly causes posterior glenoid wear and anterior capsular contracture. Anterior capsulectomy is vital in balancing the soft tissues. It is rare for posterior capsular plication or release to be needed. A 360° subscapularis release is also important to ensure external rotation is gained post-operatively following subscapularis repair. A small proportion of patients will have anterior glenoid wear and consequent posterior capsular contracture. The posterior capsule needs to be released in these patients to balance the soft tissues.
- Patients with osteoarthritis may have osteophytes on the humeral head. These need to be removed to prevent impingement of the prosthesis.
- Patients with rheumatoid arthritis generally require cemented components due to osteopenia.
- The outcome in patients with post-traumatic arthritis is less satisfactory due to soft tissue scarring and malunion of the tuberosities which need to be left in situ. CT scan with 3D reconstruction can help give an indication if the tuberosities are in an acceptable position to consider anatomic TSR. Alternative options would include reverse total shoulder arthroplasty or hemiarthroplasty with tuberosity osteotomy and fixation.

Glenoid Replacement in Shoulder Osteoarthritis

The advantage is more reliable pain relief, especially if glenoid erosion is noted at the time of shoulder surgery. If the glenoid articular surface does not exhibit significant erosion at the time of surgery, the results of hemiarthroplasty are comparable to total shoulder arthroplasty.

The disadvantages are

- Technically difficult—the glenoid is often retroverted with posterior erosion and it requires reaming of the anterior rim to provide circumferential bone support.
- Excess retroversion of the replaced component may predispose to posterior instability.
- In relatively young, high-demand patients, there is a high risk of loosening and glenoid replacement should be avoided.
- Osteolysis from polyethylene debris can lead to loosening of the glenoid component with consequent risk of failure.
- Increases operative time and blood loss.

Indications for Hemiarthroplasty

Total shoulder replacement provides significantly superior results compared to hemiarthroplasty for glenohumeral osteoarthritis. Hemiarthroplasty is occasionally indicated in young patients with preserved glenoid anatomy, for example, in patients with avascular necrosis. Hemiarthroplasty can also be used in severe glenoid bone loss when glenoid fixation is not possible. This commonly occurs in the presence of cuff deficiency. The use of a cuff tear arthropathy (CTA) head, a modular head with an addition superior articulation to articulate with the acromion, can be used in these circumstances.

Radnay CS et al. Total shoulder replacement compared with humeral head replacement for the treatment of primary glenohumeral arthritis. A systematic review. J Shoulder Elbow Surg 16(4); 396–402: 2007. Review of 23 studies, 1952 patients, mean follow up 43 months. Total shoulder provided better pain relief, forward elevation, external rotation and patient satisfaction. Revision rate of total shoulder was 6.5% compared to 10.2% for humeral head replacements.

Replacement of Both Shoulder and Elbow in Rheumatoid Arthritis

Patients with rheumatoid arthritis can commonly have degenerative joint disease of both the shoulder and elbow. Reconstructive options are compromised even further due to the increased incidence of rotator cuff insufficiency due to the inflammatory arthropathy. When considering arthroplasty for both joints it is important to either have short humeral stems for both allowing at least a 6 cm gap of normal humerus or have a cement mantle that is in continuity between each stem. Some contemporary reverse TSR designs have stemless humeral components which are helpful in managing these challenging patients when cuff insufficiency is a feature.

In a study with long follow-up, total shoulder replacement in patients with rheumatoid disease resulted in preserved ROM and no pain in most patients after a mean of 20 years.

Betts HM, Abu-Rajab R, Nunn T, Brooksbank AJ. Total shoulder replacement in rheumatoid disease. A 16 to 23 year follow up. J Bone Joint Surg Br 2009;91(9):1197–200. 58 shoulders, 19.8 year follow up. Most patients had preserved movement range and no pain.

Complications of Total Shoulder Replacement

Early Complications

Early complications can be subscapularis failure, instability, infection, nerve injury, impingement and humeral fracture.

Subscapularis repair will depend on the release performed at surgery. Healing must occur whichever method is used, unless a subscapularis sparing method is utilized. Subscapularis sparing approaches are theoretically very appealing but surgically very challenging. Different types of healing are required for the different releases:

1. Tenotomy—Requiring tendon-tendon healing
2. Peel—Requiring tendon-bone healing
3. Lesser tuberosity osteotomy (LTO)—Requiring bone-bone healing

Clinical outcomes remain similar for all the above techniques with better strength demonstrated for LTO in biomechanical studies. Fixation methods include simple sutures, transosseus sutures, anchors or screws.

Early subscapularis failure is a significant concern and early postoperative rehabilitation needs to be mindful to protect the subscapularis repair until healing occurs (6–12 weeks).

Instability can be due to poor component alignment, poor soft tissue repair or deficient bone stock.

The routine use of perioperative antibiotic prophylaxis is recommended. Cultibacterium (previously called Proprionobacterium) acnes is a common skin commensal that is found around the shoulder and axilla. It is a common pathogen in shoulder infections causing a low grade infection that can go undetected. Inflammatory markers are often normal and biopsies require extended cultures to be positive. There should be a high index of suspicion for patients with unexplained pain following total shoulder arthroplasty. Multiple biopsies through arthroscopic cannulae taken with different instruments are required to prove or disprove *C acnes* infection.

Other infections, including Gram-negative organism can cause acute infection. It is reasonable to manage early infections with debridement and retention of implants (DAIR) with a strong emphasis on obtaining positive culture results and sensitivities to direct antibiotic management.

Late infection is commonly haematogenous. A two-stage revision with use of antibiotic-loaded cement is considered to be the most reliable method of managing infection. Antibiotic cement spacers are useful in maintaining soft tissue tension in first stage revisions.

Impingement can occur with improper sizing or positioning of components. An inferiorly placed humeral component will lead to impingement of the greater tuberosity against the acromion.

Risk of humeral fracture is less than 1%. Fractures of the humeral shaft are more often intraoperative as opposed to postoperative. Excessively forceful external rotation of the arm to gain exposure or excess force while reaming or pressurising cement are common causes of humerus shaft fractures. The removal of well-cemented humeral stems can be difficult and may lead to iatrogenic fracture. If detected intraoperatively, fractures around the stem should be stabilised with struts and cerclage wires or by using a long stem implant. Fractures distal to the tip of the stem can be managed by plate fixation. Glenoid fractures are rare and are caused by retraction or over-reaming in osteoporotic bone. Bone grafting is an option.

Most nerve injuries are neurapraxias (usually neurapraxia of the brachial plexus due to stretching) and should be followed up with electromyography to monitor recovery. Direct injuries to axillary nerve, radial nerve (in patients with humeral shaft fracture) and musculocutaneous nerve are also reported, albeit rarely.

Late Complications

1. Loosening of humeral or glenoid component

There is generally a low risk of humeral loosening causing clinical symptoms (1–2%), and cemented and cementless components have similar survival.

Radiolucent lines around stems are more common around cementless stems than cemented stems, but do not necessarily indicate loosening. The subsidence rate of cementless stems is higher than that of cemented stems.

Causes of glenoid loosening include humeral head translation leading to glenoid edge loading. This may be evident radiographically as progressive lucency, migration of the component, fracture of cement and lucency at the prosthesis–cement interface. Asymptomatic radiolucent lines are not an indication in themselves for revision.

2. Radiolucent lines

Radiolucent lines are seen in two-thirds of the glenoid components in the early postoperative period. Despite this high incidence, clinical failure of the glenoid component is relatively infrequent.

3. Instability

Instability may be early or late. Table 2.13 outlines the directions and causes of instability.

Table 2.13 Directions and causes of instability

Direction of instability	Cause
Anterior	Subscapularis rupture (most common cause) Anteverted humeral component Rupture of anterior fibres of deltoid Oversized humeral head
Posterior	Rupture of rotator cuff Retroverted humerus or glenoid Laxity of posterior capsule
Superior	Rupture of rotator cuff Unopposed pull of deltoid against weak rotator cuff Deficient coracoacromial arch
Inferior	Deltoid dysfunction Inferior placement of the humeral head Excess removal of proximal humerus

4. Rotator cuff tears

Rotator cuff tear incidence increases with age. This remains an issue with patients having total shoulder replacement. Careful consideration of cuff function should have been performed prior to initial surgery to determine whether an anatomic or reverse total shoulder replacement is more appropriate. Early or late failure of the rotator cuff, however, is a significant complication causing pain and loss of function.

Rotator cuff repairs are challenging in these patients due to humeral components preventing adequate fixation for anchors with generally unsatisfactory results. Decompensated cuff tears lead to incongruency of the arthroplasty and accelerated glenoid loosening. If symptoms warrant treatment, revision surgery to reverse total shoulder replacement is the gold standard.

5. Wear

Glenoid polyethylene components are subject to surface wear as well as to fatigue failure.

6. Heterotopic ossification

Heterotopic ossification is seen in up to 40% patients after total shoulder replacement. Generally the ossification is not severe enough to restrict movements or require removal of the prosthesis.

7. Stiffness

Stiffness can be due to oversized components or poor soft tissue balance. A full 360° release of subscapularis is usually adequate to negate stiffness. Occasionally, lengthening of the subscapularis tendon can be performed to improve external rotation.

Periprosthetic Humeral Fractures

There are three types of periprosthetic humeral fracture:

- Type A—extends proximally from the tip of the prosthesis.
- Type B—fractures around the tip of the humeral stem.
- Type C—fractures distal to the tip of the humeral stem.

Type A fractures are likely to require revision of the humeral component. Type B and C fractures can be managed non-operatively if adequate alignment is achieved, or by open reduction and internal fixation.

Revision Total Shoulder Replacement

Loosening of the glenoid component is managed by removal of the glenoid component. In patients with an intact rotator cuff and good bone stock, it may be possible to implant another glenoid component.

Revision of the humeral component may be needed in patients with infection or loosening. Removal of a well-fixed humeral component carries the risk of loss of bone stock of the proximal humerus; accepting a malpositioned component and taking advantage of modularity is an option.

Resection Arthroplasty of the Shoulder

Resection arthroplasty is indicated in patients with persistent infection or inadequate bone stock for revision.

Loss of the fulcrum of the shoulder leads to loss of abduction and functional results are generally unsatisfactory.

Shoulder Replacement in Rotator Cuff Tears

The absence of a functioning rotator cuff causes the humeral head to migrate superiorly and put pressure on the superior rim of the glenoid. This edge loading, known as the 'rocking horse phenomenon' is a factor in early loosening of the glenoid component.

A total shoulder replacement should be avoided in individuals with rotator cuff tears unless the cuff tear is reparable. A shoulder hemiarthroplasty obviates the possibility of glenoid loosening.

Hemiarthroplasty is possibly the most viable option. The prosthetic humeral head depends on the intact coracoacromial arch to prevent unrestricted upward migration and a functioning deltoid is essential.

The reverse shoulder prosthesis is an option for patients with massive cuff tears.

The Reverse Shoulder Prosthesis

Developed in France in the 1980s based on a concept by Prof. Grammont, the reverse shoulder prosthesis (also known as the Delta shoulder) is a semiconstrained implant.

Matsen FA 3rd, Boileau P, Walch G, et al. The reverse total shoulder arthroplasty. J Bone Joint Surg Am 2007;89:660–7.

In the reverse shoulder prosthesis, the centre of rotation is in the scapula (Fig. 2.16). The humeral head is a socket instead of a ball. The convex articular surface (ball) is mounted on the scapula. Hence the centre of rotation is moved medial and inferior. The deltoid gets a longer fulcrum, hence a mechanical advantage.

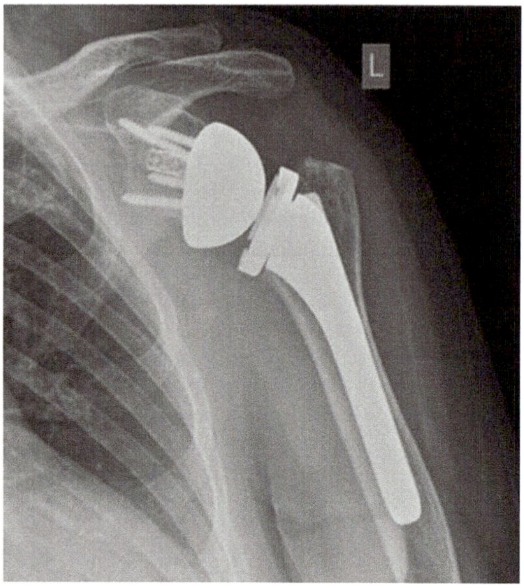

Fig. 2.16 Reverse total shoulder replacement

These prostheses have been used in patients with large rotator cuff tears in an effort to reduce the shear forces on the glenoid and improve the lever arm for deltoid. Absence of deltoid function is a contraindication for the reverse shoulder.

The Centre of rotation (COR) in rTSR is medialised and is often more inferior than an anatomic shoulder joint. This creates a larger distance between the deltoid and centre of rotation and therefore a longer moment arm, reducing the work required of the deltoid muscle to move the shoulder. In addition to improving deltoid efficiency, stability and loosening should be taken in to consideration. The closer the COR is to the glenoid bone/prosthesis interface the less loosening there will be at this site. Medialised glenospheres have a COR close to the glenoid bone, while lateralised glenospheres have a COR of over 5 mm from the glenoid bone. Lateralisation of the glenosphere aims to bring the joint surface away from the glenoid and therefore reduce notching. Glenosphere lateralisation may also lateralise the humeral component and therefore the deltoid, increasing moment arm and improving efficiency.

The humeral component can also be divided in to lateralised or medialised. A line is drawn vertically down the centre of the humerus and a parallel line transects the midpoint of the humeral sided prosthetic articular surface. If the distance between the two lines is less than 15 mm the design is "medialised humerus", and if greater than 15 mm is "lateralised humerus". A lateralised humerus design aims to increase deltoid wrapping around the proximal humerus and therefore improve stability. Deltoid-COR distance will also be increased and efficiency improved.

The beneficial effects of lateralisation and inferiorly displacing the articulation must be balanced against overtensioning of soft tissues and chance of acromial fracture.

The reverse total shoulder arthroplasty. Matsen FA. J Bone Joint Surg Am 89;660–667: 2007.

Complications of reverse shoulder include scapular notching (Table 2.14), dislocation, glenoid loosening, fracture of the acromion, fracture of scapular spine and nerve injury.

Ten years survival has been reported as 93% with an overall complication rate of 29%. NJR data

Bacle G, Nové-Josserand L, Garaud P, Walch G. Long-term outcomes of reverse total shoulder arthroplasty: a follow-up of a previous study. J Bone Joint Surg Am. 2017;99(6):454–461.

Reverse total shoulder arthroplasty has traditionally been reserved for elderly patients. The promising results seen in these patients has expanded the indications to younger patients. Sershon reported a success rate of 75% in patients under 60 at 2.8 years but long term studies are awaited.

Sershon RA, Van Thiel GS, Lin EC, McGill KC, Cole BJ, Verma NN, Romeo AA, Nicholson GP. Clinical outcomes of reverse total shoulder arthroplasty in patients aged younger than 60 years. J Shoulder Elbow Surg 2014;23(3):395–400.

Table 2.14 Classification of scapular notching by Sirveaux

Grade	Feature
Grade 1	Notching limited to scapular pillar
Grade 2	Extending to inferior screw of base plate
Grade 3	Beyond the inferior screw
Grade 4	Approaching the central peg.

NJR data has confirmed a rapid increase in the use of reverse total shoulder arthroplasty. 35% were performed in 2013 rising to 56% in 2017 [NJR UK annual report 2018]. The indications for surgery have remained the same, thus confirming that reverse total shoulder arthroplasty is being used for patients with primary osteoarthritis. Patients over the age of 70 particularly appear to be more likely to undergo reverse total shoulder arthroplasty, presumably due to the increased risk of cuff insufficiency.

Hemiarthroplasty using a cuff tear arthropathy (CTA) head, which articulates with the acromion as well as the glenoid can be used in patients with severe glenoid erosions where glenoid fixation is not possible.

Further Reading

Matsumura N, Ogawa K, Kobayashi S, Oki S, Watanabe A, Ikegami H, Toyama Y. Morphologic features of humeral head and glenoid version in the normal glenohumeral joint. J Shoulder Elbow Surg. 2014;23(11):1724–30.

Welsch G, Mamisch TC, Kikinis R, Schmidt R, Lang P, Forst R, Fitz W. CT-based preoperative analysis of scapula morphology and glenohumeral joint geometry. J Comput Aided Surg. 2003;8:264–8.

Jaggi A, Lambert S. Rehabilitation for shoulder instability. Br J Sports Med. 2010;44:333–40.

Zacchilli MA, Owens BD. Epidemiology of shoulder dislocations presenting to the emergency departments in the United States. J Bone Joint Surg Am. 2010;92:542–9.

Robinson CM, Shur N, Sharpe T, Ray A, Murray IR. Injuries associated with traumatic anterior glenohumeral dislocations. J Bone Joint Surg Am. 2012;94:18–26.

Robinson CM, Howes J, Murdoch H, Will E, Graham C. Functional outcome and risk of recurrent instability after primary anterior shoulder dislocation in young patients. J Bone Joint Surg Am. 2006;88:2326–36.

Bankart AS. Recurrent or habitual dislocation of the shoulder joint. BMJ. 1923 Dec 15;2(3285):1132–3.

Burkhart SS, De Beer JF. Traumatic glenohumeral bone defects and their relationship to failure of arthroscopic Bankart repairs: significance of the inverted-pear glenoid and the humeral engaging Hill-Sachs lesion. Arthroscopy. 2000;16(7):677–94.

Neviaser TJ. The anterior labroligamentous periosteal sleeve avulsion lesion: a cause of anterior instability of the shoulder. Arthroscopy. 1993;9(1):17–21.

Brownson P, Donaldson O, et al. BESS/BOA Patient care pathways. Traumatic anterior shoulder instability. Shoulder and Elbow. 2015;7(3):214–26.

Smith TO, Drew BT, Toms AP. A meta-analysis of the diagnostic test accuracy of MRA and MRI for the detection of glenoid labral injury. Arch Orthop Trauma Surg. 2012;132:905–19.

Platzer P, Thalhammer G, Oberleitner G, et al. Displaced fractures of the greater tuberosity: a comparison of operative and nonoperative treatment. J Trauma. 2008;65:843–8.

Miller BS, Sonnabend DH, Hatrick C, O'leary S, Goldberg J, Harper W, Walsh WR. Should acute dislocations of the shoulder be immobilized in external rotation? A cadaveric study. J Shoulder Elbow Surg. 2004;13(6):589–92.

Harris JD, Gupta AK, Mann NA, et al. Long-term outcomes after Bankart shoulder stabilization. Arthroscopy. 2013;29:920–33.

McLaughlin HL. Posterior dislocation of the shoulder. J Bone Joint Surg Am. 1952;24:584–90.

Kim SH, Park JS, Jeong WK, Shin SK. The Kim test: a novel test for posteroinferior labral lesion of the shoulder – a comparison to the jerk test. Am J Sports Med. 2005;33:1188–92.

Kim SH, Ha KI, Yoo JC, Noh KC. Kim's lesion: an incomplete and concealed avulsion of the posteroinferior labrum in posterior or multidirectional posteroinferior instability of the shoulder. Arthroscopy. 2004;20:712–20.

Zuckerman JD, Rokito A. Frozen shoulder: a consensus definition. J Shoulder Elbow Surg. 2011;20(2):322–5.

Bunker TD, Anthony PP. The pathology of frozen shoulder. A Dupuytrens like disease. J Bone Joint Surg Br. 1995;77:677–83.

Hand GC, Athanasou NA, Matthews T, Carr AJ. The pathology of frozen shoulder. J Bone Joint Surg Br. 2007;89:928–32.

Hannafin JA, Chiaia TA. Adhesive capsulitis. A treatment approach. Clin Orthop Relat Res. 2000;372:95–109.

Nicholson JA, Slader B, Martindale A, Mckie S, Robinson M. Distension arthrogram in the treatment of adhesive capsulitis has a low rate of repeat intervention. Bone Joint J. 2020;102(5):606–10.

Quraishi NA, Johnston P, Bayer J, Crowe M, Chakrabarti AJ. Thawing the frozen shoulder. A randomised trial comparing manipulation under anaesthesia with hydrodilatation. J Bone Joint Surg Br. 2007;89(9):1197–200.

Thomas WJ, Jenkins EF, Owen JM, Sangster MJ, Kirubanandan R, Beynon C, Woods DA. Treatment of frozen shoulder by manipulation under anaesthetic: does the timing of treatment affect the outcome? J Bone Joint Surg Br. 2011;93(10):1377–81.

Woods DA, Loganathan K. Recurrence of frozen shoulder after manipulation under anaesthetic (MUA); the results of repeating the MUA. Bone Joint J. 2017;99(6):812–7.

Mehta SS, Singh HP, Pandey R. Comparative outcome of arthroscopic release for frozen shoulder in patients with and without diabetes. Bone Joint J. 2014;96(10):1355–8.

Collins DN, Harryman DT 2nd, Wirth MA. Shoulder arthroplasty for the treatment of inflammatory arthritis. J Bone Joint Surg Am. 2004;86:2489–96.

Bryant D, Litchfield R, Sandow M, et al. A comparison of pain, strength, range of motion, and functional outcomes after hemiarthroplasty and total shoulder arthroplasty in patients with osteoarthritis of the shoulder: a systematic review and meta-analysis. J Bone Joint Surg [Am]. 2005;87-A:1947–56.

Louwerens JK, et al. Prevalence of calcific deposits within the rotator cuff tendons in adults with and without subacromial pain syndrome: clinical and radiologic analysis of 1219 patients. J Shoulder Elbow Surg. 2015;24(10):1588–93.

Dong W, Goost H, Lin XB, Burger C, Paul C, Wang ZL, Zhang TY, Jiang ZC, Welle K, Kabir K. Treatment for shoulder impingement syndrome: a PRISMA systematic review and network meta-analysis. Medicine (Baltimore). 2015;94(10):e510.

Beard DJ, et al. Arthroscopic subacromial decompression for subacromial shoulder pain (CSAW): a multicentre, pragmatic, parallel group, placebo-controlled, three-group, randomised surgical trial. The Lancet. 2018;391(10118):329–38.

Matthews TJW, et al. In-vivo measurement of tissue metabolism in rotator cuff tendons: implications for surgical management. J Bone Joint Surg Br. 2007;89:633–8.

Khatri C, Ahmed I, Parsons H, Smith NA, Lawrence TM, Modi CS, Drews SJ, Bhabra G, Parsons NR, Underwood M, Metcalfe AJ. The natural history of full-thickness rotator cuff tears in randomized controlled trials: a systematic review and meta-analysis. Am J Sports Med. 2019;47(7):1734–43.

Carr A, Cooper C, Campbell MK, Rees J, Moser J, Beard DJ, Fitzpatrick R, Gray A, Dawson J, Murphy J, Bruhn H, Cooper D, Ramsay C. Effectiveness of open and arthroscopic rotator cuff repair (UKUFF): a randomised controlled trial. Bone Joint J. 2017;99(1):107–15.

Maman E, Harris C, White L, Tomlinson G, Shashank M, Boynton E. Outcome of nonoperative treatment of symptomatic rotator cuff tears monitored by magnetic resonance imaging. J. Bone Joint Surg Am. 2009;91(8):1898–906.

Mall NA, Kim HM, Keener JD, Steger-May K, Teefey SA, Middleton WD, Stobbs G, Yamaguchi K. Symptomatic progression of asymptomatic rotator cuff tears: a prospective study of clinical and sonographic variables. J. Bone Joint Surg Am. 2010;92(16):2623–33.

Hossain S, Jacobs LG, Hashmi R. The long-term effectiveness of steroid injections in primary acromioclavicular joint arthritis: a five-year prospective study. J Shoulder Elbow Surg. 2008;17(4):535–8.

Kay SP, Dragoo JL, Lee R. Long-term results of arthroscopic resection of the distal clavicle with concomitant subacromial decompression. Arthroscopy. 2003;19(8):805–9.

Gurnani N, van Deurzen DF, Janmaat VT, van den Bekerom MP. Tenotomy or tenodesis for pathology of the long head of the biceps brachii; a systematic review and meta analysis. Knee Surg Sports Traumatol Arthrosc. 2016;24(12):3765–71.

Radnay CS, et al. Total shoulder replacement compared with humeral head replacement for the treatment of primary glenohumeral arthritis. A systematic review. J Shoulder Elbow Surg. 2007;16(4):396–402.

Betts HM, Abu-Rajab R, Nunn T, Brooksbank AJ. Total shoulder replacement in rheumatoid disease. A 16 to 23 year follow up. J Bone Joint Surg Br. 2009;91(9):1197–200.

Matsen FA 3rd, Boileau P, Walch G, et al. The reverse total shoulder arthroplasty. J Bone Joint Surg Am. 2007;89:660–7.

Matsen FA. The reverse total shoulder arthroplasty. J Bone Joint Surg Am. 2007;89:660–7.

Bacle G, Nové-Josserand L, Garaud P, Walch G. Long-term outcomes of reverse total shoulder arthroplasty: a follow-up of a previous study. J Bone Joint Surg Am. 2017;99(6):454–61.

Sershon RA, Van Thiel GS, Lin EC, McGill KC, Cole BJ, Verma NN, Romeo AA, Nicholson GP. Clinical outcomes of reverse total shoulder arthroplasty in patients aged younger than 60 years. J Shoulder Elbow Surg. 2014;23(3):395–400.

3 Adult Pathology: Knee

Sanjeev Agarwal and J. S. Jayadeep

Osseous Anatomy

The knee has three compartments—the medial tibiofemoral compartment, the lateral tibiofemoral compartment and the patellofemoral joint. The tibiofemoral compartments are bi-condylar, while the patellofemoral joint is a saddle joint. The proximal tibia has a convex lateral plateau and a concave medial plateau. The lateral tibial plateau is at a higher level than the medial plateau. The intercondylar area provides attachments to the cruciates and the menisci. The cruciate ligaments are intraarticular but extrasynovial structures.

There is approximately 3 degrees varus alignment of the proximal tibia in relation to the anatomical axis, and an average of 7 degrees posterior slope. As a result of proximal tibial varus alignment, the joint line is 3 degrees varus in bipedal stance. During normal gait, the feet are closer to the midline compared to the standing position. This results in the joint line being more parallel to the ground during walking.

The distal femoral condyles are shaped distinctively as the medial femoral condyle is larger and distal; whereas the lateral femoral condyle is wider but smaller. The lateral distal femoral angle (LDFA) indicates the valgus alignment of the distal femoral condyles. The valgus is 3 to 7 degrees, making the LDFA 83 to 87 degrees (Fig. 3.1).

The articular surface of patella has three facets—medial, lateral and an odd facet. A longitudinal ridge separates the medial and lateral facets. The lateral facet is larger. The odd facet is at the distal end of the medial facet and articulates with the trochlea in deep flexion. The joint reaction force (JRF) on the patellofemoral joint can be up to five times body weight when an individual is weight bearing with the knee flexed.

The proximal fibula contributes to the superior tibio fibular joint but is extraarticular for the knee joint. The fibular styloid process provides attachment to the fibular collateral ligament and the biceps tendon, which are important lateral stabilising structures.

The knee has a rich vascular anastomosis contributed by medial and lateral branches of superior and inferior geniculate artery. In addition to these, the popliteal artery also gives a middle geniculate artery. The femoral artery supplies the knee through a descending geniculate artery. The anterior tibial contributes the anterior tibial recurrent arteries.

The femoral, obturator and sciatic nerves innervate the knee joint. The infrapatellar branch of the saphenous nerve supplies the skin over the patella and proximal tibia. Branches of this nerve are often divided in a midline approach to the joint.

S. Agarwal (✉)
University Hospital of Wales, Consultant Orthopaedic Surgeon, Cardiff, UK

J. S. Jayadeep
Consultant Orthopaedic Surgeon, North Cumbria NHS Foundation Trust, Cumbria, UK

S. Agarwal (ed.), *Current Orthopaedic Practice*, https://doi.org/10.1007/978-3-030-78529-1_3

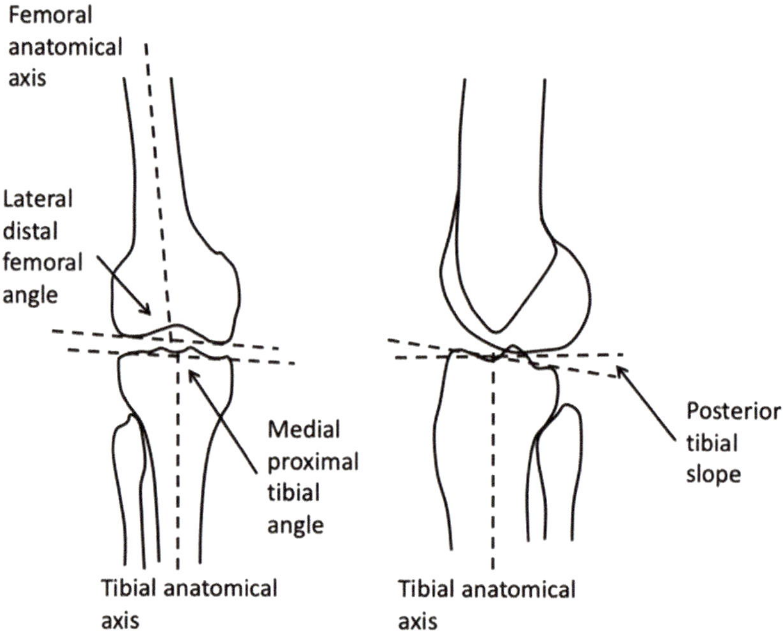

Fig. 3.1 Alignment of distal femur and proximal tibia in relation to mechanical axis

Meniscal Injuries

The medial and lateral menisci are fibrocartilaginous structures that function to transmit the load of weight bearing, increase contact area, and act as shock absorbers. They may also have a proprioceptive role, and act as secondary stabilisers in the absence of anterior cruciate ligament. Under normal loading, menisci transmit 50% load in extension.

The medial tibial plateau is concave and has greater congruence with the femoral condyle compared to the lateral plateau. Hence, loss of lateral meniscus leads to higher peak contact stress. The high contact stress on the lateral side is the cause for poor results in the long term after lateral meniscectomy compared to medial meniscectomy.

McNicholas MJ, Rowley DI, McGurty D, et al. Total meniscectomy in adolescence: a thirty-year follow-up. J Bone Joint Surg Br 2000;82:217–21. 80% patients had a good result after medial meniscectomy compared to 47% following lateral meniscectomy.

The menisci are composed of type I collagen with longitudinal and radial fibres. Longitudinal fibres help dissipate hoop stresses. The extracellular matrix has proteoglycans, elastin and glycoproteins. Proteoglycans regulate water content of the meniscus. Water moves out on loading and rehydration occurs on removal of load.

The medial meniscus is about 10 mm wide and is C shaped. The lateral meniscus is 12 mm wide, and is more rounded and mobile compared to medial meniscus. The medial meniscus is attached to the capsule via the coronary ligaments. The deep fibres of the medial collateral ligament (MCL) attach to the medial meniscus, and this limits the anteroposterior mobility of the medial meniscus. The lateral meniscus is not attached at the posterolateral area and hence is more mobile. The intermeniscal ligament connects the two menisci anteriorly. Medial meniscal tears are twice as common as lateral meniscal tears.

The meniscofemoral ligaments of Humphreys and Wrisberg arise from the lateral meniscus and pass anterior and posterior to the posterior cruciate ligament (PCL) respectively to attach to the femur (Fig. 3.2).

The medial, lateral and middle geniculate arteries vascularise the meniscus via the perivascular capillary plexus (PCP). At birth, the entire meniscus is vascular. By the second decade,

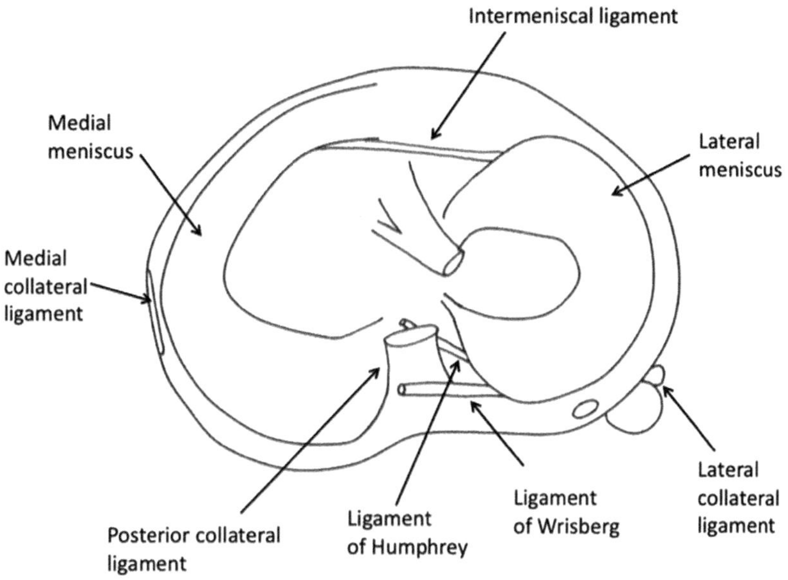

Fig. 3.2 Structures along the intercondylar area of tibia

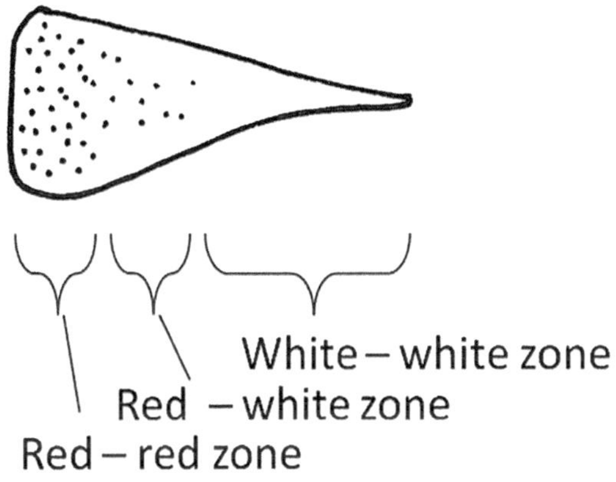

Fig. 3.3 Zones of vascularity of the meniscus

vascularity is limited to the outer third of the meniscus. Blood vessels are present in the outer 20–30% of the medial meniscus and the peripheral 10–25% of the lateral meniscus. The rest of the meniscus derives its nutrition from the synovial fluid.

Meniscal zones have been described which indicate the extent of blood supply and consequently influence repair and healing of meniscal tears. Zone 1 is red-red, Zone 2 is red—white and Zone 3 is white—white (Fig. 3.3). Red zone indicates presence of blood supply, while a white zone is inadequate blood supply. In zone 2, the tear is at the watershed with one side having blood supply and the other side being deficient. The prognosis is best when tears are within 4 mm from the periphery. This is the red-red zone, which corresponds to adequate blood supply.

Arnoczky SP, Warren RF. Microvasculature of the human meniscus. Am J Sports Med. 1982;10:90–5. Description of the blood supply to the meniscus.

Removal of the meniscus leads to a reduced contact area and increased pressure on the articular surfaces. This is manifested as loss and disaggregation of proteoglycans, and increase in hydration of the cartilage. In the long-term, it predisposes to loss of hyaline articular cartilage layer and degenerative arthritis.

McDermott, ID, Sharifi F, Bull AMJ, Gupte CM, Thomas RW, Amis, AA. The consequences of meniscectomy. J Bone Joint Surg Br 2006;88:1549–56.

Roos H, Lauren M, Adalberth T, et al. Knee osteoarthritis after meniscectomy: prevalence of radiographic changes after twenty-one years, compared with matched controls. Arthritis Rheum 1998;41:687–93. 107 patients studies 21 years after meniscectomy. The relative risk for developing arthritis was 14.

Classification of Meniscal Tears

Various classification systems have been proposed. They are based on the morphology and location of tear. A descriptive classification is illustrated in Fig. 3.4. In addition, complex tears may occur which do not bear resemblance to any described pattern.

Radial tears disrupt the circumferential collagen fibres, which are perpendicular to the direction of the tear. Loss of these fibres leads to loss of function of the meniscus as it is unable to withstand hoop stress.

The ISAKOS (International Society of Arthroscopy, Knee surgery and Orthopaedic Sports medicine) classification has been reported to have a good inter and intra observer reliability. The features evaluated are tear depth, location, radial location, central popliteal hiatus, tear pattern, quality of tissue, length of tear, amount and percentage of meniscus excised. It is a good research tool, although is limited in clinical usage.

Clinical Features

Meniscal tears present with intermittent pain and swelling of the knee. Patients may present with acute locking in bucket handle tears. Some may have symptoms in the past which settle and then recur. There is no history of trauma in most patients presenting with degenerate tears.

The clinical features are joint line tenderness corresponding to the site of meniscal tear. Various provocation tests like Apley compression test, Thessaly test or McMurray's test can be helpful. Some patients present with localised swelling adjacent to the joint line from a parameniscal cyst.

In acute anterior cruciate ligament injuries, lateral meniscal tears are more common, while medial meniscal tears are more often seen with chronic ACL injuries.

Imaging

Weight bearing x rays are helpful to check for underlying arthritis. The diagnostic modality of choice is an MRI scan.

Management of Meniscal Tears

The majority of degenerate meniscal tears are managed nonoperatively. The ESSKA (European Society of Sports Traumatology, Knee Surgery and Arthroscopy) meniscus consensus project laid recommendation for management of degenerate meniscal tears (Fig. 3.5).

The FIDELITY trial demonstrated the lack of benefit of arthroscopic meniscectomy over nonoperative management in degenerate meniscal tears. As a result, most of these are managed through nonoperative measures. Indications for

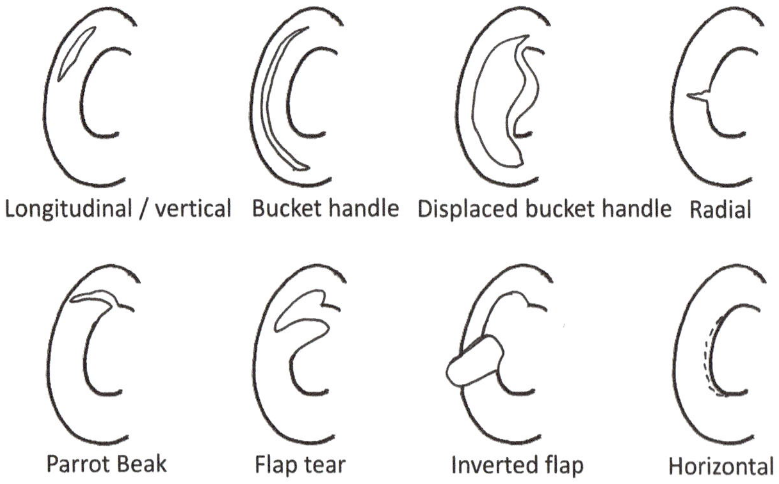

Fig. 3.4 Morphological types of meniscal tears

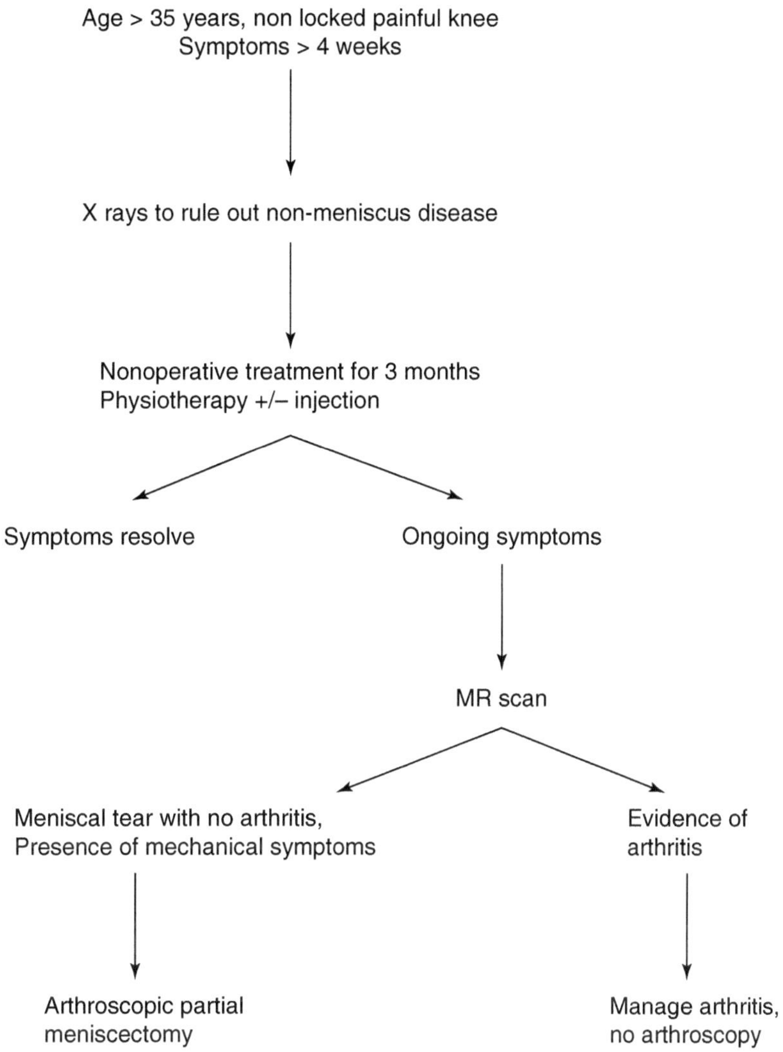

Fig. 3.5 Summary of ESSKA guidelines for management of degenerate meniscal tears

surgery are symptoms persisting beyond 3 months despite nonoperative management and absence of arthritis on radiographs.

Sihvonen R, Paavola M, Malmivaara A, Järvinen TL. Finnish Degenerative Meniscal Lesion Study (FIDELITY): a protocol for a randomised, placebo surgery controlled trial on the efficacy of arthroscopic partial meniscectomy for patients with degenerative meniscus injury with a novel 'RCT within-a-cohort' study design. NEJM 2013;369(26);2515–24. Multicentre, placebo surgery controlled trial for 146 patients. No difference in 12 months on knee scores with either arthroscopic partial meniscectomy or diagnostic arthroscopy without excision of meniscus. All clinical scores showed equal improvement in both groups.

Meniscal Repair

Indications for meniscal repair are acute peripheral tears in young active patients. Concomitant injuries to the cruciate ligament should be addressed at the same time to protect the meniscal repair.

The success rate of meniscal repair with ACL reconstruction is about 90% compared to 30% without ACL reconstruction.

The various techniques for arthroscopic repair have been described. These are—'inside-out' repair, 'outside-in' repair and the 'all inside' repair. Open repair is rarely done. The 'inside-out' vertical mattress suturing provides a secure repair and is the gold standard.

Haklar U, Donmez F, Basaran SH, Canbora MK. Results of arthroscopic repair of partial- or full-thickness longitudinal medial meniscal tears by single or double vertical sutures using the inside-out technique. Am J Sports Med 2013;41(3):596–602. 112 repairs, inside out technique. 1 to 4 year follow up. 88% healed.

All inside repair technique have become popular following the development of various suture devices and anchors. The pullout strength of the sutures is similar to mattress sutures. These are increasingly used due to easy applicability and avoidance of additional incisions.

Meniscal repair is technically difficult, carries a longer rehabilitation and higher reoperation rate, but better functional outcome compared to meniscectomy.

A variety of adjuncts have been tried to enhance healing of meniscus after repair. These include autologous blood clot, fibrin clot, needling, trephining, platelet rich plasma, stem cells, fibrin glue etc. None of these have robust scientific evidence to recommend general usage.

Meniscal Replacement

Meniscal replacement is possible through synthetic collagen scaffolds, or with the use of allografts. Collagen scaffolds replace the meniscus and are sutured to the remaining anterior and posterior horn, and along the meniscal rim. Collagen Meniscus Implant (CMI) can be performed arthroscopically. The chondroprotective ability of these implants remains unproven.

Dhollander A, Verdonk P, Verdonk R. Treatment of Painful, Irreparable Partial Meniscal Defects With a Polyurethane Scaffold: Midterm Clinical Outcomes and Survival Analysis. Am J Sports Med 2016;44(10):2615–21. 44 patients. 62% implants survived at 5 years follow up.

Meniscal Allograft Transplantation (MAT) can be used even when the anterior and posterior horns are absent. Indications for MAT are unicompartmental pain in the presence of total or functional meniscectomy, along with ACL reconstruction to aid joint stability in meniscus deficient knee, and along with articular cartilage repair in meniscus deficient knee. Significant arthritis is a contraindication for meniscal transplant.

The graft can be fixed with or without bone plugs. Fresh viable and fresh frozen allografts are used. These surgical interventions have the best results with specialised surgical teams where such procedures are performed regularly. Evidence for long term efficacy of MAT is awaited.

Elattar M, Dhollander A, Verdonk R, Almqvist KF, Verdonk P. Twenty-six years of meniscal allograft transplantation: is it still experimental? A meta-analysis of 44 trials. Knee Surg Sports Trauma Arthrosc 2011;19(2):147–57. Satisfactory outcomes reported with meniscal allografts.

Sizing of the graft is crucial for outcome and the size selected should be within 5% of size of the original meniscus. Undersized grafts do not transmit load effectively and oversized grafts are prone to extrusion.

Root Tear of the Meniscus

Root tears were first described by Pagnani in 1991. These involve detachment of the meniscus from the anterior or posterior aspect of the tibial plateau. The MR scan shows the 'ghost sign'—absence of posterior root on sagittal images; and meniscal extrusion may be evident. The effect of a root tear is equivalent to a total meniscectomy as all the circumferential fibres are interrupted.

Root repair is indicated for acute tears and symptomatic tears. Transosseous pull out sutures are needed for repair.

Ramp Lesions

Ramp lesions are peripheral tears of the posterior horn of medial meniscus at the menisco-capsular junction or injury to the menisco-tibial attachment of the posterior horn of medial meniscus (Fig. 3.6). These were initially described in 1988 by Strobel and may be associated with ACL injuries (9–16% of all ACL injuries). They are difficult to visualise arthroscopically, unless a posteromedial portal is used. There is low sensitivity for detection on MR scans. A thin fluid signal between the posterior horn of the medial meniscus and the posterior capsule may suggest a ramp lesion.

The posterior horn of the medial meniscus is a restraint to anterior translation of the tibia. Ramp lesions can increase the force on the ACL and increase rotatory instability.

In chronic ACL deficiency, ramp lesions are repaired although in acute ACL injuries, there is an option to manage these nonoperatively as the tear may be a stable injury. Repair can be done by all inside or inside out technique.

Meniscal Injuries in Children

Meniscal injuries in children are relatively rare, with children accounting for just 5% of all meniscal injuries. Discoid lateral meniscus may, however, predispose to meniscal tears.

The clinical presentation and signs of meniscal tears in children may not be typical and an MR scan is useful for diagnosis.

Treatment is based on the symptoms and preservation of the meniscus is the goal. Repair in the vascular area of the meniscus can be accomplished with suturing techniques. Every attempt should be made to preserve the rim of the meniscus.

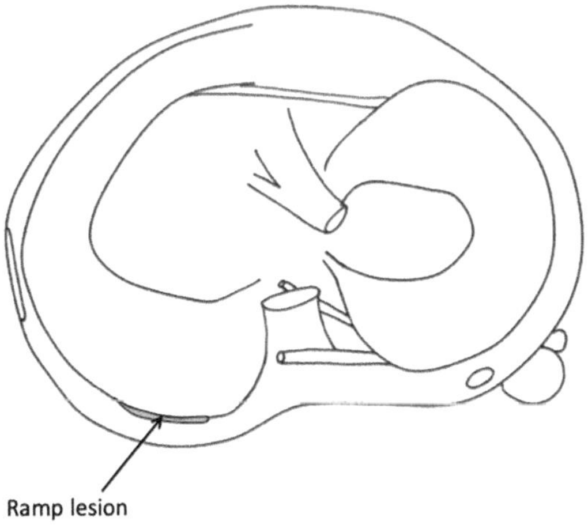

Fig. 3.6 Ramp lesion

Meniscal Cysts

Meniscal cysts often form in relation to meniscal tears, where the joint fluid is sequestered thorough a valve mechanism. The exact aetiology is unknown. These are often filled with a gelatinous fluid. Presentation can be due to localised pain, or swelling. The pain may be the consequence of associated meniscal tear. Usually, the cysts can be decompressed into the joint at the time of meniscal trimming.

Discoid Lateral Meniscus

A discoid lateral meniscus presents as a 'snapping knee' in children. It occurs in 1–3% of the population. The cause may be linked to failure of resorption of central part of the meniscus.

Discoid meniscus is grouped according to the Watanabe classification (1969). There are 3 types as shown in Fig. 3.7. In the Wrisberg ligament type, the meniscocapsular or the meniscopopliteal ligament is deficient. The only stabilising structure is the meniscofemoral ligament. This is associated with instability of the posterior horn of the meniscus, and may present with the 'snapping knee' syndrome.

Clinically, the symptoms are clicking and 'snapping' in the joint. The age of onset of symptoms is around 10 years. Pain is a late feature and represents a meniscal tear. Patients with type III lesions can have symptoms of instability. A clunk may be appreciable at 10 degrees flexion or

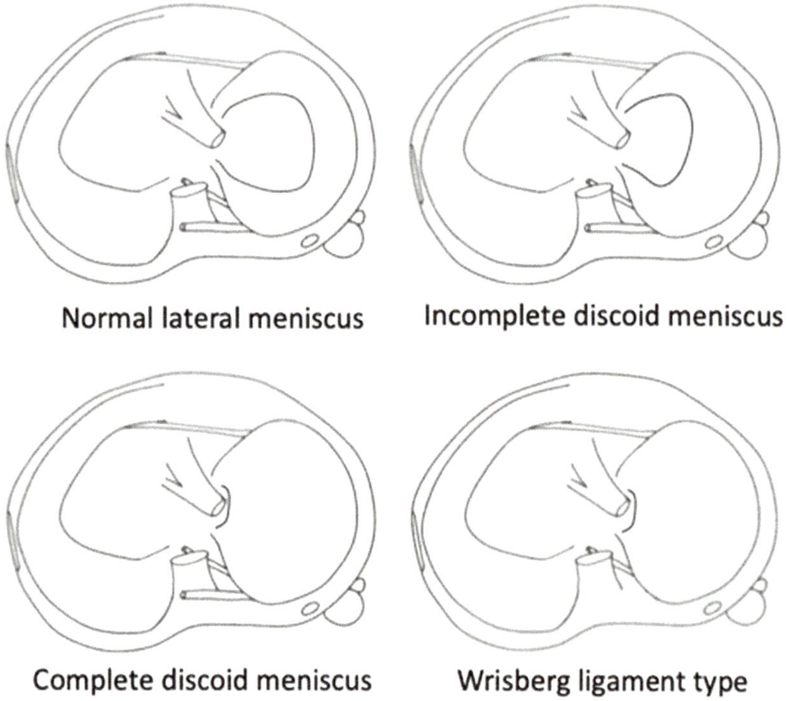

Fig. 3.7 Types of discoid lateral meniscus

beyond 90 degrees flexion. A 'pop' is sometimes felt on McMurray's test.

On plain radiographs, discoid lateral meniscus appears as widening of the lateral joint space, squaring of the femoral condyle and concavity of the lateral tibial plateau. An MR scan is diagnostic. On coronal images, the meniscal width is over 15 mm; or the ratio of minimal meniscal width to maximal tibial width is over 20%. On sagittal images, the meniscal body is seen in 3 or more consecutive standard images.

Management

Asymptomatic discoid menisci do not require treatment and do not predispose to arthritis. Treatment in symptomatic patients is aimed at trimming the meniscus to a relatively normal shape and repairing or excising the meniscal tears. Patients with instability symptoms in type III lesions are managed with a capsular suture to stabilise the meniscus or stabilising the meniscus to the tibial plateau. Meniscus preservation is preferable to total meniscectomy. Meniscal transplant may have some role if excess meniscus is removed.

Anterior Cruciate Ligament Injuries

No other ligamentous structure has been the subject of comparable volume of orthopaedic literature as the anterior cruciate ligament (ACL).

Anatomy

Measuring, on average, 33 mm × 11 mm, the ACL has two bundles, anteromedial (AM) bundle and the posterolateral (PL) bundle and this nomenclature is based on the attachment on the tibia. The AM and the PL bundle attach to the posteromedial aspect of the lateral femoral condyle—also known as the lateral wall of the inter-

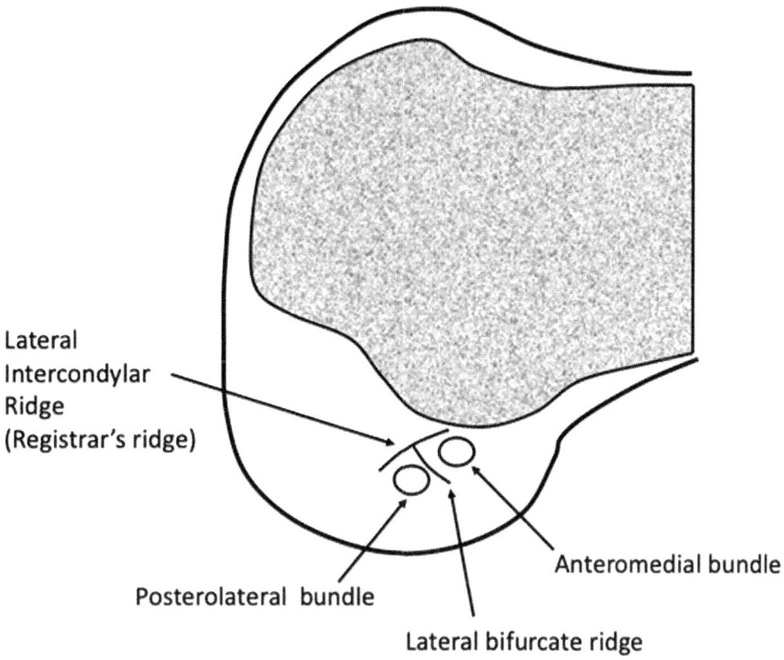

Fig. 3.8 ACL attachment on the femur

condylar notch. The anterior edge of the attachment is demarcated by the lateral intercondylar ridge and the bifurcate ridge separates the PL bundle from the AM bundle (Fig. 3.8). The tibial attachment is a wide area in the anterior tibia in between the intercondylar eminences.

It derives its blood supply from the middle geniculate artery and mechanoreceptors found in the ligament have proprioceptive function. It is predominantly Type 1 collagen with a tensile strength of around 2000 Newtons.

Function

The ACL is the primary restraint to anterior tibial translation (anteromedial bundle) and a secondary restraint to varus and valgus stress. It restricts internal rotation of the tibia (posterolateral bundle). Posterolateral bundle has an additional function of preventing hyperextension of the knee. The anterolateral ligament (ALL) restricts internal rotation of the tibia beyond 35 degrees flexion. ALL originates anterior to the lateral epicondyle and inserts at the anterolateral margin of tibia.

Mechanism of Injury

The anterior cruciate ligament is typically injured with a quick deceleration, hyperextension or a twisting injury, and is not classically a contact injury. It is more common in females, which may be due to a narrow notch, thinner ligament or valgus knee alignment. ACL injury may be associated with medial collateral and medial meniscal injury (unhappy triad of O'Donoghue). More commonly, the lateral meniscus is injured in acute injuries, while the medial meniscus injuries are seen in chronic ACL injuries.

History and Examination

In acute injuries the classic history of a "pop "should suggest an ACL tear. The injury is followed immediately by haemarthrosis and inability to weight bear.

Lachman test is 95% sensitive and specific (Table 3.1). The quality of the end point—firm or soft—is noted. Drawer test may be false negative in ACL injury because of the 'door stop' action (wedging) of the posterior third of the medial

Table 3.1 Grading for the Lachman test

Lachman test	Anterior translation
Grade 1	3–5 mm
Grade 2	5–10 mm
Grade 3	More than 10 mm

Table 3.2 Patterns of pivot shift

Pivot shift test	
Grade 1	Tibial glide
Grade 2	Clunk
Grade 3	Gross instability

meniscus against the medial femoral condyle at 90 degrees of flexion. An associated PCL injury may give a false positive anterior drawer. This is due to posterior sag of the tibia in the starting position of the test.

Pivot shift test is best avoided in an acute setting. The test is done as the knee is moved from extension to flexion. In the starting position of extension, the tibia is subluxed and internally rotated because of ACL laxity. The lateral tibial plateau is subluxed anteriorly. As the knee is flexed, the iliotibial band (ITB) moves posteriorly. This causes the tibia to rotate back to neutral position as the ITB pulls the lateral plateau posteriorly with flexion. The relocation of tibia at 20–40 degree flexion indicates a positive pivot shift.

An intact iliotibial band, intact medial collateral ligament and ability to fully extend are prerequisites for a positive pivot shift test. Different grades of pivoting have been described (Table 3.2).

KT 1000 arthrometer and other newer devices like Kinematic Rapid Assessment device which measure the laxity in conjunction with a mobile phone app can be used for objective assessment of laxity.

Acute injuries associated with ACL injury include meniscal tears, injury to medial collateral ligament, posterolateral corner injuries, chondral lesions, and increasingly diagnosed 'ramp' lesions. Ramp lesions are tears at the posterior meniscocapsular junction or tears of the posterior meniscotibial ligament.

Posterolateral corner (PLC) injuries are associated with ACL injury in 10% patients. These have to be recognised and addressed early.

Investigations

On plain radiographs, Segond fracture is classically associated with an ACL injury and such a finding on an AP radiograph indicates an avulsion of the anterolateral ligament from the tibial attachment.

MRI-Sagittal view on a T2 weighted image shows discontinuous fibres or absent fibres. There is bone bruising on the posterior third of the lateral tibial plateau and middle third of the lateral femoral condyle due to the pivot action at the time of injury. Coronal images show an 'empty notch sign' and discontinuity of fibres. Concomitant meniscal and other ligamentous injuries should be assessed.

Management

Role of non-surgical and surgical options are considered depending on the clinical requisites.

An ongoing multicentre trial (ACL SNNAP) has been designed to compare operative vs. non-operative treatment of non-acute ACL deficiency.

In a classic paper in 1983, Noyes proposed a rule of thirds for chronic ACL deficiency—one third patients do not require reconstruction and resume normal activities; one third adjust their activity level on account of instability; and a third require reconstruction.

Conservative option with rehabilitation for a low demand patient leads to acceptable outcomes. The operative option aims to achieve a stable knee and enable return to sports and high level activity.

There is evidence to suggest that reconstruction prevents repetitive instability and rapid onset of knee arthrosis.

While reconstruction of the ligament is the gold standard, ACL augmentation and repair is being tried.

The surgical options for reconstruction use autografts (hamstrings, bone patella tendon, quadriceps tendon graft), allograft or synthetic options.

All of these have their unique advantages and disadvantages.

Bone patella tendon bone (BPTB) graft has a strength of 2500 N is an excellent option for the active athlete with lower rate of re-rupture rates. The grafts incorporate faster (bone to bone healing) but there is greater incidence of anterior knee pain (30%), patella baja, fracture patella, patellar tendonitis and patellofemoral OA.

Hamstrings commonly used are semitendinosus and gracilis and various methods like single bundle, double bundle techniques have been described. The tensile strength is 4500N and is almost double that of a native ACL. These have slower healing (up to 12 weeks). Tunnel widening is a long-term problem especially with use of suspensory fixation. Harvest of hamstring risks injury to saphenous nerve.

Quadriceps grafts have a bone plug, and offers bony incorporation on one side. The graft strength is 4000N. The value of quadriceps is in a revision scenario where instead of using an allograft, a quadriceps autograft can be utilised.

Commonly used Allografts are Achilles tendon, BPTB and Quadriceps tendon. Freeze dried grafts are better as irradiated grafts rapidly lose their mechanical properties. Apart from absence of graft donor site morbidity, allografts are useful for multiligament reconstructions.

Synthetic grafts like LARS, Dacron etc. have poor evidence base to recommend in isolated ACL reconstruction. These have a higher failure rate compared to autograft, and generally find application in revision situations.

Chronic ACL insufficiency with instability can lead to degenerative changes in the knee, but there is little evidence to suggest that ACL reconstruction delays or avoids these changes. The chondral injury at the time of the impact is considered to be the precursor to degenerative changes.

The timing of surgery is debatable. Most surgeons operate once the acute pain has settled and the knee has regained full extension. Surgery in the acute phase has a higher risk of stiffness (arthrofibrosis). Better pre- and postoperative exercise programs, and more accurate placement of grafts have reduced the incidence of arthrofibrosis.

The presence of a locked knee due to a coexisting bucket-handle tear of the meniscus is an indication for early repair. Delays would lead to a fixed flexion deformity from a persistently locked knee. Associated posterolateral corner injuries also require early repair.

Kennedy J, Jackson MP, O'Kelly P, Moran R. Timing of reconstruction of the anterior cruciate ligament in athletes and the incidence of secondary pathology within the knee. J Bone Joint Surg Br 2010;92:362–6. 300 patients, higher incidence of meniscal tears if surgery was delayed for more than one year from injury. Degenerative changes were higher in the group operated more than 6 months after the injury compared to those operated earlier.

Principles of ACL Surgery

Standard anterolateral portal and low anteromedial portals are employed for anterior cruciate ligament reconstruction to achieve anatomic placement of femoral and tibial tunnels. Transtibial tunnel placement for the femur is now obsolete. Tunnels are placed commonly 'inside out' but advances in instrumentation accommodate for accurate placement of bone conserving 'outside in' tunnels which take the minimum bone necessary for adequate intra tunnel length of grafts.

Femoral tunnel and tibial tunnels in single bundle reconstruction are placed at the anatomic centre of the native ACL footprint (Fig. 3.9). The femoral tunnel is marked using a microfracture awl at the middle of a line over the anatomic site of the ACL. This can be assisted by an ACL ruler or intra operative radiography utilizing the Hertel's grid (Fig. 3.10); or through commercial software.

The tibial tunnel is positioned between the anterior horn of lateral meniscus and the medial tibial spine. The tunnel length is typically 40–50 mm and is within 15 degrees of the vertical axis. The tunnel is drilled followed by graft passage and fixation.

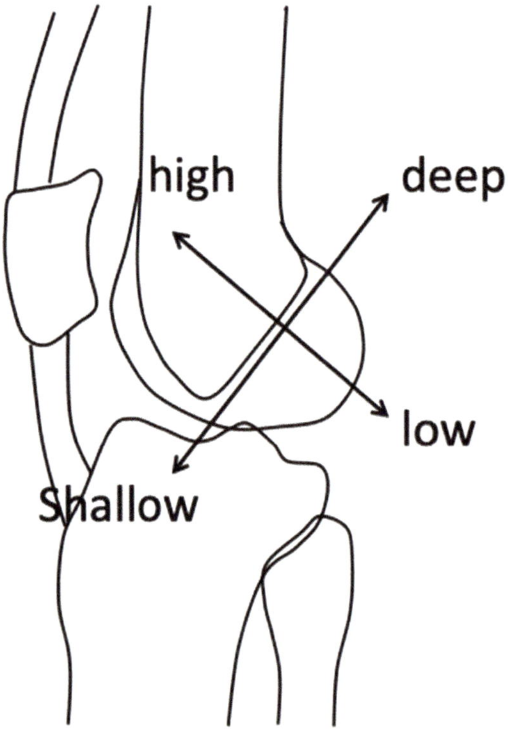

Fig. 3.9 Nomenclature of graft placement on the femoral attachment

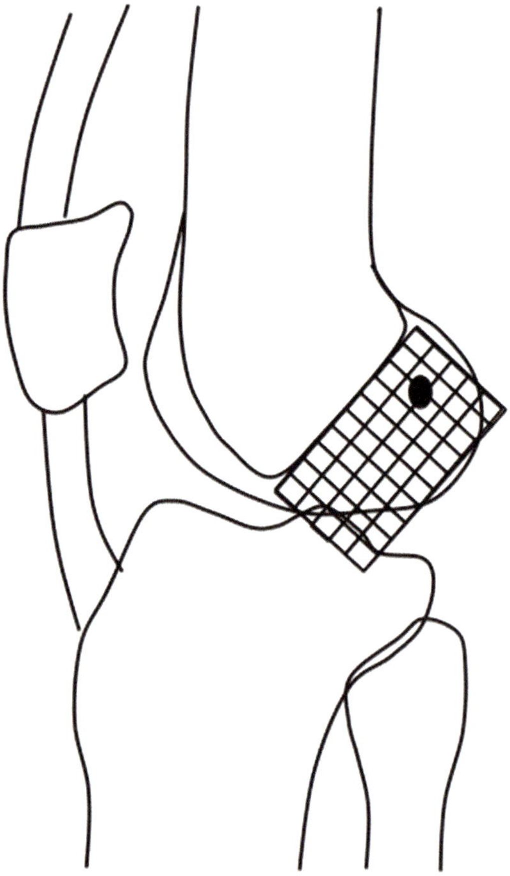

Fig. 3.10 Bernhard and Hertel grid for assessing femoral placement of ACL graft

The fixation can be achieved by aperture fixation or suspensory fixation. Femoral fixation can be with either a suspensory device like endobuttons, cross pins or with interference screws which allow the reconstructed graft to be stabilized at the joint level. Tibial fixation devices are mainly interference screws, staples, screws as posts or spiked washers.

The Bernhard and Hertel grid helps to quantify the placement of graft. This is a 5 × 10 grid and graft placement is 24–27% deep and 28–34% high.

The tibial tunnel placement is assessed in the lateral view (Fig. 3.11). The entire tibial tunnel should be posterior to the line drawn along the intercondylar notch (Blumensaat's line). The position of the tibial tunnel can also be described as a percentage of tibial width on the lateral radiograph.

An anteriorly placed graft will impinge in extension and lead to fixed flexion deformity. An excessively posteriorly placed graft will not provide adequate stability and will impinge on the PCL. An excessively vertical graft will not provide rotatory stability.

Rehabilitation

The post-operative rehabilitation is extremely important after surgery and is considered as important as the surgical procedure.

There is no role for bracing. Full weight bearing, and cryotherapy immediately postoperatively is of value. The emphasis is to gain range of movement with closed chain exercises with proprioceptive training. Return to 'pivoting' sport is permissible nine months following surgery. Open chain exercises and isokinetic quadriceps work are avoided for the first 6 weeks.

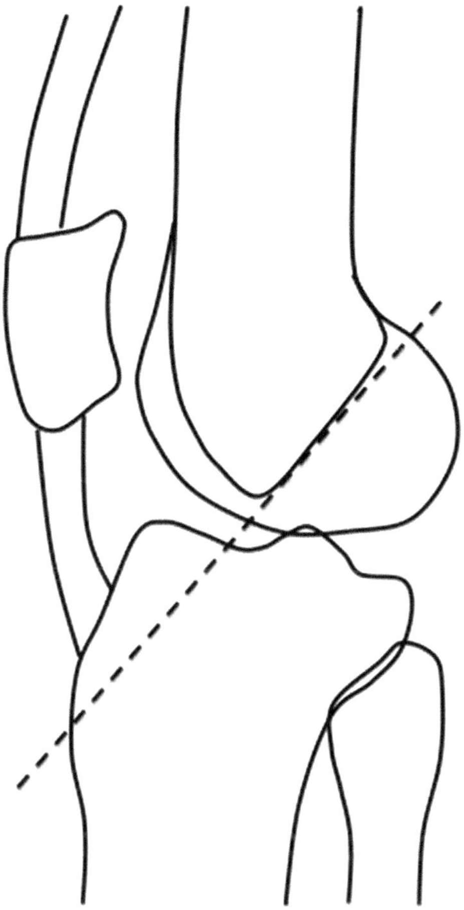

Fig. 3.11 Assessment of tibial tunnel placement on lateral radiograph in relation to Blumensaat's line

Complications

Improperly placed grafts because of tunnel malpositioning is by far the commonest cause of failure of ACL reconstruction. Graft impingement in the notch leads to loss of stiffness.

Arthrofibrosis can be a problem in acute ACL reconstructions where full mobility of the knee was not present preoperatively.

Cyclops lesion is the scar from the ACL remnant on the tibia.

Harvesting patellar tendon graft risks patellar fracture and infra patellar contracture.

There is a risk of re-rupture if patients regain contact or pivoting sport too early in the rehabilitation period.

Hamstring harvest can risk injury to branches of the saphenous nerve.

ACL Reconstruction in Paediatric Age Group

ACL injuries are uncommon in children. The incidence is increasing, however, with greater participation in high-level sports.

The cruciate ligaments in children are stronger than the physis. The fibres attach directly to the perichondrium of the articular cartilage (as opposed to in adults, where they attach by Sharpey's fibres).

Operative treatment is advised for symptomatic instability and in patients with meniscal tears that require repair. Iatrogenic damage to the growth plate is a concern, and techniques have been developed to minimise the risk.

Techniques employed are- intra articular (physis sparing), transphyseal and combined intra and extra articular reconstruction.

Recent advances have enabled repair procedures like bridge-enhanced ACL repair (BEAR) which utilises a bioactive scaffold with suture repair.

Double Bundle ACL Reconstruction

Double bundle ACL reconstruction is reconstruction of the two bundles of ACL individually. At present, the evidence for superiority of this technique is debatable. The revision rate was not different in Scandinavian registry compared to single bundle procedures. Studies have shown better stability but do not show better functional outcome with double bundle technique.

Revision ACL Reconstruction

Thorough evaluation is necessary before any further surgery is considered. The cause of failure should be determined. In patients with malalignment, osteotomies to recreate the anatomic alignment are performed along with reconstruction. A staged approach is needed if previous graft tunnels need bone grafting before surgery can be undertaken successfully.

Posterior Cruciate Ligament Injuries

Anatomy

The Posterior Cruciate Ligament (PCL) has 2 bundles—the anterolateral bundle (AL) and the posteromedial (PM) bundle. The AL bundle is stronger and is tight in flexion, the PM bundle is tight in extension. On average, the ligament measures 39 mm × 13 mm. The PCL has a tensile strength of 3000 N and is a third larger than the ACL.

The tibial attachment is the posterior tibial sulcus and the femoral attachment is a broad crescent shaped area on the anterolateral aspect of medial femoral condyle.

PCL derives its blood supply from the middle geniculate artery. The vascularity is abundant, and PCL tears heal better than ACL tears. The PCL is situated in between the Humphrey's ligament (runs anterior to PCL) and Wrisberg ligament (runs posterior to PCL). These meniscofemoral ligaments originate from the posterior horn of the lateral meniscus.

Function

The role of the PCL is to provide a restraint to posterior tibial translation and acts as a secondary stabilizer to varus-valgus stress.

Mechanism of Injury

Typically, dashboard injuries during motor vehicle accidents account for the majority of PCL tears. Other causes are motorcycle accidents, athletic injuries and falls where a posteriorly directed force on the flexed knee causes the ligament rupture. Gymnasts who land on the plantar flexed foot can be at risk of injuring the PCL.

History and Examination

The history should raise suspicion of PCL injury. Bruising in the front of the knee or femoral shaft fractures may point towards a PCL injury.

A large number of PCL injuries are missed initially. High energy injuries may be associated with neurovascular compromise, and a complete evaluation is essential.

A posterior drawer test, posterior sag sign, dial test, reverse pivot test and a quadriceps active test are useful in making a clinical diagnosis.

The dial test helps differentiate PCL injury and associated posterolateral corner (PLC) injury. Passive external rotation of the tibia is assessed at 30 degrees and 90 degrees. Increased external rotation at 30 degrees only indicates PLC injury. Increased external rotation at 30 and 90 degrees indicates combined PCL and PLC injury.

Investigations

Stress view radiographs are useful in deciding the mode of treatment and MR scans are conclusive.

Management

Management depends on the grade of injury. Nonoperative treatment is protected weight bearing rehabilitation focusing on quadriceps strengthening. The management is summarised in Table 3.3.

Table 3.3 Management of PCL injuries

Grade of injury	Management option
Grade I-partial 1–5 mm posterior translation	Nonoperative
Grade II-complete isolated injuries 6–10 posterior translation	Nonoperative
Grade III-Combined PCL and capsuloligamentous rupture—have associated injuries of PLC/ACL >10 mm posterior translation	Nonoperative/ Operative Immobilization in extension for a period/ extension bracing and surgical repair

Combined PCL and posterolateral corner (PLC) injuries result in significant instability and usually require surgery. Bony avulsions should be fixed primarily.

Surgery for PCL Injuries

The presence of combined injuries and an unstable knee requires surgery. The choices in surgery are—single or double bundle; autograft or allograft; tibial inlay or transtibial methods.

Chronic PCL injuries may require high tibial osteotomy to correct the varus malalignment. Increasing the posterior slope of proximal tibia helps reduce the posterior sag associated with PCL injuries.

Hamstring autografts are often short and synthetic grafts like LARS PCL graft have some role in PCL reconstruction.

Rehabilitation

Mainstay is intense quadriceps rehabilitation. During rehabilitation any stress on the graft by hamstring is kept at a minimum by avoiding activation of hamstrings.

Complications

The popliteal artery is in close proximity when the tibial tunnel is drilled and the risk during PCL surgery has been reported as 1%. It is a catastrophic injury and potentially limb threatening.

The Posteromedial Corner of the Knee

The ligaments and tendons around the knee form a complex stabilising mechanism. It is helpful to understand the exact relationships of the various structures.

The posteromedial corner (PMC) extends from the posterior border of the MCL up to the PCL attachment. Injuries to PMC cause anteromedial rotatory instability (AMRI). AMRI is excess anterior translation and external rotation of the medial tibial condyle due to lack of posterior restraint.

PMC injuries are usually associated with cruciate ligament injuries and if unrecognised, can lead to cruciate ligament graft failure.

The oblique popliteal ligament (OPL) is a thickening of the posterior capsule of the knee joint. It extends from the intercondylar area of femur just above the lateral femoral condyle to the proximal tibia (Fig. 3.12). The OPL forms the floor of the popliteal fossa and the popliteal artery lies on the OPL. The middle genicular vessels and the posterior division of obturator nerve pierce the OPL. The OPL is a restraint to hyperextension of the knee.

The posterior oblique ligament (POL) or ligament of Winslow is thickening of the posteromedial capsule and forms the deep layer of PMC (Fig. 3.13). The origin is distal and posterior to the adductor tubercle. It extends distally and divides into 3 sections. The central part inserts into the posteromedial tibial margin and back of

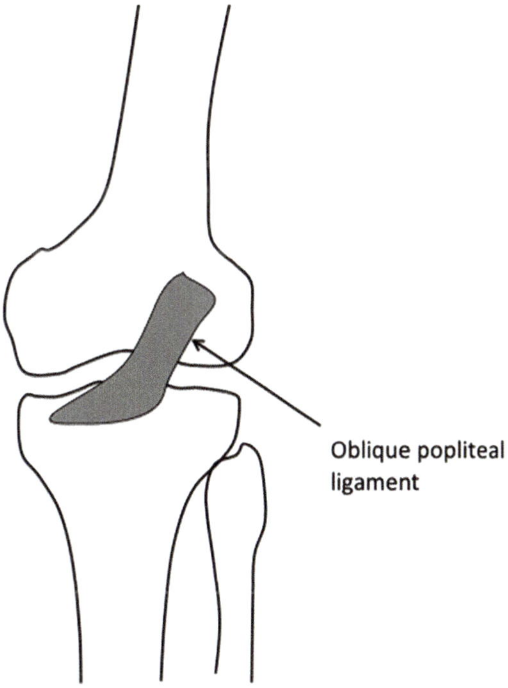

Fig. 3.12 The oblique popliteal ligament on the posterior aspect of knee

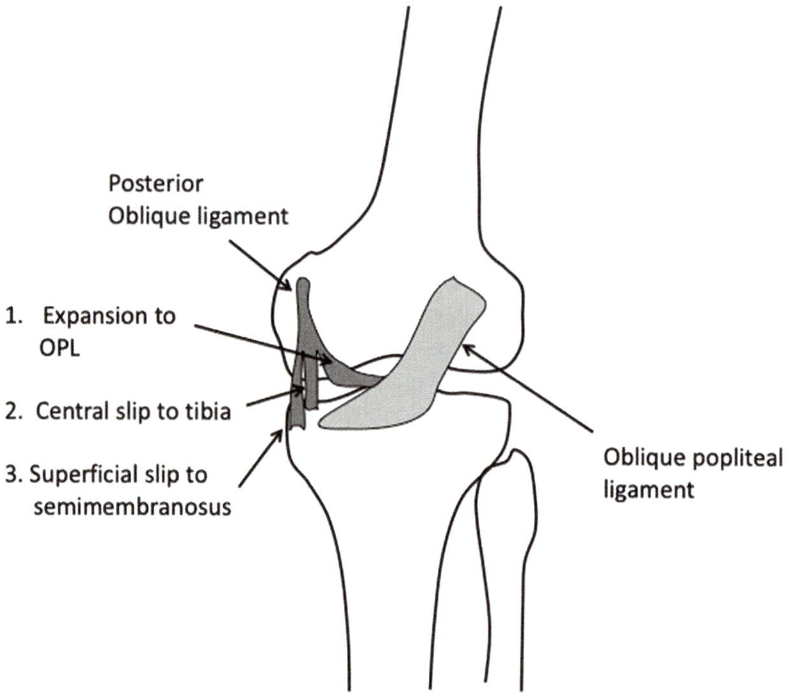

Fig. 3.13 The Posterior oblique ligament

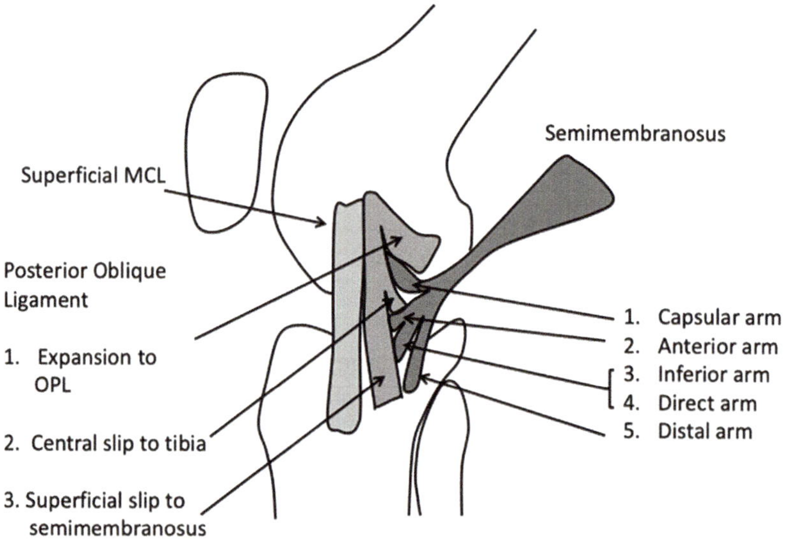

Fig. 3.14 Medial aspect of knee showing semimembranosus attachment

medial meniscus. One slip merges with the OPL and the third part merges with semimembranosus. The POL provides restraint to valgus stress and anterior/posterior translation. It may provide some anteroposterior stability in patients with ACL injury, as well as medial stability in patients with MCL injury.

The semimembranosus has 5 attachments distally as shown in Fig. 3.14. These arms interdigitate with the attachment of the POL. The tendon has a direct arm which attaches to a tubercle on the posteromedial tibial margin. Capsular arm merges with the posteromedial capsule. Anterior arm passes under POL to insert on the tibia.

Inferior and distal arms attach to the tibia. In addition, there is a reflection to OPL, which arises 2 cm proximal to the insertion of tendon, and merges with the OPL.

External rotation of the tibia tightens the PMC. In addition to the ligaments described above, the pes anserinus and the semimembranosus provide support to the PMC.

AMRI is suspected in patients with valgus instability at 30 degrees knee flexion, along with excess passive external rotation of the tibia. Opening of the medial joint on valgus stress in full extension indicates combined MCL and PMC injury. The rotatory component differentiates it from pure MCL injuries.

Isolated PMC injuries are managed nonoperatively. When combined with other injuries, reconstruction of the POL should be considered.

Medial Collateral Ligament

The medial collateral ligament (MCL) is the commonest ligamentous structure injured in the knee (40%). MCL and ACL injury are the commonest multi-ligament injury pattern.

Anatomy

Medial collateral ligament has two components. The superficial MCL is the primary restraint to a valgus strain of the knee throughout the range of motion of the knee. The deep MCL is a secondary stabilizer and contributes to the knee stability in full extension.

Superficial MCL originates from the medial femoral epicondyle and inserts distally 5–10 cm from the joint line into the periosteum of tibia, deep to pes anserinus. The deep layer is the thickening of the medial capsule and the meniscofemoral and meniscotibial ligaments.

The Layers on the Medial Aspect of Knee

The static stabilisers on the medial side are superficial and deep MCL, and the posterior oblique ligament. The dynamic stabilisers are semimembranosus, pes anserinus, medial retinaculum and the VMO.

The medial structures can be considered in three layers (Table 3.4).

Table 3.4 Layers on the medial side of the knee

Superficial layer	**Patella retinacular fascia, sartorius and its fascia**
Middle	Superficial MCL, POL
Deep layer	Semimembranosus, medial capsule and the deep MCL

History and Examination

The mechanism of injury is through contact or noncontact valgus stress. Contact injuries are through an impact on the lateral aspect of the knee.

A medial opening of the knee on valgus stress applied in 30 degrees flexion indicates an MCL tear and laxity in extension indicates involvement of ACL, grade 3 strain of MCL and posteromedial corner injury.

Tears of MCL are graded based on opening of the medial joint line on valgus stress.

Imaging

Routine AP and lateral views are obtained. In a skeletally immature patient, stress radiographs may reveal physeal separation. Calcification at the femoral attachment in chronic injuries is Pellegrini Stieda disease.

MRI scans helps delineate the extent of the injury and associated injuries. Distal lesions and "Stener" like lesions (distal avulsion) guide the need for surgical repair in Grade III injuries.

Treatment

Treatment plan is suggested in Table 3.5. Proximal tears have better healing potential compared to distal lesions.

In acute proximal avulsions, repair is performed with anchors in the medial epicondyle.

Table 3.5 Treatment plan for MCL injuries

Grade of injury	Laxity	Treatment plan
Grade I	3–5 mm	Rehab and return to sport in a week
Grade II	6–10 mm	Bracing and return to sport by 4 weeks
Grade III	>10 mm	Bracing and return to sport by 8 weeks or consider surgery

Table 3.6 Layers on the lateral aspect of knee

Superficial layer	Biceps femoris and ITB
Middle layer	Patellofemoral ligament, lateral patellar retinaculum
Deep (superficial layer)	Lateral collateral ligament, fabellofibular ligament
Deep (deep layer)	Popliteus tendon, Arcuate, Coronary and popliteofibular ligament and the lateral capsule

Chronic MCL tears are reconstructed using tendon autograft with tunnels at isometric points. Achilles tendon allograft can also be used.

Lateral Collateral Ligament and Posterolateral Corner Injuries

Anatomy

The static stabilisers of the posterolateral corner (PLC) are the LCL, popliteus tendon, arcuate ligament and the capsule. The Dynamic stabilisers are biceps femoris, popliteus muscle, iliotibial band (ITB) and lateral head of gastrocnemius. The layers comprising different structures are shown in Table 3.6.

The popliteus has its origin from the proximal tibia and courses superolaterally under the arcuate ligament and the LCL to insert into the lateral aspect of lateral femoral condyle. Popliteomeniscal fibres may connect the popliteus to the lateral meniscus.

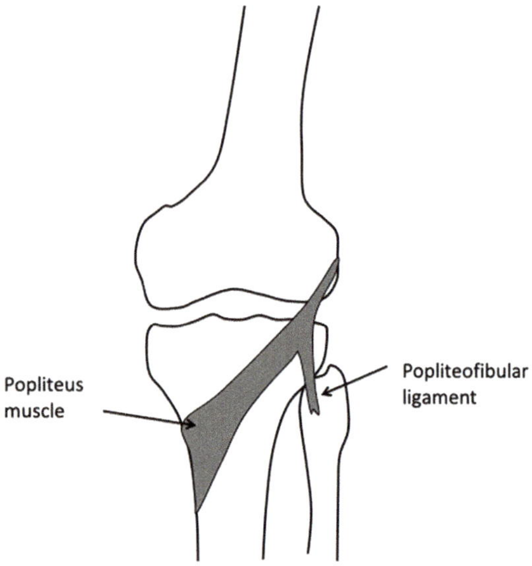

Fig. 3.15 The popliteofibular ligament

The popliteofibular ligament attaches the popliteal tendon to the fibular head (Fig. 3.15) and is considered an important stabiliser of the PLC.

The arcuate ligament is Y shaped. It arises from the fibular head, arches over the popliteus and inserts into the posterior capsule and the OPL (Fig. 3.16). The vertical limb attaches to the posterior aspect of lateral femoral condyle.

The fibular attachment is adjacent to the fabellofibular ligament at the tip of the fibular styloid. The fabellofibular ligament is superficial to the lateral femoral attachment limb of the arcuate ligament.

The lateral collateral ligament arises from the lateral femoral epicondyle and attaches to the fibular head. It may join with the biceps tendon to form a conjoint tendon (Fig. 3.17).

The LCL is the primary restraint to varus stress at 5–30 degree of flexion. It is also the primary restraint to external rotation of the tibia. The LCL is extraarticular structure. The arrangement of the structures on the fibular head is illustrated in Fig. 3.18. The fabellofibular ligament, popliteofibular ligament and the arcuate ligament attach on the fibular styloid.

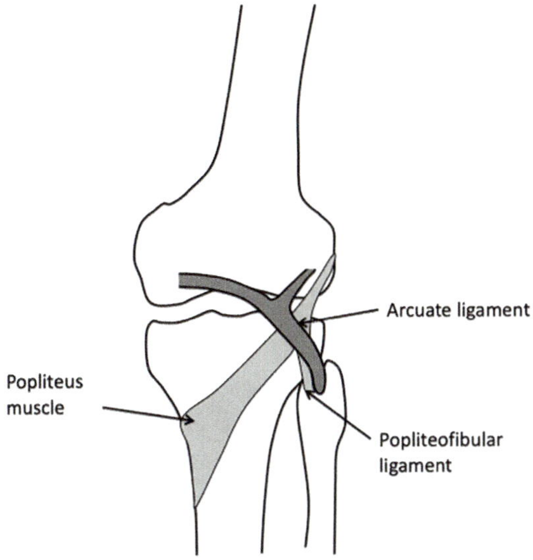

Fig. 3.16 The arcuate ligament superficial to the popliteus muscle

Mechanism of Injury

Varus stress to the extended knee or an impact on the anteromedial aspect of the knee stresses and injures the structures of the PLC and the LCL. PLC injuries are often associated with injury to cruciate ligaments, menisci and medial structures.

Examination

Varus instability at 30 degrees indicates a pure LCL injury whereas instability at 0 degree and 30 degrees is due to LCL and PCL injury. Lateral injuries are a combination of multiple structures as a pure LCL injury is rare.

Fig. 3.17 Ligaments of the posterolateral corner of the knee

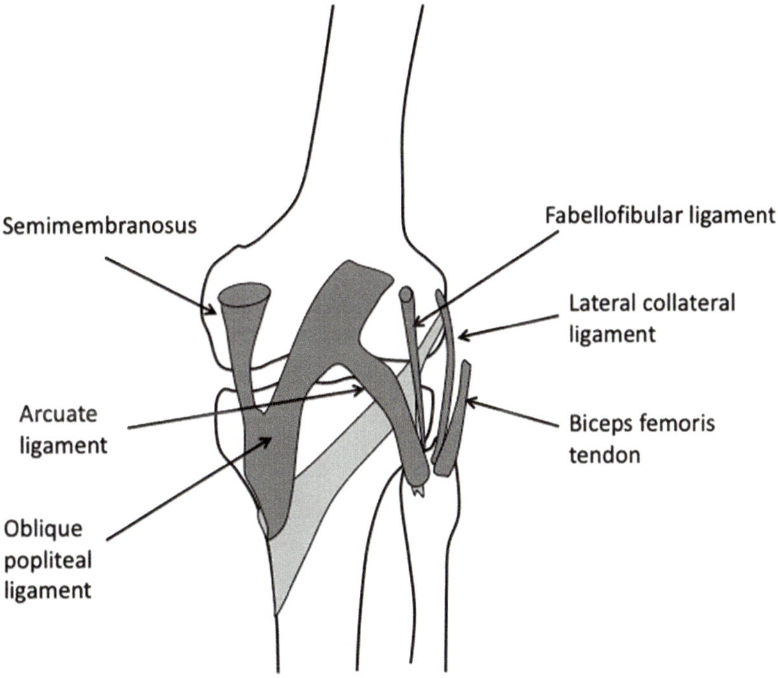

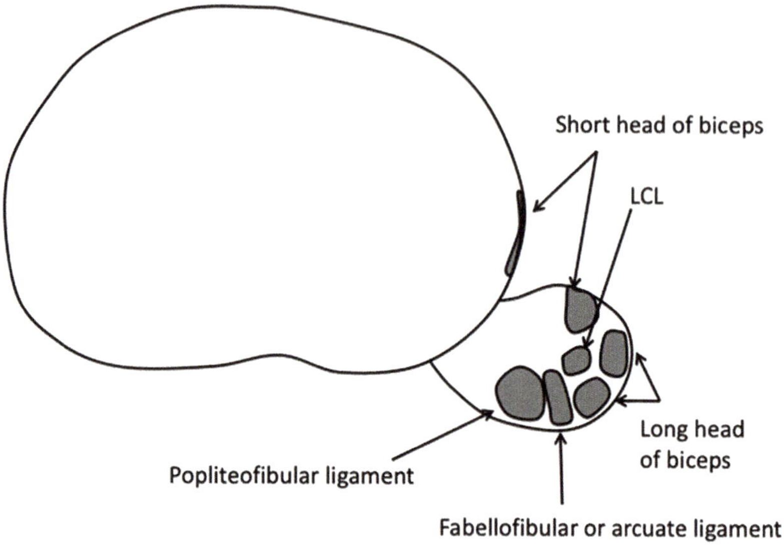

Fig. 3.18 Attachments on the proximal fibula

Table 3.7 Grading of posterolateral corner (PLC) injury

Grade 1	0–5 mm opening on varus strain	Pain along joint line. Minimal laxity
Grade 2	5–10 mm opening	Mild laxity. Definite end point
Grade 3	>10 mm opening	Rupture of the capsulo-ligamentous structure

The dial test is performed at 30 degree and 90 degrees. Increased external rotation of tibia at 30 degrees indicates PLC injury. Increase external rotation at 30 and 90 degrees indicates PLC and PCL injury.

Grading of PLC was proposed by Hughston (Table 3.7).

Imaging

Arcuate sign is a small avulsion at the tip of fibular styloid. It indicates an LCL avulsion. MR scan is diagnostic and essential for posterolateral corner injuries.

Management

Nonoperative management is appropriate for a Grade 1 or 2 laxity encouraging rehabilitation to achieve range of movement. The physiotherapy helps improve quadriceps strength and proprioception.

Grade 3 injuries should be repaired surgically within 3 weeks. Further delay leads to dense scar tissue which makes the repair difficult.

Acute surgery could involve repair of the torn ligaments employing suture anchors. Direct end-to-end open repair is also possible.

Reconstruction involves lateral structure repair using autografts/allografts/synthetic ligaments aiming to achieve fixation at isometric points for the various structures repaired.

There are many extra articular procedures described in specialised texts.

Multiligament Knee Injuries

Multiligament injury implies injury to two or more major stabilising structures of the knee. These can be high or low energy injuries and the knee becomes potentially unstable. These may be associated with a knee dislocation (Table 3.8). The low energy group is identified as an 'ultra low velocity multi ligament injury'. These individuals are often morbidly obese, have high rates of neurovascular injury, and a poor prognosis.

Table 3.8 Schenk classification of knee dislocation

I	Injury to ACL or PCL
II	Injury to ACL and PCL
IIIM	Injury to ACL, PCL, MCL and posteromedial corner
IIIL	Injury to ACL, PCL, LCL and posterolateral corner
IV	Injury to ACL, PCL, MCL, LCL, posteromedial corner and posterolateral corner
V	Multiligament knee injury with periarticular fracture

Associated injuries in high energy mechanisms require trauma management and multi-speciality care.

Based on direction, knee dislocation can be anterior, posterior, medial, lateral or rotatory.

Risk of vascular injury with knee dislocation is 3–4% and varies widely based on energy of injury and degree of ligamentous disruption. Arteriography is not routine, but any suspicion of vascular injury; or ankle brachial index less than 0.8; or an expanding popliteal hematoma should trigger a full investigation and urgent vascular surgery intervention. Prognosis of knee dislocations with vascular injury is poor with high rate of eventual amputation. The amputation rate is 11% with repair within 8 hours, rising to 86% with repair after 8 hours.

Anterior dislocations are associated with intimal injury to popliteal artery as a result of stretching. Posterior dislocations may be associated with direct tear in the popliteal artery. The popliteal artery has limited mobility due to tethering at the adductor hiatus and the soleal hiatus.

Common peroneal nerve injury may be associated with knee dislocation. Recovery of nerve function is poor and a nerve conduction study should be done within 3 weeks. Neurolysis can be considered. Nerve repair, grafting or tendon transfers are options in the event of a disabling deficit.

Imaging

On X-ray, the presence of the lateral capsular sign (avulsion in the lateral tibial condylar region) indicates a severe injury. MR scan is essential and stress radiography may give additional useful information.

Management

Immediate management is urgent reduction and assessment of neurological and circulatory status. Bracing should be done in 10–20 degrees of flexion while imaging is obtained and surgical plan is formulated.

There is lack of consensus on surgical management as well as timing for these injuries. Multiligament knee injuries are a spectrum and comparison between case series is not straightforward.

Acute repair of all injured structures is an option. If done early then the collateral ligaments can be repaired rather than reconstructed. Early repair may require ligament augmentation or substitution. There is a higher risk of stiffness with acute reconstruction of cruciate ligaments as the range of movement of the knee is compromised perioperatively.

Mook WR, Miller MD, Diduch DR, Hertel J, Boachie-Adjei Y, Hart JM. Multiple-ligament knee injuries: a systematic review of the timing of operative intervention and postoperative rehabilitation. J Bone Joint Surg Am 2009;91(12):2946–57. Early repair of cruciate ligaments is associated with higher risk of stiffness.

Staged reconstruction is repair of extraarticular structures (collaterals and posterolateral corner) within 2 weeks and then allowing range of movement. Cruciate reconstruction is undertaken once range of movement is restored. This appears to be the optimal approach based on existing literature.

Delayed repair addresses specific instability complications once the patient starts mobilising the knee. Delayed reconstruction of all structures is associated with poor outcome scores.

Cruciate ligament reconstruction is done preferentially using autograft. Extraarticular repair is augmented with allograft. The choice of autograft/allograft/single bundle/double bundle and specific techniques will depend on surgeon preference, injury pattern and available tissue.

Lachman JR, Rehman S, Pipitone PS. Traumatic Knee Dislocations: Evaluation, Management, and Surgical Treatment. Orthop Clin North Am. 2015;46(4):479–93.

Articular Cartilage Injury

Articular cartilage has no vascular supply or neural innervation. It allows low frictional movement of the joint, and derives its nutrition from the synovial fluid. It is predominantly composed of type 2 collagen.

The articular cartilage has three zones with differing properties as summarised in Fig. 3.19 and Table 3.9.

Management

Treatment of articular cartilage effects depends on the size of defect and available expertise.

Microfracture is an option for smaller full thickness defects. Typical defect size is under 4 cm^2. A chondropic (awl) is used to make multiple holes penetrating into the subchondral bone. Typically, there are 3–4 holes per cm^2. Stem cells from the bone marrow help to reconstitute the cartilage, but form predominantly type 1 collagen. The mechanical properties of the new cartilage are inferior to native cartilage. A period of 6 weeks of protected weight bearing is recommended postoperatively.

Autologous Chondrocyte Implantation (ACI) is useful for larger defects. It involves obtaining a 12 × 5 mm articular cartilage sample arthroscopically as the first procedure. The sample contains

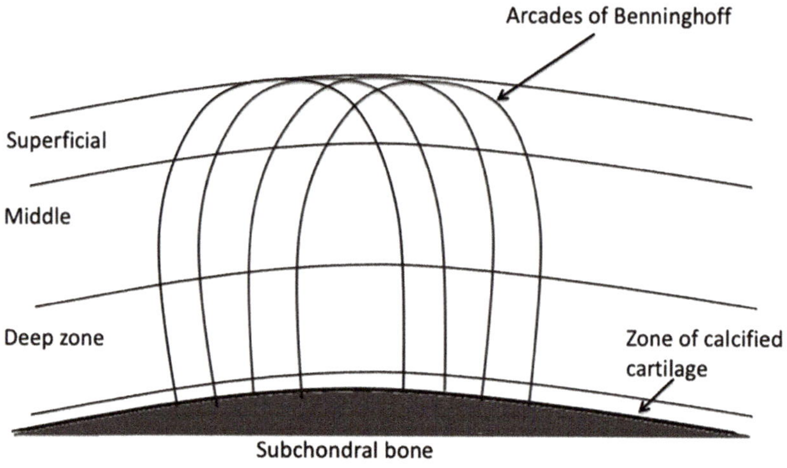

Fig. 3.19 Illustration of zones of articular cartilage

Table 3.9 Features of zones of articular cartilage

	Superficial zone	Middle zone	Deep zone
Orientation of collagen fibres	Parallel to joint surface	Oblique	Perpendicular to joint surface
Shape of chondrocytes	Flattened	Round	Round, arranged in columns
Proteoglycans	Sparse	Abundant	Highest
Collagen concentration	Highest		

about 250,000 cells, and is taken from the superior aspect of the medial femoral condyle. The cartilage cells are cultured for 3 weeks to make 12 million cells. This is then inserted back into the knee joint, usually through an open approach. The cartilage graft is covered with a periosteal flap harvested from the medial tibia. Fibrin glue can be used to hold the surface together.

In MACI (Matrix Induced Autologous Chondrocyte Implantation), the chondrocytes are embedded onto a collagen membrane, which is implanted into the knee. This technique does not lead to normal cartilage collagen composition.

AMIC (Autologous Matrix Induced Chondrogenesis) is a single stage operation where microfracture is done for a full thickness defect and a collagen membrane is placed to stabilise the initial clot. It is contraindicated in kissing lesions and patients with generalised arthritis.

Mosaicplasty is harvesting osteochondral cylindrical plugs from relatively non-weight bearing areas of the joint and transferring them to the defect. It can be used in small defects and carries the problems of donor site morbidity. The intercondylar notch and the lateral portion of the distal femur are potential donor sites in the knee. Plugs are 2.5 mm long and 2.7–8.5 mm wide. This technique leads to hyaline cartilage in the plugs with interspersed fibrous repair tissue. The donor areas, however, may not be totally free of pressure.

Larger defects can be addressed by osteochondral allografts. Accurate size and shape match may be difficult and the procedure is expensive, with risk of disease transmission.

A hemicap is a metal implant to cover localised defects. Results are still being evaluated.

Spontaneous Osteonecrosis of the Knee (SONK)

SONK affects commonly the medial femoral condyle and is characterised by insidious onset of knee pain in middle age individuals. The pain is worse on activity, can be severe, and may be associated with effusion.

It is also linked to subchondral insufficiency fracture (SIF). Extensive bone marrow oedema in fluid sensitive sequences on MR is diagnostic. Typical MR appearance is serpentine lesions with well demarcated borders.

SONK resolves with activity modification, analgesia, and in some situations, an offloading brace may help. Bisphosphonates remain unproven in efficacy. Late stages with collapse may require joint replacement or osteotomy. Satisfactory results have been obtained with medial unicompartmental knee replacement in medial femoral condyle SONK.

Langdown AJ, Pandit H, Price AJ, Dodd CAF, Murray DW, Svärd UCG, Gibbons CLMH. Oxford Medial Unicompartmental Arthroplasty for Focal Spontaneous Osteonecrosis of the Knee. Acta Orthop 2005;76(5):688–92. 29 knees compared to 28 knees with arthritis. Mean 5 year follow up. No implant failure, no significant difference in Oxford knee score.

Secondary osteonecrosis in the knee involves more than one condyle and can have multiple sites of involvement. Underlying risk factors are similar to osteonecrosis of the hip. The lesions can extend into the diaphysis.

Osteochondritis Dissecans

Osteochondritis dissecans (OCD) is an idiopathic, focal abnormality of subchondral bone causing instability and detachment of bone fragment, with or without overlying articular cartilage changes.

Possible contributory etiological factors may be traumatic, recurrent traumatic events, vascular or hereditary, although no conclusive link has been established. Microtrauma from the anterior tibial spine combined with a narrow intercondylar notch may be a possible cause. OCD is bilateral in 15% patients.

Common presentation is mechanical pain during sports. The age of presentation influences the prognosis, with better outcome in younger age. Pappas classification is based on age of presentation—under the age of 12 years, 12–20 years and over 20 years.

Sometimes OCD is picked up incidentally, and some patient may present with pain, swelling and locking of the joint. Wilson's test is elicited by extending the knee from a flexed position with foot rotated internally, and then repeating the manoeuvre with the foot rotated externally. If the pain resolves when foot is turned externally, it suggests a medial femoral condyle OCD.

A tunnel radiograph can demonstrate the lesion. MR scan is diagnostic. Criteria of instability of the fragment on MR scan are high signal line at the fragment—host bone interface; cyst at the interface; high signal intensity through the articular cartilage; and focal articular cartilage defect.

Poor prognostic factors include age at presentation over 12 years, lesion area over 240 mm^2 and presence of a cyst of diameter over 1.3 mm on MR scan.

Cahill and Berg divided the AP view of the knee into 5 segments from medial to lateral. Harding divided the lateral view into 3 areas—anterior, middle and posterior based on the Blumensaat's line between A and B, and the tangent along the posterior femoral cortex between B and C. These help in defining the area of involvement (Fig. 3.20).

The Guhl arthroscopic classification helps describe the lesion (Table 3.10).

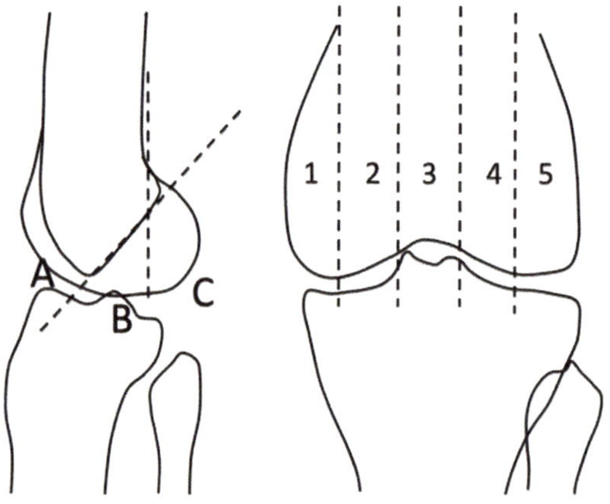

Fig. 3.20 Segments for classification of OCD

Table 3.10 Guhl classification of OCD lesions

Stage	Features
Stage 1	Intact cartilage, but soft and ballotable lesion
Stage 2	Early separation with interruption of cartilage
Stage 3	Partially detached lesion
Stage 4	Complete detachment within bed or displaced

Treatment

Incidental lesions can be followed up. Pivoting and recurrent impact sports are avoided if these aggravate symptoms.

Persistent symptoms, especially in children over the age of 12, with intact cartilage cover can be managed by drilling through the cartilage using a 1.2 mm K wire (transarticular drilling) at the time of arthroscopy. Multiple drill holes encourage revascularisation of the lesion. This carries the disadvantage of penetration of normal cartilage.

Extraarticular drilling can be done under image guidance to penetrate the lesion from the metaphyseal side. This avoids articular cartilage injury, but involves radiation exposure and is technically demanding.

Unstable fragments can be fixed using metal or bioabsorbable screws or nails. Bone graft from proximal tibia can be used to reconstruct subchondral bone defects where the cartilage is intact.

In situations where the fragment is not fixable, options are cancellous bone grafting and chondrocyte implantation; or mosaic osteochondral transplantation.

Patellofemoral Joint

Stabilisers of the patella can be dynamic or static (Table 3.11).

Clinical Assessment

The commonest symptoms due to patellofemoral pathology are anterior knee pain and patellar instability. A thorough history and examination is essential.

Table 3.11 Stabilisers of patella

Dynamic stabilisers	Static stabilisers
Components of the quadriceps femoris	Depth of the trochlear groove Shape of patellar facets Patellar tendon length Quadriceps tendon direction (Q angle) Trochlear groove–tibial tubercle distance Medial patellofemoral ligament Lateral retinaculum

Evaluation includes causes above the knee, at the knee and below the knee which could account for anterior knee pain. Referred pain from the hip or spine should be ruled out.

Specific features to note on examination are varus or valgus alignment of the leg, recurvatum, muscle atrophy, gait, patellar tracking, mediolateral displacement of the patella, the J sign, the Q angle, patellar mobility and glide. For the Q angle, line is drawn from the anterior superior iliac spine to centre of patella and a second line from the centre of patella to the tibial tubercle (Fig. 3.21). A high Q angle correlates with patellar instability.

Torsional deformities of the femur and tibia and leg length inequality should also be assessed, as well as foot disorders such as pes planus.

A positive J sign is the lateral movement of the patella when a flexed knee is extended. Beighton score will guide the surgeon when management options are considered.

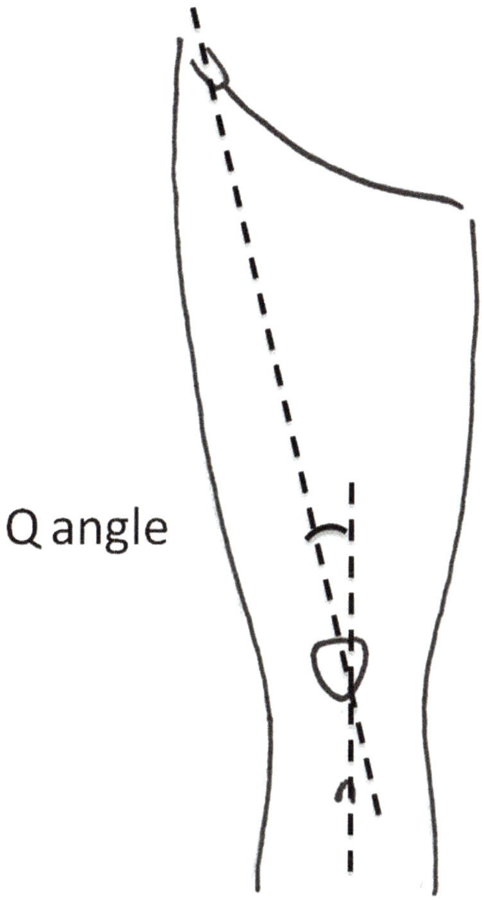

Fig. 3.21 The 'Q' or quadriceps angle

Hyperlaxity

The Beighton score is commonly used for assessing hyperlaxity (Table 3.12). The maximum score is 9. A score of 4 or more indicates hyperlaxity. The diagnosis of benign joint hypermobility syndrome takes into account the Beighton score, the presence of arthralgia for more than 3–4 months and several minor factors such as subluxation of joints and the presence of tendonitis, bursitis, abnormal skin striae and marfanoid habitus, among others.

Table 3.12 The Beighton score for assessing hyperlaxity

Finding	Score (points)
Ability to place palms on the floor on bending forward with knees extended	1
Tip of thumb can touch flexor surface of forearm on passive stretching (one point for right and one for left side)	2
Knee hyperextension over 10 degrees (one point for right and one for left side)	2
Elbow hyperextension over 10 degrees (one point for right and one for left side)	2
Passive hyperextension of the little finger MCP joints to 90° (one point for right and one for left side)	2

Imaging

Standard radiographic assessment of patella includes AP, lateral and skyline views. Long leg alignment view is helpful for evaluation of patella pathology.

A crossover sign on lateral view indicates trochlear dysplasia.

Different ratios have been described for diagnosis of patella alta (Fig. 3.22).

Patella alta is quantified by the Insall–Salvati index or the Blackburne–Peel index

The Insall–Salvati index is the ratio of the length of the patellar tendon to the diagonal length of the patella on a lateral radiograph. The normal ratio is 1.0, while a ratio of 1.2 indicates patella alta.

The Blackburne–Peel index is the ratio of the length of the articular surface of the patella to the perpendicular distance between the articular surface of the tibia and the inferior pole of the patella. The normal ratio varies from 0.54 to 1.06.

The Blumensaat's line is an anterior extension of the intercondylar notch line on the lateral view. The inferior pole of the patella should be at the level of this line when the radiograph is obtained with the knee at 30° flexion.

The lateral radiograph of the knee and axial view is used to diagnose trochlear dysplasia. The 'crossing sign' indicates a shallow trochlear groove. Cross-sectional imaging on CT and MR scans also demonstrates the trochlear groove, the shape of patella and the condition of the retinacular attachments.

MR scan can delineate trochlear dysplasia and measure tibial tubercle trochlear groove (TTTG) distance. Normal TTTG is less than 15 mm. A distance of over 20 mm predisposes to patellar instability. MRI also helps evaluate the ligamentous, cartilage and extensor mechanism integrity.

Patella Morphology Classification

The Wiberg classification of patellar shape describes three types with a fourth type added by Baumgartl (Table 3.13).

Patella Dislocation

Acute dislocation results from a significant injury. Recurrent dislocations may indicate an underlying cause for patellar instability.

Assessment

Generalised causes of laxity should be assessed. The features are summarised in Fig. 3.23.

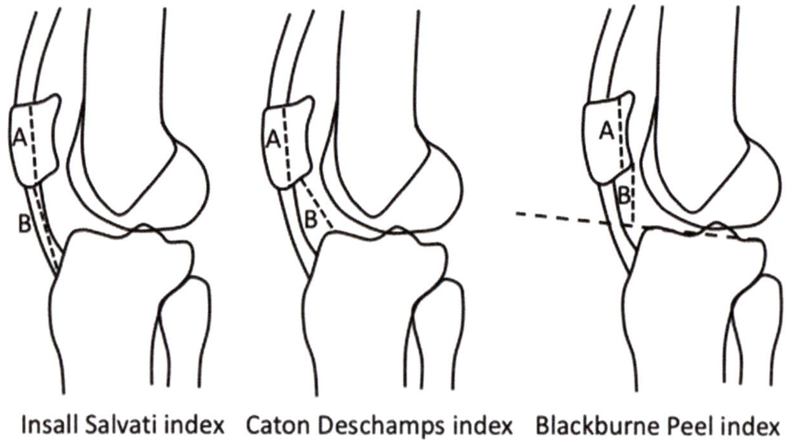

Fig. 3.22 Indices of patellar height

Treatment

Acute dislocations are commoner in teenage and young adults. Most of these are managed with simple relocation of the patella. Post-reduction radiographs should be carefully assessed for osteochondral fragments. Osteochondral fragments can be fixed using absorbable nails through an arthroscopic or mini-open approach.

A skyline view of the patella should be performed to rule out bony avulsion of the patellofemoral ligament. An avulsion fracture is amenable to reduction and fixation.

Table 3.13 Wiberg classification

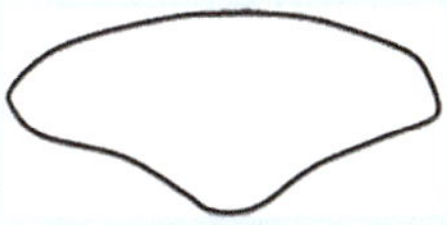	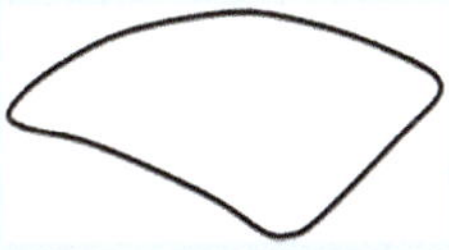
Type I—The medial and lateral facets are symmetrical and equal in size.	Type II—The medial facet is smaller than the lateral
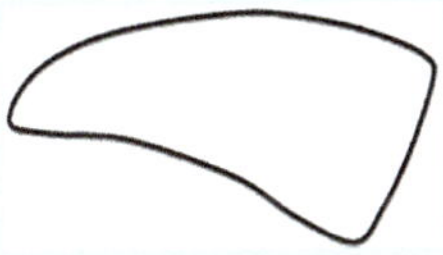	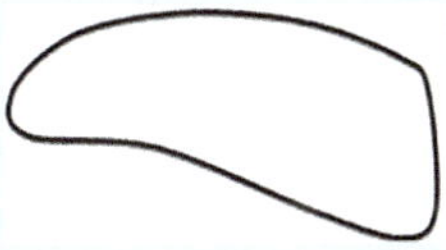
Type III—The medial facet markedly smaller than the lateral	Type IV—No medial facet and consequently no median ridge

Recurrent Dislocation

Finding the underlying cause is essential. An attempt at non-operative management with strengthening of the vastus medialis muscle is justified in patients with recurrent dislocation. The frequency of dislocation reduces as patients progress beyond the teenage years. Patients who do not respond to non-operative treatment are candidates for stabilisation procedures. A variety of options exist and the treatment is tailored to correct the underlying cause.

Reconstruction of the Medial Patellofemoral Ligament (MPFL)

Reconstruction of the MPFL is done using single hamstring (gracilis or semitenidinosus) autografts, and fixation at isometric position in the femur and patella.

The MPFL acts a restraint to lateral subluxation of patella in the initial 30 degrees of flexion. Beyond that, the trochlea helps to stabilise the patella. The femoral attachment lies between the adductor tubercle and the medial epicondyle (Fig. 3.24). The point of attachment for reconstruction is posterior to the line projected along the posterior femoral cortex.

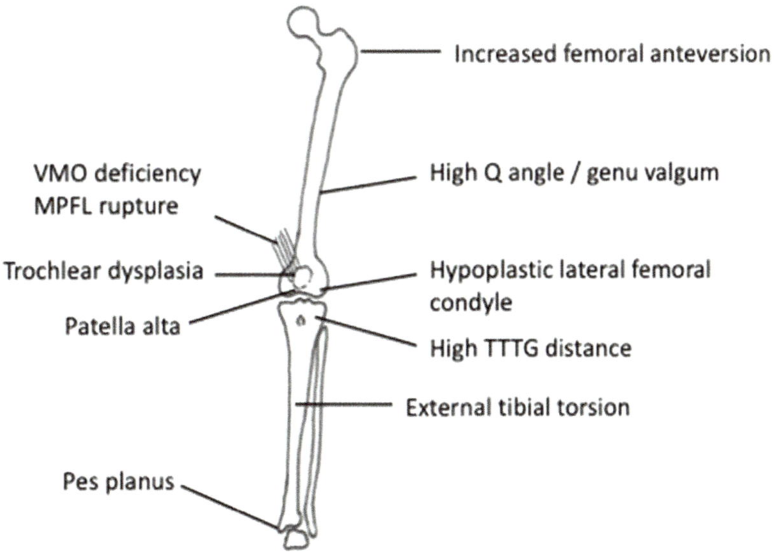

Fig. 3.23 Factors leading to patellar instability

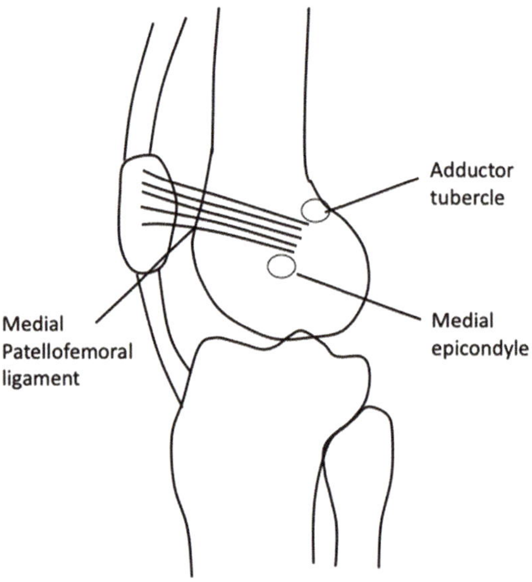

Fig. 3.24 Anatomy of the MPFL

Common injuries to the MPFL are femoral avulsions. Optimum tensioning of the graft is essential.

Realignment

Realignment of the extensor mechanism can be proximal, distal or combined. Proximal realignment is based on reefing or advancing the medial retinaculum and release of the lateral side. It can be performed in skeletally immature patients with no significant distal malalignment problems. Any bony alignment features noted needing correction are treated with femoral derotation osteotomy or a combination of ligament reconstruction and osteotomy.

Proximal realignment using a soft tissue procedure involves advancing the vastus medialis, or releasing the lateral retinaculum, or a combination of the two. This is effective if the Q angle is less than 20°. For a higher Q angle, distal realignment is required.

The lateral release may be helpful in patients with patellar tilt and clinically demonstrable tightness of the lateral retinaculum. The adequacy of release should be checked to maximise efficacy. On its own, lateral release is rarely a solution for patellar maltracking.

Distal realignment is commonly the Fulkerson osteotomy, or anteromedial tibial tubercle transfer. The osteotomy is a biplanar resection of the tibial tubercle and allows medial and anterior displacement of the tibial tubercle. The medial displacement improves Q angle and provides stability. Anteriorisation reduces patellofemoral joint reaction force and is helpful in patients with arthritic symptoms.

Various other osteotomies have been described around the tibial tubercle but are rarely done now.

Trochlear dysplasia is described separately.

Trochlear Dysplasia

Trochlear dysplasia is flattened trochlea or prominence of trochlea relative to femoral condyles leading to patellar instability and reduced patellofemoral contact area.

In a normal knee, on the lateral radiograph, the line representing the deepest part of the trochlea does not cross the line representing the anterior aspect of the femoral condyles. In a dysplastic trochlea, the two lines cross. This is known as the 'crossing sign' (Fig. 3.25).

Trochlear bump is the distance between the anterior femoral cortical line and a parallel line drawn from the anterior aspect of the trochlear prominence (Fig. 3.26). Trochlear dysplasia has been classified by Dejour (Fig. 3.27).

Treatment of trochlear dysplasia is through deepening the trochlea—trochleoplasty. Various techniques have been described. Dejour technique was an osteotomy of both femoral condyles to create a V shaped trochlea. In the Bereiter technique—a thin osteochondral flap is raised and a bony sulcus is created using burrs. The osteochondral flap is repositioned into the newly formed sulcus and can be fixed with headless screws or absorbable sutures.

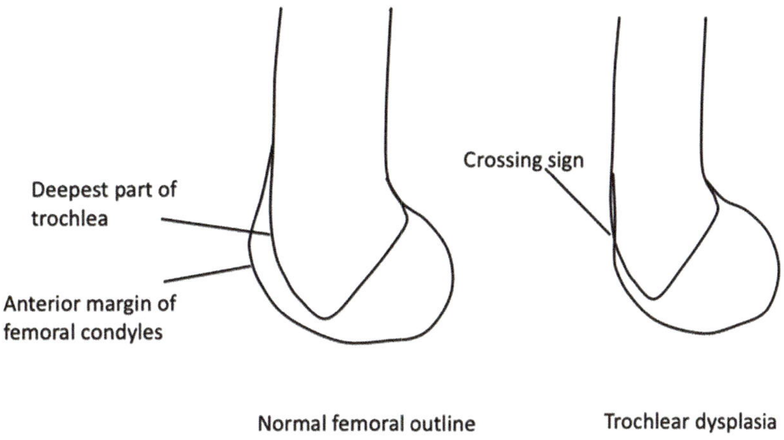

Fig. 3.25 The 'crossing sign' in trochlear dysplasia

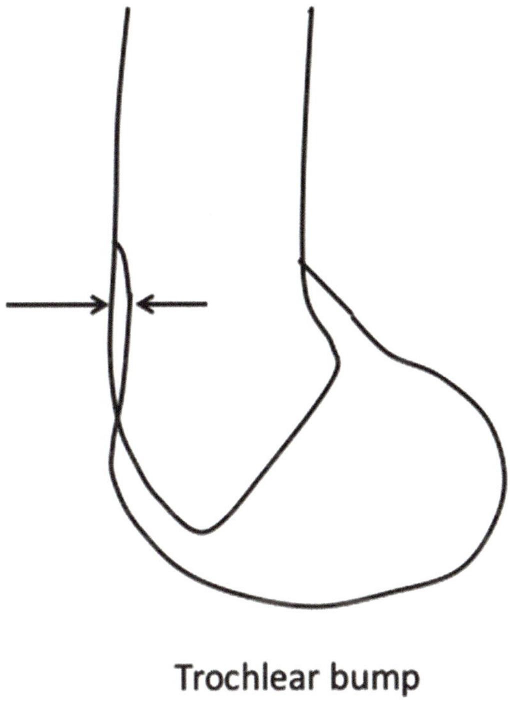

Fig. 3.26 The trochlear bump sign

Complications of trochleoplasty include loss of viability of osteochondral flap, anterior knee pain, stiffness of the knee, recurrent patellar instability and need for further stabilisation procedures. MPFL reconstruction can be combined with trochleoplasty.

Plica Syndrome

Plicae are folds of synovium present normally in the knee. Plicae can occasionally become symptomatic, however, presenting as anterior or anteromedial knee pain; or a snapping band in the knee.

On arthroscopy, changes in the articular surface adjoining the plicae should raise suspicion of plica syndrome. In the absence of any changes, the plicae are unlikely to be the cause of symptoms. Arthroscopic resection of symptomatic plicae has a good success rate.

Prepatellar Bursitis

Prepatellar bursitis presents as swelling anteriorly and may be related to a history of trauma or recurrent irritation. Non-operative treatment involves avoidance of the aggravating activity and anti-inflammatory medication. Persistent swelling is treated by excision of the bursa.

Shin Splints

Also known as medial tibial stress syndrome, shin splints is characterised by pain along the middle and distal third of medial border of the

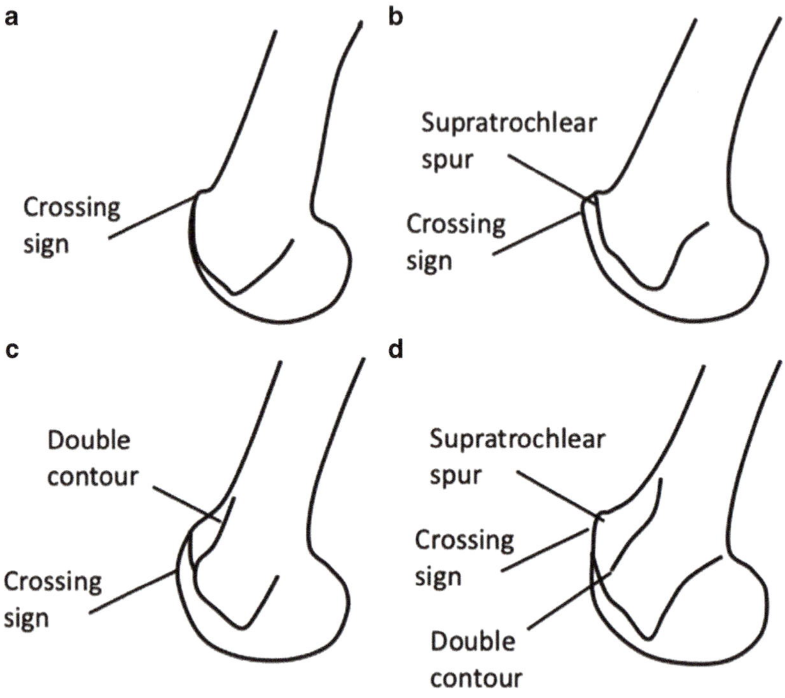

Fig. 3.27 Dejour classification of trochlear dysplasia (Type **a**–**d**)

tibia at the junction of the middle and distal third. There is local tenderness and the symptoms are aggravated by activity.

Plain radiographs are normal, and a Tc-99 bone scan may show increased linear activity along the medial border of the tibia.

Management is largely non-surgical: rest, stretching and a gradual return to activity. Surgical intervention in patients with persistent symptoms involves release of the fascial insertion in the posteromedial border of the tibia. This has a good success rate.

Iliotibial Band Syndrome

The iliotibial band arises from the fascia of the tensor fascia lata and inserts into the Gerdy's tubercle on the anterolateral aspect of the proximal tibia. The band lies anterior to the lateral femoral condyle in full extension and slips posterior to the condyle at 30° of flexion. Excessive friction between the iliotibial band and the lateral femoral condyle leads to the iliotibial band syndrome.

The presenting feature is lateral knee pain on activity. The pain is typically worse on the heel strike. There is local tenderness over the lateral femoral condyle. Pressure with the examiner's thumb over the epicondyle and active knee flexion and extension will reproduce the pain. The Ober test is used to assess tightness of the iliotibial band.

Management of iliotibial band syndrome is based on rest, NSAIDs and stretching exercises. The activity level should be adjusted to avoid aggravating the pain. A lateral heel raise or an orthosis to provide medial arch support may help. Surgical release of posterior fibres, or a Z plasty of the iliotibial band is an option for persistent symptoms.

Non-Arthroplasty Treatment for Osteoarthritis of Knee

NICE has provided guidance on management of osteoarthritis (CG177).

General Health

Exercise is recommended. Weight loss is advised for those who are overweight. Acupuncture is not effective. Walking sticks and other aids may be helpful.

Medication

Paracetamol is the first line of treatment. NSAIDs, COX-2 inhibitors and opioids are second line, and are extensively used to alleviate pain from knee arthritis. Topical Capsaicin or NSAIDs are also helpful.

Cyclo-oxygenase-2 inhibitors have less gastrointestinal side effects. Etoricoxib and NSAIDs are prescribed along with proton pump inhibitors. Renal safety profile and effect on liver function tests for COX-2 inhibitors is similar to diclofenac.

Oral Glucosamine

Oral glucosamine has some benefit, although the degree of improvement is debatable. A recent report in BMJ showed no difference compared to placebo in terms of pain relief. NICE does not recommend oral glucosamine.

Wandel et al. Effects of glucosamine, chondroitin or placebo in patients with osteoarthritis of hip or knee: network mata-analysis. BMJ 2001;341:4675.

Intra-Articular Steroids

Steroids act by reducing neutrophil migration; reducing phagocytosis, lysosomal enzyme release and inflammatory mediator release; and increasing the hyaluronic acid concentration and viscosity of synovial fluid.

Triamcinolone is longest-acting and least soluble steroid.

Side effects are suppression of the hypothalamic–pituitary axis, a reduced stress response to hypoglycaemia, steroid arthropathy (fibrillation, fissure and thinning of cartilage), patellar tendon rupture and osteonecrosis.

Intra-Articular Hyaluronic Acid

Exogenous hyaluronic acid is incorporated into articular cartilage and may have a direct effect on chondrocytes through CD44 receptors.

Intra-articular hyaluronate is usually prescribed once a week for 3–5 weeks, although newer preparations allow a single injection. It is thought to improve chondrocyte density and reduce inflammation. It may have a role in active patients aged older than 60 years and with moderate to severe arthritis. NICE does not recommend intraarticular hyaluronan injection.

Akmal et al. The effects of hyaluronic acid on articular chondrocytes. J Bone Joint Surg 2005;87(8):1143–9. Experimental study on bovine articular chondrocytes. Increased matrix deposition of chondroitin-6-sulphate and type II collagen was found in response to exposure to hyaluronic acid in vitro.

Synovectomy

Synovectomy may be recommended for patients with rheumatoid arthritis, and is indicated if there is no loss of joint space and no deformity. It leads to joint swelling and recovery is slow. The good short-term results of synovectomy deteriorate with time, but this treatment does help to remove mechanical blocks to motion and debris.

Arthroscopic synovectomy has 83% good results improved outcome at 3 years and 46% good results. Patients report improvement at 8 years. Recovery is faster with the arthroscopic procedure.

Valgus Bracing

Valgus bracing may be used to reduce the load on the medial compartment. It is indicated for active patients with unicompartmental disease, who are considered too young for arthroplasty. Long term compliance with the brace is low.

Arthroscopic Lavage

A study has shown some benefit for arthroscopic debridement. From 110 patients who were followed-up for 34 months after the procedure, 90% of patients with mild arthritis, normal alignment and more than 3 mm joint space were improved after arthroscopy. However, only 25% of knees with severe arthritis and less 2 mm joint space showed improvement.

Aaron RK, Skolnick AH, Reinert SE, Ciombor D McK. Arthroscopic debridement for arthritis of the knee. J Bone Joint Surg Am 2006; 88(5):936–43. 110 patients followed up for 34 months after arthroscopic debridement. 90% patients with mild arthritis, normal alignment and >3 mm joint space were improved after arthroscopy while only 25% of knees with severe arthritis and <2 mm joint space showed improvement.

Microfracture, Mosaicplasty and ACI

Described earlier in section on articular cartilage injury.

Osteotomy

A normal mechanical axis drawn from the centre of the hip to the centre of the ankle passes the medial to tibial spine. In High Tibial Osteotomy (HTO), the mechanical axis is shifted laterally such that it passes through the lateral compartment, hence offloading the medial compartment. A distal femoral osteotomy (DFO) is an option for patients with lateral compartment arthritis. HTO and DFO are described in the next section.

High Tibial Osteotomy

Osteotomies around the knee have staged a comeback in popularity. Better fixation methods and reproducible correction techniques have made them a viable option in many situations.

High tibial osteotomy (HTO) is procedure to shift the weight bearing axis towards the lateral side of the knee in order to reduce the load on the medial compartment. This can be achieved through a medial opening wedge or a lateral closing wedge osteotomy. HTO can be done in reverse direction to increase the varus in some very rare situations, but for the sake of simplicity, the following description refers to a valgus HTO for correction of tibia vara.

Varus knees undergo a varus thrust during weight bearing and this will not correct with HTO.

Pre-requisites for HTO are medial compartment arthritis with an intact lateral compartment, preserved flexion over 100 degrees, and non-smokers (Table 3.14). The upper age limit is 60 years (ISAKOS criteria). The knee should be stable (intact MCL). ACL deficient knee is not a contraindication, as changing the slope of proximal tibia to relatively anterior slope tends to provide stability. Similarly, in PCL deficient knees, increasing the posterior slope of the tibia improves stability. ACL reconstruction can be combined with HTO and leads to satisfactory outcome.

'Pagoda type deformity' of the proximal tibia, obesity, preoperative flexion deformity of 15 degrees or more, smoking, underlying chondral changes in the lateral compartment and unrealistic expectations are contraindications to HTO.

A tibia vara of over 5 degrees corresponds to over 90% success at 10 years.

The Miniaci method is used for planning the osteotomy. The mechanical axis (centre of hip to centre of ankle) is drawn on the long leg radiograph. The mechanical axis correction is planned so as to pass through 'Noyes point'. Noyes point lies in the lateral tibial plateau at 62% width con-

Table 3.14 Indications and contraindication for high tibial osteotomy

Indications	Contraindications
Age <60 years Single-compartment arthritis 10–15° varus 90° ROM Flexion contracture <15°	Loss of joint space on the lateral side Lateral tibial subluxation >1 cm Medial compartment loss >2–3 mm Ligamentous instability Inflammatory arthritis

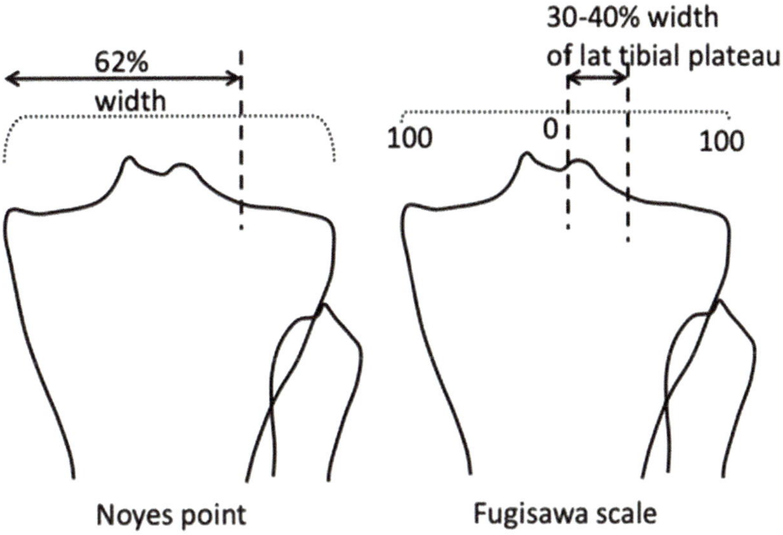

Fig. 3.28 Determining the correction point for HTO

sidering medial margin of tibia as 0 and lateral margin as 100. Fugisawa described a scale and correction should be done to 30–40% width of lateral half of plateau. In Fugisawa scale, the zero is in centre of tibia (Fig. 3.28).

Undercorrection, leaving the limb alignment in varus corresponds to poor result. Overcorrection in excess valgus leads to overload on the lateral compartment and lateral compartment arthritis. Releasing the MCL is required to reduce the pressure on the medial compartment in HTO and a slight valgus overcorrection is desirable.

The first line drawn is the mechanical axis. The second line is from centre of hip, through Noyes point and ends at the level of the ankle. The third line is from centre of ankle to Noyes point. Angle between line 2 and line 3 gives the angle of correction (Fig. 3.29). Generally, in open wedge tibial osteotomies, 1 mm opening corresponds to 1 degree of correction. Alternatively, the following calculation can be used to determine the thickness of the wedge

$$\text{Maximum wedge thickness} = 0.02 \times (\text{diameter of plateau}) \times (\text{angle of correction})$$

Fixation of osteotomy is through a locking plate applied to the medial aspect of tibia.

Both medial opening and lateral closing wedge osteotomies are popular. In a randomised study, no difference or superiority was demonstrated with either technique.

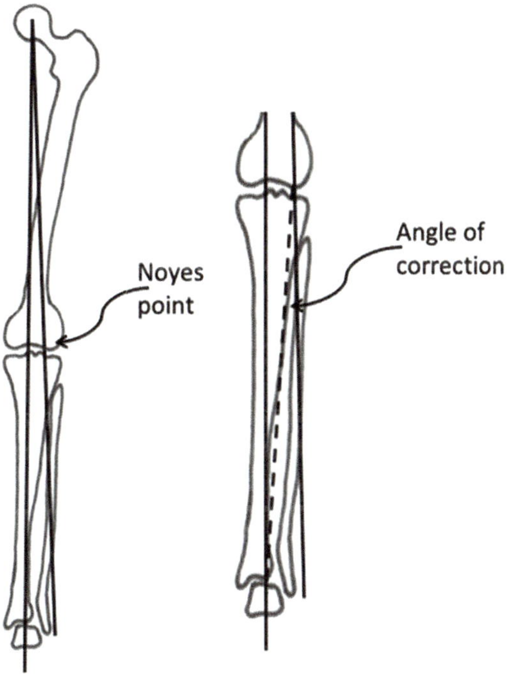

Fig. 3.29 Planning HTO

Brouwer RW, Bierma-Zeinstra SMA, Raaij TM, Verhaar JAN. Osteotomy for medial compartment arthritis of the knee using a closing wedge or an opening wedge controlled by a

Puddu Plate. J Bone Joint Surg Br. 2006;88(11):1454–9. No difference was found at 1 year follow up.

Naudie D, Bourne RB, Rorabeck CH, Bourne TJ. The Install Award. Survivorship of the high tibial valgus osteotomy. A 10- to -22-year follow up study. Clin Orthop Relat Res. 1999;367:18–27. 94 lateral closing wedge osteotomies fixed with staples and cast. Survivorship was 75% at 5 years, 51% at 10 years and 39% at 15 years.

Flecher X, Parratte S, Aubaniac JM, Argenson JN. A 12–28-year follow up study of closing wedge high tibial osteotomy. Clin Orthop Relat Res. 2006;452:91–6. 85% survivorship in 301 patients at 20 years.

Lateral closing requires a staple (less stability) or a lateral plate (more stable fixation). Lateral closing wedge has been the gold standard in literature. Advantages of lateral closing wedge osteotomy are large contact area for healing. Disadvantages are need for lateral approach and risk of peroneal nerve injury, need for fibular osteotomy, shortening, and a lateralised offset of proximal tibia, which can complicate future knee replacements.

The medial opening wedge allows easier titration of correction intraoperatively, and is becoming more popular. There is no need for fibular osteotomy and there is no shortening as a result of the osteotomy (Fig. 3.30). The offset of the tibial canal is not altered. The osteotomy can be planned as a biplanar cut for more stability. The second cut can be cranially directed or caudally directed (Fig. 3.31). Caudal direction preserves

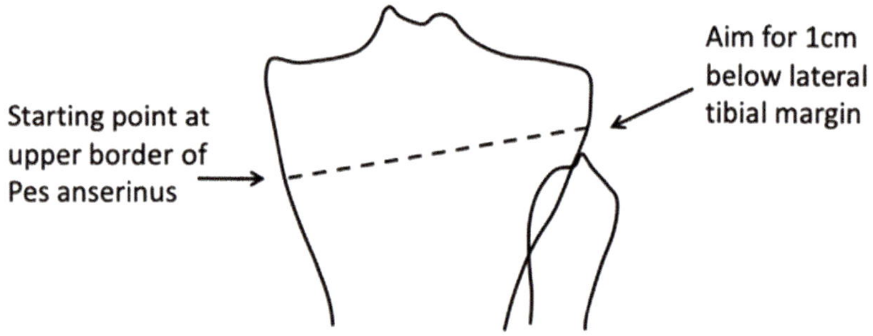

Fig. 3.30 Direction of medial opening HTO in the AP view

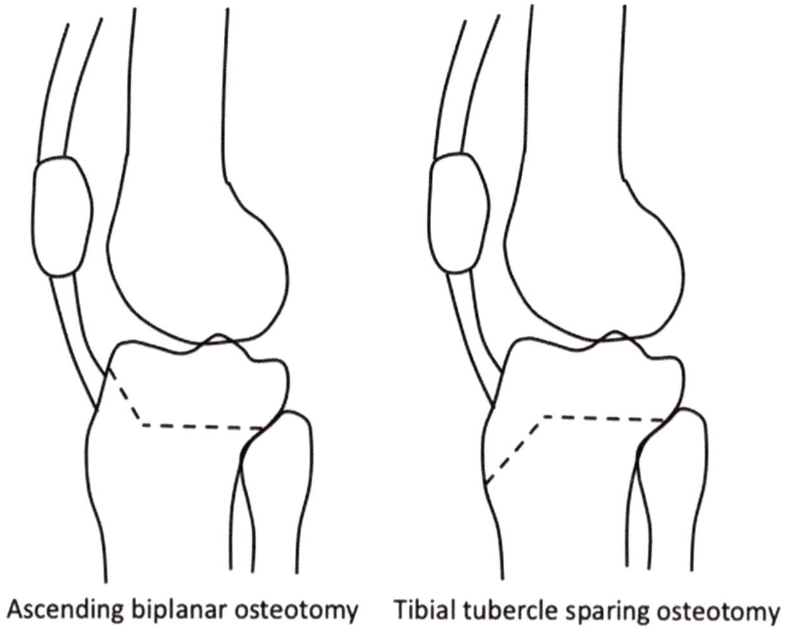

Fig. 3.31 Direction of medial opening HTO in the lateral view

the tibial tubercle and prevents patella baja where large corrections are undertaken. The disadvantage of medial opening wedge is low initial contact area for healing. There is no evidence that using an absorbable calcium filler in the gap improves or interferes with healing of the osteotomy.

Locking plates on the medial aspect of tibia provide the most stable fixation for medial closing wedge osteotomies. Dynamic Locking Screws (DLS) may further improve healing rate in medial open osteotomies.

Gaasbeek RD, Sonneveld H, van Heerwaarden RJ, Jacobs WC, Wymenga AB. Distal tuberosity osteotomy in open wedge high tibial osteotomy can prevent patella infera: a new technique. Knee 2004;11:457–61. Description of descending anterior cut for medial open wedge osteotomy.

Hopwood S, Khan W, Agarwal S. The biplanar open wedge high tibial osteotomy preserving the tibial tubercle. J Orthop Sci 2016;21(6):786–90. Results of tibial tubercle preserving high tibial osteotomy. No nonunion in the study group.

Woodacre T, Ricketts M, Evans JT, Pavlou G, Schranz P, Hockings M, Toms A. Complications Associated With Opening Wedge High Tibial osteotomy--A Review of the Literature and of 15 Years of Experience. Knee 2016;23(2):276–82. 115 patients, 8 year follow up. 80% 5 year survival. Nonunion 4.3%, deep infection 3.5%, plate removal needed in 7%.

Total knee replacement after high tibial osteotomy does not appear to be adversely affected. There can be technical challenges, as discussed in Chap. 14.

Distal Femoral Osteotomy

Distal femoral osteotomy (DFO) is indicated for correction of valgus malalignment associated with isolated lateral compartment arthritis of the knee. This can be achieved by medial closing wedge or lateral opening wedge. As with HTO, patients should be under the age of 60, relatively active, and non-smokers.

Typically, patients have a tibiofemoral angle of more than 12° and a valgus joint-line tilt of more than 10°. The knee should have at least 90° range of movement with less than 10° flexion contracture. The aim is to correct to a tibiofemoral angle of 4–6°.

Obesity, smoking, medial compartment arthritis, or a fixed flexion deformity greater than 10 degrees are contraindications for DFO.

An oblique, biplanar medial closing wedge, leaving the lateral bone bridge intact leads to a stable osteotomy (Fig. 3.32). The goal of correction is to restore the mechanical axis through the middle of the knee, or slightly medial to the midpoint (Fig. 3.33).

Advantages of medial closing wedge are a stable osteotomy with large contact area, and inherent stability due to the biplanar component preventing flexion of the distal fragment. Injury to femoral vessels is a rare but major risk with this approach.

Lateral opening wedge osteotomies require a plate on the lateral aspect of distal femur. This allows controlled opening and accurate correction. The plate can cause irritation of the iliotibial band requiring removal once the osteotomy is healed.

Current literature on DFOs is largely level IV evidence with small number of patients. Open versus closed wedge have similar outcomes.

Backstein D, Morag G, Hanna S, Safir O, Gross A. Long-term follow-up of distal femoral varus osteotomy of the knee. J Arthroplasty 2007;22:2–6. 40 patients with medial closing wedge osteotomy and plate fixation, 123 month mean follow up. 60% good result. 20% had been converted to total knee replacement.

Kosashvili Y, Safir O, Gross A, Morag G, Lakstein D, Backstein D. Distal femoral varus osteotomy for lateral osteoarthritis of the knee: A minimum ten-year follow-up Int Orthop 2010;34:249–54. 33 osteotomies. Almost half needed total knee replacement by 15 years.

Pigmented Villo Nodular Synovitis

Pigmented Villo nodular Synovitis (PVNS) of the knee presents with pain and swelling The knee is the commonest joint affected in PVNS. The disease can be localised or diffuse. (See PVNS Hip in Adult hip chapter).

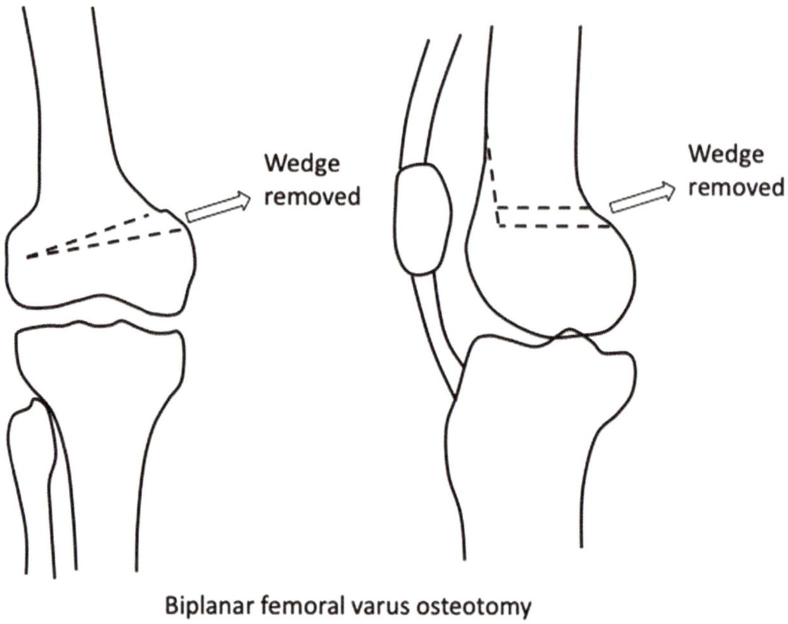

Fig. 3.32 Biplanar femoral varus osteotomy

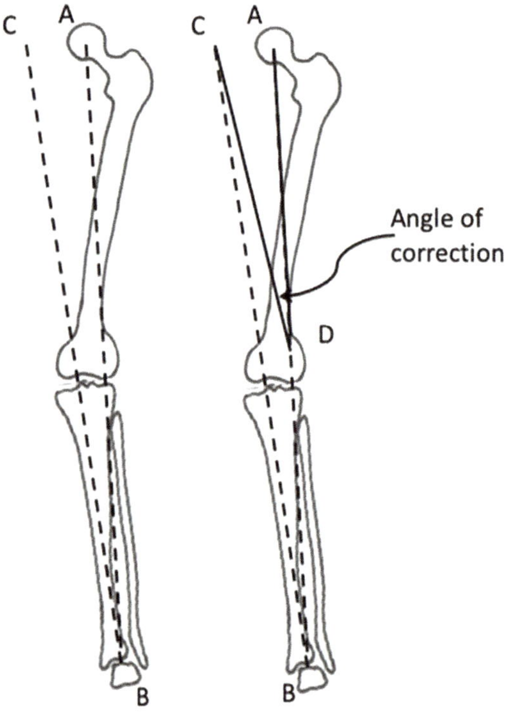

Fig. 3.33 Planning a DFO. Line **ab** is mechanical axis. Line **bc** passes through the intended correction point on the tibial plateau. The amount of translation needed is from **a** to **c**. An angle is projected onto the hinge point on lateral femoral cortex from **a** and **c** to give the angle of correction

Diagnosis is through an MR scan. STIR sequence shows a high signal. The Gradient Echo (GE) has a low signal and may show 'blooming'. Blooming is a 'susceptibility artefact' on MR due to presence of paramagnetic substances. In the case of PVNS, blooming is due to the iron in haemosiderin which gets deposited in the synovium. Blooming means the lesions appear larger than their actual dimensions.

Management is arthroscopic or open synovectomy. Diffuse disease is difficult to remove completely and there is a high risk of recurrence.

Synovial Chondromatosis

This is a condition of cartilaginous metaplasia of the synovium leading to multiple loose bodies within the joint. If symptomatic, arthroscopic or open removal is done.

Baker's Cyst

Baker's cyst or a popliteal cyst is a bulging of the synovium though the posterior capsule in the popliteal area. These are usually the result of excess synovial fluid in the joint. It causes local pain, swelling, discomfort on flexion and a feeling of tightness. The cyst can be related to underlying arthritis or gout.

Baker's cysts in patients undergoing knee replacement for arthritis tend to persist and can be symptomatic in 30% patients after knee replacement.

Imaging to determine the underlying cause is helpful. Aspiration and steroid injection can be attempted but has a high rate of recurrence. Large cysts causing persistent symptoms can be excised through a posterior approach. Vascular surgery support is advisable for the procedure.

Quadricepsplasty

Quadricepsplasty is releasing the quadriceps muscle to alleviate knee stiffness. Judet's quadricepsplasty is the preferred technique as it minimises extensor lag. Thomson technique is lengthening of the quadriceps leading to very high incidence of extensor lag, limiting its popularity.

The procedure is indicated for restricted knee flexion following tethering or scarring of the quadriceps muscle. In modern orthopaedic practice, it is usually following external fixation in the thigh. High energy femoral fractures managed with internal fixation may sometimes develop stiffness and quadricepsplasty can be considered to improve flexion in these patients.

The Judet technique is a long lateral incision from the lateral border of patella to the greater trochanter. The patella, lateral retinaculum and quadriceps are lifted off the femur releasing all the adhesions. A second medial parapatellar incision releases the medial patellar retinaculum and intraarticular adhesions. Continuous passive motion is employed postoperatively to maintain range of movement.

Ahmad A, Villafuerte J Hashmi M, Saleh M. Judet's Quadricepsplasty, Surgical Technique, and Results In Limb Reconstruction. Clin Orthop Relat Res 2003;415:214–20. 10 patients, Average preoperative 33 degrees flexion improved to 88 degrees at 24 months.

Further Reading

McNicholas MJ, Rowley DI, McGurty D, et al. Total meniscectomy in adolescence: a thirty-year follow-up. J Bone Joint Surg Br. 2000;82:217–21.

Arnoczky SP, Warren RF. Microvasculature of the human meniscus. Am J Sports Med. 1982;10:90–5.

McDermott ID, Sharifi F, Bull AMJ, Gupte CM, Thomas RW, Amis AA. The consequences of meniscectomy. J Bone Joint Surg Br. 2006;88:1549–56.

Roos H, Lauren M, Adalberth T, et al. Knee osteoarthritis after meniscectomy: prevalence of radiographic changes after twenty-one years, compared with matched controls. Arthritis Rheum. 1998;41:687–93.

Sihvonen R, Paavola M, Malmivaara A, Järvinen TL. Finnish Degenerative Meniscal Lesion Study (FIDELITY): a protocol for a randomised, placebo surgery controlled trial on the efficacy of arthroscopic partial meniscectomy for patients with degenerative meniscus injury with a novel 'RCT within-a-cohort' study design. NEJM. 2013;369(26):2515–24.

Haklar U, Donmez F, Basaran SH, Canbora MK. Results of arthroscopic repair of partial- or full-thickness longitudinal medial meniscal tears by single or double vertical sutures using the inside-out technique. Am J Sports Med. 2013;41(3):596–602.

Dhollander A, Verdonk P, Verdonk R. Treatment of painful, irreparable partial meniscal defects with a polyurethane scaffold: midterm clinical outcomes and survival analysis. Am J Sports Med. 2016;44(10):2615–21.

Elattar M, Dhollander A, Verdonk R, Almqvist KF, Verdonk P. Twenty-six years of meniscal allograft transplantation: is it still experimental? A meta-analysis of 44 trials. Knee Surg Sports Trauma Arthrosc. 2011;19(2):147–57.

Kennedy J, Jackson MP, O'Kelly P, Moran R. Timing of reconstruction of the anterior cruciate ligament in athletes and the incidence of secondary pathology within the knee. J Bone Joint Surg Br. 2010;92:362–6.

Mook WR, Miller MD, Diduch DR, Hertel J, Boachie-Adjei Y, Hart JM. Multiple-ligament knee injuries: a systematic review of the timing of operative intervention and postoperative rehabilitation. J Bone Joint Surg Am. 2009;91(12):2946–57.

Lachman JR, Rehman S, Pipitone PS. Traumatic Knee Dislocations: Evaluation, Management, and Surgical Treatment. Orthop Clin North Am. 2015;46(4):479–93.

Langdown AJ, Pandit H, Price AJ, Dodd CAF, Murray DW, Svärd UCG, Gibbons CLMH. Oxford Medial Unicompartmental Arthroplasty for Focal Spontaneous Osteonecrosis of the Knee. Acta Orthop. 2005;76(5):688–92.

Wandel S, et al. Effects of glucosamine, chondroitin or placebo in patients with osteoarthritis of hip or knee: network mata-analysis. BMJ. 2001;341:4675.

Akmal M, et al. The effects of hyaluronic acid on articular chondrocytes. J Bone Joint Surg. 2005;87(8):1143–9.

Aaron RK, Skolnick AH, Reinert SE, Ciombor DM. Arthroscopic debridement for arthritis of the knee. J Bone Joint Surg Am. 2006;88(5):936–43.

Brouwer RW, Bierma-Zeinstra SMA, Raaij TM, Verhaar JAN. Osteotomy for medial compartment arthritis of the knee using a closing wedge or an opening wedge controlled by a Puddu Plate. J Bone Joint Surg Br. 2006;88(11):1454–9.

Naudie D, Bourne RB, Rorabeck CH, Bourne TJ. The install award. Survivorship of the high tibial valgus osteotomy. A 10- to -22-year follow up study. Clin Orthop Relat Res. 1999;367:18–27.

Flecher X, Parratte S, Aubaniac JM, Argenson JN. A 12-28-year follow up study of closing wedge high tibial osteotomy. Clin Orthop Relat Res. 2006;452:91–6.

Gaasbeek RD, Sonneveld H, van Heerwaarden RJ, Jacobs WC, Wymenga AB. Distal tuberosity osteotomy in open wedge high tibial osteotomy can prevent patella Infera: a new technique. Knee. 2004;11:457–61.

Hopwood S, Khan W, Agarwal S. The biplanar open wedge high tibial osteotomy preserving the tibial tubercle. J Orthop Sci. 2016;21(6):786–90.

Woodacre T, Ricketts M, Evans JT, Pavlou G, Schranz P, Hockings M, Toms A. Complications associated with opening wedge high tibial osteotomy--a review of the literature and of 15 years of experience. Knee. 2016;23(2):276–82.

Backstein D, Morag G, Hanna S, Safir O, Gross A. Long-term follow-up of distal femoral varus osteotomy of the knee. J Arthroplasty. 2007;22:2–6.

Kosashvili Y, Safir O, Gross A, Morag G, Lakstein D, Backstein D. Distal femoral varus osteotomy for lateral osteoarthritis of the knee: a minimum ten-year follow-up. Int Orthop. 2010;34:249–54.

Ahmad A, Villafuerte J, Hashmi M, Saleh M. Judet's quadricepsplasty, surgical technique, and results in limb reconstruction. Clin Orthop Relat Res. 2003;415:214–20.

4 Adult Pathology: Hip

Sanjeev Agarwal

Avascular Necrosis of Hip

Avascular necrosis (AVN) or osteonecrosis implies death or necrosis of bone due to loss of blood supply. Most common patient population for AVN of the hip are men in second to fifth decade of life.

Etiology

Impairment of blood supply can be due to extraosseous compression of arteries, intraosseous blockage of end arteries or intraosseous compression of arteries.

In many cases cause may not be known. Common causes are oral steroid intake, alcohol, post traumatic and sickle cell disease. Uncommon causes are smoking, radiation, pregnancy, vasculitis, hyperlipidaemia, coagulopathies and decompression sickness.

The common causes are shown in Fig. 4.1.

Osteocyte apoptosis is considered a key factor in steroid induced AVN. Alcohol, steroids and hypercoagulable states lead to altered coagulation, reduced osteogenesis and impaired lipid metabolism. This leads to enthothelial disruption and thrombus formation. AVN can happen in 9–40% patients on long term steroid therapy, and can also happen with short term treatment as well as intraarticular injections. Apoptotic osteocytes cannot be phagocytosed, and do not participate in bone remodelling, leading to collapse on weight bearing.

Hypertrophy of the fat cells in the femoral head can lead to pressure on the intraosseous vessels leading to obstruction. This could be a contributing factor in glycogen storage diseases and alcoholism.

The blood supply to the femoral head is derived from the medial and lateral circumflex arteries which arise from the profunda femoris artery. The internal iliac system contributes the internal pudendal artery, which supplies part of the femoral head around the fovea through the artery of ligamentum teres. The lateral epiphyseal branch of the medial circumflex artery is the key source for the weight bearing part of the femoral head.

The circumflex arteries form an extrasynovial arterial ring at the base of the femoral neck and retinacular vessels ascend on the surface of the neck to form a subcapital arterial ring and supply the femoral head.

The blood supply is demonstrated in Fig. 4.2.

Classification

A widely used classification was proposed by Ficat and Arlet in 1964 (Table 4.1). The original system had 3 stages and a fourth stage was added in 1980.

S. Agarwal (✉)
University Hospital of Wales, Consultant Orthopaedic Surgeon, Cardiff, UK

S. Agarwal (ed.), *Current Orthopaedic Practice*, https://doi.org/10.1007/978-3-030-78529-1_4

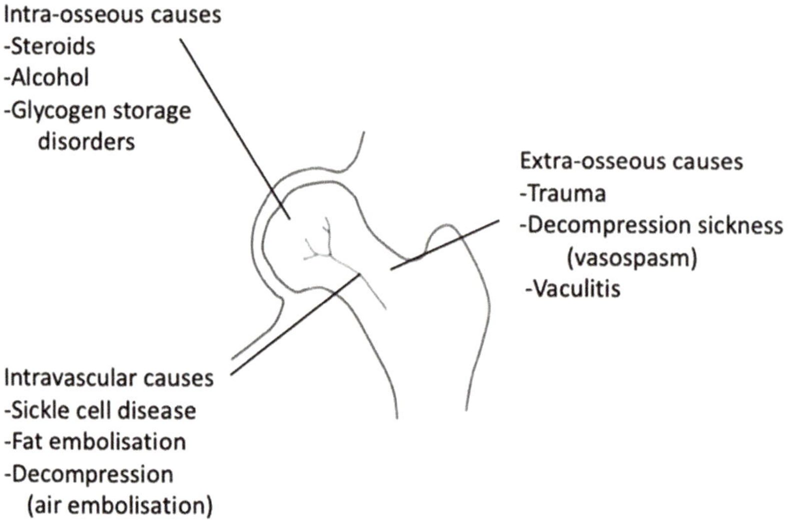

Fig. 4.1 Causes of AVN of femoral head

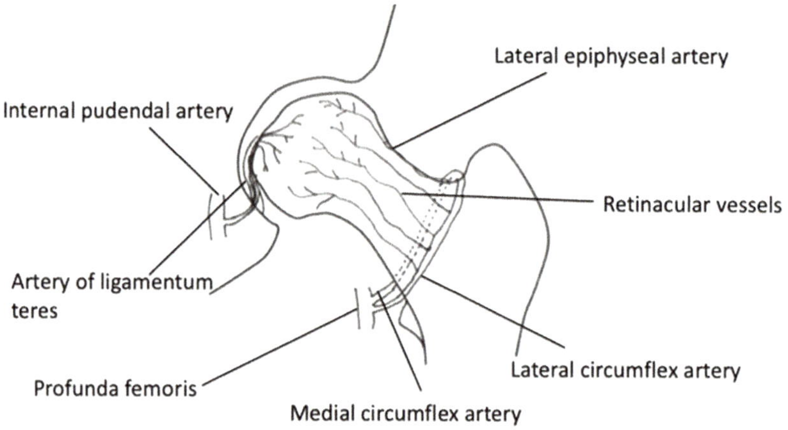

Fig. 4.2 Blood supply to the femoral head

Table 4.1 Ficat and Arlet classification for hip AVN

Stage 1	Normal X ray, MR scan changes present
Stage 2	Sclerosis and cyst formation
Stage 3	Subchondral collapse, crescent sign
Stage 4	Extensive femoral head collapse, joint destruction

A stage 0 to indicate preclinical changes with normal imaging was added in 1985. In stage 0, the other hip is involved. The Ficat classification predates MR scans.

The Steinberg / University of Pennsylvania classification considers MR scan changes and proposed 7 stages (Table 4.2 and Fig. 4.3).

Clinical Presentation

Usual presentation is with history of groin pain and restricted rotation of the hip.

Imaging

Plain radiographs are normal in the stage 0 and 1. MR scan is the gold standard for diagnosis. A single density line on T1 demonstrates the margin of ischaemic bone. A double density on T2 (double line sign) is typical for AVN and represents the hypervascular granulation tissue. Large

Table 4.2 Steinberg Classification for Hip AVN

Stage 0	Normal X ray, MR and Bone scan	
Stage 1	Normal X ray, abnormal MR and bone scan	A—<15% head involvement on X rays / MR
Stage 2	Subchondral sclerosis and cysts	B—15-30% C—>30% head involved
Stage 3	Subchondral collapse (crescent sign) without flattening	A—Crescent <15% of articular surface B—Crescent 15–30% C—Crescent >30%
Stage 4	Flattening of femoral head	A—Less than 15% head collapse and less than 2 mm depression B—15-30% collapse and 2-4 mm depression C—>30% collapse or > 4 mm depression
Stage 5	Joint space narrowing	
Stage 6	Advanced degenerative disease	

lesions in the superolateral quadrant of femoral head are more likely to lead to collapse. The percentage of femoral head involvement is a predictor for collapse of the femoral head.

In transient osteoporosis, the oedema extends in the femoral neck and metaphysis, which is not common in AVN. This helps differentiate the two conditions on MR scan.

The Kerboull angle is the combined angle subtended by the area of necrosis in the femoral head on AP and lateral view. An angle greater than 200 degrees correlates with poor outcome with hip preservation surgery.

Treatment

Nonoperative measures include analgesia, use of walking aids and physiotherapy, which do not influence the natural course, but may provide symptomatic relief. Statins may help reduce adipocyte swelling, but there is little evidence regarding their efficacy in hip AVN.

Bisphosphonates have been tried in early stage localised avascular necrosis. The evidence for their efficacy, despite multiple RCTs and meta-analysis is weak.

Luo RB, Lin T, Zhong HM, Yan SG, Wang JA. Evidence for using alendronate to treat adult avascular necrosis of the femoral head. A systematic review. Med Sci Monit 2014;20:2439–47. Eight studies with 788 hips analysed. Most studies showed reduction in pain, improvement in function and delayed need for hip replacements with the use of bisphosphonates. Overall evidence still considered weak.

Hyperbaric oxygen (HBO) over a prolonged period of time has been tried. The availability of HBO and its doubtful efficacy preclude its usage.

Core decompression can be considered in stage 1 and 2. It helps reduce intra-osseous pressure and may encourage revascularisation. The lesion is localised through preoperative MR scans and drilled under image intensification using a dynamic hip screw (DHS) reamer, or specific drills. Core decompression after femoral head collapse has poor outcome.

Fairbank AC, Bhatia D, Jinnah RH, Hungerford DS. Long term results of core decompression for ischemic necrosis of the femoral head. J Bone Joint Surg 1995;77:42. 10 year follow up of 128 hips. Survival rate in Ficat stage 1, 2 and 3 were 96, 74 and 35% respectively.

Mont MA, Jones LC, Pacheco I, Hungerford DS. Radiographic predictors of outcome of core decompression for hips with osteonecrosis stage III. Clin Orthop 1998;354:159.

Bone graft or bone marrow cells can be packed into the channel. Results of this are based on short term studies. Tantalum rod can be inserted into the channel to provide structural support. Removal of these rods can lead to fracture and results are equivocal. Multiple percutaneous drilling has been tried which involves making multiple holes with a small diameter (3.2 mm) drill or pin. Outcome is similar to core decompression.

Mont MA, Ragland PS, Etienne G. Core decompression of the femoral head for osteonecrosis using percutaneous multiple small

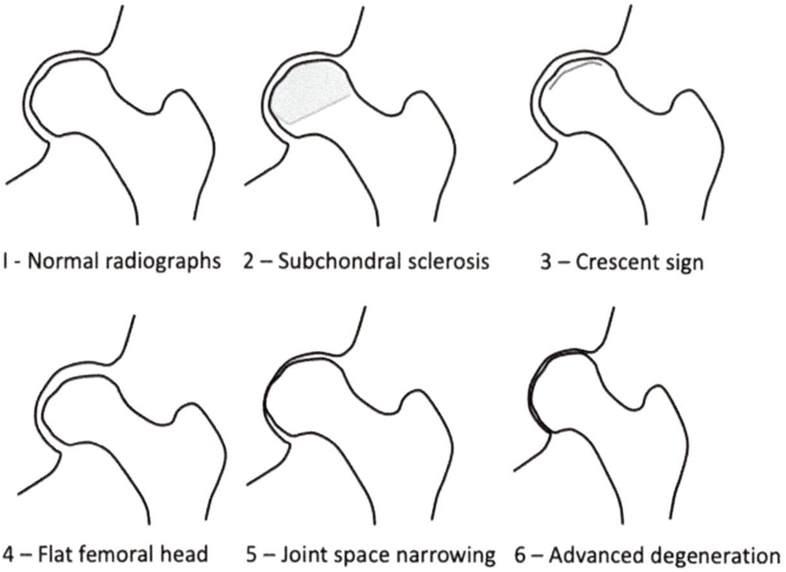

Fig. 4.3 Diagrammatic representation of Steinberg classification

diameter drilling. Clin Orthop 2004;429:131–8. 3 mm Steinmann pin used. 24 out of 30 Stage 1, and 8/15 stage 2 hips had successful result at 2 years.

Vascularised fibular bone graft, originally popularised by Urbaniak, can be considered in stage 1 and 2. The ascending lateral circumflex vessels provide the vascular pedicle. Results are good in some centres, but not reproduced elsewhere. This technique can also be used in Stage 3 and 4 (post collapse, pre-arthritis) and success rate has been reported at over 80%.

Korompillas AV, Lykissas MG, Beris AE, Urbaniak JR, Soucaros PM. Vascularised fibular graft in the management of femoral head osteonecrosis: twenty years later. J Bone Joint Surg Br 2009;91(3):287–93.

Femoral neck rotational osteotomy is an option in stage 1 to 3. It is technically difficult, and the results are not universally reproducible. The procedure is done through a transtrochanteric approach and aims to bring a non-affected part of femoral head into the weight bearing zone.

Sugioka Y. Transtrochanteric anterior rotational osteotomy of the femoral head the treatment of osteonecrosis affecting the hip; a new osteotomy operation. Clin Orthop 1978;130:191–201.

Conversion to total hip replacement at a later stage may be more challenging after osteotomy, although results of hip replacement after rotational osteotomy are comparable to hip replacement for osteoarthritis.

Total hip replacement is the treatment of choice for stage 3 and beyond. Cemented, cementless and metal on metal hips have been shown to have good outcomes.

Cheung KW, Chiu KH, Chung KY. Long term result of cementless femoral stem in avascular necrosis of the hip. Hip Int 2015;25(1):72–5. 117 patients with AVN treated with uncemented hip. Mean age 51, mean follow up 14.7 years. 19 years survival with aseptic loosening as end point was 97.1%, which was comparable to hip replacement for non AVN indications.

Kim YH, Oh SH, Kim JS, Koo KH. Contemporary total hip arthroplasty with and without cement in patients with osteonecrosis of the femoral head. J Bone Joint Surg Am 2003;85(4):675–81. 50 patients with simultaneous bilateral hip replacement for AVN, cemented on one side and cementless on the other side. Mean age 47.3 years and mean follow up 9.3 years. All acetabular components were cementless. No aseptic loosening in either group.

Amstutz HC, LeDuff MJ. Hip resurfacing for osteonecrosis: two to 18 year results of the

Conserve Plus design. Bone Joint J 2016;98:901–9. 82 patients, mean age 40.8 years, mean follow up 10.8 years. Four femoral and 2 acetabular loosening. 90% 15 year survival.

Hip fusion is very rarely done, even in young patients (see Chap. 12).

Bone Marrow Oedema Syndrome

Bone Marrow Oedema Syndrome (BMES) presents with transient nontraumatic hip pain. BMES is a generic term, which includes conditions like transient osteoporosis of the hip. The condition may involve the knee or bones of the foot. About 40% patients may have transient migratory osteoporosis.

MR scan shows high signal in T2 sequence. Absence of focal subchondral changes favours a diagnosis of BMES, as opposed to AVN. The changes extend into the intertrochanteric area.

Treatment of this is nonsurgical through protected weight bearing, physiotherapy and analgesia.

Hip Dysplasia

Patients with dysplastic hips often exhibit a shallow, lateralized, retroverted acetabulum. On the femoral side, there is excess femoral anteversion, valgus neck shaft angle, narrow canal, small head size and shortening (Fig. 4.4).

Excess femoral anteversion may be evident by increased range of internal rotation of the hip on clinical examination. Limb lengths, and signs of impingement should be accurately assessed. Hip replacement is needed in dysplastic hips with secondary osteoarthritis.

Radiological parameters (Fig. 4.5) to consider include

1. Lateral Centre edge angle of Wiberg—normal angle is over 25 degrees. Angle between 20 and 25 is considered borderline and angle under 20 degrees indicates dysplasia. A high angle is seen in pincer impingement.
2. Tonnis angle—measures inclination of the weight bearing dome of the acetabulum. Normally, this should be less than 10 degrees. The weight bearing part or sourcil of the acetabulum is the dome of the acetabulum, usually evident as a zone of thick trabeculae.
3. The ventral (anterior) centre edge angle of Lequesne is measured on the false profile view of the pelvis and should be over 25 degrees. An angle of less than 20 degrees indicates anterior subluxation.
4. Cross over sign indicates a retroverted acetabulum. Visualisation of the ischial spine on the AP view is also a possible indicator of acetabular retroversion.
5. Acetabular angle of Sharp. This is the angle between the line connecting the tear drops and another line from the tear drop to the supero-

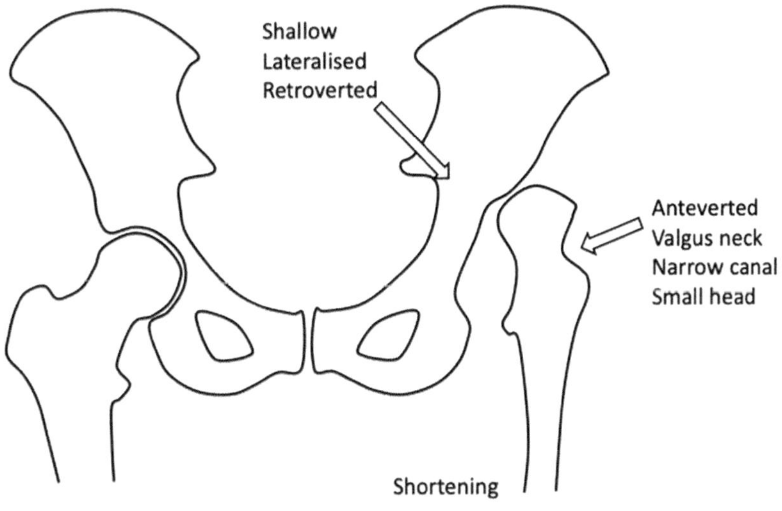

Fig. 4.4 Anatomical changes in hip dysplasia

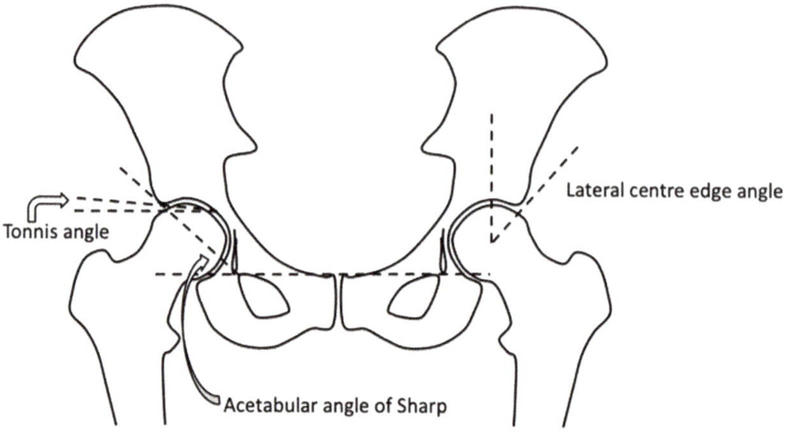

Fig. 4.5 Angles for assessment of acetabular dysplasia

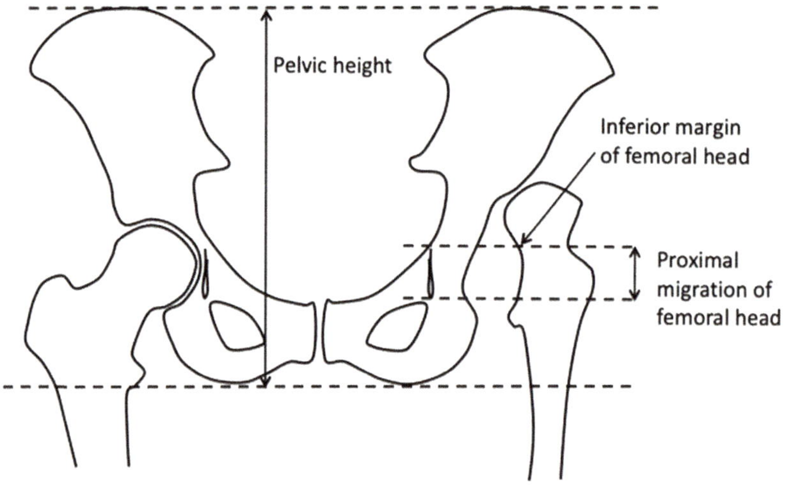

Fig. 4.6 Crowe classification of femoral dysplasia

lateral margin of the acetabulum. An angle over 40 degrees is suggestive of dysplasia.

Hip replacement is needed in dysplastic hips with secondary osteoarthritis. The degree of dysplasia is classified by the Crowe method.

Crowe JF, Mani J, Ranawat CS. Total hip replacement in congenital dislocation and dysplasia of the hip. J Bone Joint Surg Am 1979;61(1):15–23.

The junction of the head and neck of the femur on the medial aspect is identified. A horizontal line is drawn along the inferior border of the teardrop. The proximal migration of the junction point is assessed in relation to the inter-teardrop line. The femoral head diameter is 20% of the vertical height of the pelvis on the AP radiograph.

Table 4.3 Grading of hip dysplasia (Crowe)

Grade	Degree of proximal subluxation as a percentage of femoral head height	Degree of proximal subluxation as a percentage of pelvic height
I	<50%	Less than 10%
II	50–75%	10–15%
III	75–100%	15–20%
IV	>100%	More than 20%

The proximal migration is measured in relation to the femoral head diameter, or 20% of the vertical pelvic height (Fig. 4.6).

The Crowe grading of hip replacement dysplasia is shown in Table 4.3.

An alternative classification was proposed by Hartofilakidis (Table 4.4).

Table 4.4 Hartofilakidis classification of hip dysplasia

Type A	**Mild dysplasia. Head contained within acetabulum.**
Type B	Low dislocation. The false acetabulum is in continuity with the true acetabulum.
Type C	High dislocation. False acetabulum not contiguous with the true acetabulum.

Hip arthroscopy has limited use in dealing with labral pathology, which can coexist with hip dysplasia.

Joint preserving surgery (periacetabular osteotomy) is the mainstay where the secondary degenerative changes are minimal. This corrects the underlying problem and improves coverage of the femoral head. A femoral osteotomy can be combined with the acetabular osteotomy if adequate coverage cannot be achieved with the acetabular osteotomy on its own.

The modern technique of PAO preserves the posterior column and the abductors, allowing early mobilisation and weight bearing. The complication rate is lower compared to previous techniques where the posterior column was divided. Currently, it is offered to symptomatic patients with low CE angle and a well preserved hip joint.

For hip arthroplasty, accurate preoperative planning using templates is essential. The aim of arthroplasty is to restore the hip centre and achieve adequate coverage of the acetabulum. The surgical approach can be through trochanteric osteotomy, posterior approach or the Smith Peterson approach.

The technical problems encountered in the dysplastic hip include anteversion or retroversion of the acetabulum, deficient anterior and superior support, an oblong and shallow acetabulum, and formation of a false acetabulum with a high hip centre. Identification of the true level of acetabulum may be difficult. The ideal position of the prosthetic acetabulum is at the anatomical level.

The capsule and iliopsoas are thickened, and there is tightness of the adductors and hamstrings. The abductors are aligned more transversely than normal.

70 to 80% coverage of a cementless acetabulum is adequate for stability. The component can be medialised to an extent to improve coverage. A shelf graft using the femoral head can be done to augment the superolateral aspect of the acetabulum. Alternatively, tantalum (trabecular metal) augments can be used to buttress the superior acetabular deficiency.

A high hip centre (proximally placed acetabulum) is an option, but not desirable. High hip centre leads to excess shear and high rate of loosening of the acetabulum. Additionally, the acetabular component which can be used is often small, and a small head size has to be used. This can increase the risk of dislocation.

The sciatic nerve is congenitally shorter, and a leg length discrepancy of up to 2.5 cm can be corrected without significant stretching of the nerve. An effort is made to restore hip centre. If the hip is shortened preoperatively such that planned lengthening would compromise the sciatic nerve (more than 2.5 cm lengthening) then a subtrochanteric osteotomy to shorten the femur should be considered (Fig. 4.7). The subtrochanteric shortening osteotomy prevents overlengthening of the limb, while allowing the proximal femoral metaphysis to be moved distally for fixation of femoral component. A fully coated cementless stem that allows the version to be adjusted as required is used.

If sciatic nerve is lengthened by over 3 cm, intraoperative 'wake up test' should be considered.

The femoral canal is narrow and smaller stems are often needed. The version of the neck is abnormal and cannot be used as a guide for femoral component version. Uncemented stems allow modularity and adjustment of version. Such stems may not be part of standard implants and preoperative planning will help the surgeon have these stems available.

*Nagoya S, Kaya M, Sasaki M*et al. *Cementless total hip replacement with subtrochanteric femoral shortening for severe developmental dysplasia of the hip. J Bone Joint Surg Br 2009;91:1142–7. 20 patients, Crowe grade IV,*

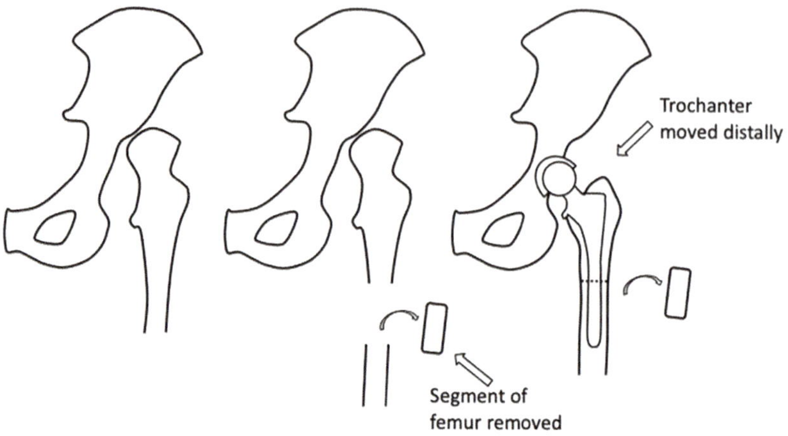

Fig. 4.7 Principle of subtrochanteric shortening osteotomy

8.1 yr follow up. All had subtrochanteric osteotomy, acetabulum placed at anatomical site.

Periacetabular Osteotomy

A Periacetabular osteotomy (PAO) is indicated for symptomatic patients with hip dysplasia. The acetabulum is repositioned to improve the congruence and contact area between the femoral head and the acetabulum. The centre of rotation is medialised, which improves the biomechanics of the hip and reduces the joint reaction force. The widely used technique is known as the Bernese osteotomy popularized by Prof. Ganz from Berne.

Ganz R, Klaue K, Vinh TS, Mast JW. A new periacetabular osteotomy for the treatment of hip dysplasias. Technique and preliminary results. Clin Orthop Rel Res 1988;232:26–36.

The advantages of the Bernese osteotomy are preservation of posterior column, allowing full weight bearing; preservation of abductors; and ease of correction as the sacrospinous ligament is not connected to the mobile fragment.

Indications are a patient under the age of 40 years with Tonnis grade 0 or 1 changes in the hip, congruence possible and preferably BMI under 30 kg/m^2 (Table 4.5).

Outcomes of PAO are defined in terms of survivorship not requiring hip replacement or arthrodesis.

Steppacher SD, Tannast M, Ganz R, Siebenrock KA. Mean 20 year follow up of Bernese periacetabular osteotomy. Clin Orthop Rel Res 2008;466:1633–44. 68 hips, mean age 29 years, minimum 19 year follow up. 60% patients did not have hip replacement surgery. Some patients had arthritis preoperatively.

Table 4.5 Tonnis grading of hip arthritis

Grade 0	No sign of arthritis
Grade 1	Sclerosis of joint with minimal joint space narrowing and osteophytes
Grade 2	Small cysts in the femoral head or acetabulum with moderate joint space narrowing
Grade 3	Advanced arthritis with large cysts, joint space obliteration and severe deformity of femoral head

Femoro-Acetabular Impingement

Femoro-acetabular impingement (FAI) is abnormal contact between the femur and acetabulum resulting in pain, labral disease and secondary osteoarthritis. The two broad mechanisms for FAI are cam lesion (aspherical femoral head with loss of femoral head—neck offset) and pincer lesion (focal or global excessive acetabular coverage of femoral head). A combination of the two may exist (Fig. 4.8). Repeated contact between the femoral neck and the acetabular margin leads to labral injury, and chondral damage.

Compression of labrum between the cam lesion and acetabular rim leads to labral detachments and detachment in the transition zone car-

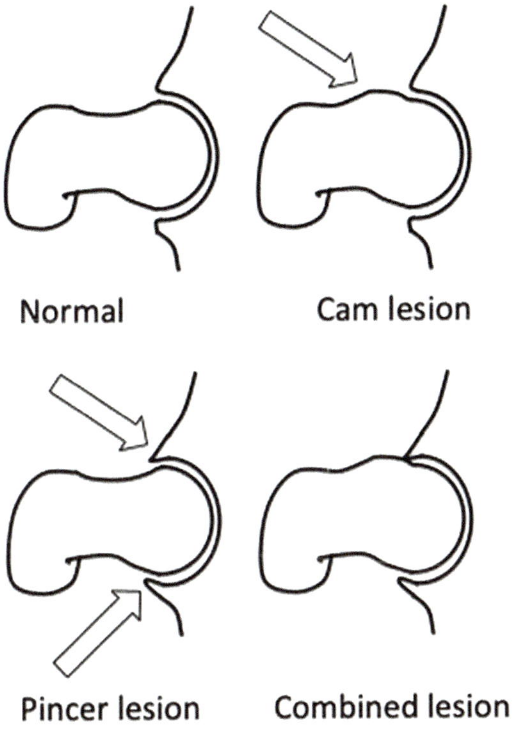

Fig. 4.8 Types of FAI

tilage layer. Damage to the acetabular cartilage is typically in the anterosuperior part of the acetabulum. Outcome following repair of these labral injuries is favourable. Cam lesions are commoner in young active males.

Retroversion of the acetabulum leading to overcoverage anterosuperiorly is commoner in women. Overcoverage can be focal or global. Retroversion may be apparent on plain radiographs as the crossover sign. This leads to degeneration of the labrum anterosuperiorly and a contrecoup posteroinferior cartilage loss on femoral head. The contrecoup injury could be due to shear forces when the femoral head is levered following abutment anteriorly. The labral injury is intra-substance and results of repair are less favourable. Heterotopic bone formation may be evident along the rim adjacent to base of labrum.

Most commonly, a mixed pattern with both cam and pincer lesion is found. A retroverted femur will exacerbate symptoms and restriction of motion resulting from FAI.

FAI can be primary or secondary. Primary FAI is likely to be genetic. Secondary FAI can be due to previous Slipped Upper Femoral Epiphysis (SUFE), previous Perthes disease, following acetabular (innominate) osteotomy, malunited femoral neck fracture, or an exostosis.

The alpha angle measures the anterior concavity of the head neck junction (Fig. 4.9). A high alpha angle correlates with a chondral defect at the rim of the acetabulum and delamination of the cartilage. The beta angle measures the concavity posteriorly. Similarly the anterior and posterior offset of the head-neck can be determined. A centre edge angle greater than 40 degrees is indicative of pincer impingement.

Cam lesions are managed by arthroscopy or open surgical dislocation and osteoplasty. Formation of new cortex at the site of resection occurs over the following 2 years. Resection of over 30% of femoral neck increases the risk of femoral neck fracture. Labral lesion can be repaired or trimmed.

Open surgical dislocation provides extensile exposure but is associated with potential complications of trochanteric nonunion, avascular necrosis of femoral head, heterotopic ossification and abductor weakness. Arthroscopic techniques can provide similar results and is the preferred option in most centres around the world for mild deformities. Moderate deformities may be better managed by open approach. The FASHIoN trial supports hip arthroscopy for FAI.

Griffin DR, Dickenson EJ, Wall PDH et al. Hip arthroscopy versus best conservative care for the treatment of femoroacetabular impingement syndrome (UK FASHIoN): a multicentre randomised controlled trial. Lancet 2018;391:2225–35. Prospective multicentre RCT. 348 patients randomised to hip physiotherapy or hip arthroscopy for FAI. Both groups improved, but hip arthroscopy group had greater improvement.

Surgical hip dislocation was popularised by Ganz. The blood supply to the femoral head is preserved through preservation of the medial circumflex femoral artery. It provides wide exposure. Potential problems are trochanteric

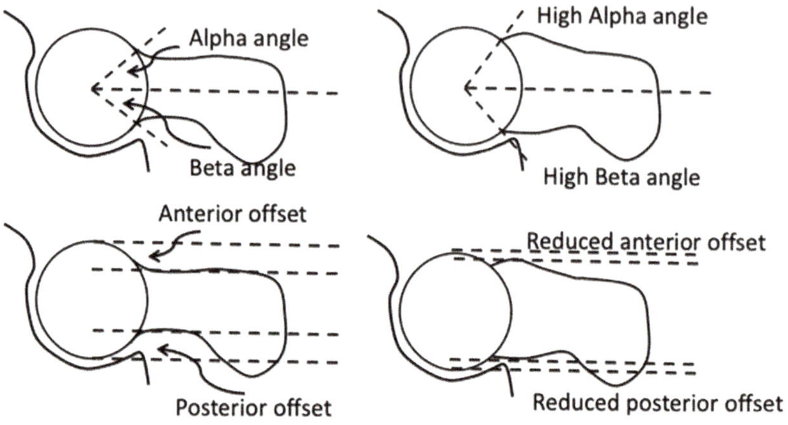

Fig. 4.9 The alpha angle, beta angle and offset in FAI

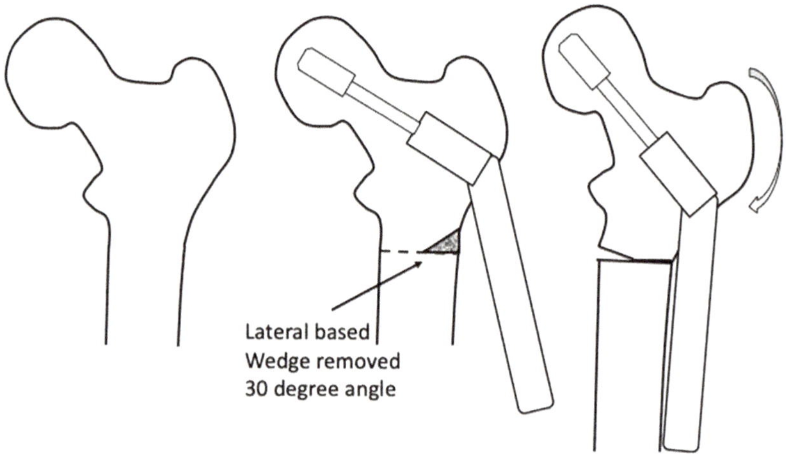

Fig. 4.10 Principle of valgus intertrochanteric osteotomy using a DHS

nonunion, avascular necrosis, retained hardware and heterotopic ossification.

Proximal Femoral Osteotomy

Proximal femoral osteotomy is an increasingly rare operation, and often confined to specialist centres.

A valgus intertrochanteric osteotomy (VITO) can be considered for nonunion of femoral neck in a young person, or femoral neck stress fractures with persistent symptoms despite internal fixation. A lateral closing wedge subtrochanteric osteotomy is planned.

Choice of internal fixation devices include Dynamic hips screw, angled blade plate or a dynamic compression screw (DCS). Blade plates are unforgiving implants although preserve bone and have less risk of damaging the femoral head blood supply.

The familiarity of most surgeons with a DHS makes it an easier implant to use in this situation (Fig. 4.10). A laterally based wedge is removed. The wedge is half the cortical diameter. The plate of DHS is reduced to the femoral shaft, which achieves 30 degree correction. The transverse osteotomy allows immediate full weight bearing with the DHS. The direction of femoral canal is not significantly altered which does not compromise a hip replacement, if needed in future.

Ozkul A, Necmioglu NS, Ziyadanogullari MO, Alemdar C, Arslan H, Uzel K. An evaluation of treating non union of femoral neck fractures with valgus angulation osteotomy using sliding hip screw. Acta Orthop Belg 2019;85:210–7. 16 patients, all united, no avascular necrosis.

A varus osteotomy is achieved by removal of a medially based wedge. Varus osteotomy leads to shortening of the limb. It is rarely undertaken.

Protrusio Acetabuli

Protrusio is the supero-medial migration of the femoral head beyond the Kohler's or ilioischial line (Fig. 4.11). The protrusion is associated with thinning of the medial wall of the acetabulum.

In the majority, the cause of acetabular protrusion may not be obvious. Known underlying cause can be conditions with reduced bone density like osteoporosis, osteomalacia, osteogenesis imperfecta or inflammatory joint disease. Paget's disease, Ehlers Danlos syndrome and Marfan syndrome can be associated with protrusio acetabuli.

The degree of protrusio is graded based on the Hirst classification (Table 4.6).

The normal thickness between the ilioischial line and medial wall of acetabulum is considered to be 2 mm in men. In women, the medial wall may be collinear with the ilioischial line or one mm medial to the line. This measurement will vary between individuals and also on the radiographic projection.

Moderate of severe protrusion can lead to impingement of the femoral neck against the acetabulum and consequent stiffness. Patients present with pain from associated arthritis, or stiffness.

Joint preservation options in young patients include valgus proximal femoral osteotomy or reverse periacetabular osteotomy.

Total hip replacement is needed for advanced symptoms or arthritis. Preoperative planning is helps achieve leg length equality.

Dislocation of the hip is difficult and the neck may have to be divided in situ to avoid fracture of the acetabular margin.

Table 4.6 Hirst classification of protrusio acetabuli

Grade	Degree of protrusion
Mild	5–10 mm protrusion
Moderate	10–15 mm protrusion
Severe	More than 15 mm protrusion

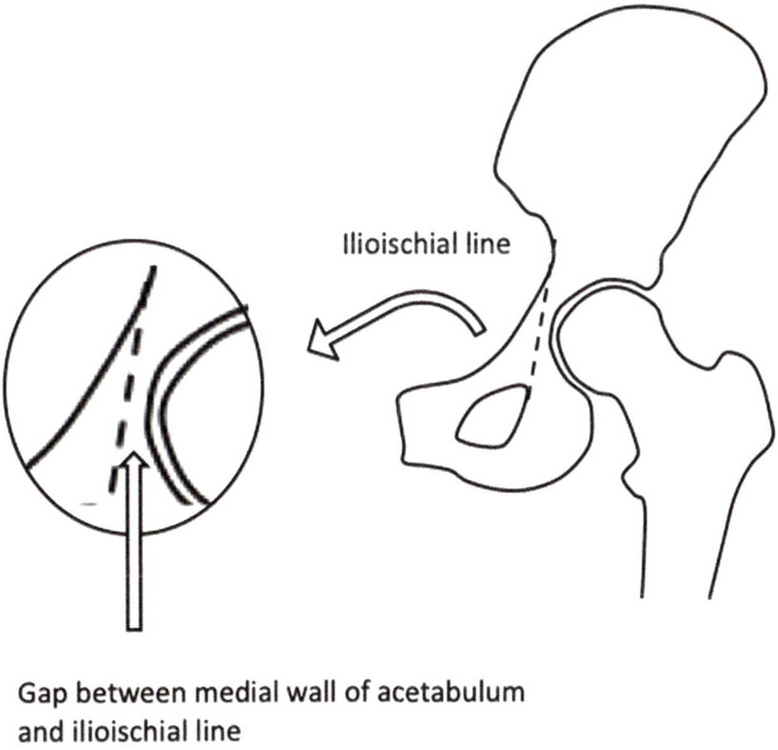

Fig. 4.11 Assessment of acetabular protrusion

The thin medial wall is not reamed and the medial wall may need bone grafting to lateralize the acetabular component to the normal hip centre. Autograft from the femoral head is ideal for this purpose. Restoration of hip centre to the anatomical positions improves survival of the acetabular component.

Pigmented Villo-Nodular Synovitis of Hip

Pigmented Villo Nodular Synovitis (PVNS) of the hip is benign proliferation of the synovium of the hip resulting in nodular and villous projections. This is a locally invasive process leading to recurrent haemarthrosis and joint damage. The condition is usually monoarticular and is common in second to fifth decade of life.

Patients present with recurrent hip pain and stiffness. Radiographs in the initial stages may be normal, but an MR scan will demonstrate the hyperplastic synovium.

Localised symptomatic disease can be managed by radiotherapy or arthroscopic synovectomy. Total hip replacement is needed for advanced joint damage.

Snapping Hip

Causes of snapping hip can be extraarticular or intraarticular.

Extra-articular causes include movement of the iliotibial band over the greater trochanter, or the anterior margin of the gluteus maximus over the greater trochanter.

The iliopsoas tendon can lead to snapping sensation as it moves over the iliopectineal eminence or the femoral head. It may also happen after total hip replacement if the acetabular component is prominent due to large size, malposition, or loss of anterior column bone stock.

Intra-articular causes of a snapping hip are loose bodies, labral tears, hip subluxation and synovial chondromatosis.

Patients are often able to localize the spot where they feel the snapping. Flexion, Adduction and Internal Rotation (FADIr) test is done to check for labral pathology. Iliopsoas snapping can be reproduced by moving the hip from a position of Flexion, Abduction and External Rotation (FAbEr) to Extension, adduction and Internal rotation. The Ober test is used to test for iliotibial band tightness.

MR scan can help detect inflammation in the tendon or thickening of the anterior fibres of iliotibial band. Dynamic ultrasonography can be used.

Management is through physical therapy, steroid injection or surgical release of the tendon. The iliotibial band can be released or lengthened by Z-plasty. The psoas tendon can be released arthroscopically or through open approach. Surgical release leads to improvement in symptoms but temporary reduction in muscle strength. Nonoperative treatment should be tried before surgical methods.

Hamstring Injuries

Hamstring injuries are common sporting injuries and can present acutely or through chronic degenerative changes. Usual mechanism is concomitant hip flexion and knee extension, such as when kicking a football, surfing, running or hurdling.

Injuries can be intratendinous, or at the musculotendinous junction and usually involve the biceps femoris.

Clinical Presentation

Patients present with sharp stabbing pain in the local area, pain on range of movement of the hip and knee, and are unable to continue the sporting activity. Chronic tears present with ongoing pain and reduced range of movement.

Imaging

Plain radiographs of the pelvis may show an avulsion from the ischial tuberosity. MR scan is the imaging of choice and shows high signal, tendon avulsions and fluid collection. The severity of injury on the MR scan correlates with return to sports. Ultrasound may be helpful, but is operator dependant.

Classification

The Wood classification is commonly used for proximal hamstring avulsions (Table 4.7).

Excision of avulsion fractures is recommended due to problems of hardware if fixation is chosen. Elite athletes with type 2 injuries can be considered for repair.

Another system—the British Athletics Muscle Injury Classification (BAMIC) is useful for classifying the extent of injury. It is based on the grade of tear, site and the gap between the ends of the tear.

Treatment

Myofascial injuries account for over 80% of hamstring injuries and can be managed nonoperatively. Treatment follows RICE (rest, ice, compression and elevation) with protected weight bearing. High grade injuries often involve the central tendon or musculotendinous junction. High grade injuries and proximal tendon avulsions have better outcomes following surgical repair in terms of function, restoration of strength and reducing recurrence of injury. If repair is planned, early repair has better results. Sciatic nerve entrapment in the scar tissue requires neurolysis, excision of scar and repair of tendinous attachment.

Bony avulsions are managed by excision of the fragment and reattachment of the tendons to the osseous bed using suture anchors.

Table 4.7 Wood classification

Type	Pathology	Treatment
1	Osseous avulsion	Excise avulsed fragment and reattach tendon
2	Musculotendinous junction Injury	Usually nonoperative
3	Incomplete / partial avulsion	Nonoperative initially. Consider repair in chronic presentation
4	Complete avulsion with minimal retraction	Repair recommended. Nonoperative for low demand individuals
5	Complete avulsion with tendon retraction	Repair recommended
6	Complete avulsion with tendon retraction and sciatic nerve tethering	Repair recommended with sciatic neurolysis

Further Reading

Amstutz HC, LeDuff MJ. Hip resurfacing for osteonecrosis: two to 18 year results of the conserve plus design. Bone Joint J. 2016;98:901–9.

Cheung KW, Chiu KH, Chung KY. Long term result of cementless femoral stem in avascular necrosis of the hip. Hip Int. 2015;25(1):72–5.

Crowe JF, Mani J, Ranawat CS. Total hip replacement in congenital dislocation and dysplasia of the hip. J Bone Joint Surg Am. 1979;61(1):15–23.

Fairbank AC, Bhatia D, Jinnah RH, Hungerford DS. Long term results of core decompression for ischemic necrosis of the femoral head. J Bone Joint Surg. 1995;77:42.

Ganz R, Klaue K, Vinh TS, Mast JW. A new periacetabular osteotomy for the treatment of hip dysplasias. Technique and preliminary results. Clin Orthop Rel Res. 1988;232:26–36.

Griffin DR, Dickenson EJ, Wall PDH, et al. Hip arthroscopy versus best conservative care for the treatment of femoroacetabular impingement syndrome (UK FASHIoN): a multicentre randomised controlled trial. Lancet. 2018;391:2225–35.

Kim YH, Oh SH, Kim JS, Koo KH. Contemporary total hip arthroplasty with and without cement in patients with osteonecrosis of the femoral head. J Bone Joint Surg Am. 2003;85(4):675–81.

Korompillas AV, Lykissas MG, Beris AE, Urbaniak JR, Soucaros PM. Vascularised fibular graft in the management of femoral head osteonecrosis: twenty years later. J Bone Joint Surg Br. 2009;91(3):287–93.

Mont MA, Jones LC, Pacheco I, Hungerford DS. Radiographic predictors of outcome of core decompression for hips with osteonecrosis stage III. Clin Orthop. 1998;354:159.

Mont MA, Ragland PS, Etienne G. Core decompression of the femoral head for osteonecrosis using percutaneous multiple small diameter drilling. Clin Orthop. 2004;429:131–8.

Nagoya S, Kaya M, Sasaki M, et al. Cementless total hip replacement with subtrochanteric femoral shortening for severe developmental dysplasia of the hip. J Bone Joint Surg Br. 2009;91:1142–7.

Ozkul A, Necmioglu NS, Ziyadanogullari MO, Alemdar C, Arslan H, Uzel K. An evaluation of treating non union of femoral neck fractures with valgus angulation osteotomy using sliding hip screw. Acta Orthop Belg. 2019;85:210–7.

Steppacher SD, Tannast M, Ganz R, Siebenrock KA. Mean 20 year follow up of Bernese periacetabular osteotomy. Clin Orthop Rel Res. 2008;466:1633–44.

Sugioka Y. Transtrochanteric anterior rotational osteotomy of the femoral head the treatment of osteonecrosis affecting the hip; a new osteotomy operation. Clin Orthop. 1978;130:191–201.

Luo RB, Lin T, Zhong HM, Yan SG, Wang JA. Evidence for using alendronate to treat adult avascular necrosis of the femoral head. A systematic review. Med Sci Monit. 2014;20:2439–47.

Spinal Disorders

5

Iqroop Chopra and Abdul Nazeer Moideen

Spinal Anatomy

The main ligaments connecting the vertebrae are the anterior and the posterior longitudinal ligaments, which run along the anterior and posterior aspect of the vertebral bodies. The ligamentum flavum runs between the laminae and the supraspinous and interspinous ligaments connect the spinous processes (Fig. 5.1).

Disc Disease

The intervertebral disc has a central avascular portion called the nucleus pulposus and a peripheral portion called the annulus fibrosus. The outer third of annulus has neural innervation, and tears in the annulus can cause backache in degenerative disc disease. The annulus is primarily composed of type I collagen. The nucleus has a proteoglycan matrix with a framework of type II collagen fibres. Fragmentation of the nucleus is considered to be one of the initial events in disc disease, but is largely asymptomatic.

The lifetime prevalence of low back pain is 80–85%. In a small percentage of patients (approximately 2%) low backache is associated with radiating pain down the leg (sciatica). Overall, 80% of these patients will recover.

Bigos S, Bowyer O, Braen G, et al: Acute Lower Back Problems in Adults. Clinical Practice Guideline No 14. AHCPR Publication No 95–0642. Most cases of low back pain (90%) will improve within a month of onset, although recurrence is common.

Nomenclature for Abnormal Discs

There is no standardised nomenclature for disc herniation. One system of classification is described in Table 5.1.

Spitzer WO, LeBlanc FE, Dupuis M, et al. *Scientific approach to the assessment and management of activity-related spinal disorders. A monograph for clinicians. Report of the Quebec Taskforce on Spinal Disorders. Spine (Phila Pa 1976) 1987;12(Suppl.): S16–2. Proposed the classification system for disc herniation.*

Based on the site of herniation (Fig. 5.2), the extrusion can be central (in the midline posteriorly), posterolateral (the most common form), lateral (foraminal) or far lateral (extraforaminal).

On computed tomography (CT) discography, the tears are graded as shown in Table 5.2.

The sequence of events in lumbar disc disease is fragmentation of the nucleus followed by annular tears, leading to herniation of the nucleus. Annular tears are associated with backache, and

I. Chopra (✉) · A. N. Moideen
University Hospital of Wales, Cardiff, UK
e-mail: ichopra@doctors.org.uk;
abdul.moideen@wales.nhs.uk

S. Agarwal (ed.), *Current Orthopaedic Practice*, https://doi.org/10.1007/978-3-030-78529-1_5

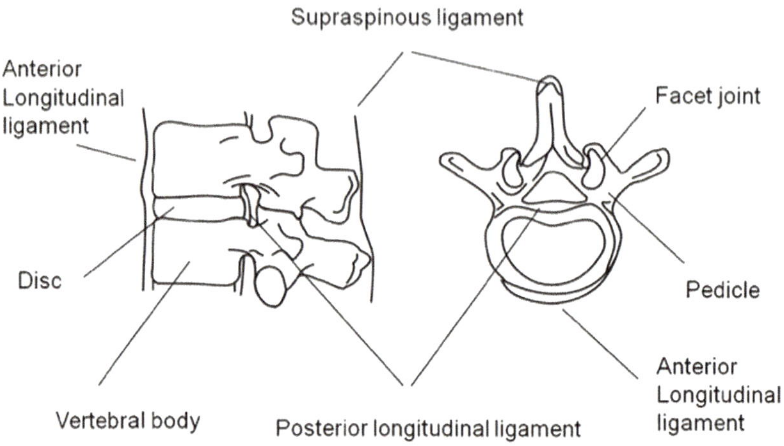

Fig. 5.1 Spinal anatomy

Table 5.1 A classification system for disc herniation (Spitzer et al)

Type	Description
Degenerate disc	Deterioration of the internal disc structure, often with loss of hydration and reduced disc height
Bulging disc	Circumferential symmetrical outpouching of the disc beyond the end plates Maybe a normal variant
Protruded disc	Focal, often asymmetric extension of the disc beyond the disc space, with a broad connection with the herniated part and the parent disc
Extruded disc	A more extreme extension of the protruding disc, with narrow or no connection to the parent disc
Sequestration	A subset of the extruded disc, where the disc material is contained by the posterior longitudinal ligament
Migrated disc	The extruded material is displaced above or below the edge of the disc space
Contained disc	Disc herniation where a part of the annulus is intact

the herniation may cause nerve root symptoms or cauda equina syndrome.

Central and posterolateral herniation involve the nerve root below the level of herniation. For instance, the L4/5 disc will cause pressure on the L5 root as the L4 root exits just above the disc. A lateral or far-lateral herniation will press on the root of the same level. For instance, the L4/5 lateral or far-lateral herniation will press on the L4 root (Table 5.3).

The composition of the disc changes with age: Proteoglycan synthesis, chondroitin sulphate, water content and elastin are all reduced; and collagen content increases in the nucleus and annulus. The loss of water and increase in collagen make the discs stiff. The outer third of the annulus has sensory nerve endings, which may explain the pain of disc disease.

Herniation is a feature of degenerate discs. A normal disc with an annular tear will not herniate due to cohesiveness of the nucleus pulposus.

Clinical Features

Patients with disc prolapse usually present in the third to fifth decade. Disc prolapse is rare in the young and the elderly.

Degenerative disc disease may cause intermittent low backache over a period of time.

Pressure on the nerve roots results in radicular pain (sciatica). The pain is dermatomal, and radiates from the lower back to the legs. The pain may be worse with coughing, sneezing or sitting for long periods. The sitting position is associated with higher intradiscal pressure compared to standing and lying.

Wilke H, Neef P, Caimi M, et al. *New In Vivo Measurements of Pressures in the Intervertebral Disc in Daily Life. Spine 1999;24:755-62.*

Some patients will present with radicular pain without significant backache. Large disc

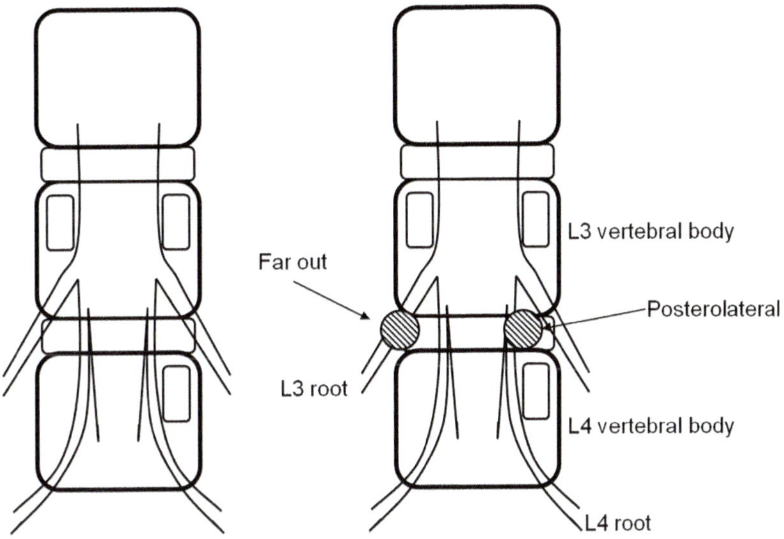

Fig. 5.2 Anatomical sites for disc herniation, showing the difference between posterolateral and far-out compression

Table 5.2 Grading of tears

Grade 0	no evidence of tear
Grade 1	Tear in the inner third of the annulus
Grade 2	Tear in the middle third of the annulus
Grade 3	Tear in the outer third of the annulus

herniations may present as spinal stenosis and can cause cauda equina.

Clinical examination will demonstrate an antalgic gait and lateral curvature in the lower lumbar spine. In posterolateral disc herniation, patients tend to list away from the side of herniation; in axillary presentation, on the other hand, the list is towards the side of herniation. Forward bending may aggravate the radicular pain.

The straight leg raising (SLR) test is valuable, especially in young patients. The deformation of the L5 and S1 nerve roots, at the level of the foramen, is maximal with 35–70° of leg elevation. Reproduction of radicular pain with a leg elevation of 35–70° is highly suggestive of disc herniation.

The crossover SLR test (Fajersztajn's sign) is elicited by raising the contralateral leg, which causes pain in the affected leg. This is more specific for disc herniation. The SLR test can also be performed by flexing the hip and knee of the affected side to 90° and then extending the knee. This reproduces the radicular pain. Once the pain is elicited, the knee is flexed by a few degrees to relax the stretching of the nerve root. Pressure in the popliteal fossa in this knee position may reproduce the radicular pain.

The femoral stretch test is used to check for pressure on the L2–L4 nerve roots. It can be performed in the prone or lateral position. The affected hip is extended, keeping the knee flexed. Reproduction of pain in the front of the thigh and knee is suggestive of femoral nerve root involvement.

A full neurological examination is mandatory. The sensory areas of innervation of lumbar nerve roots are shown in Fig. 5.3.

L4 root involvement causes weakness in the tibialis anterior and loss of the patellar tendon reflex. L5 root involvement causes weakness of the extensor hallucis longus and extensor digitorum longus. S1 root involvement causes weakness of the peronei and the gastro-soleus. The ankle deep tendon reflex will also be weak.

Thoracic disc prolapse is rare and malignancy and infections should be ruled out. Most patients are in their fourth decade and presents with signs of cord compression and radicular back pain. These are usually below the T8 level.

Patients with cauda equina present with acute onset of perianal sensory loss (saddle anaesthesia), loss of ankle reflex, sensory loss in the L4,

Table 5.3 Nerve roots affected by prolapsed discs

	L3–4 disc	L4–5 disc	L5–S1 disc
Posterolateral disc herniation	L4 root	L5 root	S1 root
Far-lateral disc herniation	L3 root	L4 root	L5 root
Pain	Anterior thigh/leg	Posterior leg/front of foot	Posterior/lateral foot
Motor weakness	Quadriceps and tibialis anterior	Extensor hallucis longus (EHL) and tibialis anterior	Gastrocnemius
Reflex involved	Knee jerk	Medial hamstring jerk	Ankle jerk
Incidence	3–10%	40–45%	45–50%

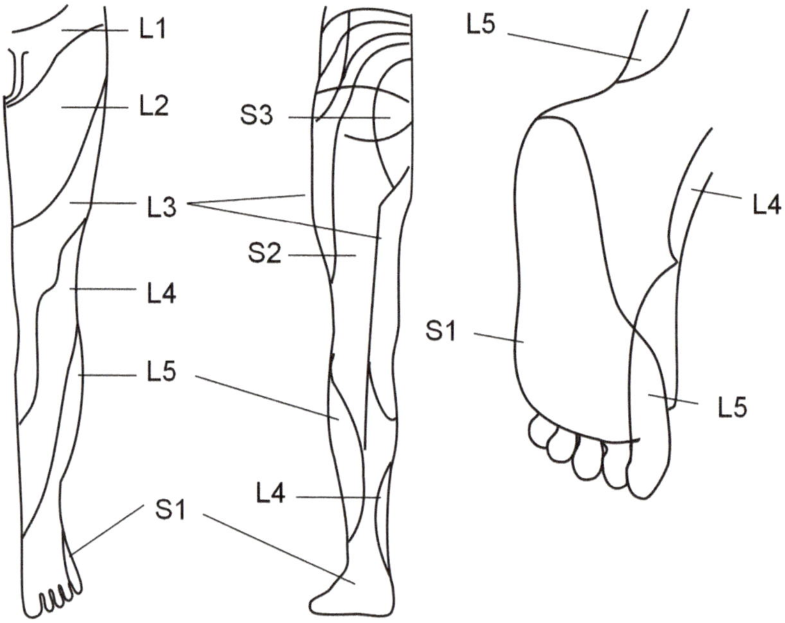

Fig. 5.3 Sensory areas of innervation

L5 or S1 dermatome, weakness of anal tone, urinary retention or overflow incontinence, or a combination of these. Immediate diagnosis and decompression are essential to prevent permanent neurologic deficit.

Imaging

Magnetic resonance (MR) scanning is the imaging modality of choice. The size of the herniation correlates with the improvement following surgery. Large disc protrusions fare better. High resolution CT or CT myelography is an option for patients who are unable to have an MR scan.

Differential Diagnosis

In the adolescent patient, consider spondylolisthesis, infections and spinal tumours. In the elderly, consider vertebral compression fractures, infections, spinal metastasis, myeloma and primary malignancies.

Management

Non-operative management is appropriate in the initial phase of acute disc herniation. Bed rest for 3–4 days is advised, but longer periods of bed rest do not help recovery.

In the acute phase, non-steroidal anti-inflammatory drugs (NSAIDs) or opioid analgesics are useful. Epidural steroid injection or nerve root blocks are sometimes used to resolve leg pain.

Physiotherapy is helpful in promoting a gradual increase in activity levels.

Most patients (90%) do not have a relapse following an episode of radicular pain. Those with an increasing number of episodes have a poorer prognosis and many will require surgical intervention.

Surgical treatment is open or micro-discectomy and is indicated for patients with unrelenting pain or cauda equina syndrome.

Patients with cauda equina require an urgent MR scan and discectomy. Loss of neurologic function is permanent after 48 hours and decompression should be achieved within 8–12 hours of symptom onset.

Todd N. Cauda equina syndrome: The timing of surgery probably does influence outcome. Brit J Neurosurg 2009;19:301–6.

Outcomes

A classic paper on the natural history of a herniated disc is by Weber. This study followed 280 patients with lumbar disc herniation proven on myelography. All patients received 14 days of in-patient treatment, followed by randomisation to surgical or non-surgical treatment. Sixty percent of the non-surgical group improved, meaning they would have undergone unnecessary surgery. A 3-month wait before surgery did not compromise the outcome. Symptoms should be allowed to resolve if there is no cauda equina or progressive neurologic deficit. The quality of the surgical result decreases after 12 months of onset of leg symptom.

Weber H. Lumbar disc herniation. A controlled, prospective study with ten years of observation. Spine (Phila Pa 1976) 1983:8:131–40.

A further study found that patients with an uncontained herniated disc had shorter symptoms and better functional outcomes. Sciatica for more than 12 months correlated with a less favourable outcome.

Ng LC, Sell P. Predictive value of the duration of sciatica for lumbar discectomy. A prospective cohort study. J Bone Joint Surg Br 2004;86(4):546-9.

Finally, a recent prospective study randomised 501 patients to open discectomy or non-operative care. At 4 years, patients receiving surgery had significantly better outcomes. There was a high cross-over between the two study arms.

Weinstein JN, Lurie JD, Tosteson TD, et al. *Surgical versus nonoperative treatment for lumbar disc herniation: four-year results for the Spine Patient Outcome Research Trial (SPORT). Spine (Phila Pa 1976) 2008;33:2789–800.*

Lumbar Disc Replacement

Lumbar disc replacement has been proposed as a method to preserve motion at the disc space and minimise adjacent segment disease, which follows immobility of the diseased segment.

The evidence for benefit is debatable, and a review found no evidence to suggest better functional outcomes with disc replacement than with fusion surgery for discogenic disc disease.

Resnick DK, Watters WC. Lumbar disc arthroplasty: a critical review. Clin Neurosurg 2007;54:83–7.

Some recent studies have shown benefit with disc replacement.

Gornet MF, Burkus JK, Dryer RF, Peloza JH. Lumbar Disc Arthroplasty With Maverick Disc Versus Stand-Alone Interbody Fusion: A Prospective, Randomized, Controlled, Multicenter Investigational Device Exemption Trial. Spine (Phila Pa 1976),36 (25), 2011. 577 patients were treated in either the investigational group (405), receiving lumbar disc arthroplasty, or the control group (172), receiving anterior lumbar interbody fusion. Better function, pain and return to work with disc arthroplasty.

A Cochrane review from 2012 found no benefit in Lumbar disc replacement.

Back Pain

Back pain is thought to affect 60–80% people in their lifetime. About 90% of cases are self-limiting and resolve with non-operative measures.

The causes of back pain vary with the age of presentation. In children, the common causes are congenital malformation, spondylolisthesis, infections of the spine and spine tumours such as eosinophilic granuloma, Ewing's sarcoma and neuroblastoma.

In adults, trauma and disc disease are more prevalent, along with Scheuermann's disease and ankylosing spondylitis.

Metastatic tumours and spinal stenosis are common in middle-aged and elderly patients, as are osteopenic fractures and infections.

Osteopenic Vertebral Collapse

Osteopenic vertebral collapse is a common feature in patients with osteoporosis. The number of reported cases is rising every year.

Most of these are managed nonoperatively and 85% patients have resolution of symptoms within 3 months of onset of pain. Patients with persistent pain can be considered for percutaneous vertebroplasty (PVP). It involves injection of PMMA (Poly Methyl Meth Acrylate) into the inter-trabecular marrow spaces of the fractured vertebra. Prerequisites for PVP are persistent pain, localised tenderness and edema on MRI Scan. Potential problems relate to leakage of cement causing nerve root or cord compression and cement embolisation. Evidence for efficacy of PVP is still scant.

Muijs SPJ et al. *Treatment of painful osteoporotic vertebral compression fractures. J Bone Joint Surg Br 2011;93(9):1149-53. No randomised prospective trial available to prove usefulness of PVP.*

Waddell's Inappropriate Signs

In 1980, Waddell and colleagues proposed a set of signs that indicate a non-organic aetiology of back pain.

- Tenderness to a light touch or pinch in a wide part of the lumbar area.
- Non-anatomic deep tenderness in a wide area.
- Pain on axial compression—pressing down on the head of the patient causes pain.
- Pain on pelvic rotation when the shoulder and pelvis are rotated in the same direction.
- Findings disappear when the patient is distracted.
- Non-anatomic voluntary motor release or giving way of muscle groups.
- Non-dermatomal sensory loss.
- A disproportionate verbal or physical response to examination.

The presence of more than three signs is considered to be significant.

Waddell G, McCulloch JA, Kummel E, Venner RM. Nonorganic physical signs in low-back pain. Spine (Phila Pa 1976) 1980;5:117–25.

Cervical Disc Disease

Cervical disc disease and nerve compression are seen in the fourth and fifth decades of life and are more common in women.

Compression can be caused by disc prolapse (soft disc) or osteophytes in the uncovertebral joint (hard disc). The C7 root is most often involved.

The presenting features are neck pain, pain in the inter-scapular region and radiating pain down the arm. This may be accompanied by sensory and motor deficit. Distribution of sensory and motor changes in dermatomal and myotomal patterns indicates cervical spine involvement,

Table 5.4 Clinical features of cervical nerve root compression

Disc herniation	Root	Motor involvement	Sensory loss	Pain location	Deep tendon reflex	%
C3–4	C4	None	Shoulder Arm, upper	Neck, upper	Normal	<1
C4–5	C5	Shoulder abduction Elbow flexion	Arm, upper lateral	Neck; shoulder Scapula Arm, anterior	Biceps Brachioradialis	2
C5–6	C6	Elbow flexion Wrist extension Forearm pronation	Forearm, lateral Hand, thumb and second/index finger	Neck; shoulder Scapula Arm, lateral Hand, lateral	Biceps Brachioradialis Pronator	19
C6–7	C7	Extension Elbow	Forearm, dorsal and lateral Hand, third/middle finger	Neck Shoulder Scapula, medial Forearm, extensor	Triceps	69
C7-T1	C8	Hand, intrinsic	Forearm, medial Hand, fourth/ring and fifth/little fingers	Neck Scapula, medial Arm, medial Forearm, medial Hand, fourth and fifth fingers	None	9

while a deficit in the distribution of specific nerves indicates nerve entrapment syndromes (Table 5.4).

Levin KH, Maggiano HJ, Wilbourn AJ. Cervical radiculopathies: comparison of surgical and EMG localization of single-root lesions. Neurology 1996;46:1022–5.

Spurling's compression test is helpful in diagnosing cervical spine problems. The head is tilted to the symptomatic side and the neck extended; downward pressure on the head reproduces the pain.

In the shoulder abduction test, radicular symptoms disappear or are reduced on lifting the hand above the head.

Lhermitte's sign is the occurrence of an electric-shock-like sensation radiating down the spine and limbs on flexing the neck.

Imaging

Plain radiographs of the cervical spine may show osteophyte formation and reduced joint space. The herniated cervical discs often have a preserved disc height. MR scanning is the imaging modality of choice for detecting nerve root compression. Foraminal narrowing is better illustrated on a fine-slice CT scan, although a CT myelogram is an alternative for soft tissue imaging if MR imaging is contraindicated.

Management

Non-operative measures include rest, NSAIDs and nerve root blocks. Most patients will improve with these measures, but there is a high incidence of pain recurrence.

Indications for operative interventions are neurological deficit and unremitting pain.

The operation involves decompression of the nerve root/osteophytes, which can be achieved through the anterior (anterior cervical discectomy and fusion—ACDF) or posterior approach (foraminotomies). Along with decompression, interbody fusion of the involved cervical disc is performed using an iliac crest bone graft or spinal cage.

Potential complications of ACDF include injury to recurrent laryngeal nerve, which can lead to hoarseness. Other problems are non-union of the graft, graft migration, and progression of disease in adjacent levels.

Posterior foraminotomy preserves motion but can lead to instability and cervical kyphosis.

Cervical disc replacement has shown some promising results, but continued motion at the posterior facet joints may lead to ongoing pain. A recent meta-analysis showed better results with Total Disc Replacement (TDR) compared to ACDF.

Findlay C, Ayis S, Demetriades AK. Total Disc Replacement Versus Anterior Cervical Discectomy and Fusion: A Systematic Review With Meta-Analysis of Data From a Total of 3160 Patients Across 14 Randomized Controlled Trials With Both Short- And Medium- To Long-Term Outcomes. Bone Joint J 2018;100-B:991-1001. In the short-term, patients who underwent TDR had better patient-reported outcomes than those who underwent ACDF, but at two years this was typically not significant. Results between four and seven years showed significant differences in Neck Disability Index (NDI), 36-Item Short-Form Health Survey (SF-36) physical component scores, dysphagia, and satisfaction, all favouring TDR.

Cervical Myelopathy

Cervical myelopathy is the commonest manifestation of cervical spine disease in the elderly. Cervical myelopathy results from spinal cord compression due to osteophytes, hypertrophied ligamentum flavum or prolapsed disc.

The clinical presentation is with upper motor neuron signs. More general symptoms include unsteady gait, difficulty in fine movements of hands, poor handwriting, difficulty in balance and bladder and bowel symptoms. Cervical radicular symptoms maybe associated with myelopathy. Hyperreflexia, positive Babinski and Hoffmann signs, unsteady gait, wasting of intrinsic muscles of hand, positive Romberg's test are other features.

Romberg's test is for sensory ataxia resulting from impaired proprioception. The cerebellum maintains truncal stability (equilibrium) from three sensory inputs—visual, vertibular and proprioception. A minimum of two of these is needed to maintain equilibrium. In patients with cervical myelopathy, proprioception is impaired due to cord compression. If the visual input is removed by closing eyes, balance is impaired. Tandem Romberg's test involves tandem walking with eyes open and then eyes closed, and noting the degree of instability.

ACDF is the mainstay of surgical treatment for cervical myelopathy.

Ankylosing Spondylitis

The common seronegative spondyloarthropathies are ankylosing spondylitis, Behçet's syndrome, psoriasis and inflammatory bowel disease.

Ankylosing spondylitis (AS) is a common spondyloarthropathy that is predominantly seen in men. It is related to human leukocyte antigen (HLA) B27, with 90% of patients positive for HLA B27 (HLA B27 is present in 5–10% of the general population). HLA is a surface antigen encoded by the major histocompatibility complex on chromosome 6.

Ankylosing spondylitis causes synovitis of the diarthrodial joints (e.g., costovertebral joints) and inflammation of the enthesis and fibro-osseous junction of the syndesmotic joints such as intervertebral discs, the sacroiliac joint and pubic symphysis.

The inflammation leads to granulation tissue, bone destruction and formation of fibrous tissue. The calcification of fibrous tissue causes stiffness and syndesmophytes (marginal) can be seen on radiographs.

Clinical Presentation

Most patients present in adolescence with recurrent episodes of back pain accompanied by reduced chest expansion. Thoracic kyphosis develops in due course and spinal movements are grossly restricted. Involvement of the peripheral joints is a late feature and affects the shoulders, hips and knees.

Uveitis and conjunctivitis are seen in about 20% of patients, while other extraskeletal manifestations (pulmonary fibrosis and carditis) are rare.

Table 5.5 New York Criteria for diagnosis of Ankylosing Spondylitis

Sacroilitis visible on imaging; and
Two out of these 3
– Low back pain and stiffness for over 3 months that improves with exercise but not relieved by rest
– Limited sagittal and frontal plane movement of lumbar spine
– Limited chest expansion

The New York criteria (Table 5.5) are used for diagnosis of AS.

Imaging

Radiographs in the early stages show sacroiliitis, which progresses to fusion of the sacroiliac joint. Spine radiographs demonstrate squaring of the vertebral bodies and formation of syndesmophytes. Ankylosis of the spine gives the appearance of 'bamboo spine' or 'rugger-jersey spine'. Ankylosis of the hips can be seen in late stages.

Treatment

In the initial phases, the mainstay of treatment is maintenance of activity through physiotherapy and exercises, along with NSAIDs. Surgical intervention is needed in the later stages to correct spinal deformity through a spinal osteotomy, or for joint arthroplasty of the hips, knees or shoulders.

Fractures of the spine in patients with ankylosing spondylitis are often unstable and patients are at higher risk of neurological injury. Surgery has a higher risk of failure of instrumentation and progression of deformity.

Diffuse Skeletal Idiopathic Hyperostosis

Diffuse skeletal idiopathic hyperostosis (DISH), also known as Forestier's disease, is a condition of ossification of the ligaments and tendon insertions. It is more common in men. Type I involves the anterior longitudinal ligament, Type II is characterised by diffuse changes and type III involves the posterior longitudinal ligament. Type I is classically known as Forestier's disease.

Rheumatoid Cervical Spine Disease

Involvement of the cervical spine is common in rheumatoid disease. The spine may be affected in various ways:

- Atlantoaxial subluxation.
- Basilar invagination.
- Involvement of the lower cervical spine joint.
- Cervical spine myelopathy.

Atlantoaxial Subluxation

Atlantoaxial subluxation is the most common manifestation and is due to destructive pannus at the synovial joint between atlas and odontoid process. This leads to destruction of the transverse ligament and anterior subluxation of the atlas on axis.

The Ranawat classification for clinical presentation is shown in Table 5.6.

Physicians should maintain a high index of suspicion in patients with upper cervical spine pain. Upper motor neuron signs may be present. Radiographs of the cervical spine are obtained to assess the atlanto dens interval (ADI) and the posterior atlas and dens interval (PADI).

Ranawat CS, O'Leary P, Pellicci P, et al. Cervical spine fusion in rheumatoid arthritis. J Bone Joint Surg Am 1979;61:1003–10.

Table 5.6 Ranawat classification of atlanto axial instability

Class I	Pain, no neurological deficit
Class II	Subjective weakness, hyperreflexia and dysaesthesia
Class III	Objective weakness and long tract signs IIIA—ambulatory IIIB—non-ambulatory

Atlanto Dens Interval

Flexion–extension X-rays of the spine show an increase in the distance between the posterior aspect of anterior arch of the atlas and the anterior margin of the odontoid process (Fig. 5.4). An increase of 3 mm indicates instability and more than 6 mm indicates disruption of the alar ligament. Further increases correlate with a high risk of neurological injury.

There is a weak correlation between ADI and neurological deficit (Table 5.7).

Weissman BN, Aliabadi P, Weinfeld MS, et al. *Prognostic features of atlantoaxial subluxation in rheumatoid arthritis patients. Radiology 1982;144:745–51.*

Posterior Atlas and Dens Interval

The PADI is the distance between the posterior border of the odontoid process and the anterior aspect of the posterior arch of the atlas (Fig. 5.4).

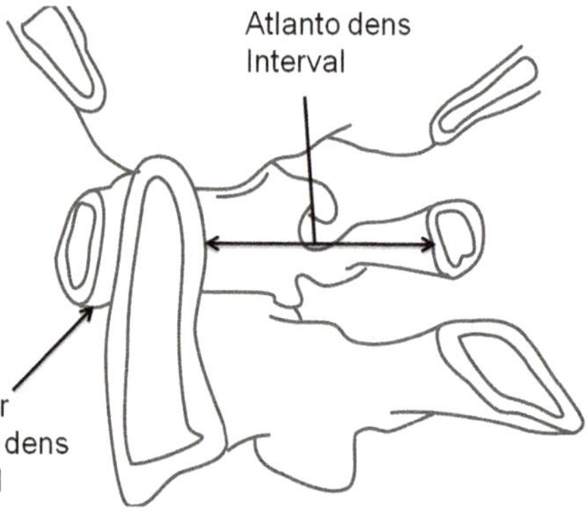

Fig. 5.4 The anterior atlanto dens interval (ADI) and Posterior atlanto dens interval (PADI)

Table 5.7 Relationship between atlantoaxial subluxation and neurological injury

<3 mm	normal ADI
>3 mm	Anterior AA subluxation
3–6 mm	Transverse ligament damage
>6 mm	Alar ligament damage
>9 mm	Surgical intervention (cord compression likely)

The normal PADI is more than 14 mm, and a space of less than 10 mm indicates a risk of neurologic compromise.

A minimum of 10 mm space is needed for the cord, 2 mm for the CSF and 2 mm for the dura.

A PADI of 14 mm or less yields 97% sensitivity for predicting cord compression and paralysis.

Predictors for recovery:

(a) Ranawat classification
(b) Preoperative PADI
- ≤10 mm Poor chance of recovery.
- ≥14 mm significant motor recovery

(c) Sub axial diameter < 14 mm less chance of recovery

Boden SD, Dodge LD, Bohlman HH, Rechtine GR. Rheumatoid arthritis of the cervical spine. A long-term analysis with predictors of paralysis and recovery. J Bone Joint Surg Am 1993;75:1282–97.

Treatment

Surgical treatment of atlantoaxial subluxation is indicated when the ADI is more than 6 mm or the PADI is less than 14 mm, in the presence of neurologic impairment or instability.

The indications for surgery are shown in Table 5.8.

Stabilisation can be achieved by posterior fusion between C1 and C2 (Gallie/Brooke's technique) or with a transarticular screw (Magerl technique) or Harm's fusion.

Table 5.8 Indications for surgery in patients with atlantoaxial subluxation

Asymptomatic	Ranawat class I	Ranawat class II or III
PADI <10 mm (MR scan) PADI 10–14 mm + pannus on MR scan AADI >8 mm	PADI <12 mm PADI >12 mm + pannus on MR scan	Medically fit Includes some IIIb patients

MR magnetic resonance; *PADI* posterior atlas and dens interval

Basilar Invagination

Basilar invagination is cranial migration of the dens. Diagnosis is based on measurement in radiographs and an occiput—C2 fusion is performed to stabilise this. Further anterior decompression maybe required through a transoral odontoidectomy.

Involvement of the Lower Cervical Spine Joint

In the lower cervical spine, rheumatoid disease involves the facet joint and the uncovertebral joints. This can lead to subluxation, which is managed by posterior fusion with lateral mass screws (Roy–Camille or Magerl techniques).

Cervical Spine Myelopathy

Cervical spine compression can be present in patients with rheumatoid disease due to pressure on the cord from the bony instability of directly from rheumatoid pannus.

Torticollis

Torticollis (from the Latin *torti* meaning twisted and *collis* meaning neck) is a condition where the head is tilted to one side and the chin is elevated and turned to the opposite side.

Torticollis can be congenital or acquired. Congenital causes are Klippel–Feil syndrome and congenital muscular torticollis. Acquired causes may or may not be related to the cervical spine (Table 5.9).

Congenital muscular torticollis is the result of contracture of the sternomastoid muscle on one side. The contracture may be related to intrauterine pressure, as this condition is often associated with a breech presentation and dysplasia of the hip.

Table 5.9 Acquired causes of torticollis

Related to the cervical spine	Not related to the cervical spine
Trauma: Atlanto-axial subluxation Inflammatory conditions: Rheumatoid arthritis and ankylosing spondylitis Infections: Pyogenic, tubercular and sometimes following upper respiratory tract infection (known as Grisel's syndrome) Tumours: Osteoid osteoma causing painful torticollis	Contractures of the neck Paralysis of the superior oblique muscle resulting in compensatory head tilt Posterior fossa tumours

The deformity is obvious by the age of 1–2 years and the sternomastoid muscle feels hard and fibrotic. The heat tilt leads to asymmetric development of the face.

Congenital muscular torticollis is managed by division of the lower end of the muscle (unipolar release) and rarely by division of both the lower and upper ends (bipolar release), followed by stretching exercises.

Klippel–Feil syndrome is a failure of segmentation resulting in multiple fused cervical vertebrae. The classic triad of a low posterior hairline, short webbed neck and restricted cervical movements is seen in less than half of patients. The syndrome is associated with congenital scoliosis, renal aplasia, Sprengel's deformity, congenital heart disease and brain-stem abnormalities.

Scoliosis

Scoliosis is lateral curvature of the spine associated with rotational malalignment. On the basis of Hueter–Volkmann law, the compressive forces restrict growth while tensile forces increase growth. This leads to progression of the deformity.

Etiology

Scoliosis has several possible etiologies:

- Genetic.
- Tissue deficiency—fibrous dysplasia, Marfan's syndrome, Duchenne muscular dystrophy.
- Vertebral growth abnormality theory—anterior spinal growth outpaces posterior growth, leading to buckling of the vertebral column.
- Disorders of the brain or spinal cord—syringomyelia, Chiari malformation.
- Melatonin deficiency in children leads to scoliosis.

Based on its etiology, scoliosis can be idiopathic or secondary. Secondary causes of scoliosis include congenital malformations, neuromuscular disorders, degenerative diseases, trauma, tumours, infections and improper posture.

Clinical Evaluation

Specific features to discuss in the history are perinatal history, developmental milestones, family history, growth spurt, menstrual history and pain. The age of onset and rate of progression should be noted, along with the presence of any neurological symptoms. The family history is relevant and should be documented.

Examination includes the following:

- General—neurofibromas, café-au-lait spots, axillary freckling, spinal cord dysraphism (tuft of hair, naevus, skin dimple), cavus feet, Ehlers–Danlos syndrome.
- Trunk—symmetry is determined by the level of the shoulders, the waist crease, the level of the iliac crest crease and the prominence of the loin.
- Balance and rib deformity—a rib hump is the major cause of cosmetic disability. The balance of the curve is determined by the relationship of the occiput to the sacrum.
- Limb length.
- Correction of curve on bending forward and side bending—a plumb line from the vertebra prominens demonstrates decompensation of the curve.
- Neurologic examination—to check abdominal reflexes (to rule out syrinx) and other reflexes such as Hoffmann, clonus and Babinski.
- SLR—reduced in hamstring tightness due to spondylolisthesis or a spinal tumour.
- Sitting and standing heights.
- Neuromuscular scoliosis—balanced curves have a square pelvis while unbalanced curves have a tilted pelvis. For balanced curves—see gait (broad-based in Friedreich's ataxia).
- Sitting patient—sit the patient on the edge of the bed and assess head control and sitting ability.

Investigations

A standing PA view is the standard radiograph to assess the deformity. Side bending and lateral views are obtained if surgery is being considered.

The Cobb angle is measured and the Risser sign graded. The superior and inferior end vertebrae are identified for measurement of the Cobb angle. The end vertebrae are those that are tilted maximally towards the concavity of the curve being measured. A line is drawn along the superior end plate of the superior end vertebra and the inferior end plate of the inferior end vertebra. The angle between these lines, or the perpendiculars drawn to these lines, is the Cobb angle (Fig. 5.5).

The Risser sign is based on appearance and progressive fusion of the iliac apophysis. The fusion progresses from lateral to medial and the iliac crest is divided into four segments. Grade 0 is when the apophysis has not appeared, while grades 1–4 indicate the segments where the apophysis is visible. In grade 5, the entire apophysis is fused.

The triradiate cartilage and X-rays of wrist can be used to estimate bone age.

Peak height velocity (PHV) is thought to be a more accurate assessment of maturity than the Risser sign, and consequently a better indicator of curve progression. The average PHV is approximately 8 cm/year in girls and 9.5 cm/year in boys.

MRI

MR imaging is indicated for all preoperative patients, for left thoracic curves and in patients with painful scoliosis.

In boys, a bone scan is used to screen for painful scoliosis and a single-photon emission CT (SPECT) scan is useful for detection of spondylolysis.

Idiopathic scoliosis (a curve >10°) is found in 0.5–3% of the adolescent population. Curves of greater than 30° are present in 0.3%.

Classification

Scoliosis is commonly classified based on the age diagnosis is made: early onset (<10 years) or late onset (>10 years of age). The alveoli are not fully developed before the age of 4 years and a deformity before the age of 5 years seriously limits its pulmonary function.

Idiopathic scoliosis can be of three types, based on the age at which the curve is noticed.

- Infantile, <3 years of age.
- Juvenile, 3–10 years.
- Adolescent, >10 years.

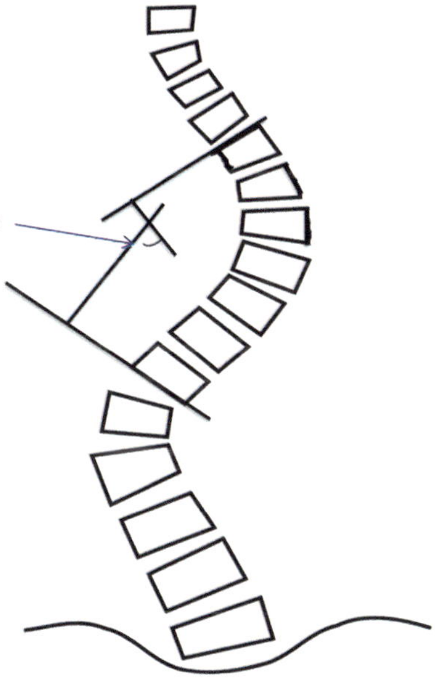

Fig. 5.5 Measurement of Cobb angle

Infantile Scoliosis

Infantile scoliosis is more common in boys, and typically presents as thoracic curves, convex to the left. It can be associated with mental retardation, developmental dysplasia of the hip, congenital heart problems and plagiocephaly.

It has been suggested that scoliosis may be preventable if infants are laid prone. Infants tend to lie on the right side, causing plastic deformation of the thorax.

Wynne Davies R. Infantile idiopathic scoliosis. Causative factors, particularly in the first six months of life. J Bone Joint Surg Br 1975;57(2):138-141.

Infantile curves can be progressive or resolving. Resolving curves are usually detected before 1 year of age. There are no compensatory curves, and these curves are associated with plagiocephaly (intrauterine moulding defect).

The rib–vertebral angle difference (RVAD) is an important measurement in scoliosis (Fig. 5.6). A line is drawn perpendicular to the apical vertebral endplate. Another line is drawn from the mid neck to the mid head of the convex rib and concave rib. The RVAD is the difference in angles between the two sides. If the convex rib head overlaps the vertebral body, or if the angle is more than 20°, there is a high chance of curve progression.

Fig. 5.6 Measurement of the rib vertebral angle difference

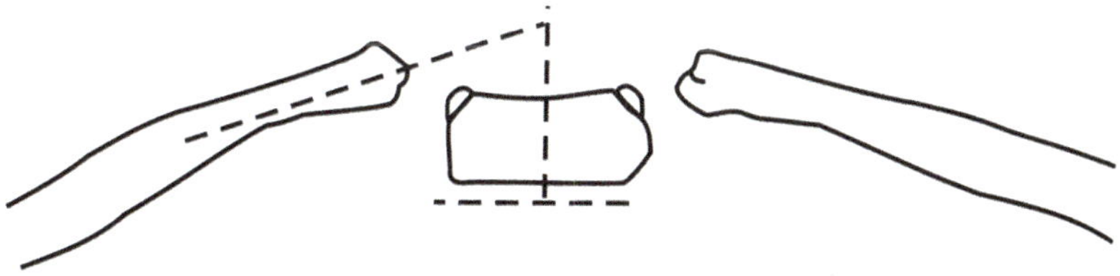

Mehta MH. The rib–vertebra angle in the early diagnosis between resolving and progressive infantile scoliosis. J Bone Joint Surg Br 1972;54:230–43.

Infantile curves can be progressive if –

(a) Cobb angle >20^0
(b) RVAD >20^0
(c) Rib head overlaps vertebral body

Treatment

Treatment of infantile scoliosis is indicated if the RVAD is more than 20° or cobb angle >30^0 and there is a rigid curve on examination.

Bracing is advised for small, flexible curves and can be a thoracolumbosacral or cervicothoracolumbosacral orthosis (Milwaukee brace). The brace is continued until the curve has been stable for 2 years.

A cast can be applied for children who are too young to brace. The cast is changed every 2–3 months.

Surgical treatment involves insertion of growing rods if cobb angle >50^0 or there is a failure of bracing. Fusion is delayed until skeletal maturity.

Juvenile Scoliosis

Juvenile scoliosis usually presents as a right thoracic curve and is more common in girls. For the diagnosis of scoliosis, the curve should be more than 10° on standing PA radiographs.

About two thirds of these curves are progressive. Progression occurs in 100% of cases where the curve is more than 20°.

An MR scan is indicated for patients with a left thoracic curve, pain, neurological deficit or rapid progression.

Treatment

For curves less than 20°, a standing PA X-ray is obtained every 4–6 months. A 10° increase in the RVAD indicates curve progression. Bracing is advised if the curve progresses by 5–7°on follow up. Bracing is also advised for curves between 20° and 50°, while curves of more than 50° require operative treatment. Observation to check for curve progression continues until skeletal maturity.

A Milwaukee brace or thoracolumbosacral orthosis is given for curves with an apex below T8. The brace is worn for 23 out of 24 hours. If the curve improves after 1 year, bracing is reduced gradually to night-time wear.

In the crankshaft phenomenon, solid posterior fusion stops growth of the posterior elements, but the vertebral body continues to grow. This anterior growth causes the vertebral bodies to bulge laterally towards the convexity, leading to recurrence of the rib hump and loss of correction.

Moe advised subcutaneous Harrington rod without fusion in juvenile scoliosis. Surgery is required every 6 months to lengthen the construct, before final fusion.

The amount of shortening as a result of fusion is calculated by the following formula:

Shortening = 0.07 cm × (no. of segments fused) × (no. of growth years remaining).

If the child is aged more than 9–10 years then combined anterior and posterior fusion is often needed. Anterior release with fusion and no instrumentation is performed along with posterior multihook segmental instrumented fusion.

Growing rod treatment has been used for early onset scoliosis but has a high complication rate related to implant and wound problems.

Bess S et al. *Complications of growing rod treatment for early onset scoliosis. J Bone Joint Surg Am 2010;92(15);2533-43.*

Adolescent Scoliosis

Adolescents present with lateral curvature plus rotation. Lordosis or hypokyphosis is seen in the dorsal region.

The etiology is may be genetic (there is a high concordance in monozygotic twins) or hormonal (related to growth hormone).

Overall, 2–3% children aged less than 16 years have curves of more than 10°, but only 10% need treatment.

Probability of Progression

The probability of progression is indicated by several features:

- A 5° increase in the Cobb angle over two visits in one year.
- Rapid growth in girls prior to their first menses.
- Risser sign 0, 36–68% will progress; Risser sign 4, 11–18% will progress.
- A double curve; single thoracic curves progress more than single lumbar.
- Curve magnitude (20% of 20° curves progress vs 90% of 50° curves).

Overall, 3% of curves resolve (usually if <11°).

Radiographs

The following radiographs should be taken:

- Standing PA radiograph (reduced radiation to breast), including iliac crest and cervical spine.
- Spot lateral of the lumbosacral junction to check for listhesis.
- Stagnara lateral view—corrects for rotational malalignment.
- Side bending only if considering surgery or bracing.

Assessment of Skeletal Maturity

Skeletal maturity should be assessed:

- Clinical assessment of secondary sexual characteristics.
- Risser sign.
- Bone age at hand and wrist.
- Maturation of vertebral ring apophysis.
- Peak height Velocity (PHV).

PHV is based on serial measurement of height. It is 8 cm/year in girls and 9.5 cm/year in boys. Growth stops 3.6 years after PHV in 90% of people, and also indicates cessation of curve progression.

Curve Measurement

The curve can be measured with the Cobb angle and vertebral rotation. Nash and Moe recommended measuring the distance of the pedicle from the centre of the vertebra.

Nash CL, Moe JH. A study of vertebral rotation. J Bone Joint Surg Am 1969;51(2);223-9.

A Perdriolle torsionmeter measures rotation on an AP X-ray.

Sagittal balance should also be measured. A vertical line is drawn from the dens passes anterior to thoracic spine, posterior to lumbar spine and through the posterosuperior corner of the S1 vertebral body. In a positive sagittal vertebral axis, the line passes anterior to the body of S1; in a negative axis, the line passes posterior to S1.

Lumbar lordosis should be 20–30° more than thoracic kyphosis to maintain sagittal balance. Thoracic kyphosis is measured from T4 or T5, and 14° (±8°) is added to the figure for kyphosis from T1 to T4 or T5. T1 is not normally seen on the lateral spine view.

Lumbar lordosis is mostly in the disc. L5 and S1 cause 60% of lumbar lordosis cases. The thoracolumbar junction is normally straight.

A structural curve is over 25 degrees on the PA view and does not correct to under 25 degrees on side bending radiographs. Nonstructural curves will reduce on side bending radiographs to less than 25 degrees.

Curve Patterns

Ponseti and Friedman have identified five types of curve pattern, with a sixth added by Moe:

- Single major lumbar curve—apex between L1 and L4. Causes an asymmetric waist line and prominent hip.
- Single major thoracolumbar curve—apex at T12 or L1. Causes disbalance and severe cosmetic disability.
- Combined thoracic and lumbar curves (double major curves)—usually well balanced.
- Single major thoracic curve—convex right. Produces prominence of ribs on the convex side and elevation of the shoulder causing cosmetic deformity.
- Single major high thoracic curve—causes an unsightly deformity due to an elevated shoulder. Curves from C7 to T5.
- Double major thoracic curve—A short upper thoracic curve from T1 to T6 and a lower curve from T6 to L1. The upper curve is convex to the left. Deformities are not severe.

Curve Types

Lenke *et al* developed a classification system for adolescent idiopathic scoliosis based on radiographs made on coronal and sagittal planes (Table 5.10).

A diagrammatic representation of the curves is shown in Fig. 5.7.

In Type 2, the proximal thoracic curve is minor and structural.

In Type 3, the main thoracic curve is the major curve and is greater than, equal to, or no more than 5° less than the Cobb measurement of the thoracolumbar/lumbar curve.

In Type 6, the thoracolumbar/lumbar curve is the major curve and measures at least 5° more than the main thoracic curve, which is structural.

For a structural curve, side bending Cobb's angle should be greater than 25 degrees and Kyphosis should be more than 20 degrees.

The location of apex for thoracic curve is from T2 to T11-12 disc; for Thoracolumbar curve is T12 to L1; and for Lumbar curves, it is from L1-2 disc to L4.

A lumbar spine modifier (Fig. 5.8) has been added to the curve pattern. A vertical line is drawn from the centre of sacrum and the relation of the lumbar apical vertebra is assessed in relation to the vertical line. In A, the line passes

Table 5.10 Lenke Classification for scoliosis curves

Curve Type	Proximal thoracic	Main Thoracic	Thoracolumbar / lumbar	Description
1	Nonstructural	Structural	Nonstructural	Main thoracic
2	Structural	Structural	Nonstructural	Double thoracic
3	Nonstructural	Structural	Structural	Double major
4	Structural	Structural	Structural	Triple major
5	Nonstructural	Nonstructural	Structural	Thoracolumbar/ Lumbar
6	Nonstructural	Structural	Structural	Thoracolumbar/ lumbar main thoracic

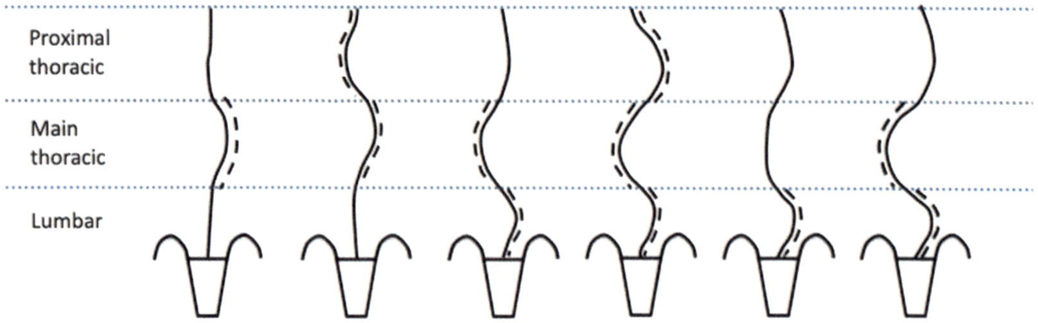

Fig. 5.7 Curve patterns as described by Lenke. The structural curve in each pattern has been highlighted with a dotted line

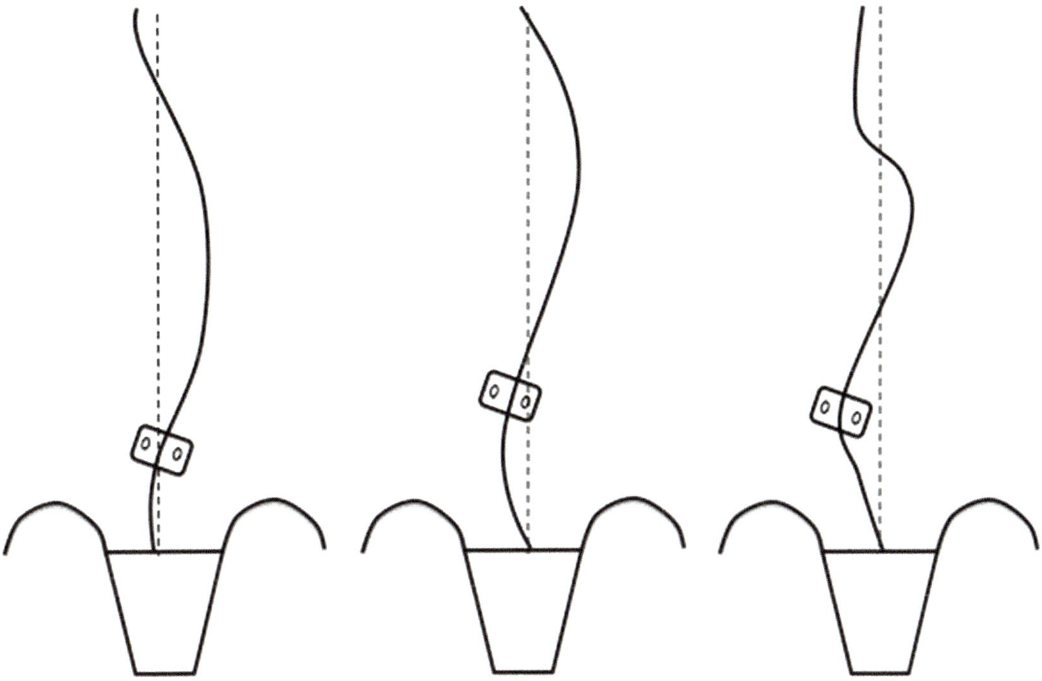

Fig. 5.8 Lumbar Spine modifiers as part of Lenke classification

between the pedicles of the lumbar apical vertebra; in B it is within the body; and in C, it is beyond the body of the vertebra.

Treatment

Initial treatment is often with observation. X-rays of the spine are regularly obtained to document curve size and progression.

A flowchart for management is shown in Fig. 5.9.

A Milwaukee brace will improve curves by 50% within 6 months, but the results of bracing are the same as no bracing after 5 years.

Other braces are the Boston underarm brace and Wilmington brace. Patient adherence is a problem. Patients may be more likely to adhere to part-time brace wear (16 hours), but this is less effective in preventing curve progression.

Surgery is indicated for -

- An increasing curve in a growing child.
- Over 50° deformity in a mature patient.
- A curve of more than 40–50° in a skeletally immature patient.
- Uncontrolled pain.
- Thoracic lordosis.

Cotrel–Dubousset instrumentation allows distraction and compression on the same rod. A rod rotation manoeuvre is performed to translate the apex of the curve to a normal position.

Anterior release and fusion are performed for curves over 75°. For rigid curves, bending correction is less than 50° and has a risk of crankshaft phenomenon. Crankshaft phenomenon only occurs in immature patients (Risser grade 0 or 1).

Anterior disc excision increases disc flexibility and bone graft leads to stable fusion. Anterior vertebral body screw fixation and anterolateral rod constructs can be used, but an iatrogenic flat back should be avoided.

For children with aggressively progressive curves, a subcutaneous rod and limited fusion at the proximal and distal hook sites is an option. Sequential distraction should be performed every 6 months and the patient protected with brace throughout. Formal fusion is eventually performed.

The treatments for various curve types are shown in Table 5.11.

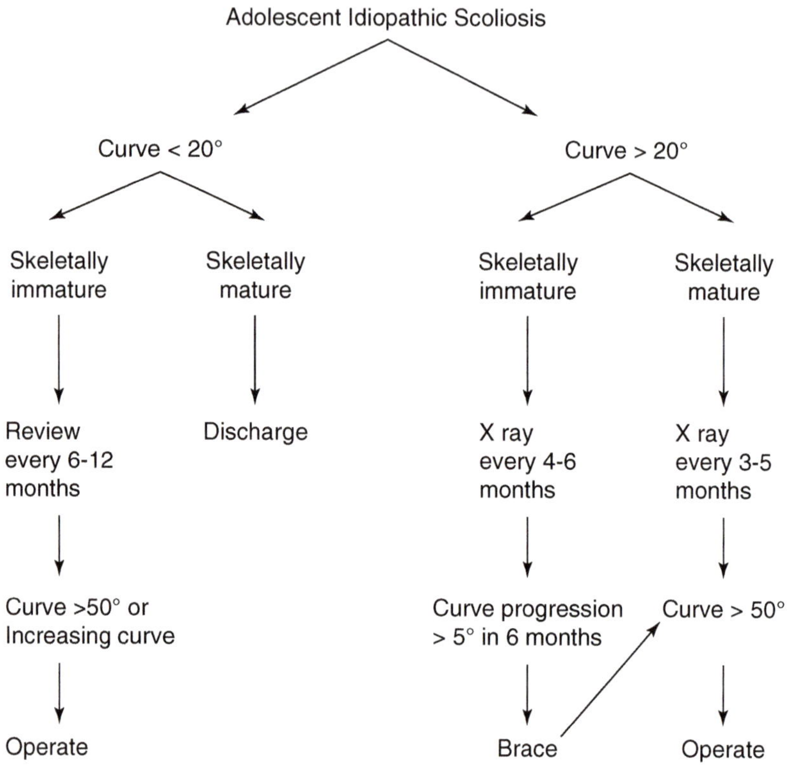

Fig. 5.9 Management plan for AIS

Outcomes

Harrington rods provide 48% coronal correction on long-term follow-up. These are no longer in use in most centres.

The Cotrel–Dubousset instrument gives 61% coronal plane correction.

An anterior lumbar approach gives 67–98% correction, but maintaining lumbar lordosis is a challenge.

Anterior thoracic correction is comparable with posterior correction, but has a higher incidence of rod breakage.

Table 5.11 Treatments for different curve types

Curve	Treatment
Right thoracic curve	Posterior instrumentation and fusion Distal hook—One level above the stable vertebra Multiple hooks or sublaminar wires on concave side Can also do anterior correction—Fuse all vertebrae within the cobb angle
Right thoracic, left lumbar	Usually thoracic is primary Can fuse only the thoracic, but avoid decompensation Trunk may decompensate to left if the lumbar curve is 45–50° and only the thoracic is corrected If both are instrumented—Extend fusion to L3 or L4 or up to the stable vertebra
Double thoracic—Elevated left shoulder	Correct both curves. An elevated right shoulder means an isolated right thoracic curve Correct both curves
Left lumbar—Isolated fusion of the lumbar curve	Limited anterior fusion is more effective in controlling rotation Posterior fusion with pedicle screws is acceptable

Congenital Scoliosis

Several abnormalities of vertebral shape cause deviation, which leads to congenital scoliosis. These can cause isolated scoliosis, kyphosis or lordosis, or a combination of the three.

Examination

It is easiest to examine the child dressed in a nappy, sitting on a parent's lap and facing the parent.

Note:

- The size of the child.
- Alertness level.
- Head and neck control.
- Nourishment.
- Comfort.
- Palpate the spine.
- Deformity—note the number of curves.
- Shape of head—plagiocephaly, plagiothorax.
- Bat ear, wry neck or adducted hip.
- Sternomastoids (examine for stiffness).
- Short neck and low hair line
- Sprengel's deformity—the height of the scapula
- Use of all muscle groups.
- Leg lengths and hip range of motion.
- Lower-limb wasting, signs of spinal dysraphism.

Imaging

Asymmetric size or number of pedicles, absent rib and unsegmented bars maybe seen.

Natural History

Thoracic curves progress the most. Multiple hemivertebra indicate a poor prognosis. Block vertebrae do not require surgery—progress is less than 1°/year. Hemivertebrae progress at 1–2.5°/year. An unsegmented bar progresses at 6–9°/year. An unsegmented bar with contralateral hemivertebra progresses at more than 10°/year.

Treatment

Regular radiographic follow-up is needed. Brace treatment is not very effective.

Preoperative evaluation includes an ultrasound of the genitourinary tract and MR imaging of the spine.

It may be possible to correct the curve, but this can cause neurologic damage. A safe approach is to fuse *in situ*.

Treatment options are—posterior fusion; anterior fusion; partial fusion, hemiepiphysiodesis—fuse only on the convex side; or hemivertebra excision—for lower lumbar vertebrae with truncal decompensation.

Neuromuscular Scoliosis

The neuromuscular causes of scoliosis include cerebral palsy, Duchenne's muscular dystrophy, syringomyelia, Marfan's syndrome, myelodysplasia and polio.

The onset of deformity is early and it is generally severe and progressive. Cerebral palsy is associated with a long C curve, while curves in neurofibromatosis often involve few vertebrae.

Bracing is commonly needed and surgical stabilisation of curves should be performed to prevent progression. The principle of surgery is multiple-level long fixation and fusion to the pelvis.

In neurofibromatosis, the vertebral foramen is widened and there is scalloping of the vertebrae, pencilling of the ribs and cervical kyphosis.

Postural Scoliosis

Postural scoliosis is non-structural and is not associated with rotational malalignment. It may be a result of leg-length discrepancy or of a painful lesion in, or adjacent, to the spine.

Scheuermann's Disease

Scheuermann's disease is kyphosis of the spine. For the diagnosis, at least three adjacent vertebrae must be wedged by 5° each.

Normal sagittal curvature of thoracic kyphosis spine is 20–40°. Two types of Scheuermann's disease are recognised:

- Type I—lower thoracic.
- Type II—lumbar Scheuermann's or apprentice kyphosis.

Type II is more commonly seen in athletic adolescent boys and with heavy lifting. There is no increased kyphosis, but severe endplate irregularity and Schmorl's nodes.

Etiology

The etiology of Scheuermann's disease is unknown. It is not related to osteonecrosis of the apophysis, disc herniation or a persistent anterior vascular groove.

Mechanical factors include tight hamstrings, which prevents anterior pelvic tilt.

Incidence

The incidence varies from 1% to 8%. The age of presentation is 8–12 years, and the usual presentation is with pain and deformity.

Natural History

Pain is present in 50% of patients and gradually subsides with skeletal maturity. It is debated as to whether the deformity causes disabling back pain.

Treatment

A brace is advised for kyphosis of less than 65°, if there is growth remaining.

The indications for surgery are controversial and depend on the patient's choice. Surgery may be indicated for kyphosis of more than 75° with pain.

Posterior Harrington compression instrumentation produces good initial correction, but this is lost over time.

Posterior spinal fusion using pedicle screw construct improve the correction and prevent late loss of correction. This is indicated if the patient has severe kyphosis of more than 75° or more than 50° kyphosis on an extension lateral radiograph. Fusion from T3 to L2 is generally necessary. Smith-Peterson or Ponte's osteotomy can be performed at apex to achieve good correction. Anterior release, though uncommon, indicated in larger curves which are rigid.

Junctional kyphosis at the superior and inferior end of the fusion is seen with all instrumentations. To avoid this, correction is limited to 50% of the initial deformity.

Spinal Stenosis

Spinal stenosis is a narrowing of the spinal canal, leading to compression of the neural elements. The stenosis may be localised to one level or may be diffuse.

Classification

Spinal stenosis can be congenital or acquired. Causes of congenital stenosis are idiopathic narrowing of the spinal canal or achondroplasia causing developmental stenosis.

Acquired causes include degenerative changes, Paget's disease, tumours, infections. Spinal stenosis can also occur following trauma and surgery.

Depending on anatomic location within the spinal canal, stenosis can be central, lateral recess or foraminal (Fig. 5.10). Central is in the region of the dural sac. The lateral recess is the region lateral to the dural sac and the longitudinal line along the medial border of the pedicles. Foraminal is in the region of the pedicles. This is based on the grid pattern whereby each level is divided into three segments from the cephalad to the caudad: pedicle, intermediate and disc. In the coro-

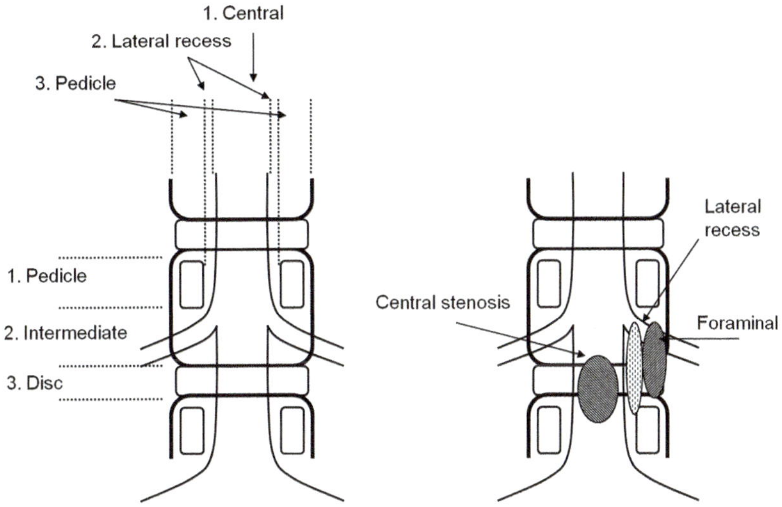

Fig. 5.10 Spinal stenosis

nal plane, there are five zones: one central zone, two lateral recesses and two pedicle zones.

Pathology

Degenerative changes in the facet joints with osteophyte formation cause narrowing of the spinal canal. The inferior articular process causes central canal narrowing, while the superior articular process causes narrowing of the lateral recess and the intervertebral foramen. Cyst formation in the synovial joints contributes to narrowing and activity-related pain.

Central stenosis leads to compression of the dural sac and the cauda equina, while lateral and foraminal stenosis cause pressure on the nerve root. Facet hypertrophy, congenital narrowing of the canal, spondylolisthesis, central disc herniation, trauma and surgery can lead to central spinal stenosis. Lateral stenosis is predominantly due to disc protrusion, facet hypertrophy or ligamentum flavum hypertrophy.

Clinical Features

Spinal stenosis causes neurogenic claudication symptoms that are worse with standing, activity or extension of the lumbar spine. The pain radiates to the thigh or leg and may be associated with sensory symptoms such as burning or numbness. Flexion of the spine, sitting and lying tend to relieve the symptoms.

Patients with lateral stenosis have more night pain, but better walking ability compared to those with central stenosis.

Vascular claudication can mimic neurogenic claudication. Associated signs of vascular insufficiency—skin changes and weak pulses—point to a vascular cause. Standing makes the pain worse in neurogenic claudication, but relieves it in vascular claudication. Riding a stationary bicycle with the spine flexed will exacerbate the pain from vascular causes, but not neurogenic pain.

Imaging

Plain radiographs of the lumbar spine are helpful in diagnosing coexisting scoliosis and degenerative spondylolisthesis. A CT scan will provide good osseous detail and MR scans provide soft tissue delineation. Myelography is invasive and is less frequently employed. The use of electromyography and somatosensory evoked potentials is limited to differentiation of neuropathy from spinal compressive lesions.

Treatment

The symptoms of spinal stenosis can be non-progressive and may resolve with time. Non-operative treatment is therefore considered in the first instance. The mainstays are NSAIDs, physiotherapy, bracing, activity modification and epidural steroid injections.

Operative treatment is aimed at decompression and can be achieved by removing the lamina and ligamentum flavum at the affected level. The nerve roots are decompressed up to their exit from the neural foramen. Total laminectomy should be avoided. Medial facetectomy is helpful in lateral recess stenosis to remove the part of facet joint causing pressure on the nerve root.

More limited resection techniques have been described. These involve removal of the anterior part of the lamina, foraminotomies, multiple laminotomies, partial laminectomy or laminoplasty. Soft stabilisation with interspinous spacers offers an alternative in both central and foraminal stenosis. Limited decompression is effective in patients where the involved level can be accurately diagnosed on the basis of clinical examination and imaging.

The early results of decompression are generally good, but symptoms may recur in the long-term, where limited resection has been carried out.

Spondylolisthesis is a complication of laminectomy where posterior fusion is not performed and can result in an unsatisfactory outcome. Removal of single facet joints may not significantly compromise spinal stability, but removal of both facet joints is an indication for concomitant fusion, although this is not universal practice. The use of internal fixation avoids progression of spondylolisthesis after laminectomy. Patients with scoliosis and spinal stenosis should be managed by concomitant stabilisation to prevent deformity progression.

Spine Infections

Spine infections can broadly be classified into pyogenic (bacterial) or non-pyogenic (commonly tubercular).

Pyogenic Osteomyelitis of the Spine

Bacterial spread to the spine is along the end arteriole in the region of the vertebral end plate. These are low-flow vessels and bacterial seeding leads to destruction of the end plate and involvement of the intervertebral disc. The destruction and collapse of the disc is one of the first signs of the disease. The infection spreads to adjacent discs through the posterior spinal arterial anastomoses. The spread of infection along Batson's venous plexus is unlikely.

Risk Factors

Immune deficiency is a risk factor for the development of vertebral osteomyelitis. Smoking, diabetes, malignancy, irradiation, intravenous drug abuse and trauma can predispose to infection. It is more common in older people and prevalence is equal in men and women.

Infective Organisms

Staphylococcus aureus is the most common organism causing pyogenic osteomyelitis. Gram-negative infections are increasingly common, with the spine secondarily infected from the genitourinary tract, chest or foot ulcers. Infecting organisms include *Escherichia coli* and *Pseudomonas*, *Proteus* and *Enterococcus* species. MRSA is on the increase.

Clinical Features

The first symptom is back pain. This may be pain at night and associated with muscle spasm, causing hip flexion or torticollis depending on the site of infection. The lumbar spine is the most common site of infection.

Infection in the spine can lead to abscesses and tracking of the infection along the tissue planes. Cervical epidural abscesses are often anterior and can track into the mediastinum causing pressure symptoms. Lumbar and dorsal spine abscesses are usually posterior.

Approximately 15–20% patients have neurological deficit. Various causes of neurologic deficit are pressure on the neural structures from pus, scar tissue, an extruded disc, vertebrae or oedema. Ischaemic damage to the cord from septic emboli or phlebitis can also cause neurologic deficit.

Differential Diagnosis

Pyogenic osteomyelitis of spine must be differentiated from granulomatous osteomyelitis, primary and secondary neoplasms, degenerative disease, trauma, osteoporotic vertebral fractures and multiple myeloma.

Vertebral discitis can produce localised pain and restricted movements in the back in young patients. Patients are typically not systemically unwell and radiographs show a reduced disc height.

The erythrocyte sedimentation rate and C-reactive protein level are elevated in acute infections and serve as a marker to response to treatment. They are non-specific, however, and elevation of these markers by itself does not imply infection. Blood cultures are useful, if positive, to identify the responsible organism, but a negative blood culture has a poor predictive value.

Imaging

The first sign on plain radiographs is diminution of the joint space, which may appear 2–4 weeks after the onset of infection. In addition, osteolysis and haziness of the end plate may be seen. Obliteration of the psoas shadow indicates a possible abscess. A prevertebral shadow or widened mediastinum may appear in patients with a paraspinal abscess.

Destruction of the intervertebral disc space is a late feature of malignant disease and generally indicates an infective process.

A gallium-67 scan is more sensitive and specific than the Tc-99 m scan. It is positive earlier than the Tc-99 m scan in infection and the return to normal is also quicker following treatment. SPECT scanning increases the accuracy.

An MR scan is the modality of choice. Gadolinium enhancement is useful in differentiating postoperative scarring from acute infection changes. Significant oedema in the bone is evident in T2-weighted images.

CT-guided biopsy is useful to obtain tissue and fluid for cultures and identification of the organism. Antibiotic therapy diminishes the positivity of samples. Histology should be obtained routinely along with cultures from the tissue samples. Cultures are performed for aerobes, anaerobes, mycobacteria and fungi.

Management

The aim of treatment is to maintain spinal stability and eradicate infection. The management of spinal infections can be surgical or non-surgical.

The trend of inflammatory markers—erythrocyte sedimentation rate and C-reactive protein level—is useful to monitor response to treatment. An adequate immune system and age less than 60 years are associated with an improved prognosis.

Non-surgical treatment is aimed at correcting malnutrition, initiating appropriate antibiotics and using an orthosis to prevent deformity and control pain.

The indications for surgical intervention are as follows:

- Failure of response to non-surgical treatment.
- Acute onset of neurologic deficit.
- Management of spinal instability.
- Systemic sepsis.
- Formation of a paraspinal or epidural abscess.

Surgery achieves debridement of the infected tissue, decompression and reconstruction. Reconstruction can be performed with an iliac crest bone graft, fibular graft, allograft or instrumentation. Anterior instrumentation achieves good debridement, but carries the risk of persistent infection due to direct contact between the metalwork and the infected tissue. Debridement of infected tissue from an anterior approach, with posterior instrumentation, is an option.

Granulomatous Osteomyelitis

Mycobacterium tuberculosis is the predominant organism responsible for granulomatous infection of the spine. This has been widespread in developing countries and is staging resurgence in developed countries in immune-compromised hosts.

Percival Pott described the paraplegia associated with tuberculosis of the spine in 1779.

Pathology

Tuberculous osteomyelitis can affect the paradiscal, anterior, posterior or central part of the vertebral column. This is based on the site of initial infection in the spine. The mode of spread is usually haematogenous, from a primary focus. The primary focus can be in the lungs, genitourinary system or lymph nodes.

The paradiscal site is most common place for the initial infection (Fig. 5.11). The infection begins from arterial spread in the vertebral metaphysis, spreading to the adjacent vertebra under the anterior longitudinal ligament. This leads to destruction of the vertebral ends, without disc destruction. The central type causes destruction of the centre of the vertebral body and collapse. In the central type, the spread of bacteria is through the Batson's plexus and may be associated with vertebral meningitis.

The anterior type tracks under the anterior longitudinal ligament and scallops the anterior margins of multiple adjacent vertebrae. These can lead to interruption of the blood supply of the vertebra and collapse. The posterior or appendiceal type is rare, and involves the posterior elements only.

Paraspinal abscess formation can be seen in tubercular osteomyelitis. The dura acts as a barrier to spread of infection. Epidural abscess is a particularly serious complication and can lead to cord compression, or cord oedema from venous obstruction. The abscess can lead to paralysis within 3–4 days of onset. It requires urgent treatment through decompression—either from the anterior approach or via a laminectomy.

Persistent kyphosis leads to attenuation of the spinal cord over the internal gibbus. This causes irreversible myelomalacia and is a cause of late onset paraplegia.

Candida, *Aspergillus* and *Actinomyces* species can all cause granulomatous infections.

Diagnosis

Patients present with weight loss, constitutional symptoms, progressive spinal pain and deformity. Paraspinal abscess in the cervical region

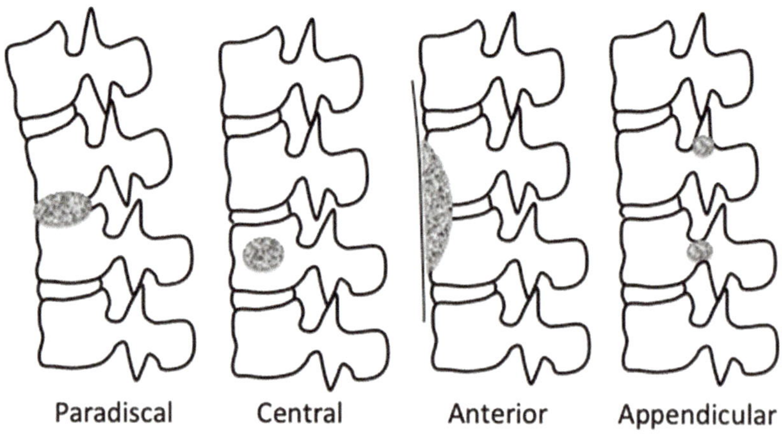

Fig. 5.11 Sites for granulomatous infection in the spine

can cause hoarseness, dysphagia or respiratory distress. Lumbar paraspinal abscess may communicate with psoas sheath and cause swelling around the inguinal area.

The diagnostic work-up for granulomatous infections is similar to that for pyogenic infection. The white cell count is often normal. Cultures for acid-fast bacilli may take up to 8 weeks.

X-ray imaging shows localised osteopenia of two adjacent vertebrae, which is an early sign. There is narrowing of the disc space. In later stages, vertebral collapse may be evident. Fusiform paraspinal abscesses are sometimes seen and may be the first radiological sign.

In tuberculous osteomyelitis the thoracic spine is involved more often than lumbar, and the disc spaces are preserved until the late stage of the disease. This helps to differentiate it from pyogenic infection.

Nuclear scan has a higher false-negative rate. MR scan with gadolinium enhancement is useful in differentiating abscess cavities from granulation tissue. CT-guided biopsy and polymerase chain reaction are the modalities of choice for a definitive diagnosis.

Treatment

The treatment mainstay of tubercular spinal infection is antitubercular drugs. The most commonly used drugs are rifampicin, isoniazid, pyrazinamide and ethambutol. The duration of treatment is 6–9 months.

Bracing may be needed to control deformity.

Surgery (in addition to medical treatment) is indicated where there is neurologic involvement, lack of response to medical treatment, a large abscess or signs of spinal instability.

The degree of kyphosis can be predicted by:

Kyphosis = total vertebral involvement × 30.5 degree +5.5 degree.

Hence, complete two vertebrae involvement will lead to 66.5 degrees kyphosis at 5 years.

The number of vertebrae involved is counted by dividing the vertebral body into tenths and adding up all the tenths from all vertebrae affected.

Surgery helps relieve cord compression, alleviate pain and improve kyphosis. For the cervical spine, anterior decompression and stabilisation is done with or without posterior instrumentation.

In thoracic spine with minimal kyphotic deformity, a costotransversectomy helps to drain the pus and relieve pressure on the spinal cord. The anterior spinal debris can be removed and a posterior fusion carried out at the same time. Severe kyphosis and cord compression can be managed by anterior decompression and reconstruction of anterior column in the lower thoracic region.

For thoracolumbar area, a posterior approach can be utilised for decompression and stabilisation using pedicle screws.

Mycobacterium does not form biofilm, and insertion of metalwork in the presence of tubercular pus is not contraindicated.

Spondylolisthesis

Spondylolisthesis is anterior translation (slipping) of a vertebra caused by a defect in the pars interarticularis. It is a common cause of low backache in adolescents.

The defect in the pars is most commonly due to a stress fracture from repeated hyperextension stresses.

Classification

Spondylolisthesis is classified with the Wiltse and Neuman classification (Table 5.12).

Wiltse LL, Newman PH, Macnab I. Classification of spondylolysis and spondylolisthesis. Clin Orthop Relat Res 1976;117:23–9.

Radiologic Measurement

Plain radiographs show the lesion in 80% patients. Oblique views of the lumbar spine improve the sensitivity and the classic sign, the

Table 5.12 Classification of spondylolisthesis

Type	Description
I	Congenital/dysplastic: • facets are malaligned or improperly developed (axially or sagittally oriented) • the cranial vertebra displaces anteriorly, but the integrity of the ring is maintained • underlying cause in 25% patients • symptoms include tight hamstrings • neurologic signs such as paraesthesia or cauda equina may be present because the canal is closed
II	Isthmic/spondylotic: • defect in the pars interarticularis • neurologic sequelae are less common than in type I • may present by the age of 5–6 years or at adolescence • this is the most common type and comprises 50% of patients with spondylolisthesis • symptoms are low back pain, tight hamstrings and possibly irritation of the fifth nerve root
IIA	Lytic/fatigue pars fracture
IIB	Elongated but intact pars
IIC	Acute fracture of pars
III	Degenerative: • due to loss of disc/structure integrity or facet joints • accounts for 20% patients
IV	Traumatic: • traumatic disruption of facets allowing anterior slip • results from a severe traumatic event
V	Pathologic: • Destruction of the pars/pedicle/facet by tumours or Paget's disease

defect in the pars, is known as the 'Scottie dog' sign.

Radiographs should be obtained in the standing position to assess the degree of slip and the slip angle.

Spondylolisthesis can be graded with the Meyerding system. Five grades of slip are described based on anterior translation of the posterior border of the vertebra in relation to the posterior border of the vertebra below. The translation distance is measured in relation to the AP dimension of the vertebra below.

- Grade I—less than 25% slip.
- Grade II—25–50% slip.

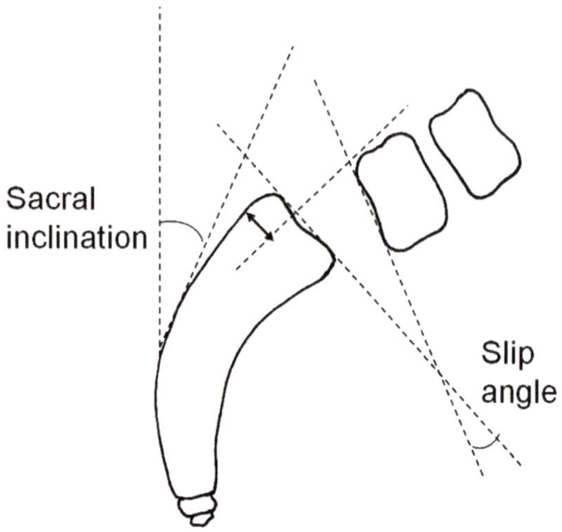

Fig. 5.12 Sacral inclination and slip angle

- Grade III—50–75% slip.
- Grade IV—75–100% slip.
- Grade V—more than 100% slip (known as spondyloptosis).

In grade V, the posterior border of the vertebra above displaces anterior to the anterior margin of the vertebra below.

Other measures are the percentage of slip (related to the upper border of S1), the lumbar index, sacral inclination, sagittal pelvic tilt and slip angle (Fig. 5.12).

Slip angle is the angle between the lower border of the vertebra above and the upper border of vertebra below. Normally the gap between the vertebra is wider anteriorly, making the slip angle positive. In spondylolisthesis the gap is wider posteriorly, making the angle negative.

Serial radiographs are helpful to document progression. Changes of less than 10% are not considered significant because of errors in radiographs.

Rothman RH, Simone FA, eds. The Spine, second edn. Philadelphia: WB Saunders, 1982.

Investigations

Useful investigations include -

- Discography.
- Bone scan—to distinguish an acute (increased uptake) from longstanding pars defect.
- CT scan—for planning.
- MR imaging—to identify the nerve roots, disc and other congenital anomalies such as a tethered cord.

Non-surgical Treatment

Isthmic

In asymptomatic children, yearly X-rays are undertaken, but no activity modification is needed. For symptomatic children, stretching exercises for the hamstrings are recommended.

In adults, a stretching program and weight control is advised. Nerve root blocks can be considered for radicular pain caused by narrowing of the foramen.

Dysplastic

In children, there is a high incidence of neurologic complications and most require surgery. A study looking at conservative treatment examined the use of a soft thoracolumbar brace in 23 children and adolescents with a pars defect. A high signal in the adjacent pedicle on a T2 MR scan and early-stage defect on CT correlated with better healing potential.

Sairyo K, Sakai T, Yasui N. Conservative treatment of lumbar spondylolysis in childhood and adolescence: the radiological signs which predict healing. J Bone Joint Surg Br 2009;91:206–9.

In adults, tight hamstrings and low back pain can be managed non-operatively. Cauda equina, however, requires an urgent operation.

Management

Non-surgical Treatment

During the acute phase, it is generally agreed that conservative management should be attempted before surgical intervention. Many studies support the non-surgical approach.

Wiltse et al. demonstrated that 12 of 17 young patients diagnosed with spondylolysis showed osseous healing with conservative treatment and no surgery.

Wiltse LL, Widell EH Jr, Jackson DW. Fatigue fracture: the basic lesion in isthmic spondylolisthesis. J Bone Joint Surg Am 1975;57:17–22.

Early diagnosis is important for a good prognosis in bone healing. Ciullo and Jackson studied gymnasts and found that longer the symptoms were present before treatment, the more likely surgical intervention became.

Ciullo JV, Jackson DW. Pars interarticularis stress reaction, spondylolysis, and spondylolisthesis in gymnasts. Clin Sports Med 1985;4:95–110.

During the acute phase of rehabilitation for patients with spondylolysis, the focus is on reducing pain. Instruction in posture and biomechanics with activities of daily living can help to protect the injured pars, thus reducing symptoms and preventing further injury. A period of rest for an average of 2–4 weeks can provide beneficial effects by modulating pain, decreasing inflammation and decreasing the risk for further progression of a pars stress reaction to a frank fracture.

Applying ice to the injured area for 20 minutes three to four times a day, in conjunction with gentle range of motion exercises and stretching of the quadriceps and hamstring muscles, is strongly advised. Activity modification is recommended. The patient is advised to stop the activity or sport that evokes the back pain for an average of 2–4 weeks. In particular, the patient should avoid any activities involving hyperextension.

Indications for the use of a brace are lack of symptom improvement by 2–4 weeks, the presence of a true fracture or spondylolisthesis, the need for pain control and lack of patient adherence with activity restrictions.

The risk factors for progression of slip are female sex, young age, high slip angle, high-grade slip, a dome-shaped sacrum and high sacral inclination.

Seitsalo S, Osterman K, Hyvãrinen H, et al. *Progression of spondylolisthesis in children and adolescents. A long-term follow-up of 272 patients. Spine (Phila Pa) 1991;16:417–21.*

Surgical Treatment

Surgical treatment is indicated in most patients with high-grade slip (≥3), progressive slip, an associated neurologic deficit or unremitting back and leg pain.

Pars interarticularis repair is indicated if the disc is normal on MR imaging, pain is arising from the defect, low back pain is increased by extension and pain relief is obtained with injection of the pars.

Ideal candidates for direct repair of the pars defect are those with early lesions, with lysis but no listhesis, and with the lytic defect between L1 and L4. L5 lytic defects have been reported to yield less predictable results because many L5 defects arise from a developmentally weakened and elongated pars.

Surgical techniques generally employ debridement of the lytic defect, application of large amounts of autogenous iliac crest cancellous bone graft and tension band wiring or screw fixation from the cephalad portion of the posterior element to the free-floating caudal fragment.

Fusion *in situ* procedures are performed in patients with low-grade spondylolisthesis that remains symptomatic despite non-operative measures or those with high-grade listhesis but acceptable sagittal balance. Decompression and fusion are indicated when severe neurologic signs of compression are present, such as radiating leg pain, numbness and weakness, with corresponding imaging studies demonstrating nerve root or thecal sac compression.

Reduction is indicated to prevent the complications of slip progression, pseudarthrosis and cosmetic deformity associated with *in situ* fusion; hence, reduction of high-grade slips is often performed. Reduction (closed or open) serves to correct lumbosacral kyphosis and diminish the sagittal translation seen in high-grade slips. For more severe slips, instrumented fusion from S1 to L4 is recommended. It may be difficult to place a pedicle screw in the L5 pedicle.

In spondyloptosis (grade 5 slip), an attempt is made to improve the slip angle and fuse L4 to S1; alternatively, a vertebrectomy may be indicated. Gaines procedure is to anteriorly remove L5 and fuse L4 to S1 posteriorly as a second stage. This has a high complication rate, with 25% iatrogenic neurological deficit.

General complications of surgery include pneumonia, urinary tract infections, deep vein thrombosis, pulmonary embolism and infection.

Further complications are as follows:

- Surgical approach:
  - Epidural scarring.
  - Nerve root injury.
  - Dural tear.
  - Great vessel injury.
  - Bowel injury.
  - Injury to the ureter.
  - Injury to the hypogastric plexus and genitofemoral nerve.
- Related to fusion:
  - Pseudarthrosis.
  - Graft extrusion or subsidence.
  - Accelerated degeneration of adjacent discs.
  - Donor-site morbidity.
- Related to the metalwork:
  - Implant failure.
  - Misplaced/fracture of pedicle screws.
  - Nerve root injury.

Further Reading

Bess S, et al. Complications of growing rod treatment for early onset scoliosis. J Bone Joint Surg Am. 2010;92(15):2533–43.

Bigos S, Bowyer O, Braen G, et al: Acute Lower Back Problems in Adults. Clinical Practice Guideline No 14. AHCPR Publication No 95–0642.

Boden SD, Dodge LD, Bohlman HH, Rechtine GR. Rheumatoid arthritis of the cervical spine. A long-term analysis with predictors of paralysis and recovery. J Bone Joint Surg Am. 1993;75:1282–97.

Ciullo JV, Jackson DW. Pars interarticularis stress reaction, spondylolysis, and spondylolisthesis in gymnasts. Clin Sports Med. 1985;4:95–110.

Findlay C, Ayis S, Demetriades AK. Total disc replacement versus anterior cervical discectomy and fusion:

a systematic review with meta-analysis of data from a Total of 3160 patients across 14 randomized controlled trials with both short- and medium- to long-term outcomes. Bone Joint J. 2018;100-B:991–1001.

Gornet MF, Burkus JK, Dryer RF, Peloza JH. Lumbar disc arthroplasty with maverick disc versus stand-alone interbody fusion: a prospective, randomized, controlled, multicenter investigational device exemption trial. Spine (Phila Pa 1976). 2011;36:25.

Levin KH, Maggiano HJ, Wilbourn AJ. Cervical radiculopathies: comparison of surgical and EMG localization of single-root lesions. Neurology. 1996;46:1022–5.

Mehta MH. The rib–vertebra angle in the early diagnosis between resolving and progressive infantile scoliosis. J Bone Joint Surg Br. 1972;54:230–43.

Muijs SPJ, et al. Treatment of painful osteoporotic vertebral compression fractures. J Bone Joint Surg Br. 2011;93(9):1149–53.

Nash CL, Moe JH. A study of vertebral rotation. J Bone Joint Surg Am. 1969;51(2):223–9.

Ng LC, Sell P. Predictive value of the duration of sciatica for lumbar discectomy. A prospective cohort study. J Bone Joint Surg Br. 2004;86(4):546–9.

Ranawat CS, O'Leary P, Pellicci P, et al. Cervical spine fusion in rheumatoid arthritis. J Bone Joint Surg Am. 1979;61:1003–10.

Resnick DK, Watters WC. Lumbar disc arthroplasty: a critical review. Clin Neurosurg. 2007;54:83–7.

Rothman RH, Simone FA, editors. The spine. 2nd ed. Philadelphia: WB Saunders; 1982.

Sairyo K, Sakai T, Yasui N. Conservative treatment of lumbar spondylolysis in childhood and adolescence: the radiological signs which predict healing. J Bone Joint Surg Br. 2009;91:206–9.

Seitsalo S, Osterman K, Hyvãrinen H, et al. Progression of spondylolisthesis in children and adolescents. A long-term follow-up of 272 patients. Spine (Phila Pa). 1991;16:417–21.

Spitzer WO, LeBlanc FE, Dupuis M, et al. Scientific approach to the assessment and management of activity-related spinal disorders. A monograph for clinicians. Report of the Quebec taskforce on spinal disorders. Spine (Phila Pa 1976). 1987;12(Suppl):S16–2.

Todd N. Cauda equina syndrome: the timing of surgery probably does influence outcome. Brit J Neurosurg. 2009;19:301–6.

Waddell G, McCulloch JA, Kummel E, Venner RM. Nonorganic physical signs in low-back pain. Spine (Phila Pa 1976). 1980;5:117–25.

Weber H. Lumbar disc herniation. A controlled, prospective study with ten years of observation. Spine (Phila Pa 1976). 1983;8:131–40.

Weinstein JN, Lurie JD, Tosteson TD, et al. Surgical versus nonoperative treatment for lumbar disc herniation: four-year results for the spine patient outcome research trial (SPORT). Spine (Phila Pa 1976). 2008;33:2789–800.

Weissman BN, Aliabadi P, Weinfeld MS, et al. Prognostic features of atlantoaxial subluxation in rheumatoid arthritis patients. Radiology. 1982;144:745–51.

Wilke H, Neef P, Caimi M, et al. New in vivo measurements of pressures in the intervertebral disc in daily life. Spine. 1999;24:755–62.

Wiltse LL, Newman PH, Macnab I. Classification of spondylolysis and spondylolisthesis. Clin Orthop Relat Res. 1976;117:23–9.

Wiltse LL, Widell EH Jr, Jackson DW. Fatigue fracture: the basic lesion in isthmic spondylolisthesis. J Bone Joint Surg Am. 1975;57:17–22.

Wynne DR. Infantile idiopathic scoliosis. Causative factors, particularly in the first six months of life. J Bone Joint Surg Br. 1975;57(2):138–41.

6 Foot and Ankle

Gavin John Heyes and Lyndon Mason

Hallux Rigidus

Structural hallux rigidus refers to degenerative arthrosis of the first metatarsophalangeal (MTP) joint. This is the most common form of osteoarthritis in the foot. It is differentiated from functional hallux limitus by having a painful fixed reduction in joint motion, even when non-weight-bearing. Other clinical features include a prominent 'dorsal bunion' and synovitis, particularly dorsolaterally, altered gait due to lateral foot weight bearing to offload painful medial column.

Incidence

The incidence is 1 in 45 over the age of 65 years, however it commonly affects much younger patients.

Aetiology

Two thirds are familial and up to 90% are bilateral. Aetiological factors include acute and or repetitive trauma, gout and functional hallux limitus.

Common associations are.

- A long first metatarsal
- Flat metatarsal head
- Metatarsus Adductus
- Metatarsus Elevatus
- Hallux Valgus Interphalangeus

Coughlin MJ. Hallux Rigidus: Demographics, etiology and radiographic assessment. Foot and Ankle Int. 2003;24:731–734.

Radiological Findings

The earliest radiographic sign may be a depression in the dome of the metatarsal (MT) head. Radiographs may also show osteophyte formation and a reduction in the joint space. Lateral osteophytes are often responsible for the symptoms. The severity of hallux rigidus is determined by the radiographic appearance (Fig. 6.1).

Classification

The Coughlin and Shurnas classification is commonly used (Table 6.1).

Coughlin MJ, Shurnas PS. Hallux rigidus. Grading and long-term results of operative

G. J. Heyes
Liverpool University Hospitals NHS Foundation Trust, Aintree University Hospital, Liverpool, UK

L. Mason (✉)
University of Liverpool, Liverpool, UK

S. Agarwal (ed.), *Current Orthopaedic Practice*, https://doi.org/10.1007/978-3-030-78529-1_6

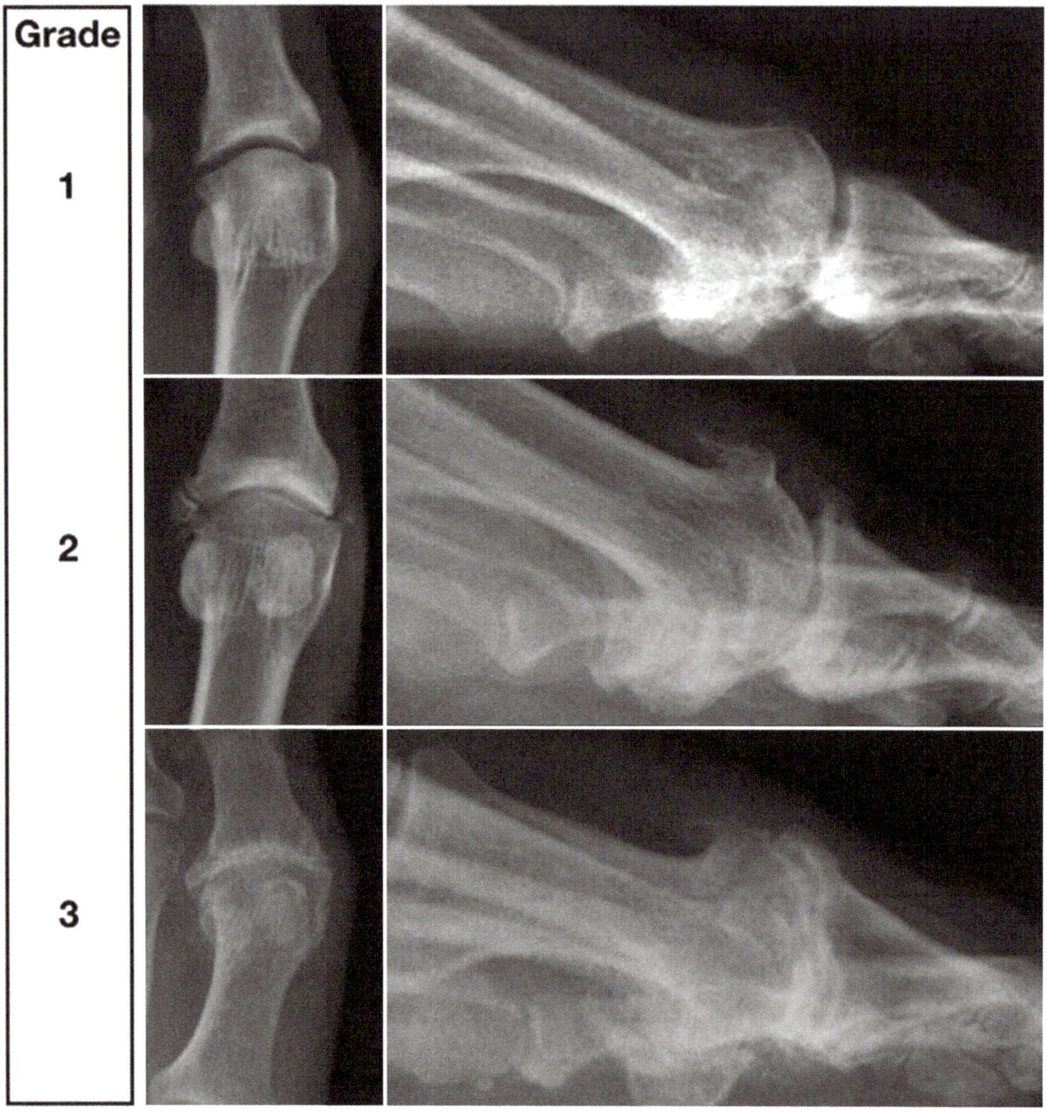

Fig. 6.1 Grades of Hallux rigidus

treatment. J Bone Joint Surg Am. 2003;85(11):2072–2088.

Conservative Treatment

Conservative measures include non-steroidal anti-inflammatory drugs (NSAIDs), an adequate toe box, a rigid or rocker-bottom sole or a Morton's extension splint (a stiff foot plate with an extension under the great toe). Weight loss, activity modification and ensuring an adequately stretched Gastro-Soleus complex are important. Steroid injections could also be considered, however their effect is often transient with reports of up to a half those injected requiring surgery within one year.

Table 6.1 Coughlin and Shurnas Classification of Hallux Rigidus

Grade	Dorsiflexion	Radiographic Findings	Clinical Findings
0	40°-60° +/or 10–20% loss compared to other side	Normal	Stiffness
1	30°-40° +/or 20–50% loss compared to other side	Dorsal osteophyte. Minimal joint space narrowing, flattening of metatarsal head and periarticular sclerosis	Stiffness and mild pain on end range of motion
2	10°-30° +/or 50–70% loss compared to other side	Dorsal, lateral +/– medial osteophyte. Flattening metatarsal head with >1/4 dorsal joint involvement. Mild to moderate joint space narrowing	Stiffness. Moderate to severe pain, occurring just before end range of motion
3	≤10° +/or 75–100% loss compared to other side. ≤10° plantar flexion	Grade 2 + substantial joint space narrowing +/– periarticular cystic change. >1/4 dorsal joint space involvement. Sesamoid enlargement/cystic change	Stiffness and constant pain except mid range motion
4	Grade 3	Grade 3	Grade 3 BUT mid range pain on passive motion

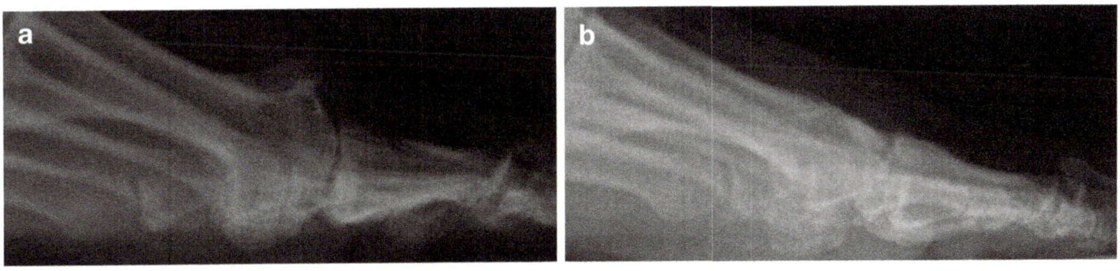

Fig. 6.2 Cheilectomy for hallux rigidus. Image (**a**) illustrates a grade 2 hallux rigidus who sustained an intraarticular fracture to the interphalangeal joint. Image (**b**) illustrates a dorsal cheilectomy to preserve the movement at the MTPJ and reduce the stress through the IPJ

Surgical Treatment

Cheilectomy

A systematic review (Roukis) reported revision rates <20% for cheilectomy in grade I, II or III provided <50% of the metatarsal head is involved; this compares to over 50% revision rate for cheilectomy in grade 4. The aim is to eliminate dorsal impingement and achieve at least 70° of dorsiflexion. This involves resection of the proliferative bone and removal of 30% of the dorsal metatarsal head and the lateral osteophytes. Cheilectomy to maintain movement is also useful to protect adjacent joints (Fig. 6.2).

Roukis TS. The need for surgical revision after isolated cheilectomy for hallux rigidus: a systematic review. J Foot Ankle Surg. 2010;49(5):465–70.

Cheilectomy + Dorsiflexion Osteotomy of the Metatarsal

This can be considered in young, active patients in order to avoid fusion. Osteotomy alone may be used in patients who lack dorsiflexion and do not have dorsal impingement. Shortening or elevation osteotomies of the first metatarsal have also been used to reduce pain, especially in the sesamoid region of the joint.

Cheilectomy + Proximal Phalanx Osteotomy

Dorsal closing wedge (Moberg) osteotomy facilitates an increase in dorsiflexion and is also thought to decompress the joint.

Regardless of the osteotomy adjunct used, the primary aim is to increase functional range of motion through alteration of current arc of movement in addition to decompression of the joint. Recent review of the literature has shown that there is currently no good quality evidence to state that one osteotomy yields superior results to another.

Polzer H, Polzer S, Brumann M, Mutschler W, Regauer M. Hallux rigidus: Joint preserving alternatives to arthrodesis—a review of the literature. World J Orthop. 2014;5(1):6–13.

Arthrodesis

To be considered in cases of advanced arthritis or failed cheilectomy. There are consistent reports of good function outcomes with arthrodesis and it remains the gold standard for many.

A standard medial or dorsomedial approach to the MTP joint is used. After releasing the capsule dorsally and plantarly, osteophytes are excised. The surfaces of the metatarsal and phalanx are prepared using congruent reamers down to bleeding subchondral bone. Small holes are drilled in the MTP surfaces to promote bony ingrowth. A guide wire is inserted just distal to the flare of the proximal phalanx and the position is checked with a foot plate or X-ray. The optimal position of fusion is 10° dorsiflexion in relation to the floor (15–25° in relation to the first MT) and 10° of valgus.

Biomechanically, Alentorn-Geli found that high dorsiflexion angles (>30 degrees) correlated with higher plantar pressures under the first metatarsal head, and low dorsiflexion angles (<15 degrees) correlated with increased plantar pressures beneath the hallux during gait.

Alentorn-Geli E, Gil S, Bascuas I, et al. *Correlation of dorsiflexion angle and plantar pressure following arthrodesis of the first metatarsophalangeal joint. Foot Ankle Int. 2013;34(4):504–511.*

Reduction in valgus puts increased strain on the interphalangeal (IP) joint and can result in arthritis. Methods of fusion vary, with high rates of fusion (>90%) seen for most techniques, with no technique shown to be superior clinically.

Harris E, Moroney P, Tourne Y. Arthrodesis of the first metatarsophalangeal joint-A biomechanical comparison of four fixation techniques. Foot Ankle Surg. 2017;23(4):268–74. Biomechanically, a compression screw combined with a dorsal locking plate was the ideal construct for fixation when comparing different methods.

Roukis TS. Nonunion after arthrodesis of the first metatarsal-phalangeal joint: a systematic review. J Foot Ankle Surg. 2011;50(6):710–3. Regardless of osteosynthesis technique, the overall non-union rate was 5.4%, mal-union rates of 6.1% (of which only 32.7% were symptomatic.

Figure 6.3 illustrates an example of plate and screw construct for deformity correction. We have found better union rates in fusions of arthritic hallux valgus with this screw and plate configuration.

Other complications include, IP joint degenerative disease developing after the fusion and hardware problems.

Replacement Arthroplasty

There are many forms of replacement arthroplasty in the literature including; hemiarthroplasty, total joint resurfacing and more constrained Silastic implants. Results are generally worse than a fusion, although recent studies of Silastic implants have been roughly on a par with joint fusion. Nevertheless, there are some who are concerned about revision options, particularly for Silastic implants. Inevitably, the mode of failure here is loosening with significant bone loss.

Morgan S, Ng A, Clough T. The long-term outcome of silastic implant arthroplasty of the first metatarsophalangeal joint: a retrospective analysis of one hundred and eight feet. Int Orthop. 2012;36(9):1865–9.

Interposition Arthroplasty

Useful in higher-demand patients and should be considered when the adjacent sagittal plane joints are also affected by degeneration. Interpositions have been reported using capsule, gracilis, fascia lata, regenerative tissue matrix and synthetic car-

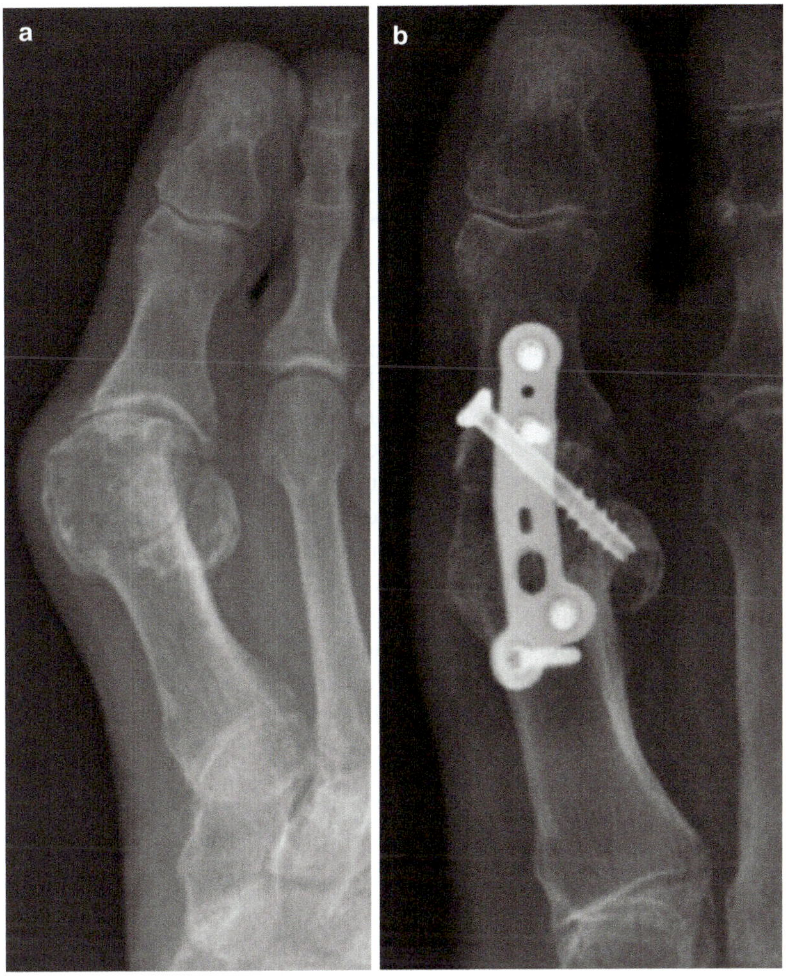

Fig. 6.3 Image (**a**) illustrates an arthritic hallux valgus deformity. Image (**b**) shows the same patient 6 months post-operative following a first metatarsophalangeal joint arthrodesis with deformity correction

tilage Implants (Polyvinyl Alcohol). Results up to 2 years of synthetic cartilage implants are similar to that of first MTPJ arthrodesis.

Baumhauer JF, Singh D, Glazebrook M, et al. *Prospective, Randomized, Multi-centered Clinical Trial Assessing Safety and Efficacy of a Synthetic Cartilage Implant Versus First Metatarsophalangeal Arthrodesis in Advanced Hallux Rigidus. Foot Ankle Int. 2016;37(5):457–69.*

This is however a relatively new implant and despite good satisfaction scores there is a revision rate of 9.2% at 2 years, slightly higher than some reported arthrodesis studies. Interestingly the outcomes of revisions to arthrodesis are similar to those that underwent primary arthrodesis in the original randomized controlled trial.

Keller's Resection Arthroplasty

This involves resection of most of the proximal phalanx of the hallux. Traditionally recommended for low demand and or frail individuals. Some report good functional scores, however up to 10% report transfer metatarsalgia (pain under the other metatarsals) and 20% are dissatisfied with cosmetic appearance. Other issues include cock up deformity, instability and reduced push-off.

Coutts A, Kilmartin TE, Ellis MJ. The long-term patient focused outcomes of the Keller's arthroplasty for the treatment of hallux rigidus. Foot (Edinb). 2012;22(3):167–71.

Currently reported short term outcomes for interposition and replacement arthroplasties are on a par with joint fusion.

Erdil M, Bilsel K, Imren Y, et al. *Metatarsal head resurfacing hemiarthroplasty in the treatment of advanced stage hallux rigidus: outcomes in the short-term. Acta Orthop Traumatol Turc. 2012;46(4):281–5.*

Hallux Varus

Hallux Varus is medial deviation of the hallux. It can be congenital, traumatic, inflammatory, neurological or most commonly iatrogenic due to previous hallux surgery. The muscle imbalance can be caused by resection of the lateral sesamoid, abductor hallucis or lateral slip of the flexor hallucis brevis. Excessive medial eminence resection, medial tightening of the capsule and lateral positioning of the metatarsal head following osteotomy can also cause it.

Patients present with deformity or painful rubbing from their footwear. Symptomatic flexible deformity can be treated by extensor hallucis longus (EHL) transfer to the base of the proximal phalanx under the intermetatarsal ligament. Alternatively Myerson et al. reported good correction with slight loss of dorsiflexion at 2 years with Extensor Hallucis Brevis (EHB) tenodesis. This can be combined with fusion of the IP joint.

Myerson MS, Komenda GA. Results of hallux varus correction using an extensor hallucis brevis tenodesis. Foot Ankle Int. 1996;17(1):21–7.

With the availability of newer devices, soft tissue reconstruction procedures are common. However positioning the implants incorrectly will adversely influence the movement of the joint. If the deformity is fixed or is associated with arthritis of the MTP joint, fusion of the first MTP joint is advisable and is the most reliable procedure for all types.

Hallux Valgus

Hallux valgus is a medial deviation of the first metatarsal joint and lateral deviation and/or rotation of the hallux, usually with medial soft tissue enlargement of the first metatarsal head. This movement is a consequence of the first metatarsal translating and rotating (pronation) medially.

Hallux valgus affects 1% of adults, with a higher incidence in women. The incidence increases with age, with rates of 3% in persons aged 15–30 years, 9% in those aged 31–60 years and 16% in those older than 60 years. There is also a genetic predisposition, with evidence to suggest familial tendencies.

Aetiology

Hallux valgus has been linked to excessive movement at the tarsometatarsal joint. Different types of joints have been described, conferring different levels of stability. Known factors are summarised in Fig. 6.4.

Mason LW, Tanaka H. The first tarsometatarsal joint and its association with hallux valgus. Bone Joint Res. 2012;1(6):99–103.

Classification

Hallux valgus is generally classified by either the severity, or the time of occurrence. For example, juvenile or adolescent hallux valgus is a different entity to adult hallux valgus, as there is a high distal metatarsal articular angle (DMAA) and usually a congruent joint (i.e. the head of the metatarsal points laterally unlike in aquired hallux valgus where the head of the metatarsal is normal position and the joint points laterally due to failure of the medial joint stabilisers).

Assessment

Clinical presentation includes deformity, shoe pressure, pain over the bunion, swelling and metatarsalgia. Lesser toe problems like MTP joint instability, pain, claw toes, transfer metatarsalgia and calluses over the heads of metatarsals occur as the first ray becomes insufficient.

It is important to assess the stability of the first tarsometatarsal joint (TMTJ), as a corrective distal or shaft osteotomy may struggle to correct or prevent recurrence in a very unstable TMTJ. It is also important to assess the passive correction of

Fig. 6.4 Etiology of hallux valgus

Etiology of hallux valgus

- Instability of the joint
  - Arthritic conditions
    - Rheumatoid arthritis
  - Neuromuscular diseases
    - Cerebral palsy
    - Charcot Marie Tooth disease
  - Hypermobility syndromes
    - Ehlers Danlos Syndrome
- Increased force on the hallux
  - Footwear
  - Pes planus
  - Second toe deformity
  - Second toe absence

the hallux and motion of the MTP joint following passive correction of the deformity, as this will give an estimate on postoperative stiffness. Adolescent hallux valgus will have a congruent MTPJ and will therefore not passively correct. Arthritis in the first MTP joint should be considered, and a positive mid-range grind test turns the surgical treatment towards fusion surgery rather than an osteotomy.

Consider the alignment of the entire limb including the medial longitudinal arch of the foot and any tightness of the triceps surae. A pes planus deformity and supinated forefoot will exacerbate the deformity. Assess any lesser toe deformities as these may require concurrent corrections. Metatarsus adductus deformity with lateral deviated lesser toes can prove to be a significant challenge when correcting any hallux valgus deformity.

Radiography continues to be the standard means with which to assess joint pathology and measure angular deformity. Weight-bearing AP, oblique and lateral projections are routinely used. The AP projection is used to determine the intermetatarsal angle (IMA), metatarsus adductus angle, hallux valgus angle (HVA), distal metatarsal articular angle (DMAA), hallux valgus interphalangeus, first metatarsal length, sesamoid position, first MTP joint condition and medial metatarsal head enlargement. Figure 6.5 shows the angles on the foot radiograph.

If lateral subluxation of proximal phalanx on metatarsal head is present then the joint is incongruent, meaning that the proximal phalanx can be rolled medially on the metatarsal head to correct the deformity.

The lateral projection is used to determine the first metatarsal sagittal plane position and the presence of dorsal exostosis or osteophytes. The lateral oblique projection is useful to evaluate the presence of dorsomedial exostosis. The sesamoid axial view can be used to detect any lateral subluxation of the sesamoids out of their respective grooves (Fig. 6.6) erosion of crista and sesamoid–metatarsal joint-space degenerative changes.

The normal angles in hallux valgus are summarised in Fig. 6.6 and Table 6.2.

The hallux valgus and inter-metatarsal angles are used to quantify the severity of hallux valgus (Table 6.3) on weight bearing radiographs.

Management

The mainstay of treatment is non-operative management in the form of patient education, footwear modification and tendo-Achilles stretching. Operative treatment is indicated if conservative methods fail.

The goals of surgery are to relieve symptoms, restore function and correct the deformity. The clinician must consider the patient's history, physical examination and radiographic findings

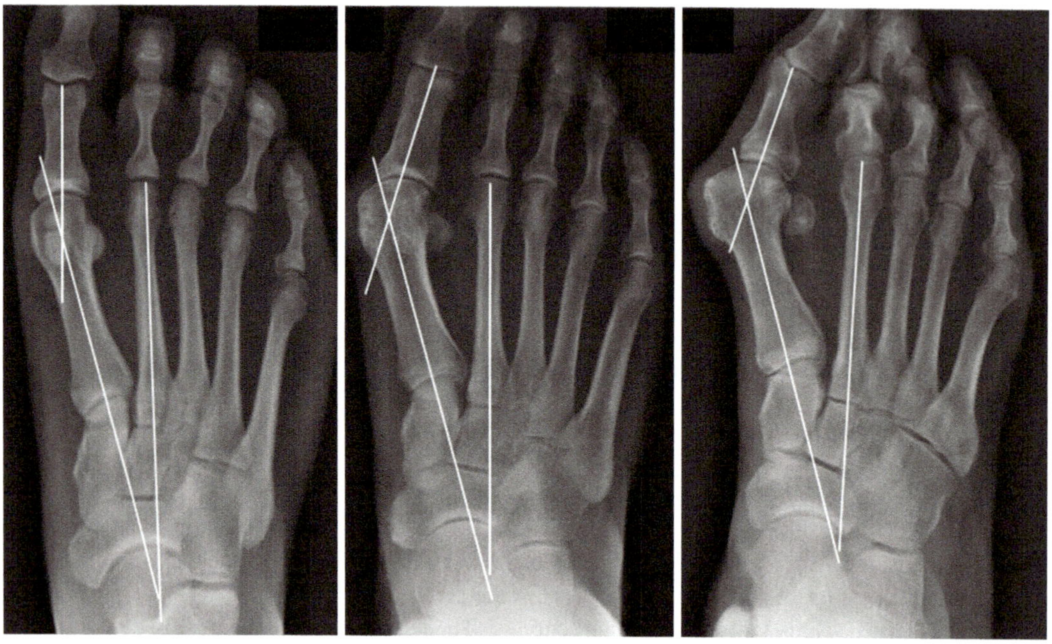

Fig. 6.5 The hallux valgus angle and intermetatarsal angles on dorsoplantar foot radiograph

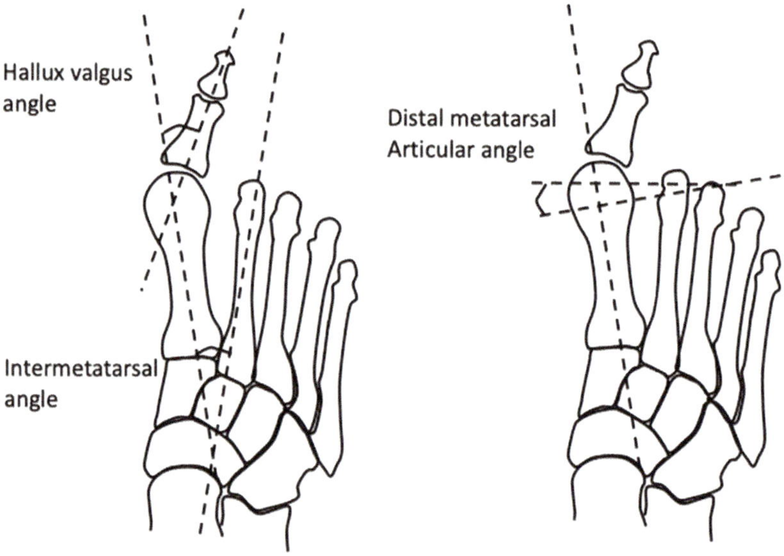

Fig. 6.6 The angles measured in hallux valgus deformity

before selecting a procedure. Occasionally, the final procedure is determined intraoperatively when the physical appearance of the joint, bone and tissue can be observed directly.

The following features of surgical repair allow successful correction of the deformity–

- Establishment of a congruous first MTP joint.
- Reduction of the intermetatarsal angle.
- Realignment of the sesamoids underneath the metatarsal head.
- Restoration of the ability of the first ray to bear weight.

Table 6.2 Normal angles in hallux valgus

Angle	Location	Importance	Normal
Hallux valgus interphalangeus	Long axis of the proximal phalanx and distal phalanx	Degree of deformity at interphalangeal joint.	<10°
Hallux valgus angle	Long axis of the proximal phalanx and first metatarsal	Degree of deformity at MTP joint.	<15°
Inter metatarsal angle	Long axis of the first and second metatarsal	Increased in metatarsus primus varus	<9°
Distal metatarsal articular angle (DMAA)	Long axis of the metatarsal, with a line through the base of the distal articular cartilage cap of the first metatarsal	Increased offset predisposes to development of hallux valgus	<10°

Table 6.3 Classification of severity of hallux valgus based on the hallux valgus and inter-metatarsal angles

	Hallux valgus angle	Inter-metatarsal angle
Mild	15° to 30°	9° to 13°
Moderate	30° to 40°	13° to 20°
Severe	Over 40°	Over 20°

- Balancing of the soft tissues
- Maintenance or increase of the first MTP joint range of motion

Osteotomy

The specific procedures used will vary depending on the surgeon's preference, the nature of the deformity and the particular needs of the patient. In 2017 a systematic review demonstrated that there was no evidence for superiority of one particular osteotomy/surgical procedure over another. Therefore, the primary aim of surgery should be to reposition the first metatarsal head over the sesamoids using the simplest method possible. Common osteotomies are depicted in Fig. 6.7.

Scarf osteotomy is a Z osteotomy from medial side with lateral translation of metatarsal head on metatarsal shaft (Fig. 6.8).

The advantage of the Scarf osteotomy is its versatility in providing a lateral shift of the first metatarsal. In addition, it can lower or elevate the metatarsal head, lengthen or shorten the first metatarsal, and even provide axial rotation.

The main disadvantage is that predictable correction is possible up to 50% of head width. It has a long learning curve and it can be difficult to rotate the head to correct DMAA. Troughing has been described which elevates metatarsal head.

Akin osteotomy is a closing wedge osteotomy of proximal phalanx. Osteotomy is completed from the medial side (Fig. 6.9).

The Akin osteotomy medial deviates the phalanx medially and reduces tension on Extensor Hallucis Longus (EHL). It also corrects interphalangeus deformity. However, it will not correct a hallux valgus deformity on its own.

Distal Chevron osteotomy is a V osteotomy from medial side with lateral translation of metatarsal head on proximal shaft (Fig. 6.10).

Advantage of the chevron osteotomy is that head rotation is easier for correction of DMAA. The osteotomy is easy to perform. As in the scarf osteotomy, 50% of head width is the predictable correction possible. AVN of metatarsal head is possible, although this is negated if a long plantar limb is used.

Proximal metatarsal osteotomy can be either an opening wedge osteotomy from the medial side, or crescentic osteotomy from the dorsal aspect. This allows lateral angular correction of metatarsal.

This allows much greater correction compared to distal metatarsal osteotomies due to a longer lever arm. The main disadvantage is a high non-union rate. Also, it is unable to correct DMAA unless combined with distal osteotomy. Opening wedge can increase metatarsal length and it requires a period of non-weight bearing after surgery. The proximal osteotomy is often used in combination with other osteotomies to correct severe deformities (Fig. 6.11).

Fig. 6.7 Common types of osteotomies for correction of hallux valgus

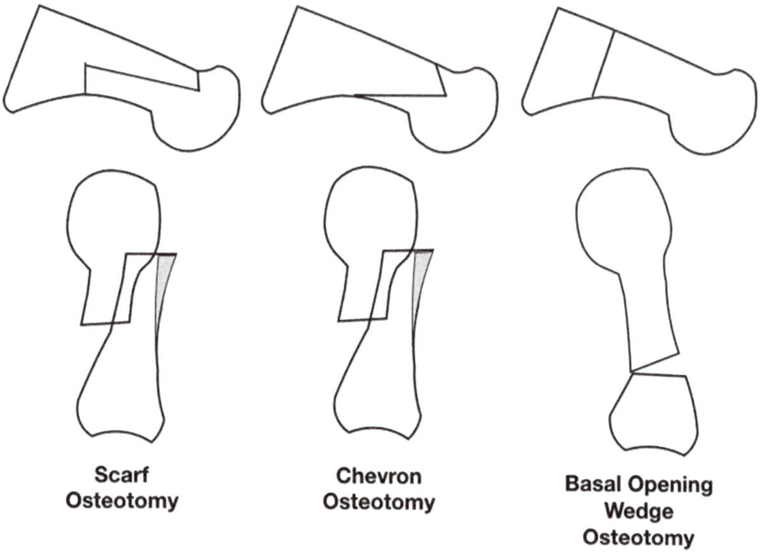

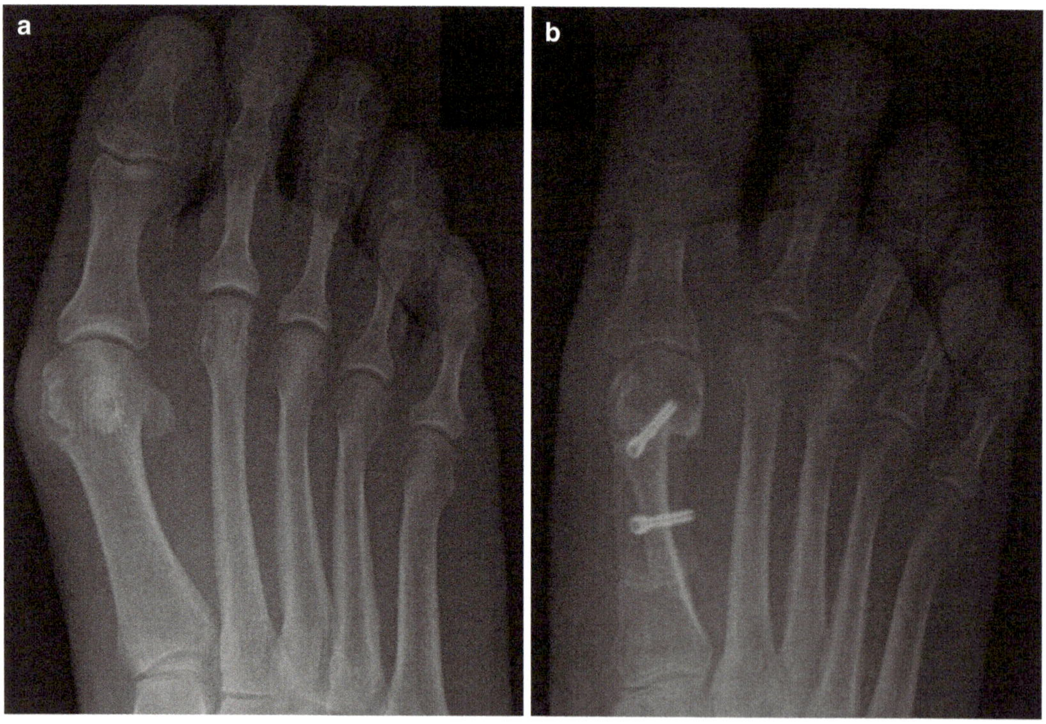

Fig. 6.8 Image (**a**) shows a hallux valgus deformity on weight bearing radiographs. Image (**b**) shows the same patient 3 months following a Scarf osteotomy for correction of hallux valgus

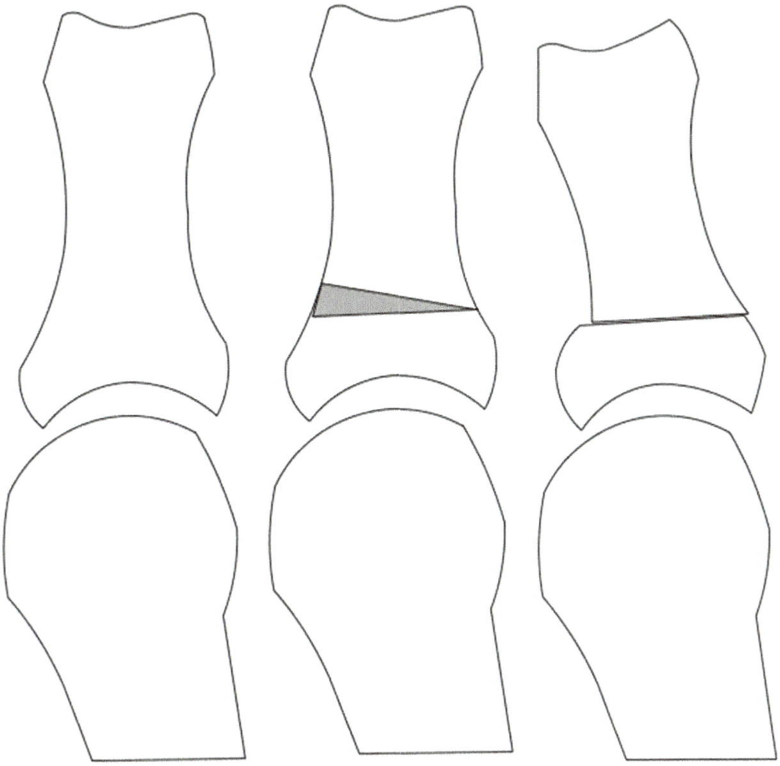

Fig. 6.9 Akin osteotomy of the proximal phalanx

All the above procedures require a soft tissue balancing procedure which will include an adductor tenotomy, lateral capsular release, and medial capsulorraphy.

Fusion Procedures

Hallux valgus correction can be achieved by either fusion of the first MTPJ or first TMTJ. In arthritis of the first MTPJ, a fusion of that joint is preferred. In large deformities with unstable first TMTJ, a fusion of the first TMTJ is preferable.

Lesser Toe Disorders

Commonly encountered lesser toe problems include deformities (claw toe, hammer toe and mallet toe), metatarsalgia, Morton's neuroma, Freiberg's disease, MTP joint instability and bunionette.

Deformities

These are usually associated with first ray deformities and insufficiencies causing the second toe to elevate or drift. Footwear is the most common and important factor in the development of lesser toe deformities.

Deformities may be flexible or fixed. Full passive correction can be achieved in flexible deformities, but not in fixed deformities. This is a key discriminator because fixed deformities require bony correction or joint fusion.

Claw Toes

Claw toes are characterised by hyperextension of the MTP joint and flexion of the IP joints, and are due to imbalance of the intrinsic and extrinsic muscles. A neuromuscular pathology is suspected if all of the lesser toes are involved. Clawing in the second or third toes only is

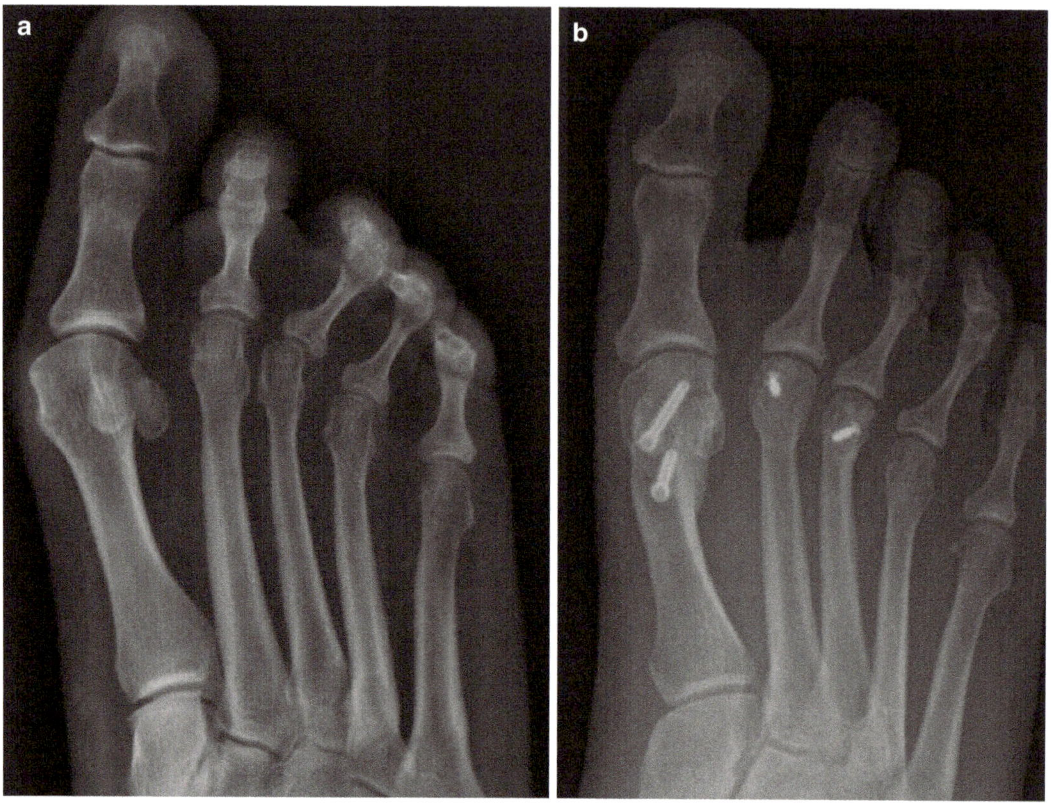

Fig. 6.10 Hallux valgus deformity on weight bearing radiographs, with clawing and lateral deviation of the lesser toes (**a**). The same patient 6 months following a chevron osteotomy for correction of hallux valgus, and lesser toe straightening with correction of the normal parabola of the metatarsal cascade using Weil osteotomies (**b**)

unlikely to be from a neuromuscular cause. Other causes include rheumatoid arthritis, previous foot compartment syndrome and a cavus foot deformity. Most, however, are idiopathic.

Deformities are initially flexible, becoming fixed as the disease advances. The plantar plate is placed under stretch, whereas the dorsal capsule becomes inflamed and contracted. The toe begins to sublux dorsally and results in downward pressure on the metatarsal head. This causes metatarsalgia and further damage to the plantar tissues. Eventually the plantar plate can rupture altogether, and the toe dislocates dorsally.

Conservative management of claw toe deformities is similar to that of other lesser toe deformities. These include accommodative footwear, protective padding and strapping. In the early stages, taping the toe down and stretching can settle the synovitis and prevent a worsening deformity. Intra-articular steroids can also help, but carry a risk of accelerating the deformity.

Surgery is considered when conservative management fails to control the symptoms. Addressing the first ray pathology is very important when treating lesser toe deformities and should be included whenever the first ray is symptomatic.

MTPJ Correction

MTP joint deformity is addressed through a dorsal longitudinal incision centered either over the MTPJ or over an intermetatarsal space if both adjacent toes require correction. It is common to perform an Extensor Digitorum Longus (EDL)

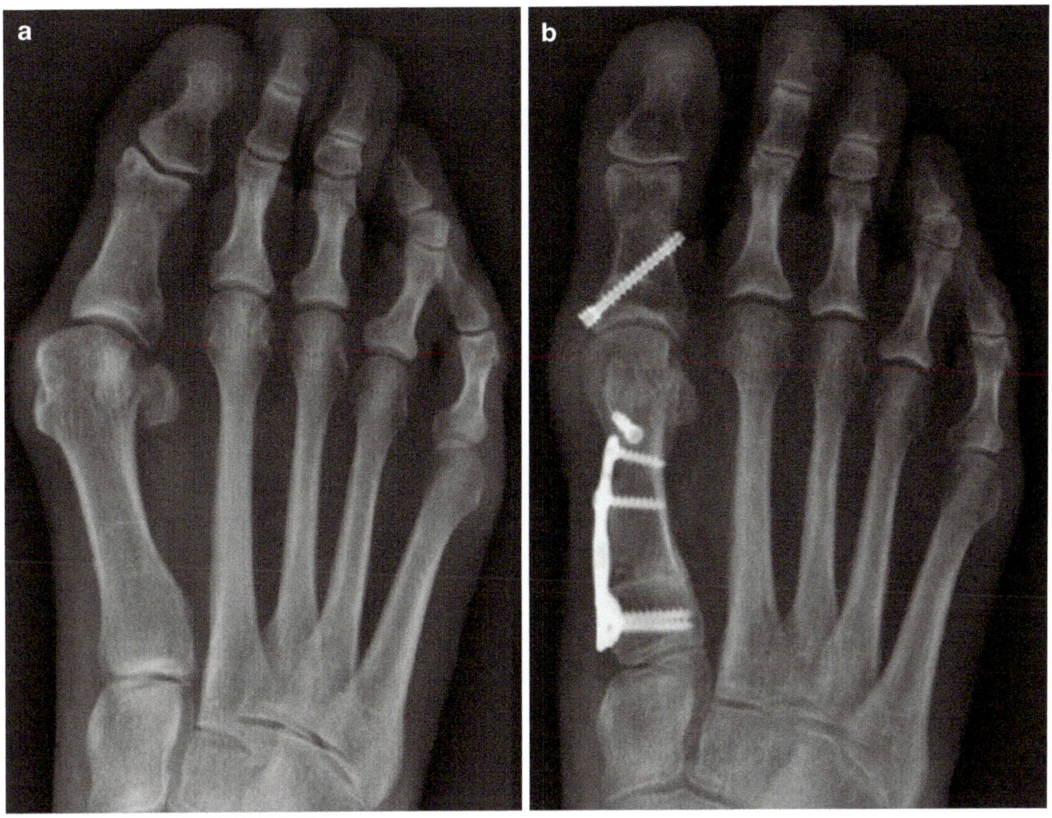

Fig. 6.11 A hallux valgus deformity on weight bearing radiographs (**a**). The same patient 6 months following a combination of basal metatarsal osteotomy, chevron osteotomy and Akin osteotomy (**b**)

Z-lengthening, Extensor digitorum Brevis (EDB) release and dorsal capsulotomy. If contracture still persists, release of collaterals can be considered. If MTPJ is performed in isolation consider immobilizing MTPJ with a transarticular K wire. There is a small risk of wire breakage in the MTPJ with the use of transarticular wire.

If the MTPJ is subluxed or dislocated then a soft tissue release on its own may not be sufficient. To maintain a reduction the intrinsics may need to be relatively lengthened and their line of pull directed plantar to the centre of rotation of the joint. This can be done by performing a shortening metatarsal osteotomy. Weil osteotomies are often considered to achieve this. Weil osteotomies can be performed through the same dorsal approach to the MTPJ described earlier. Once metatarsal head is reduced and subperiosteal dissection of the distal dorsal metatarsal shaft is done, an osteotomy is performed. The cut should be made on the dorsal surface at the edge of the metatarsal head. The osteotomy should be parallel to plantar surface in the frontal plane and slight dorsal oblique in sagittal plane. This is supplemented by a double parallel cut to avoid directing the metatarsal head more plantarly as it shortens. The osteotomies should exit the plantar surface proximal to joint capsule. Stabilisation of the osteotomy is done with a screw (Fig. 6.12).

In order to even load the metatarsal heads and minimize the risk of transfer metatarsalgia Maestro's parabola must be obeyed (Fig. 6.13). The length of first two metatarsals must be the same or second can be up to 2 mm longer than first but the first should never be longer. The metatarsals should then decrease incrementally in length. The third metatarsal is 4 mm shorter than first, the fourth metatarsal is 6 mm shorter than the first and the fifth metatarsal is 12 mm shorter than the first.

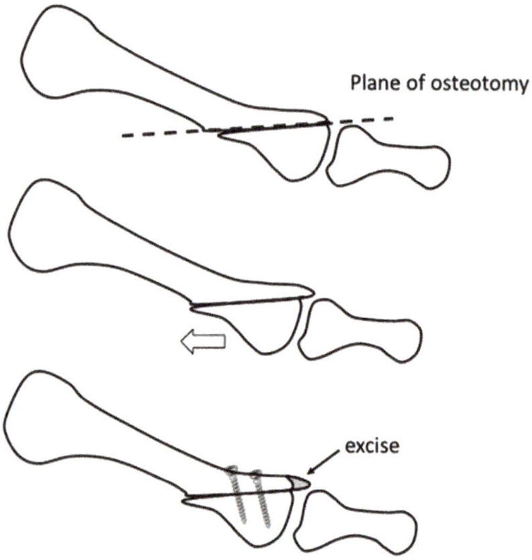

Fig. 6.12 Weil's osteotomy

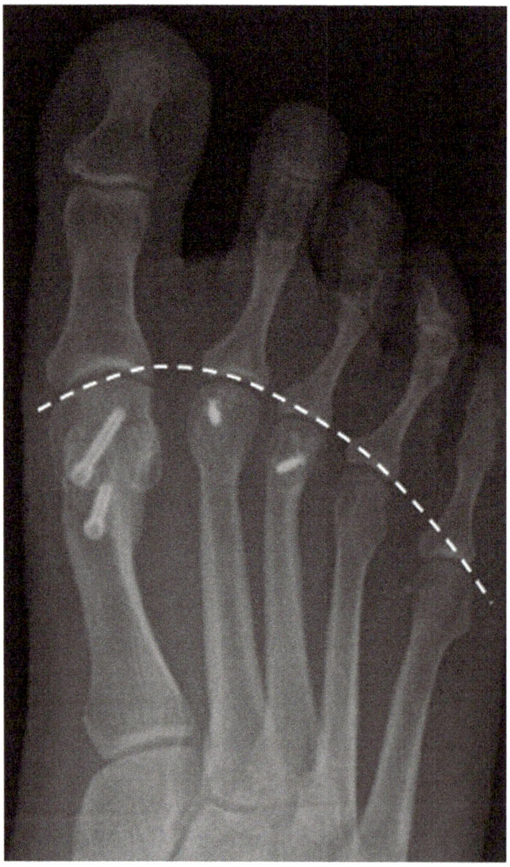

Fig. 6.13 The metatarsal parabola as depicted by the curved line

For flexible deformities, Girdlestone flexor to extensor tendon transfer of the FDL is useful but the toe can become stiff and swollen. Fixed flexion deformity of the IP joint is addressed by resection arthroplasty or fusion of the proximal interphalangeal (PIP) joint. Severe deformities require temporary stabilisation with K wire for 4–6 weeks, with taping and physiotherapy beyond that to reduce the risk of recurrence.

Hammer Toes

Patients with hammer toes have an abnormal flexion posture of the PIP joint and a compensatory extension of the distal interphalangeal (DIP) joint. The second toe is most commonly affected. Here there is no rotational deformity as in curly toes. If conservative measures fail then milder deformities are treated with flexor tenotomy or flexor to extensor transfer. In severe deformities, resection arthroplasty of the PIPJ is necessary, with or without DIPJ fusion.

Mallet Toes

In mallet toes there is an isolated flexion deformity of the DIP joint. The underlying pathology is a spastic FDL. The involved digit may be elongated. Surgically, smaller deformities are treated with flexor tenotomy alone. For more severe deformities, however, tenotomy alone is associated with high rate of recurrence. In these patients, resection arthroplasty or fusion of the DIP joint is advisable. This may be combined with flexor tenotomy. Amputation of the distal phalanx is reserved for very severe deformities involving the nail.

Crossover Toe

Crossover toe describes a deformity in which the second toe lies dorsomedial relative to the hallux.

This is caused by rupture of the collateral ligament and disruption of the plantar plate of the 2nd metatarsophalangeal joint. There may be attrition of the lateral capsule and first dorsal interosseous tendon. The medial structures, such as the capsule, collateral ligament, lumbricals and interosseous tendon, become tight and contracted. The deformity may be initially correctable passively. As the disease advances, the deformity becomes fixed.

Conservative treatment consists of strapping to the third toe and accommodative footwear. In mild deformities, surgical correction consists of soft tissue release of the medial structures, extensor tendon and dorsal capsule. Flexor to extensor tendon transfer can be performed to stabilise the toe. Alternatively, the EDB tendon can be used as a dynamic stabiliser.

In severe deformities, resection arthroplasty or metatarsal shortening osteotomies are advised. It is important to address the hallux deformity as well because the recurrence rate is high, especially in the presence of a deforming force from a deviated hallux.

Metatarsalgia

Metatarsalgia is a symptom rather than a diagnosis. It is pain on the plantar aspect of the lesser metatarsal heads. It can generally be divided into primary metatarsalgia (due to a problem with the metatarsals) or secondary metatarsalgia (the result of a non-metatarsal based problem).

Primary Metatarsalgia

This is further categorized by aetiology:

(a) *First ray insufficiency*

The first ray bears 40% of the weight distribution of the forefoot, the lesser four rays share the remaining 60%. Bearing in mind that the first, fourth, and fifth metatarsal-tarsal articulations allow considerable flexibility compared with the more rigid second and third metatarsal-tarsal articulations, any factor that lessens the ground force of the first metatarsal can increase the pressure applied to the lesser metatarsal heads. Conditions that can cause first ray insufficiency are a shortened first metatarsal (congenital or acquired), elevation of the first metatarsal (congenital or acquired) or hypermobility of the first ray.

Jahss MH. The abnormal plantigrade foot. Orthop Review. 1978;7:31–37.

(b) *Metatarsal prominence*

Metatarsal length discrepancy or plantar protrusion can similarly cause overload of one or more of the metatarsal heads. These cause different pathologies, and can be split into the phase of gait it occurs. Firstly, propulsive phase metatarsalgia (e.g. excessively long second metatarsal) is due to the prominence of the metatarsal head when moving from flat foot stance to toe off, which causes a diffuse plantar swelling. Secondly, a stance phase metatarsalgia (e.g. plantar flexed metatarsalgia), occurs in the foot flat position and causes a discrete callosity.

Secondary Metatarsalgia

(a) *Intractable Plantar Keratosis (IPK)*

An IPK is a localized callosity occurring on the plantar aspect of the foot. An isolated keratotic lesion typically develops beneath a bony prominence as a direct result of increased pressure or friction. Establishing the correct diagnosis is essential to treatment. Care must be taken to distinguish an IPK from other lesions of the plantar skin such a viral infections.

(b) *Midfoot abnormality*

Midfoot flexibility and alignment can have a considerable effect on the distal metatarsals. A cavus midfoot is characterized by decreased flexibility and is associated with a high incidence of metatarsalgia.

(c) *Equinism*

An equinus contracture is defined as the inability to dorsiflex through the tibiotalar joint. It causes excessive forefoot loading and early loading of the forefoot in the normal gait cycle. This repetitive stress can lead to functional and painful problems of the forefoot. Equinus contracture can be related to Achilles tendon or an isolated gastrocnemius contracture. Silfverskiold described a method to differentiate between the two, by dorsiflexing the ankle with and without the knee flexed.

Silfverskiold N. Reduction of the uncrossed two-joints muscles of the leg to one-joint muscles in spastic conditions. Acta Chir Scand. 1924;56:315–30.

Other secondary causes of metatarsalgia, such as referral of pain from tarsal tunnel, Morton's Neuroma, or Freiberg's disease, are described subsequently in this chapter.

MTP Joint Synovitis and Instability

Instability and synovitis of the lesser MTP joints is a common cause of forefoot pain. This topic has already been covered to an extent in the previous toe deformity section. The most common reason for this problem is a mechanically induced synovitis with damage to the plantar plate. However, as previously seen in hallux valgus deformity, the causation can be linked to both mechanical overload (first ray instability, tight gastrocnemius etc.) or to an inherent problem with the plantar plate (rheumatoid arthritis, injury to plantar plate etc.).

On examination there is puffiness around one or more MTP joints, divergence of the toes and tenderness around the joint, especially under the plantar plate. The fat pad under the metatarsal heads deteriorates with age. In patients with severe overload this deterioration is accelerated, resulting in easily palpable and painful metatarsal heads. Patients may have associated hallux valgus, hammer toes, crossover toe deformity and instability, subluxation or dislocation of the MTP joint.

Conservative measures of management include NSAIDs, functional taping to limit dorsiflexion, steroid injection and footwear modification. Knowledge of the cause (as above, first ray instability, tight gastrocnemius etc) allows not only treatment but prevention of recurrence. Steroid injection risks causing complete rupture of the capsule and plantar plate, increasing the deformity, and thus should be avoided in most instances. The metatarsalgia becomes less responsive to conservative measures with dislocation of the joint.

Surgical options are aimed at treatment of the problematic MTP joint and the underlying cause. When subluxation is not severe then synovectomy, extensor tenotomy, dorsal capsulotomy and immobilization in the corrected position for 6 weeks is advised. For severe deformities, in addition to the above procedure the collateral ligaments and plantar plate are released, as they can become reattached in a dislocated position. Any associated hammer toe deformity is also corrected with proximal IP resection arthroplasty or fusion. The MTP joint can be stabilised with flexor to extensor transfer and K wire fixation of the joint in flexion for 4 weeks. Irreducible dislocations can require metatarsal neck osteotomy and holding the toe in the corrected position with K wires for 4 weeks. In acute ruptures to the plantar plate, there has been an increasing vogue for plantar plate repair using new devices on the market.

Elmajee M, Shen Z, A'Court J, Pillai A. A Systematic Review of Plantar Plate Repair in the Management of Lesser Metatarsophalangeal Joint Instability. J Foot Ankle Surg. 2017;56(6):1244–8.

Overload and Plantar Keratosis

The overload of the lesser metatarsals can be broadly classified into stance phase metatarsalgia (the metatarsal head is too far plantarward as compared to the other metatarsals) and propulsive phase metatarsalgia (the metatarsal is too long). The second toe is most often affected with overload under the second MT head. This is evidenced by a plantar keratosis on the skin overlying the second metatarsal head. It is particularly common if there is a defunctioned first metatarsal due to medial drift or a long second metatarsal. Diffuse plantar keratosis suggests that the overload is affecting all the metatarsals; this is particularly common in pes cavus.

A discrete intractable plantar keratosis can be due to a plantar wart (verruca plantaris). These can be very painful and the lesion under the skin is often larger than what is visible on the surface. Plantar warts can be identified by a dark discolouration due to capillaries and can be very large. They are easily treated with liquid nitrogen, but occasionally require excision.

Other causes of a discrete intractable plantar keratosis include a prominent metatarsal head fibular condyle. This is best viewed on a sesamoid-view X-ray and is especially common on the fourth metatarsal. Treatment is with condylectomy if it fails to settle with orthotics. The medial sesamoid is often subject to overload. This can be treated very successfully with accommodative insoles. If this fails, the superior half can be removed to decompress and elevate the sesamoid. Sesamoidectomy is associated with a high risk of complications, including pain and deformity.

Pedobarography can be helpful in orthotic design and modification, and in surgical planning. The fourth and fifth metatarsals (the so-called lateral column) are mobile, and the risk of transfer metatarsalgia to them is therefore low if the second and third metatarsals have been addressed. The second and third metatarsals are reasonably immobile, and therefore if the second MT is addressed in isolation there is a risk of transfer metatarsalgia. Operating on an asymptomatic metatarsal is controversial and it is more important to be sure preoperatively that this is not already overloaded.

Surgery to the metatarsal neck is commonly performed using a Weil osteotomy. This aims to shorten and elevate the metatarsal head. Swelling and stiffness are common. Other risks include recurrence, nerve or vessel injury and deformity.

Morton's Neuroma

The condition was initially described by Durlacher in 1845, but the attributed eponym derived from T.G. Morton (1876) who described the symptoms but wrongfully attributed the problem to the fourth MTPJ articulation. It is not a neuroma (i.e. a nerve unorganised growth when cut), although we will continue to refer to it as such for ease of reading, but a nerve swelling dut to fibrosis. The neuroma most commonly involves the third interdigital nerve; less commonly, the second interdigital nerve; and rarely the first and fourth interdigital nerves. Symptoms most commonly occur in middle-aged women (78% of cases are in women). It also appears to be more common in those who wear narrow toe box shoes and those who hyperextend their MTP joints. This may be due to the nerve being brought against the unyielding transverse intermetatarsal ligament.

Durlacher L. Corns, bunions, the diseases of nails and the general management of the feet. 1845:72.

Morton TG. A peculiar and painful affection of the fourth metatarso-phalangeal articulation. Am J Med Sci. 1876;71:37–45.

Wu KK. Morton's interdigital neuroma: a clinical review of its etiology, treatment, and results. The Journal of foot and ankle surgery 1996;35(2):112–119.

It is theorized that the predilection to the third intermetatarsal space was because the third common digital nerve was thicker than the other nerves and in a position of potential entrapment between the immobile third metatarsal and mobile fourth metatarsal. Anastomotic branches between the medial and lateral plantar nerves in the third intermetatarsal space may also tether the nerve risking a traction neuritis.

Diagnosis

Diagnosis is primarily based on history and examination. Patients complain of pain, burning and tingling down the interspace of the involved toes. The pain is usually made worse by walking in high-heeled shoes with a narrow toe box and is relieved by rest, removing the shoe and or wearing open toe sandals. The pain will radiate to the toes or vague pain may radiate up the leg. This condition can be very non-specific.

The whole foot should be examined, looking for any other factors likely to produce metatarsalgia. Patients may have local tenderness and swelling in the intermetatarsal space. There may be reproduction of pain or, less reliably, a Mulder's click (click between the metatarsal heads at site of pain, indicating an enlargement of nerve) on metatarsal compression. Local anaesthetic injection into the affected space may relieve symptoms and support the diagnosis. The gastrocnemius-soleus complex should also be examined. Significant tightness, a common finding, is often a contributing factor.

Naraghi R, Bremner A, Slack-Smith L, Bryant A. The relationship between foot posture index, ankle equinus, body mass index and intermetatarsal neuroma. J Foot Ankle Res. 2016;9:46.

Standing AP, lateral and oblique forefoot films should be obtained if other forefoot pathology is suspected. Ultrasounds and MRIs can be used if the clinical situation is atypical. Ultrasound-guided injections and pain monitoring increase the diagnostic accuracy.

Management

Conservative measures of management are footwear modification, NSAIDs and local steroid injection. Footwear modification is by avoiding high heels and narrow toe boxes. Metatarsal bars and pads placed proximally to the painful area decompress the nerve by widening the intermetatarsal space during weight bearing. Local steroid injection brings initial pain relief in about 80% of patients, but the recurrence rate is high (50%).

Surgery for Morton's Neuroma

Surgical management is indicated if conservative measures fail to adequately relieve symptoms. Contraindications are poor circulation, diabetes mellitus, reflex sympathetic dystrophy, atypical symptoms and hysterical personality disorders.

The standard operation is a digital neurectomy, which is most often performed through a dorsal approach (although a plantar incision has also been advocated). The nerve is divided 2–3 cm proximal to the bifurcation and excised. The deep transverse metatarsal ligament may be wholly or partially released. Surgery has a success rate of 80%. Recurrent symptoms can be caused by inadequate resection of the nerve, recurrent neuroma formation and an initial wrong diagnosis.

Histologically, the nerve is thickened with perineural fibrosis and severe degeneration of the neuritic elements.

Freiberg's Disease

Freiberg's disease is an 'infarction' of the dorsal part of one of the lesser metatarsal heads. It is a condition of young adults, occurring during puberty, mostly in girls. Repetitive trauma with micro-fractures is one attributed cause. Two-thirds of lesions occur in the second metatarsal, and a quarter in the third. The metatarsal head partially collapses, with later degenerative changes in the joint. The inferior part of the head is normally well preserved. It is more common in those with relatively long second metatarsals.

Helal B, Gibb P. Freiberg's disease: a suggested pattern of management. Foot Ankle. 1987;8(2):94–102.

Gauthier and Elbaz described five stages (Table 6.4).

Patients present with pain in the forefoot localised to head of the second metatarsal. Wearing high heels aggravates the pain. There may be localised swelling and a limited range of movement in the involved MTP joint, as well as signs of synovitis.

Table 6.4 Stages of Freiberg disease

Stage 0	Subchondral fracture
Stage 1	Osteonecrosis without deformation
Stage 2	Deformation by crushing of the osteonecrotic segment
Stage 3	Cartilaginous tearing
Stage 4	Arthrosis

Radiographs initially show sclerosis of the epiphysis and widening of the joint space. Subsequently epiphysis becomes fragmented with formation of bone spurs, giving the appearance of osteoarthritis. In late stages the metatarsal head becomes irregular, widened and flattened.

Initial management includes proper footwear with a metatarsal bar or pad and limitation of activity for 4–6 weeks. For more troublesome joints, a steroid injection, local anaesthetic and immobilising the foot in short-leg walking cast for 4 weeks can help resolve symptoms.

Failure of conservative measures is an indication for surgery. Surgical options are debridement with excision of osteophytes and or loose bodies, debridement with dorsiflexion osteotomy, metatarsal shortening osteotomy, interposition arthroplasty and joint replacement. The evidence for choice of surgery is based on small case series. Both extraarticular and intraarticular dorsal closing wedge osteotomies and metatarsal shortening osteotomies report satisfactory/good results in over 90%. Similarly for later stage Freiberg's disease there is fair evidence for interposition arthroplasty demonstrating superior results to excision arthroplasty alone.

Carmont MR, Rees RJ, Blundell CM. Current concepts review: Freiberg's disease. Foot Ankle Int. 2009;30(2):167–76.

Chao KH, Lee CH, Lin LC. Surgery for symptomatic Freiberg's disease: extraarticular dorsal closing-wedge osteotomy in 13 patients followed for 2–4 years. Acta Orthop Scand. 1999;70(5):483–6.

Bunionette (Tailor's Bunion)

The bunionette deformity is a prominence of the fifth metatarsal head, usually with medial deviation of the fifth toe. This is associated with a wide fifth metatarsal head, lateral bowing of the fifth metatarsal shaft, an increased angle between the fourth and fifth metatarsal shafts (Fig. 6.14) and an increased incidence of hallux valgus. When bunionette is associated with hallux valgus and metatarsus primus varus, the deformity is called splay foot. There is usually pain over the lateral aspect of the MTP joint. Almost 50% of patients have bilateral bunionettes.

Three distinct types have been described by Coughlin (Table 6.5).

Coughlin MJ. Treatment of bunionette deformity with longitudinal diaphyseal osteotomy with distal soft tissue repair. Foot Ankle. 1991;11(4):195–203.

Besides cosmetic concerns, patients usually complain of pain over the prominent fifth metatarsal head, difficulty in finding comfortable shoes and rubbing between the fourth and fifth toes. General widening of the forefoot is often seen on examination. The deformity may be associated hallux valgus, hammer toes and congenital curly toes.

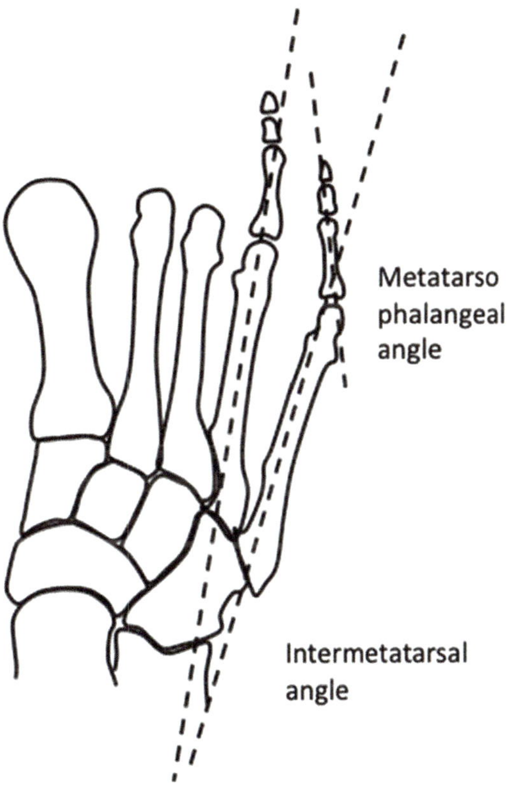

Fig. 6.14 Bunionette deformity

Table 6.5 Types of bunionette deformity

Type 1	Large, wide metatarsal head
Type 2	Lateral metatarsal shaft bowing
Type 3	Increased fourth-fifth intermetatarsal angle (>8°)

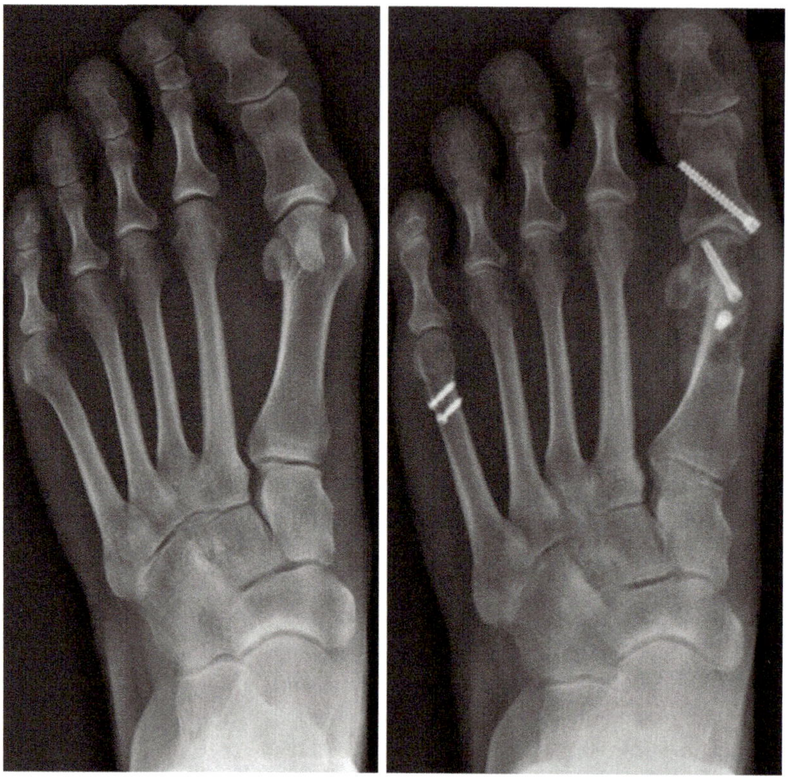

Fig. 6.15 Pre and post operative radiographs of a hallux valgus deformity with high distal metatarsal articular angle, and a type b bunionette. The hallux deformity was treated with a rotational chevron of the first metatarsal, combined with an Akin osteotomy. The bunionette was treated using a scarf osteotomy

Initial treatment is conservative and consists of shaving the symptomatic callus and footwear modification. A metatarsal pad or plantar pressure-relieving orthosis is advised if there is coexisting pes planus or if the callosity is plantar. Surgical options include distal, basal and diaphyseal osteotomies, such as the reverse Scarf osteotomy. Proximal osteotomy is avoided because of the tenuous blood supply. As a general guide, Coughlin type 1 deformities are treated with lateral condylectomy, type 2 with a distal or diaphyseal osteotomy (Fig. 6.15) and type 3 with a proximal diaphyseal osteotomy.

Rheumatoid Foot

Foot involvement is common in rheumatoid arthritis.

The pathophysiological process begins with synovitis of the metatarsophalangeal joint, leading to attenuation of joint capsule and incompetence of collateral ligaments. Subsequent joint subluxation ensues, followed by clawing, plantar fat-pad atrophy and distal migration leading to uncovering of metatarsal heads, metatarsalgia and plantar keratosis.

The changes are summarised in Table 6.6.

Forefoot changes are ten times more common than hindfoot changes.

General radiological changes include soft tissue swelling, osteopenia, erosions, and joint space widening in the early stages. In the later stages, there is joint space narrowing, subchondral cysts, subluxation/dislocation/deformity of joints and ankylosis.

Nonoperative Management

This includes–

- Optimising medical therapy
- Physical therapy to improve gastrocnemius tightness and mobility aids
- Corticosteroid injections
- Orthotics

Table 6.6 Changes in rheumatoid foot

General Findings	Forefoot changes	Hindfoot changes
Rheumatoid nodules Skin/fat atrophy and ulceration Friable tissues /poor wound healing Digital ischaemia Peripheral neuropathy	Metatarsalgia Hallux valgus MTPJ dislocation Clawing Toe separation (MTPJ synovitis) Splaying of metatarsals (weakening of intermetatarsal ligaments)	Planovalgus foot secondary to tibialis posterior tenosynovitis, attenuation and or rupture leading to destruction of subtalar joint capsule and interosseous ligaments. Tendo Achilles contracture Ankle arthritis, rare in isolation and is almost always associated with pantalar arthritic changes.

For fixed deformity, accommodative footwear, with extra depth and light-weight soft shoes are used. For flexibility deformities, UCBL (University of California Biomechanics Laboratory) insert may be used for mid and hindfoot pain. A custom ankle–foot orthoses (AFOs) can be used when instability, and midfoot or hindfoot deformities develop.

Surgical Management

In the early stages, surgical options are synovectomy and soft tissue reconstruction. Patients who present to the orthopaedic clinic with advanced disease often require formal reconstruction. Multiple procedures can be performed on one foot, but concomitant bilateral procedures are best avoided.

Rheumatoid forefoot pathology commonly presents with hallux valgus with clawing of lesser toes. The aims of surgery are to provide pain relief, restore the plantar fat pad in a more proximal position, restore alignment of the toes, unload the metatarsal heads and provide a stable medial column.

The conventional standard of treatment is fusion of the first MTP joint with preparation of both joint surfaces and fusion in approximately 10–15 degrees of valgus and 10 degrees of dorsiflexion from plantar surface, and excision arthroplasty of the lesser metatarsal heads (Fig. 6.16). Good or excellent results are frequently reported with non-union rates from 3–8%.

Bolland BJ, Sauve PS, Taylor GR. Rheumatoid forefoot reconstruction: first metatarsophalangeal joint fusion combined with Weil's metatarsal osteotomies of the lesser rays. J Foot Ankle Surg. 2008;47(2):80–88.

There is a growing body of evidence for joint preserving surgery, even in the presence of some degenerative change. Similar early functional and pain scores have been reported however long term recurrence rates for pain and deformity are not yet known.

Kushioka J, Hirao M, Tsuboi H, et al. *Modified Scarf Osteotomy with Medial Capsule Interposition for Hallux Valgus in Rheumatoid Arthritis: A Study of Cases Including Severe First Metatarsophalangeal Joint Destruction. J Bone Joint Surg Am. 2018;100(9):765–76.*

Keller's arthroplasty may be used to deal with deformity of the first MTP joint in low-demand patients. An alternative to excision of the metatarsal heads is the Stainsby procedure. This involves resecting the proximal phalanx through the neck. It is important to release and reduce the plantar plate; when all the toes are dislocated, they may all need to be released before reduction is possible.

Rheumatoid arthritis patients frequently have severe deformity and thus the soft tissues (and also the neurovascular bundle) can be very stretched after reduction. In order to address lesser MTP joint pathology, it may be preferable to do 2/3 and 3/4 web-space incision, rather than four separate but close incisions. If all toes are dislocated, some specialists advocate a single transverse incision, which can then be left to granulate.

Methotrexate and sulfasalazine therapy does not increase complication rates following surgery. These medications can be continued in the perioperative period.

Grennan DM, Gray J, Loudon J, Fear S. Methotrexate and early postoperative complications in patients with rheumatoid arthritis

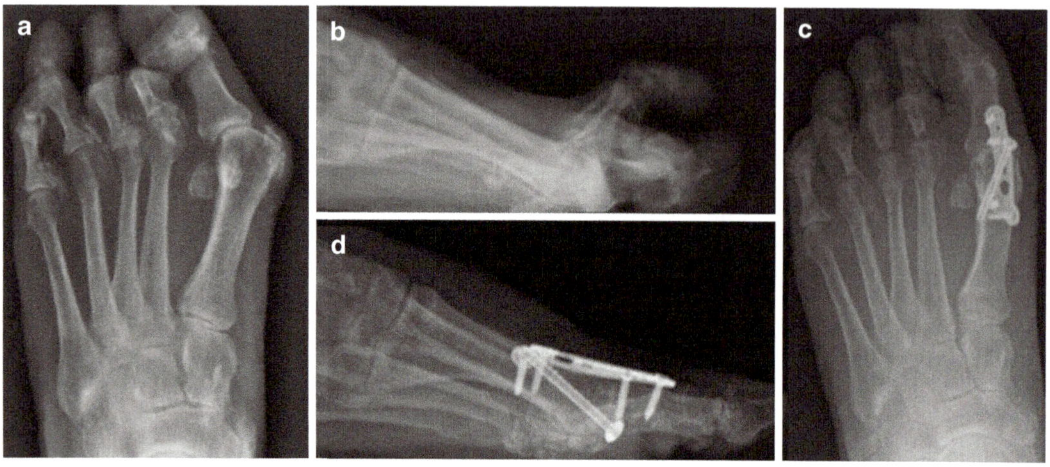

Fig. 6.16 Severe forefoot deformity from systemic sclerosis and rheumatoid disease (**a**, **b**). The same patient 6 months following a first metatarsophalangeal joint fusion and Stainsby procedure to the second, third and fourth toes (**c**, **d**)

undergoing elective orthopaedic surgery. Ann Rheum Dis. 2001;60(3):214–7.

Sreekumar R, Gray J, Kay P, Grennan DM. Methotrexate and post operative complications in patients with rheumatoid arthritis undergoing elective orthopaedic surgery--a ten year follow-up. Acta Orthop Belg. 2011;77(6):823–6.

With regards to biologics, the British Society for Rheumatology have produced guidelines stating that the risk of post-operative infection should be measured against the risk of having a significant disease exacerbation. There is currently no strong evidence to suggest that continuing biologics increases infection/wound complications. However, their use does correlate with increased risk of complications and many advocate stopping them. The length of time to stop them is dictated by the drug's half-life, for most that is 3 to 5 weeks or stopping 1.5 times the length of dosing interval.

Diaper R, Wong E, Metcalfe SA. The implications of biologic therapy for elective foot and ankle surgery in patients with rheumatoid arthritis. Foot 2017;30:53–58.

Surgical management of midfoot involvement entails fusion of the involved joints. This can be performed as an in situ fusion if there is no deformity. When a larger deformity is present, fusion is performed in the corrected position.

When hindfoot involvement is isolated to the subtalar, a subtalar fusion will suffice. When the patient has significant hindfoot varus or valgus deformity with involvement of the talonavicular and calcaneocuboid joints, double or triple arthrodesis is the preferred surgical treatment. In patients with subtalar and ankle degeneration, subtalar fusion and ankle replacement can result in excellent function. Despite often having amongst the poorest preoperative functional scores, rheumatoid arthritis patients do well with ankle arthroplasty. Provided hindfoot alignment is restored and pathology addressed, outcomes are equivocal to replacements for osteoarthritis with similar revision rates.

Pedersen E, Pinsker E, Younger AS, et al. *Outcome of total ankle arthroplasty in patients with rheumatoid arthritis and noninflammatory arthritis. A multicenter cohort study comparing clinical outcome and safety. J Bone Joint Surg Am. 2014;96(21):1768–75.*

Flat Foot

Loss of the normal medial longitudinal arch leads to pes planus or flat foot. There is a lack of distinct definition between a physiological flat foot which does not need treatment as opposed to a pathological flat foot, which needs treatment.

This can be broadly classified as congenital and acquired. The congenital variety is usually seen in children and the acquired variety in adults. The causes of both varieties are listed in Table 6.7.

A key discriminator is whether the foot is fixed or flexible. In children a fixed flat foot points to a tarsal coalition or congenital vertical talus. In adults, it points to a late stage with fixed, degenerative changes that invariably require major bony fusion surgery.

A flexible flat foot in a child is evident when the child is asked to stand on tip toes; or by passive dorsiflexion of the great toe (Jack's test). Restoration of the arch by either of these manoeuvers indicates a flexible flat foot.

Clinically the main distinction is between the following:

- Feet with a low arch, but no rotation into planovalgus. This is almost always clinically irrelevant, but the patient or parents may require reassurance that it is a normal appearance.
- Flexible, over pronated feet without any other pathology (e.g., arthritis, muscular imbalance, tendinopathy). Arch is present when non-weight bearing and flattens on standing, arch then reappears and the heel moves into varus on tiptoe or when the great toe is dorsiflexed (Jack test), as the plantar fascia tightens. Reassurance that this is a normal variant may be all that is required.
- Over pronated feet with evidence of Tibialis posterior tendinopathy.
- Stiff, over pronated feet. These may be simple flexible feet that have stiffened with age, or they may have developed arthritis or muscle imbalance.
- Arthritic flat feet may require investigation to identify a rheumatological diagnosis. Treatment is directed at controlling the arthritis and protecting the foot against deforming forces with an orthosis (either in-shoe or external devices).
- Neuromuscular flat feet may particularly occur in myelomeningocele or spastic cerebral palsy. Orthoses, usually external devices such as KAFOs, may protect against further deformity and give support to allow walking. Some of these patients will need soft tissue procedures, tendon transfers or hindfoot fusions (usually triple fusions to prevent and treat progressive deformity).

Table 6.7 Causes of flat foot

Congenital	Acquired
Normal variant/ generalised ligamentous laxity Congenital vertical talus Tarsal coalition—May present in adolescence as the midfoot ossifies or in adulthood as a flat foot with degenerative change Accessory navicular Spina bifida Cerebral palsy	Trauma—Fractures of the talus, os calcis or mid foot resulting in post-traumatic osteoarthritis of the mid- or hindfoot Rupture or stretching of the tibialis posterior tendon Muller–Weiss syndrome (avascular necrosis of the navicular) Rheumatoid arthritis Diabetes—Charcot neuropathic foot Neuromuscular disease (e.g., polio)

Clinical assessment is aimed at identifying the severity of symptoms, and particularly whether there is associated pain. Flexibility is also assessed and the underlying cause of the deformity identified.

Subtalar Fusion

In subtalar fusion, the incision is made from the tip of the fibula to the base of the fourth metatarsal. The sural nerve lies 1–2 cm beneath the distal tip of the fibula and should be protected, as should the extensors, which lie anteriorly, and the peroneal tendons, which lie posteriorly.

The extensor digitorum brevis (EDB) tendon is exposed, freed from its insertion and reflected distally. Dissection is kept subperiosteal to avoid damage to the neurovascular bundle, which enters approximately 1.5 cm medial and distal to the anterior process of the calcaneum. The EDB is delivered out of the sinus tarsi, and the fibro-fatty contents of the sinus tarsi are removed.

The calcaneocuboid joint, which is found just distal to the anterior beak of the calcaneus, is identified. The talonavicular joint lies superior and medial to the calcaneocuboid joint. The neck of the talus is identified and the extensor tendons are elevated off the neck. A retractor is inserted over the neck and under the extensor tendons, which helps to retract the neurovascular bundle. Another retractor is placed deep to the peroneal tendon and around the calcaneus at the level of the subtalar joint.

The lateral process of the talus can be removed for better exposure of the posterior facet. The joint capsule of the talocalcaneal joint is incised and a laminar spreader is inserted into the sinus tarsi to expose the entire subtalar articulation.

Articular cartilage and subchondral bone of the subtalar joint is excised. All of the articular cartilage must be removed from the anterior, middle and posterior facets, but excessive bone resection is avoided as this will decrease the subtalar joint height and disrupt the articular relationship of the talonavicular joint. Additional bone can be removed to correct fixed valgus or varus deformity.

The joint is held in a corrected position and can be stabilised with two or three 6 mm cannulated screws or staples. A variety of configurations have been described however using just 1 screw does not prevent rotation and should be avoided.

Radiographic Analysis

This is based on standing anteroposterior (AP) and lateral views.

Screen for differential diagnoses—tarsal coalition (Fig. 6.17), oblique/vertical talus and accessory navicular.

In standing lateral views, Meary's (talar—first metatarsal) line should equal 0° +/− 3° (Fig. 6.18) In the flat foot, this relationship is lost most commonly in the talonavicular or naviculocuneiform joint as these sag. The normal calcaneal pitch is 20 to 30 degrees. A reduced calcaneal pitch is seen in pes planus.

A C-shaped line created by the outline of the talar dome and the inferior margin of the sustentaculum tali can be seen.

The talocalcaneal angle is measured in standing AP views (Fig. 6.19). If the angle is more than 35° then heel valgus is said to be present. AP views also show the degree of talonavicular uncoverage and subluxation indicative of an advanced deformity.

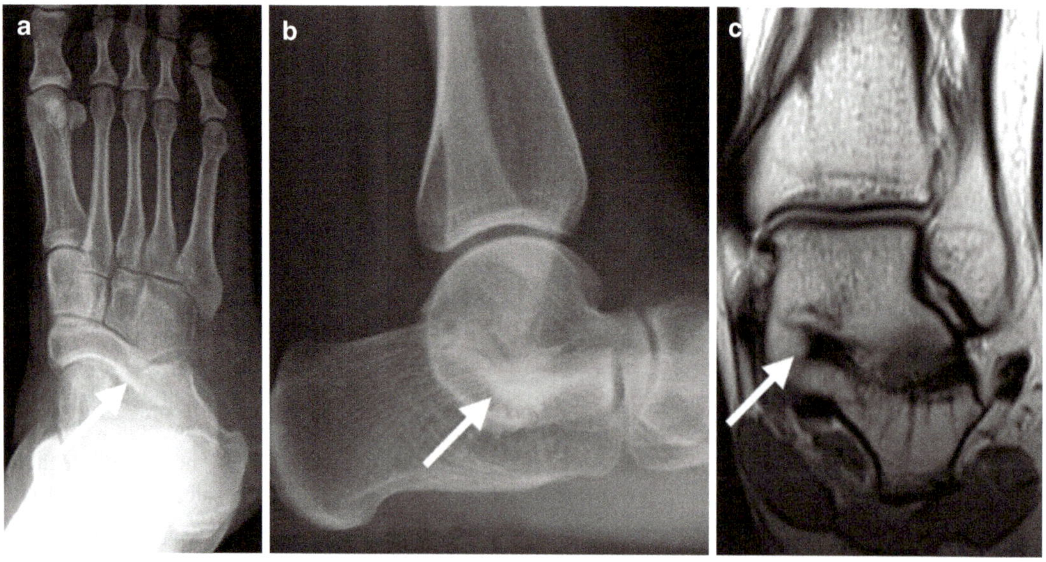

Fig. 6.17 A calcaneonavicular bony coalition (**a**). An inclined talus with a C-sign in keeping with a talocalcaneal coalition (**b**). Talocalcalcaneal coalition (**c**) in the same patient as in image (**b**)

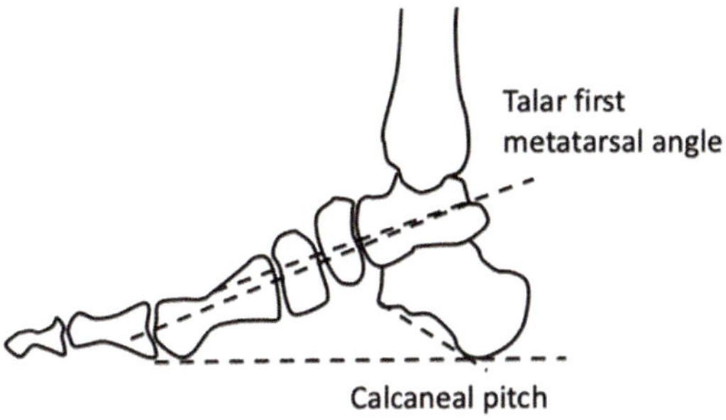

Fig. 6.18 Talar first metatarsal angle on lateral view

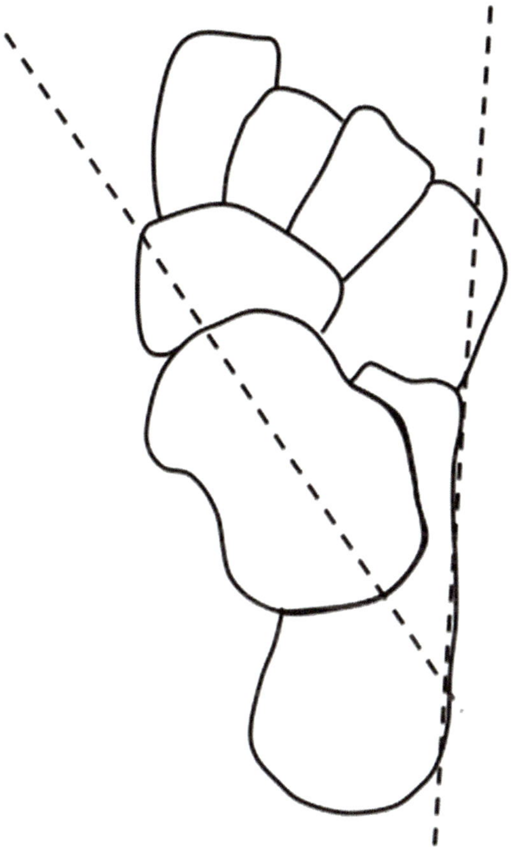

Fig. 6.19 Talocalcaneal angle on AP view

Oblique views are preferred for showing Calcaneonavicular tarsal coalition. If tarsal coalition is suspected, the extent and severity is assessed with either computed tomography (CT) or magnetic resonance imaging (MRI) for fibrous coalition.

MRI is the best modality to assess the tendon pathology, particularly in the initial stages of tibialis posterior tendon dysfunction.

Management

A flexible flat foot rarely requires treatment. If symptomatic, physiotherapy in the form of gastrocnemius stretching is useful, as the gastrocnemius is often tight. Orthotics can help to correct flexible deformity (e.g., when medial pain and lateral impingement are present). They are used to accommodate and support a fixed deformity in midfoot degeneration, but by this stage only about 50% of patients will show some improvement. Be aware that if gastrocnemius tightness is present, the application of an orthotic can cause an equinus deformity as the hindfoot corrects, and forefoot overload can occur.

Indications for surgery are a painful rigid flat foot, a painful uncontrolled or deteriorating flexible flat foot and a neuromuscular flat foot. A neuromuscular flat foot, especially in cerebral palsy associated with Tendo Achilles contracture, can be treated with subtalar fusion before midfoot breakdown occurs. Once a midfoot break (i.e., midfoot abduction) occurs, a triple or double (talonavicular and subtalar) arthrodesis maybe required. Hypermobile syndrome does not respond well to soft tissue surgery.

Treatment options are fusion of the involved joints (subtalar, triple fusion or midfoot joints) for fixed deformity. Reconstructive options—for example flexor digitorum longus (FDL) transfer, medialising calcaneal osteotomy, spring ligament reconstruction, subtalar arthroereisis and lateral column lengthening—are reserved for flexible deformities.

Posterior Tibial Tendon Dysfunction

The tibialis posterior is an invertor of the foot that originates in the deep posterior compartment of the leg. It has a complex insertion, with the main bulk of the tendon inserting to the navicular tuberosity. Its insertions, in addition to the navicular, include the cuboid, cuneiforms and bases of second third and fourth metatarsals. It functions as a dynamic stabiliser of the longitudinal arch and resists hindfoot valgus.

Posterior tibial tendon dysfunction has been described as a 'hidden epidemic', and recent evidence suggests that its incidence is as high as 6% in women over the age of 40 years. Early diagnosis and treatment is the key to preventing morbidity.

There is an area of hypovascularity 1 cm distal to the medial malleolus that could be the reason for tendon failure here.

Risk factors include:

- deterioration of a long-standing flat foot
- trauma
- inflammatory arthritis (rheumatoid and sero-negative arthritis)
- diabetes
- Obesity
- Tarsal coalition

Diagnosis

The initial clinical presentation is with pain and tenderness along the course of the tendon. The pain is aggravated by resisted active plantar flexion and inversion. There may be evidence of an objective weakness of inversion. Later, a planovalgus attitude of the foot develops with flattened longitudinal arches, forefoot abduction and 'too many toes' sign (>2 toes seen lateral to lateral malleolus) when viewed from behind the patient.

A positive single heel raise test is the best method for clinically evaluating functional loss resulting from tibialis posterior dysfunction. When the patient stands on the ball of the toe, the heel should move into a varus position. If the patient is unable to perform this fully then the test is positive, irritability or fatigue in doing this heralds tendinopathy. In late stages, when there is calcaneal impingement against the fibula, the patient experiences lateral heel pain.

Classification

The Strom and Johnson/Myerson classification is shown in Table 6.8.

Johnson KA, Strom DE. Tibialis posterior tendon dysfunction. Clin Orthop Relat Res. 1989;39:196–206.

Myerson MS. Adult acquired flatfoot deformity: treatment of dysfunction of the posterior tibial tendon. Instr Course Lect. 1997;46:393–405.

Management

Flexible Deformity

Flexible deformities that are correctable to a plantigrade position can be treated conservatively or with joint-sparing surgery.

Conservative options include–

Table 6.8 Strom and Johnson/Myerson classification of posterior tibial tendon dysfunction

Stage	Description
1	Tendon tenosynovitis and/or degeneration. No deformity, can single limb heel raise with varus of the heel.
2	Tendon degeneration and elongation Flexible and reducible pes planovalgus, hindfoot in equinus Weakness with single limb heel raise and difficulty in achieving hindfoot varus. No ankle deformity or arthritis 2a—Normal forefoot, <40% Talonavicular uncovering. 2b—'too many toes' sign positive, >40% Talonavicular joint uncovering.
3	Tendon degeneration and elongation Fixed, irreducible pes planovalgus deformity Unable to perform single limb heel raise, no inversion of hindfoot 'Too many toes' sign positive. No ankle deformity or arthritis
4	Degeneration and elongation Fixed irreducible pes planovalgus deformity Medial and/or lateral pain. 'Too many toes' sign positive Unable to perform single limb heel raise, no inversion of hindfoot Ankle deformity or arthritis, talus has started to go into valgus.

- Analgesics, including anti-inflammatory agents.
- Shoe adaptations
- Weight reduction
- Orthotics (e.g., a UCBL-type medial heel wedge device). This provides correction of hindfoot valgus, balances ankle loading and produces a demonstrable improvement in gait parameters.
- AFO-type braces.
- It is crucial to continue observation. Failure to respond requires consideration of surgery, particularly prior to the onset of fixed deformities. Otherwise bony fusion surgery rather than soft tissue reconstruction and joint salvage may need to be considered.

Tenosynovectomy is useful in early disease (stage 1, prior to rupture) if symptoms do not settle with conservative measures. Part of the flexor retinaculum is preserved to prevent subluxation of the tendon. The tendon sheath is opened and the diseased tissue is removed. The flexor retinaculum is not closed. Early synovectomy of the tendon sheath relieves discomfort and may delay rupture of the tendon.

FDL transfer is performed for stage 2 disease when there is almost full inversion at the subtalar joint. If the subtalar joint cannot be brought into nearly full inversion then FDL transfer is contraindicated; in this case, subtalar fusion is considered. The flexor hallucis longus or the tibialis anterior can also be used for transfer instead of the FDL. Tendon transfer must be combined with a medialising osteotomy of the calcaneum and/or a spring ligament reconstruction in order to protect the transferred tendon from the biomechanical abnormalities that led the much stronger tibialis posterior tendon to fail. The calcaneum is translated about 1 cm and fixed with one or more screws. The osteotomy is made 1 cm posterior and parallel to the peroneal tendons. The realignment neutralises the eversion force of the Achilles tendon, but gastrocnemius tightness is common and may need to be addressed (Fig. 6.20).

Multiple deformities often need to be addressed at the same time to give a plantigrade foot. Myerson has advocated for a more complex classification system that identifies and manages all the separate issues that are present. For instance, a supinated forefoot is a common feature of longstanding pes planovalgus; if this is

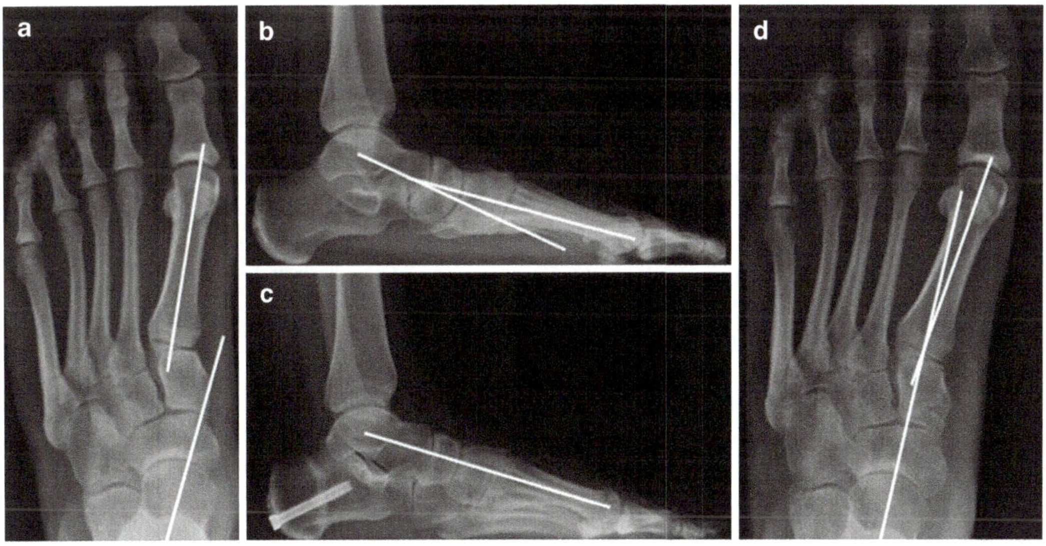

Fig. 6.20 A stage 2 acquired pes planus deformity with an increase in the talar-first metatarsal angle (**a**) and a break in Meary's angle (**b**) at the talar-navicular joint. The same patient 6 months post operative following a spring ligament reconstruction, tibialis posterior reconstruction, medialising calcaneal osteotomy and gastrocnemius release (**c**, **d**)

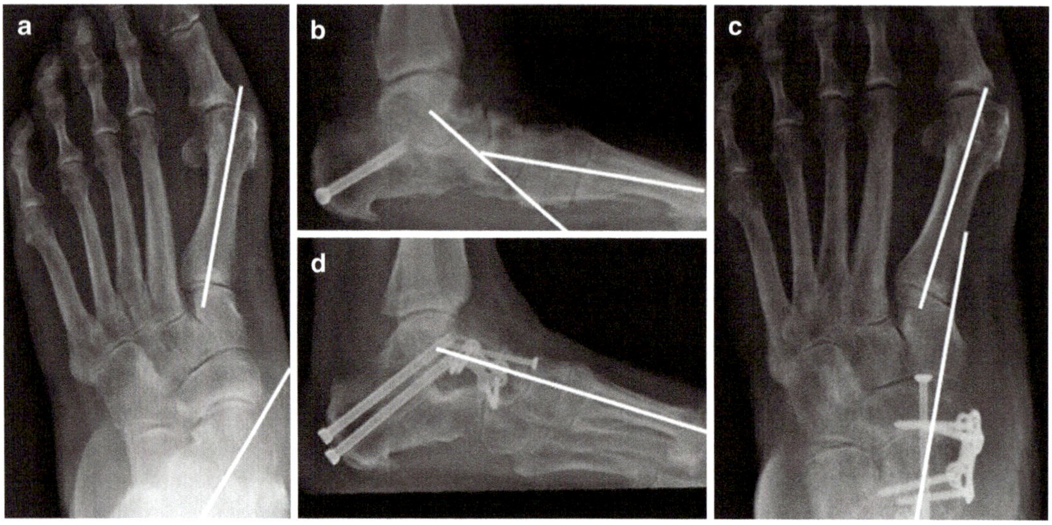

Fig. 6.21 A failed stage 2 acquired pes planus reconstruction that has developed onto stage 3. The talar-first metatarsal angle (**a**) and a break in Meary's angle (**b**) at the talar-navicular joint are both severe. The same patient 6 months post-operatively following a double fusion (talar navicular and subtalar joints) through the medial approach with correction of the deformity (**c**, **d**)

fixed then a Cotton osteotomy of the medial cuneiform may be required. A midfoot break with abduction is also common and can require a spring ligament reconstruction, Cobb tendon transfer (to medialise the pull of the tibialis anterior) or correction with a lateral column lengthening.

Fixed Deformity

Fixed deformities require surgical intervention, although a trial of accommodative orthotics may be helpful. Arthrodesis is advisable in advanced disease (stages 3 and 4). This is usually either a double or triple fusion (Fig. 6.21).

Table 6.9 shows the outcomes following isolated arthrodesis.

Concomitant Achilles tendon lengthening is often required to correct equinus deformity. Pantalar fusion is advised in cases of severe deformity and arthritis involving the tibiotalar joint, although double or triple arthrodesis with ankle replacement is an option. This is more complex and can only be performed in the presence of minor talar tilt.

A summary of management is presented in Table 6.10.

Table 6.9 Motion available following isolated arthrodesis

	ST fusion	CC fusion	TN fusion
ST motion		90%	10%
CC motion	50%		
TN motion	25%	70%	

CC Calcaneonavicular; *ST* subtalar; *TN* talonavicular.

Table 6.10 Management summary for pes planus

Stage 1	– Conservative (orthotics—Medial arch support, medial heel wedge, UCBL, AFO). – Tendon sheath divided and synovitis excised. – Gastrocnemius release
Stage 2	– FDL transfer to tibialis posterior tendon. – Plus calcaneal shift. – Plus spring ligament reconstruction. – plus gastrocnemius release. Additional procedures—Subtalar arthroereisis screw, cotton osteotomy, cobb tendon transfer, lateral column lengthening.
Stage 3	Fusion of degenerate and deformed joints
Stage 4	Pantalar fusion or ankle replacement with double/triple fusion.

Diabetic Foot

15% of diabetics will sustain a foot ulcer in their lifetime and approximately 20% of diabetic admissions are due to foot problems. The main pathologies are vasculopathy and neuropathy.

Risk factors for ulceration and poor healing include; poorly controlled diabetes, poor nutrition (albumin <30 g/l), difficulty offloading area, local infection, immunocompromised and low lymphocyte count (1500/mm^3). Caution should be exercised with normal ankle brachial pressure indices of 0.9–1.1 in the presence of atherosclerosis, as it can give a false impression of adequate perfusion.

Neuropathy, particularly sensory neuropathy, is the most common cause of foot complications in diabetic patients. However, autonomic neuropathy affecting sweating plays a key role in aetiology and progression. This causes drying of the skin, leading to fissuring and finally ulcers.

Motor involvement is less common than sensory neuropathy. The intrinsic muscles of the foot are involved initially, resulting in atrophy. This causes the plantar fat pad to shift and the plantar fascia to shorten. This, in turn, leads to cavus deformity of the foot and clawing of the toes, which stiffens the foot. The combined effect of these changes is less plantar protection of the bony prominences, callus formation and subsequent ulceration. Isolated neuropathy can involve the common peroneal nerve, resulting in foot drop. This leads to ulceration on the tips of the toes.

The sensory neuropathy is progressive from distal to proximal, beginning with a stocking distribution in the feet. An inability to perceive a 5.07 Semmes–Weinstein monofilament is a key finding, as this is associated with loss of protective sensation and hence a high risk of ulceration in the feet.

Peripheral vascular disease occurs in about 70% of people who have had diabetes for more than 10 years. Both small and large vessels are involved. Compared to non-diabetics, diabetics will typically have vascular disease below the knee. Occlusions are often longer in diabetic patients. In addition, people with diabetes have poor cellular defense because of changes in white-cell phagocytic mechanisms.

Another complication of the neuropathy in diabetic patients is Charcot arthropathy (see later).

The risk factors for major complications in the diabetic foot are:

- A history of previous ulceration.
- A long duration of diabetes.
- Poor metabolic control.
- Poor foot care.
- Ill-fitting shoes.
- Deformity.
- A tight Achilles tendon (which increases forefoot overloading).

Diabetic Ulceration

This accounts for approximately–

- 50% of admissions related to Diabetes
- 50% of all leg amputations
- 50% involve major level (BKA or AKA)
- 50% coexisting vascular disease
- 50% contralateral amputation 5 years
- 50% mortality 5 years

Examination

A useful mnemonic for structuring a diabetic foot examination is as follows:

- **D**—Deformity.
- **I**—Ischaemia.
- **A**—Atrophic nails.
- **B**—Breakdown of skin.
- **E**—Oedema.
- **T**—Temperature.
- **I**—Infection.
- **C**—Callosities.
- **S**—Sensation/Skin colour.

Focused vascular examination should include measurement of the ankle–brachial pressure index (ABPI) and absolute toe pressures. The

Table 6.11 University of Texas classification of diabetic foot ulcers

	Grade 0	Grade 1	Grade 2	Grade 3
Stage A	Pre- or postulcera-tive lesion completely epithelialis-ed	Superficial wound, not involving tendon, capsule or bone	Wound penetrating to tendon or capsule	Wound penetrating to bone or joint
Stage B	Infected	Infected	Infected	Infected
Stage C	Ischaemic	Ischaemic	Ischaemic	Ischaemic
Stage D	Infected and ischaemic	Infected and ischaemic	Infected and ischaemic	Infected and ischaemic

normal value of the ABPI is 1, and the minimum required for healing is 0.45. One should however interpret ABPIs cautiously in the presence of significant atherosclerosis. Vessel compliance will be reduced and thus readings may be falsely reassuring. The absolute toe pressure is normally 100 mmHg and the minimum required for healing is 40 mmHg. In addition, a transcutaneous oxygen measurement of toes greater than 40 mmHg is predictive of healing. Doppler scans and MR arteriograms can also be used to assess the vascular supply.

Plain radiographs will show the severity of deformities and any evidence of osteomyelitis or Charcot arthropathy. MRI is very useful in assessing abscesses and soft tissue involvement. A white blood cell (WBC) labeled or dual-image Tc scan is more sensitive and specific for osteomyelitis than standard bone scans.

Ulcer Classification

Ulcers are assessed for their location, size and depth (Fig. 6.24). Diabetic ulcers used to be classified according to Wagner but the more recent University of Texas system (Table 6.11) has modified this to include the presence of infection and ischaemia and provide a more useful validated system.

Armstrong DG, Lavery LA, Harkless LB. Validation of a diabetic wound classification system. The contribution of depth, infection, and ischemia to risk of amputation. Diabetes Care. 1998;21(5):855–859.

Table 6.12 Wagner classification

Grade	Lesion	Treatment
0	No open lesions; may have deformity or cellulitis	Extra-depth shoes Custom-moulded pressure relief insoles Serial examinations
1	Superficial diabetic ulcer (partial or full thickness)	Debridement of the ulcer Total-contact cast if vascularity is satisfactory Cast changes weekly in the initial stages and then every 2 weeks until healing is complete
2	Ulcer extension to ligament, tendon, joint capsule or deep fascia without abscess or osteomyelitis	Debridement Total-contact cast
3	Deep ulcer with abscess or osteomyelitis	Debridement Total contact cast
4	Gangrene localised to a portion of the forefoot or heel	Partial amputation, if ischaemia is present Vascular surgery consultation to decide if vascular reconstruction is possible Debridement and total contact cast
5	Extensive gangrenous involvement of the entire foot	Major amputation Consider arterial bypass for the healing of a below-knee amputation

Table 6.12 outlines the management of diabetic ulcers based on Wagner grades.

Table 6.13 Risk of amputation based on University of Texas classification

	Grade 0	Grade 1	Grade 2	Grade 3
Stage A	0%	0%	0%	0%
Stage B	12.5%	8.5%	28.6%	92%
Stage C	25%	20%	25%	100%
Stage D	50%	50%	100%	100%

Wagner FW, Jr. The diabetic foot. Orthopedics. 1987;10(1):163–172.

Table 6.13 shows the risk of amputation based on the University of Texas classification.

Medical Management

The basic principles of diabetic foot treatment require a multiple disciplinary team to implement and are as follows:

- In the diabetic foot with no infection or ulceration
- Education good blood glucose reduces incidence of neuropathy and minimises complications.
- Patient led preventative foot care
  - Daily wash with mild soap
  - Powder and moisturise to avoid fissuring
  - Cotton socks (to reduce shear), no barefoot walking.
  - Regular checks through the day
  - Report immediately at risk skin, blisters, ulceration, unilateral warmth or swelling (Charcot) and any trauma.
- Patients must have a point of contact or direct access to secondary care when concerned.
- Custom made footwear and orthotics reduce neuropathic ulcers.
- Good glycaemic control.
- For infections
- Mild cellulitis +/− ulcer
  - If no ulcer always consider Charcot's arthropathy
  - If ulcer serial x-rays +/− MRI to screen for osteomyelitis (OM)
  - If ulcer, cellulitis and no OM treat with broad spectrum antibiotics.

    Co-Amoxiclav or Cefalexin +/−Metronidazole

    Clindamycin + Ciprofloxacin (Penicillin Allergy)
  - Off load with total contact casting or custom orthotics
  - Biweekly or weekly review until settled
- Severe cellulitis +/− ulcer
  - IV broad spectrum antibiotics
  - Consider MRI to screen for abscess or osteomyelitis.
  - Offload
- Osteomyelitis +/− ulcer
  - Surface swabs or swabs from ulcer are unreliable when cultured
  - Serial x-rays are useful to monitor response. Early osteomyelitis not often apparent on x-ray.
  - MRI has a high sensitivity for osteomyelitis detection.
  - Ulcer that probes to bone have a relatively low positive predictive value (0.57) but a high negative predictive value (0.98)
  - If stable, aim for urgent deep tissue biopsy with/ without debridement prior to starting antibiotics.

Surgical Management

The primary goal in the treatment of diabetic foot ulcers is to obtain wound closure. A multidisciplinary approach should be employed because of the multifaceted nature of foot ulcers and the numerous co-morbidities that can occur in these patients. Rest, elevation of the affected foot, pressure relief and appropriate footwear are the essential components of treatment.

In the UK the National Institute for Health and Care Excellence (NICE) recommended that a pathway should be set up to assist in the management of the acute diabetic foot abscess. Subsequently the British Orthopaedic Foot and Ankle Society (BOFAS) have recommended that patients should ideally be admitted to a diabetology ward under joint care. The diabetic abscess is a surgical emergency. Time is crucial.

In the absence of a specialist foot surgeon, a general orthopaedic surgeon should perform drainage and debridement. The patient can then be referred to specialist orthopaedic foot surgeon for further inspection, debridement and planning of definitive management. Drainage should not be delayed for imaging.

Where there is significant tissue loss or destruction, limited amputations may need to be performed to aid wound closure. Where possible, agonist and antagonist muscle groups should be balanced through myotenodesis. The intention is to maintain a balanced plantigrade foot.

Charcot Arthropathy

Charcot arthropathy is a severe destructive process affecting the bony architecture and joint alignment in people who lack protective sensation. The most common cause is diabetes, although about 10% of Charcot patients have other causes such as Spina bifida, leprosy, hereditary motor/sensory neuropathy, post-traumatic sensory deficits and alcoholic peripheral neuropathy.

Charcot arthropathy can occur with or without neuropathic ulceration. In those with diabetes it typically arises in the fifth and sixth decades of life, and can occur alongside a relatively normal vascular examination. Other relatively rare aetiologies to be aware of include polio, paraplegia, syringomyelia, leprosy and syphilis.

The pathophysiology of Charcot arthropathy probably begins with either a recognised traumatic incident or multiple episodes of micro trauma. Injury to the joint is followed by rapid destruction of the joint surfaces and demineralisation. There is osteoclast overactivity, bone vascular shunting and bone breakdown. Care must be taken with foot and ankle injuries (even if fracture is not present) in patients with diabetes. An alternative hypothesis may involve a neurovascular pathway where by a neurally stimulated vascular reflex leads to stimulation of bone resorption through pro-inflammatory cytokines.

The joint destruction and demineralisation may lead to deformity, skin pressure and ulceration. Healing begins after a few weeks, and there is usually bony union associated with joint incongruity and deformity in a few months.

Charcot arthropathy is often said to be painless, but pain is in fact very common—although it may be less than expected from the degree of arthropathy and deformity.

Classification

Eichenholtz has described three stages of Charcot arthropathy.

Stage 1: Fragmentation or Destruction Stage

This process may last as long as 6–12 months. The bone fragments, the joint(s) become unstable and, in some cases, the bone is completely reabsorbed. This stage is clinically identified by significant swelling, erythema and a warm foot.

Stage 1 Charcot arthropathy can be confused with infection and the distinction may be very difficult. MRI can be helpful, and white-cell-labeled bone scans may be more reliable. The recent increased availability of positron emission tomography scanning offers hope of improved accuracy.

As the bones and joint are affected, fractures and instability develop and the joints can dislocate or shift in relation to each other. This can lead to severe deformity of the foot and ankle. Most often the midfoot joints are affected, and the result is a flattened foot, that which is wider where the normal foot narrows in the arch. Bony prominences often develop on the plantar surface of the foot and are risk factors for subsequent ulceration.

Stage 2: Coalescence

During this stage the acute destructive process slows and the body tries to begin healing. The swelling and heat begin to disappear.

Stage 3: Resolution/Consolidation

The swelling and erythema resolve. There may be residual instability.

Shibata has modified Eichenholtz's classification with a clinical Stage 0 with clinical signs of erythema and swelling without radiological changes. Treatment with a NWB cast may prevent x-ray changes.

Shibata T, Tada K, Hashizume C. The results of arthrodesis of the ankle for leprotic neuroarthropathy. J Bone Joint Surg Am. 1990;72(5):749–756.

Radiographs

In the early stages, plain radiographs show bone fragmentation. There may be joint subluxation or dislocation. Later on, resorption and coalescence of fragments occur. Periosteal new bone formation with sclerosis may be seen. In the final stages of resolution, remodelling occurs with smoothing of bone edges and reduction of the sclerosis.

Brodsky Classification

The Brodsky classification describes the site of destruction (Table 6.14).

Management

Management in the early and acute phase is non-weight-bearing followed by a total-contact cast.

Table 6.14 Brodsky classification for Charcot arthropathy of foot

Type 1	Tarsometatarsal and lesser tarsus, 60% of cases. Collapse of medial longitudinal arch with rocker bottom.
Type 2	Peritalar, 30% of cases. Often requires prolonged immobilization, developing hindfoot malalignment and frequently instability.
Type 3	(A) Ankle, often post trauma (B) posterior calcaneum, high risk of ulceration.
Type 4	Multiple sites
Type 5	Forefoot

This allows even distribution of pressure and supports areas of softening and collapse. Orthotic management is the mainstay of treatment if the residual deformities are minimal and can be braced. The Orthotic typically used is a bivalve Charcot resistant Orthotic Walker (CROW).

In severe deformities where the foot is not braceable in a plantigrade fashion, a combination of osteotomy/bone resection (particularly of a 'rocker-bottom' deformity), arthrodesis and soft tissue release are performed. Surgery is best performed once imaging shows that the disease process has settled, i.e. consolidation stage 3. General principles of surgery include using the strongest fixation possible.

Amputation may be required if ulceration and deep infection are present.

Plantar Heel Pain

Causes of plantar heel pain include the following

- Plantar aponeurosis
  - Plantar fasciopathy
  - Rupture
  - Enthesopathy
- Other soft tissues
  - Fat pad atrophy
  - Bursitis
  - Extrinsic tendinopathy
    Medial—FHL, FDL, TP
    Lateral—PL, PB
- Calcaneum
  - Calcaneal stress fracture
  - Osteomyelitis
  - Calcaneal periostitis.
  - Neoplastic—benign or malignant
  - Metabolic—osteomalacia, Paget's, hyperparathyroidism
- Neurological
  - Entrapment of Baxter's nerve
  - Medial calcaneal nerve entrapment
  - Tarsal tunnel syndrome
  - S1 radiculopathy

Plantar Fasciitis

This is the most common cause of heel pain and can affect both the active and sedentary adult population. Micro-tears at the origin (medial calcaneal tuberosity) of the plantar fascia are the likely pathology. These incite an inflammatory and repair process.

The typical presentation is with pain and tenderness under the medial aspect of the heel at the attachment of the fascia. Typically, this is worst on the first step in the morning, improving as the day goes on and then often becoming more painful towards evening. Some patients have more weight-bearing than first-step pain. The pain may radiate across the heel or down the plantar fascia.

Differential diagnoses may include symptoms suggestive of a spondyloarthropathy such as ankylosing spondylitis; or pain and tenderness of the abductor hallucis due to entrapment and inflammation of the first branch of the lateral plantar nerve. In addition, an os calcis stress fracture, subtalar osteoarthritis, retrocalcaneal bursitis and Achilles tendinopathy may cause pain in the local area.

Plantar 'spurs' seen on lateral X-rays are not relevant as they lie on the lateral part of the calcaneum away from the attachment of the fascia.

In 90% of patients, plantar fasciitis will resolve by 10 months without intervention. The triad of aetiology includes calf tightness, obesity and working in a standing job. First line management includes reducing the overload to this area, by loss of weight and reducing calf tightness. Plantar fascia specific stretches have been shown to improve pain. Other conservative measures include NSAIDs, cushioned heel inserts, night splints, and steroid injections. A meta-analysis on all conservative measures showed that only ultra sound guided pulsed radiofrequency had a high rate of improvement as compared to placebo. Low level laser therapy, dry needling and calcaneal taping had a moderate improvement compared to placebo. Shock wave therapy, orthotics, stretching exercises and pulsed radiofrequency electromagnetic field had a low level improvement as compared to placebo. Other treatments with level 1 and 2 evidence include steroid injection, autologous blood product injection and Botox injection.

Salvioli S, Guidi M, Marcotulli G. The effectiveness of conservative, non-pharmacological treatment, of plantar heel pain: A systematic review with meta-analysis. Foot (Edinb). 2017;33:57–67.

Operative management should only be considered in recalcitrant cases that have failed appropriate physiotherapy and conservative treatment. Treatment may include release of the medial third of the plantar fascia with spur resection. Excessive release has its complications with lateral column pain and flattening of the arch reported if >50% of fascia released. Neurolysis of the first branch of the lateral plantar nerve by release of deep fascia of the abductor hallucis is beneficial if nerve entrapment is suspected. Recently proximal medial gastrocnemius release has gained popularity in the treatment of plantar fasciitis. With results showing better patient satisfaction and less morbidity than partial plantar fasciotomy.

Monteagudo M, Maceira E, Garcia-Virto V, Canosa R. Chronic plantar fasciitis: plantar fasciotomy versus gastrocnemius recession. Int Orthop. 2013;37(9):1845–50.

Calcaneal Stress Fracture

Calcaneal stress fracture results from multiple compressive loads and weight-bearing activities and is most often seen in military recruits. Symptoms include pain and swelling on both sides of heel and exquisite tenderness to palpation on the lateral and medial aspects of the heel (heel squeeze test).

Plain radiographs may not become positive for 2–4 weeks. A lateral radiograph may show an area of increased density perpendicular to trabecular stress lines through the posterior aspect of the calcaneus (from the posterior–superior surface to the anterior–inferior surface). Bone scans can be useful in those with acute symptoms and negative radiographs. MRI is more specific and sensitive in the diagnosis.

Management involves reducing activity and cast or brace immobilisation until the symptoms have resolved and bone healing is evident on radiographs. This takes approximately 4–8 weeks.

Posterior Heel Pain

Common causes of posterior heel pain are

- Retrocalcaneal bursitis
- Haglund's deformity
- Achilles tendonitis
- Paratenonitis
- Inflammatory conditions like ankylosing spondyltis, psoriatic arthritis and Reiter's syndrome.

Paratenonitis

When the paratenon is inflamed, the whole area is diffusely swollen and tender and crepitation may be felt when the tendon glides. This typically occurs in distance runners and is worth identifying as an injection of saline with or without local anaesthetic can rapidly resolve the condition.

Non-insertional Achilles Tendinosis

Non-insertional tendinosis occurs approximately 2–6 cm proximal to the insertion of the tendon and a tender fusiform swelling can be palpated (Fig. 6.22). This is considered an overuse condition, leading to mucoid degeneration of tendon, hypercellularity and neovascularisation. Non-insertional Achilles tendinosis accounts for over 55% of tendoachilles disorders. Factors such as a gastrocnemius tightness, lower limb malalignment, leg length discrepancy, corticosteroid and fluoroquinolone use have been associated with increased prevalence.

Alfredson H, Ohberg L, Forsgren S. Is vasculo-neural ingrowth the cause of pain in chronic Achilles tendinosis? An investigation using ultrasonography and colour Doppler, immunohistochemistry, and diagnostic injections. Knee Surg Sports Traumatol Arthrosc. 2003;11(5):334–8.

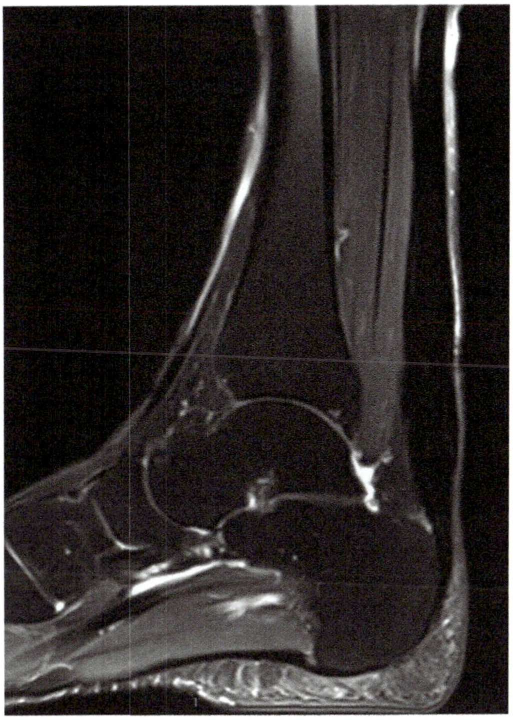

Fig. 6.22 A proton density fat suppressed MRI showing a long segment of non-insertional Achilles tendonopathy

Non-insertional Achilles tendonitis generally responds well to conservative treatment. The current balance of evidence does not support a clear recommendation of one type of exercise protocol over another for Achilles tendinopathy.

Wilson F, Walshe M, O'Dwyer T, Bennett K, Mockler D, Bleakley C. Exercise, orthoses and splinting for treating Achilles tendinopathy: a systematic review with meta-analysis. Br J Sports Med. 2018;52(24):1564–74. A level 1 meta-analysis of 22 studies on exercise as a treatment of non-insertional Achilles tendonitis, showed strength of evidence for all studies was 'moderate' for reducing pain (VAS), improving function (assessed by VISA-A) and improving quality of life (SF-36).

Boesen AP, Hansen R, Boesen MI, Malliaras P, Langberg H. Effect of High-Volume Injection, Platelet-Rich Plasma, and Sham Treatment in

Chronic Midportion Achilles Tendinopathy: A Randomized Double-Blinded Prospective Study. Am J Sports Med. 2017;45(9):2034–43. High volume injection was found to give a significant improvement as compared to placebo and platelet rich plasma, but only with short term follow up.

Orthotics do not give any benefit over placebo.

Lin MT, Chiang CF, Wu CH, Hsu HH, Tu YK. Meta-analysis Comparing Autologous Blood-Derived Products (Including Platelet-Rich Plasma) Injection Versus Placebo in Patients With Achilles Tendinopathy. Arthroscopy. 2018;34(6):1966–75. A meta-analysis of 7 level 1 RCTs showed no improvement as compared to placebo for autologous blood (including PRP) injections.

Steroid injections into or around the Achilles tendon may provoke rupture and should generally be avoided. However, there is plenty of anecdotal evidence that steroid injections can offer good relief of symptoms. Further to the use of eccentric calf strengthening, additional improvement in pain scores and patient reported outcome measures by including the use of low energy shock wave therapy.

Rompe JD, Furia J, Maffulli N. Eccentric loading versus eccentric loading plus shock-wave treatment for midportion achilles tendinopathy: a randomized controlled trial. Am J Sports Med. 2009;37(3):463–70.

Approximately 25% of cases will be resistant to conservative measures. Resistant cases are treated surgically by excision of the inflamed paratenon and debridement of the pathologic areas of tendon, followed by repair. If more than 50% of the tendon is involved then flexor hallucis longus tendon transfer is often added to support the tendon.

Success rates quoted are extremely variable with success rates upwards from 50%. This is likely due to difference in severity, operative technique and use of tendon graft.

It is also worth noting that up to a 10% complication rate has been quoted following surgery. Complications include infection, seroma, wound edge necrosis, sural nerve injury, tendon rupture and venous thromboembolism.

Paavola M, Orava S, Leppilahti J, Kannus P, Jarvinen M. Chronic Achilles tendon overuse injury: complications after surgical treatment. An analysis of 432 consecutive patients. Am J Sports Med. 2000;28(1):77–82.

Minimally invasive and endoscopic debridement with release of plantaris have been reported with similar results. However large comparative studies of open and all less invasive procedures, with and without plantaris tendon excision, are required to decide upon optimal treatment strategy.

Maffulli N, Longo UG, Spiezia F, Denaro V. Minimally invasive surgery for Achilles tendon pathologies. Open Access J Sports Med. 2010;1:95–103.

Insertional Achilles Tendonitis

Insertional Achilles tendonitis is an enthesopathy with tenderness localised to tendon insertion. Patients will often report pain and stiffness exacerbated beyond periods of immobility. Pathologies include attritional changes, tendinosis, intratendinous ossification and a bony spur. The pain is related to contact between the posterior calcaneus and the Achilles tendon, and there can be progressive enlargement of the bony prominence of the heel. Localised calcification within the Achilles tendon may be seen as a sequel of chronic insertional tendonitis. Some reports suggest radiological parameters such as the Fowler-Phillip angle >75 degrees and Bohler's angle <20 degrees and a loss of parallel pitch lines are a risk factor for the development of insertional tendonitis. More recently this has been refuted as studies of asymptomatic individuals show similar variance in radiological parameters.

Kang S, Thordarson DB, Charlton TP. Insertional Achilles tendinitis and Haglund's deformity. Foot Ankle Int. 2012;33(6):487–91.

Bulstra GH, van Rheenen TA, Scholtes VA. Can We Measure the Heel Bump? Radiographic Evaluation of Haglund's Deformity. J Foot Ankle Surg. 2015;54(3):338–40.

Conservative management is the mainstay of treatment. NSAIDs, ice, heel lifts, silicone pads

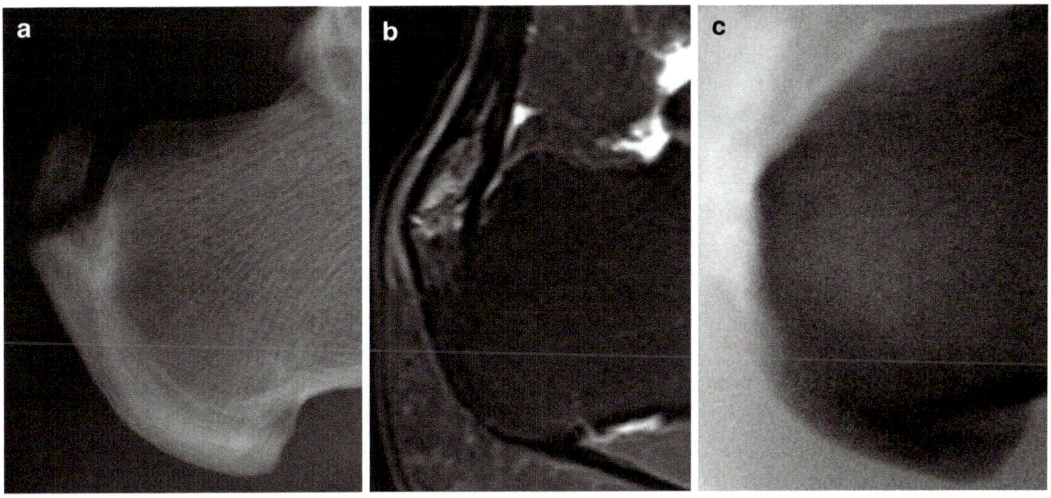

Fig. 6.23 Preoperative insertional Achilles tendonopathy radiograph (**a**) and MRI (**b**) with large intratendinous enthesophyte. Intraoperative imaging of Achilles tendon elevation, excision of enthesophyte and reattachment (**c**)

and stretching are the conservative measures, but are less successful than in non-insertional tendinosis. Surgical treatment is by excision of heterotopic bone and the degenerative part of tendons, and re-anchoring or repair of the tendon if more than 50% of the tendon is involved (Fig. 6.23). Other surgical methods, including taking a dorsal wedge (Zadek procedure) from the calcaneal tuberosity to alter the pull of the Achilles, are reporting good results.

Retrocalcaneal bursitis and Haglund's Deformity

Retrocalcaneal bursitis presents with anterior pain (deep to the tendon), with pain on palpation of the soft spot. It can occur alone or with tendinosis. When it occurs in isolation, a steroid injection can be very useful in resolving the pain.

Haglund's deformity is a normal variant and is a prominence of the posterior superior calcaneal tuberosity. Retrocalcaneal bursitis is due to inflammation of the bursa between the anterior surface of the Achilles tendon and Haglund's deformity. It is most common in women and is related to footwear, rigid heels or heel counters.

Patients present with posterolateral heel prominence, deep posterior heel pain, fullness of the tendon and increased pain with dorsiflexion of the ankle. Conservative management is similar to that for Achilles tendonitis, and consists of NSAIDs, heel-cord stretching, footwear adjustment and raising the heel out of the shoe with a heel insert, which shifts the contact against the heel.

Surgical treatment consists of debridement of the inflamed retrocalcaneal bursa and excision of the Haglund's prominence. The excision must be kept proximal to the Achilles insertion. A lateral approach is easier, but care must be taken to avoid the sural nerve. A medial incision may also be used. In this case, a vertical incision is made 1 cm anterior and parallel to the medial border of the Achilles tendon, and down onto the calcaneus. Then the posterior calcaneal tuberosity is removed, and the Achilles tendon is debrided and reattached using bone anchors. The Achilles tendon is dissected subperiosteally at the insertion of the Achilles tendon and about 50% of the tendon is elevated. The calcaneal prominence is then removed. The average size of fragment removed is 3 cm long, 3 cm wide and 6 mm thick. The ankle is subsequently immobilised for 4–6 weeks.

'Pump bump' refers to the bony prominence that is found at the back of the heel distal to the tendon insertion. Management includes padding the area, but it occasionally needs to be shaved down.

Pes Cavus

Pes cavus describes a foot with an abnormally high longitudinal arch that does not flatten with weight bearing. The forefoot is plantar flexed, which is most marked in the first ray causing apparent pronation of the forefoot. The hindfoot is usually in dorsiflexion (calcaneus) with a calcaneal pitch >30 degrees, although in some neuromuscular conditions, such as CMT, the gastrocnemius/soleus complex becomes tight or shortened and the hindfoot tilts into equinus. The heel may be neutral, but more often lies in varus creating a cavovarus foot. Figure 6.24 depicts a typical pes cavus with an apex at the Chopart joint, plantar flexed first ray, varus hindfoot with an increased calcaneal pitch and clawing of the lesser toes.

A cavovarus foot is considered pathological until proven otherwise, but in particular, beware of the unilateral pes cavus.

The causes of cavus foot are related to muscle imbalance or contracture of structures on the medial aspect. The causes include–.

- Neuromuscular:
  - Cerebral palsy.
  - Hereditary motor sensory neuropathy.
  - Multiple sclerosis.
  - Friedrich's ataxia.
  - Spinal cord tumour.
  - Syringomyelia.
  - Tethered cord.
  - Myelodysplasia.
  - Poliomyelitis.
  - Guillain–Barré syndrome.
  - Muscular dystrophy.
- Congenital.
- Residual talipes equinovarus.
- Arthrogryposis.
- Trauma.
- Fibrosis post-compartment syndrome.
- Peroneal palsy.
- Fracture malunion.
- Burn contracture.

Charcot–Marie–Tooth Disease (Hereditary Sensory Motor Neuropathy)

Charcot–Marie–Tooth disease (CMTD) or Hereditary Sensory Motor Neuropathy (HSMN) is the most common inherited neuropathy, affect-

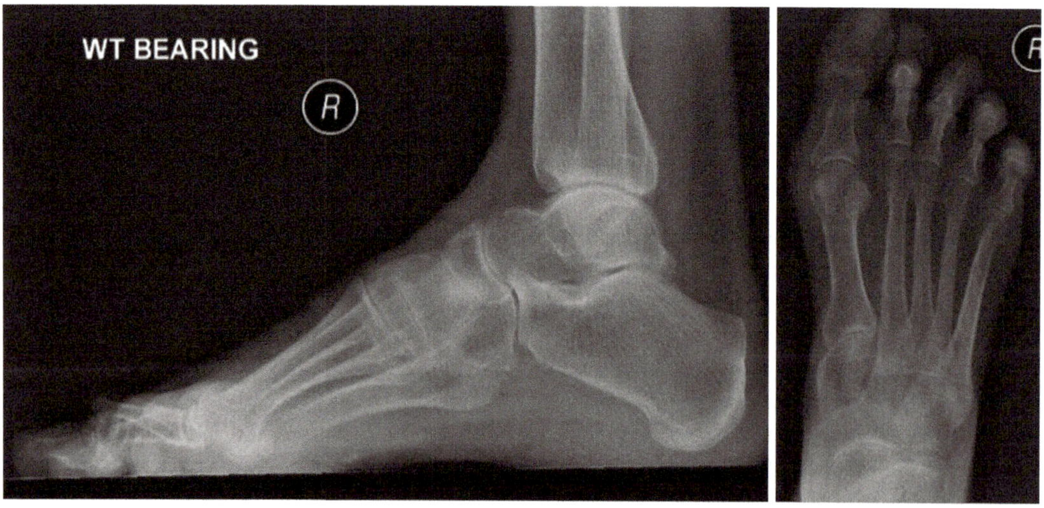

Fig. 6.24 Radiographic appearance of cavus foot

ing 1 in 2500 people. CMTD has different genetic variants with variable expressivity and clinical picture. The most common foot presentation in CMTD is the cavovarus deformity. Some patients may present with muscle cramps, recurrent ankle sprains and difficulty with gait. The upper extremities are involved in as many as two-thirds of patients with peripheral neuropathy. It is important to note, however, that up to 20% of patients show no demonstrable sensory loss at presentation. Upper-limb involvement tends to be milder than lower-extremity involvement, and becomes clinically symptomatic as the patient ages. Later, intrinsic-minus hands develop with clawing of the fingers and atrophy of the small muscles of the hand.

Type 1 CMTD

Type 1 CMTD is inherited as an autosomal dominant disease. There is hypertrophic demyelination and slow nerve conduction. Type 1 affects two thirds of CMTD patients.

Patients with type 1 CMTD have a defect in the gene encoding peripheral myelin protein-22 on chromosome 17. Clinical presentation is most common during the second decade of life. This is a progressive neuropathy in which both motor and sensory nerve function are affected. Distal muscle groups are involved first with typically weakness of lower limb intrinsic muscles at the beginning. This is followed by loss of reflexes and atrophy. Sensory loss occurs later in the disease course, although vibratory sense can be affected early. Type 1 CMTD may be associated with scoliosis and hip dysplasia.

Type 2 CMTD

Type 2 CMTD (neuronal form) is infrequently seen. Patients have an axonal neuropathy with relatively normal nerve conduction. The inheritance pattern is variable. Onset is delayed until the second or third decade of life. The reflexes are normal and there is more profound distal lower-extremity weakness than encountered in type 1. A characteristic stork-leg appearance, caused by atrophy of the distal third of the quadriceps and hamstrings, is frequently seen. Some patients develop a calcaneovalgus deformity.

Cavovarus Deformity

The underlying pathology in the development of cavovarus deformity in CMTD is muscle imbalance. The tibialis anterior and peroneus brevis weaken early on in the disease course. This may be due to their relatively small cross-sectional area compared with their antagonists. Recruitment of the long extensors of the foot can be seen in an attempt to maintain active dorsiflexion. The weakness results in plantar flexion of the first ray, resulting in hindfoot varus through the tripod effect (i.e., with a plantar flexed first ray and mobile lateral rays). For the foot to remain plantigrade, the heel must roll into varus in order to get the lateral metatarsals on the ground.

In the early stages of the disease the hindfoot is flexible. Deformities of the hindfoot involve malposition of the talus and calcaneus, with the latter inverted into a varus position. In later stages the plantar flexed position of the first ray eventually becomes rigid, which forces the heel to remain in varus and fixes the hindfoot in varus.

When deformities become rigid, neither weight bearing nor passive manipulation fully corrects the foot. The degree of rigidity is classically elicited by the Coleman block test, which confirms whether the hindfoot deformity is forefoot driven. The test is performed by placing a block under the lateral column of the foot and allowing the first metatarsal to drop. This eliminates the need for hindfoot varus. If the hindfoot is flexible, the varus will correct.

Management

Because of the progressive nature of the disease, surgical management is preferred to conservative measures such as braces, orthotics and physical therapy. In general, the treatment comprises two soft tissue releases (plantar fascia, tendo-Achilles), two tendon transfers (peroneus longus to brevis, EHL to first metatarsal or 'Jones procedure') and two osteotomies (lateralising calcaneal osteotomy, dorsiflexion osteotomy of the first metatarsal).

Sackley C, Disler PB, Turner-Stokes L, Wade DT, Brittle N, Hoppitt T. Rehabilitation interventions for foot drop in neuromuscular disease. Cochrane Database Syst Rev. 2009(3):CD003908.

Surgical management can be divided into soft tissue and bony procedures. Very rarely are they ever performed in isolation and more typically a combination of both is required for reconstruction.

Plantar fascia release ('Steindler release') is the first procedure considered, though this is seldom performed in isolation. A medial plantar approach is used to transect the plantar fascia and the fascia investing the abductor hallucis. The contracted intrinsic muscles are also released. The Achilles tendon can be released to correct the equinus.

The deforming force of the peroneus longus can be countered by transferring the longus to brevis. The clawed hallux is managed by transferring the EHL to the first metatarsal; this also increases the dorsiflexion power. This procedure can be combined with fusion of the IP joint of the big toe (Jones procedure). Clawing of lesser toes may need extensor tendon lengthening, MTP joint capsulotomies and resection of the head and neck of the proximal phalanges.

A lateralising or lateral closing wedge osteotomy of the calcaneum will help to shift the weight-bearing axis slightly medial to the midline of the calcaneum. This converts it to a stabilising force and protects the stretched lateral ligaments. The use of a Z osteotomy allows an even more powerful correction by allowing both translation and rotation of the os calcis.

Maynou C, Szymanski C, Thiounn A. The adult cavus foot. EFORT Open Rev. 2017;2(5):221–9.

A first metatarsal osteotomy is performed to correct plantar flexion deformity of the first ray. The second and third metatarsal can also be corrected if required.

Advanced fixed deformities are corrected by osteotomies and fusion of the midfoot or hindfoot, depending on the deformities (e.g., triple fusion). One should bear in mind that CMTD is a progressive disease with a risk of recurrence. The long term results of triple arthrodesis in CMTD are not as favourable as in those without CMTD. There is a higher incidence of ankle arthritis and deformity recurrence.

Management is described as 'à la carte' because the procedures are selected according to the needs of the individual foot—for example, the most severe toe clawing may be asymptomatic and can therefore be left.

Ankle Arthritis

Ankle arthritis is uncommon, contributing to 1% of all arthridities affecting weight-bearing joints, possibly because it has the largest contact area. Rare and common causes are listed in Table 6.15. Disorders that cause bleeding into the joint (e.g., haemophilia, pigmented villonodular synovitis) can also cause ankle arthritis.

Clinical symptoms can be due to mechanical block or inflammation. Inflammatory changes cause swelling, pain and stiffness, especially in the morning. Mechanical symptoms are due to anterior osteophytes causing impingement, particularly on dorsiflexion. Osteophytes develop first in the anterior tibia, with a 'kissing lesion' subsequently developing in the talus. The pain due to impingement may be relieved by the use of a heel raise.

Pain and tenderness in the anterior joint line with dorsiflexion (Molloy impingement test) suggest anterior impingement. Some patients complain of locking or giving way. This may be due to a loose body or reflex inhibition of the support-

Table 6.15 Causes of ankle arthritis

Common	Rare
Post-traumatic arthritis Inflammatory or systemic arthropathy (e.g., rheumatoid arthritis, psoriatic arthropathy, gout)	Septic arthritis Primary osteoarthritis Chronic instability Ochronosis Polyostotic fibrous dysplasia

ing muscles. Other joints are often involved in patients with arthritic ankles, which may affect the surgical option and likely outcomes.

Investigation

Preliminary investigation includes a standing AP and lateral radiograph of the ankle. This can show narrowing of the joint space, spurs, loose bodies and malalignment. The surrounding joints can also be seen and may have a bearing on the management strategy, especially if degenerate. A CT scan is useful where there is loss of bone stock due to trauma, infection and so on. An MRI is useful to assess the extent of talus osteonecrosis.

Management

Conservative management is advised if the symptoms are mild. This comprises NSAIDs, disease-modifying drug management for specific treatment of inflammatory arthropathy, splints, braces, boots and local steroid or hyaluronic acid injections. Adding a rocker bottom orthosis to the shoe will improve transition throughout the stance phase and allow a normalized gait whilst reducing painful ankle motion. The addition of a solid ankle cushioned heel will also offload the ankle during heel strike.

Surgery is an option where non-surgical treatment has failed to control the patient's symptoms and the patient's activities of daily living are seriously affected. A wide range of surgical options are available: arthroscopic debridement, arthrodesis, arthroplasty, osteotomy and joint distraction.

Arthroscopic Debridement

Arthroscopic debridement is useful when the joint is reasonably well preserved, especially if the main problem is impingement from synovitis, spurs or loose bodies. Arthroscopic debridement for impingement has a 75% success rate at 5 years in the presence of spurs, but only 50% with loss of joint space. In severely degenerated ankles there is a small risk of worsening pain due to the increased movement.

Osti L, Del Buono A, Maffulli N. Arthroscopic debridement of the ankle for mild to moderate osteoarthritis: a midterm follow-up study in former professional soccer players. J Orthop Surg Res. 2016;11:37.

Arthrodesis

Arthrodesis is the mainstay of treatment for advanced symptomatic arthritis of the ankle. It can be performed with an open technique or arthroscopically. Prior to ankle arthrodesis, it is beneficial if the patient is given the option of wearing either a below-knee cast or cam walker. A good candidate for ankle arthrodesis is a patient with documented ankle arthritis who has obtained pain relief from a cam walker. Cigarette smoking increases the risks of ankle non-union by at least three times, and may affect wound healing after any procedure.

Compression arthrodesis using internal fixation is popular. The ankle should be held in a neutral position with regard to varus/valgus and plantar/dorsiflexion, as well as in slight external rotation. The talus should be directly beneath the tibia. AP translation should be avoided, but a slight medial translation is acceptable. A variety of approaches have been described. A lateral approach excising the fibula is quite popular. Open arthrodesis allows correction of greater deformities than arthroscopic procedure (Fig. 6.25).

Arthroscopic Arthrodesis

Arthroscopic arthrodesis usually requires a correctable deformity, or less than 10° varus or valgus malalignment (Fig. 6.26). The main advantages are reduced postoperative pain and a high rate of rapid union. This is particularly useful in patients with a poor vascular supply, poor soft tissue envelope and bleeding disorders.

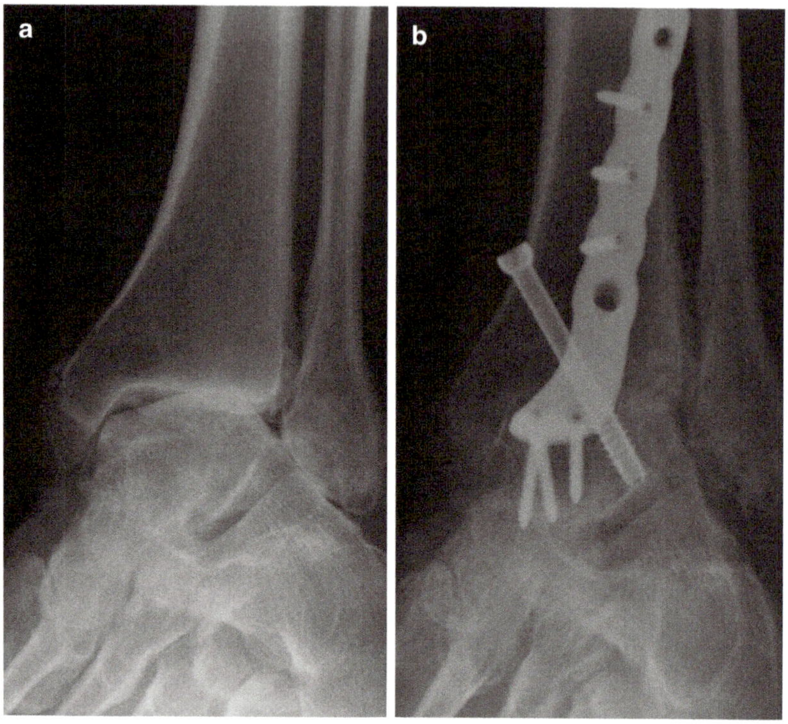

Fig. 6.25 Ankle arthritis with a severe valgus deformity (**a**). The same patient 6 months following an open ankle fusion (**b**)

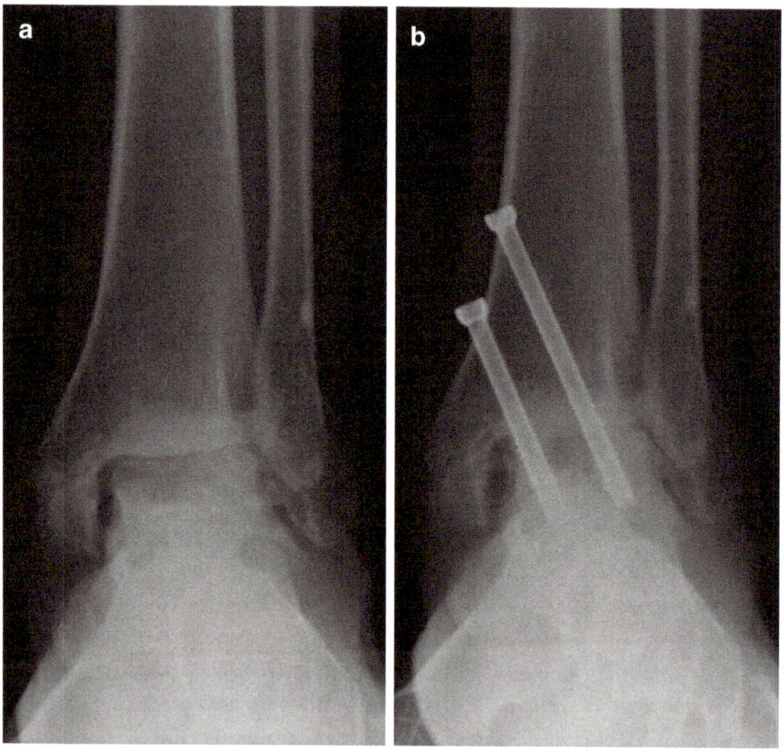

Fig. 6.26 Post traumatic ankle arthritis (**a**). The same patient 6 months following an arthroscopic ankle fusion (**b**)

With regards to long term outcomes, over a mean of 20 years, patients have a significantly greater risk of developing severe arthritis in hindfoot, midfoot and first metatarsophalangeal joint than the contralateral side without an ankle arthrodesis.

Cottino U, Collo G, Morino L, et al. *Arthroscopic ankle arthrodesis: a review. Curr Rev Musculoskelet Med. 2012;5(2):151–5.*

Coester LM, Saltzman CL, Leupold J, Pontarelli W. Long-term results following ankle arthrodesis for post-traumatic arthritis. J Bone Joint Surg Am. 2001;83(2):219–28.

Fuchs S, Sandmann C, Skwara A, Chylarecki C. Quality of life 20 years after arthrodesis of the ankle. A study of adjacent joints. J Bone Joint Surg Br. 2003;85(7):994–8.

Ankle Replacement

Early prostheses did not reproduce the biomechanics of the ankle adequately and had a very high failure rate. Second-generation prostheses have reported success in more than 90% of patients. Ankle replacement is advisable in patients with bilateral disease or rheumatoid arthritis, and when other joints around the ankle are involved. The 10 year survival is approximately 75%.

Haddad SL, Coetzee JC, Estok R, Fahrbach K, Banel D, Nalysnyk L. Intermediate and long-term outcomes of total ankle arthroplasty and ankle arthrodesis. A systematic review of the literature. J Bone Joint Surg Am. 2007;89(9):1899–905.

The latest evidence suggests superior pain relief at 2 years. However, level of return to recreation and sporting activities are the same for both arthrodesis and ankle replacements. The failure rate for revision arthroplasty is high and most patients will require a tibiotalocalcaneal fusion.

Schuh R, Hofstaetter J, Krismer M, Bevoni R, Windhager R, Trnka HJ. Total ankle arthroplasty versus ankle arthrodesis. Comparison of sports, recreational activities and functional outcome. Int Orthop. 2012;36(6):1207–14.

Saltzman CL, Mann RA, Ahrens JE, et al. *Prospective controlled trial of STAR total ankle replacement versus ankle fusion: initial results. Foot Ankle Int. 2009;30(7):579–96.*

Wood PL, Karski MT, Watmough P. Total ankle replacement: the results of 100 mobility total ankle replacements. J Bone Joint Surg Br. 2010;92(7):958–62.

Distraction Arthroplasty

In distraction arthroplasty, a distraction force is applied with an external fixator frame. Joint movement is possible through the hinges in the fixator. It is thought to improve pain by allowing cartilage to repair (fibrocartilage) in a low pressure environment. Some reports suggest sustained relief with 78% of patients having only mild to moderate discomfort up to 5 years. After that period, the benefit appears to tail off, however there is a report of one patient only requiring occasional non-steroidal anti-inflammatory drugs at 13 years following the procedure. This technique is not very popular because of the long periods required in the fixator and less than optimal improvement.

Paley D, Lamm BM, Purohit RM, Specht SC. Distraction arthroplasty of the ankle--how far can you stretch the indications? Foot Ankle Clin. 2008;13(3):471–84.

Osteotomy of the Distal Tibia

Realignment is an option if the joint is reasonably well preserved. An osteotomy should be considered when supramalleolar malalignment is present, or if there is an ankle/tibial plafond malunion. It should only be considered in non-smokers, compliant patients and in the presence of a good soft tissue envelope and blood supply. In appropriately selected patients good outcome can be sustained beyond five years, with improvement in functional scores. However one study did report a relatively high revision rate of up to 25% over intermediate follow up.

Pagenstert G, Knupp M, Valderrabano V, Hintermann B. Realignment surgery for valgus ankle osteoarthritis. Oper Orthop Traumatol. 2009;21(1):77–87.

Ankle Instability

The lateral ligament complex comprises of the Anterior Talofibular ligament (ATFL), Calcaneofibular ligament (CFL) and Posterior Talofibular ligament (PTFL). The PTFL is the strongest of the three. The ATFL is the most frequently injured and acts to prevent anterior subluxation and inversion in plantar flexion. The CFL stabilizes the ankle in dorsiflexion and is rarely injured in isolation, more typically it is injured with ATFL.

Chronic ankle instability can result from an ankle ligament sprain. Patients present with pain, stiffness, swelling, locking, 'giving-way' or repeated sprains. Tenderness is usually maximal over the lateral ligament, often in the anterior talofibular ligament only. A few patients will also have localised tenderness over the deltoid ligament, which tends to indicate more complex injuries. Tenderness or swelling over the Achilles, peroneal or tibialis posterior tendons should be identified.

There is an association between ankle instability and peroneal tendon instability. The patient will usually complain of snapping or giving way over the peroneal tendons, and instability is maximal on plantar flexion/eversion. Deficits in peroneal strength and function have been shown to impair proprioception and contribute to ankle instability and recurrent injury.

Ankle instability is demonstrated with the anterior draw and tilt tests. The anterior draw test should be performed with the ankle in 20° plantar flexion. The tibia may be pushed posteriorly against a fixed foot or the foot drawn forwards. The characteristic positive sign is a 'suction sign' as the synovium is sucked into the joint, drawing the skin inwards in the lateral gutter. In many patients, however, there is no suction sign but the talus can obviously be drawn anteriorly more than on the other side.

The talar tilt test is conventionally performed by tilting the hindfoot and looking for a suction sign or asymmetrical movement. It should be performed with the ankle plantigrade. Palpation of the talar neck will help in differentiating between movement in the ankle and the subtalar joint.

There are three common presentations of chronic ankle instability:

- Pain.
- Pain and instability symptoms.
- True mechanical instability.

Functional instability is a subjective sensation of giving way. Mechanical instability is excessive laxity of the lateral ligament complex. Clinically, the anterior drawer test is positive.

Investigation

Radiologically, instability may be demonstrated with the anterior drawer or talar tilt test (Fig. 6.27). Absolute displacement of more than 10 mm or a difference of more than 3 mm compared with the opposite side is considered positive radiographic evidence on an anterior drawer stress radiograph. A talar tilt stress radiograph should show a difference of more than 10° compared with the opposite side to be positive.

Management

Conservative treatment consists of peroneal strengthening and proprioceptive rehabilitation. This is particularly useful in functional instability. Ankle braces can also be used. Surgery is advised if symptoms persist, although generalised hypermobility is a contraindication for surgery. Patients with mechanically stable ankles and other intra-articular problems generally have good results with arthroscopic surgery. Some studies report up to 93% patients undergoing lateral ligament reconstruction also have an intra-articular pathology. Consequently many experts

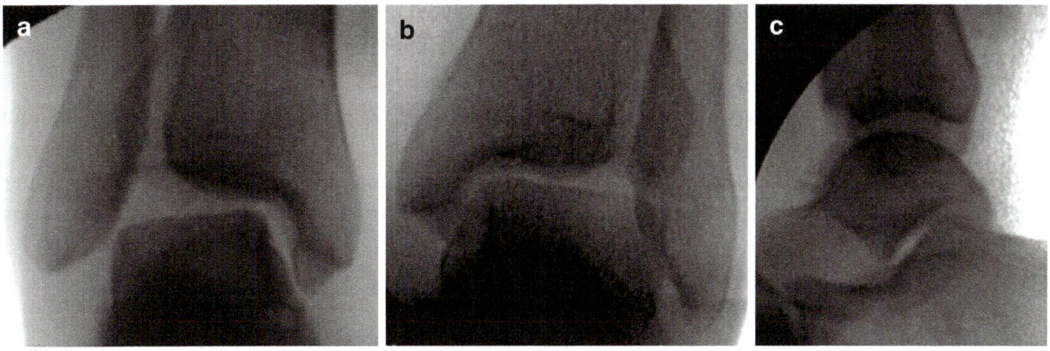

Fig. 6.27 Images of an examination under anaesthetic of an ankle with a positive anterior drawer and talar tilt test. Absolute displacement of more than 10 mm or a difference of more than 3 mm compared with the opposite side is considered positive, which is present in this patient. A talar tilt stress radiograph should show a difference of more than 10° compared with the opposite side to be positive (**a**) which this case clearly illustrates even though there was some laxity on the other ankle (**b**). The anterior drawer test is demonstrated in image c

advocate arthroscopic evaluation of the ankle routinely during lateral ligament reconstruction.

Komenda GA, Ferkel RD. Arthroscopic findings associated with the unstable ankle.

Foot Ankle Int. 1999;20(11):708–13.

The most commonly performed surgical procedure is anatomic reconstruction. Originally described by Brostrum as a mid substance ATFL repair and later modified by Gould to include detachment, shortening and reinsertion of the attenuated ATFL, with reinforcement using the extensor retinaculum. Karlsson found improved outcomes when repair of CFL was also performed.

Karlsson J, Eriksson BI, Bergsten T, Rudholm O, Sward L. Comparison of two anatomic reconstructions for chronic lateral instability of the ankle joint. Am J Sports Med. 1997;25(1):48–53.

Success is reported between 80–90% with long term follow up.

Repair with tendon allograft/autograft is considered in patients with poor tissues, patients with ongoing instability or those needing revision stabilisation.

Pagenstert G VV, Hintermann B Lateral Ankle Ligament Reconstruction With Free Plantaris Tendon Graft. Techniques in Foot and Ankle Surgery 2005;4(2):104–12.

Paterson R, Cohen B, Taylor D, Bourne A, Black J. Reconstruction of the lateral ligaments of the ankle using semi-tendinosis graft. Foot Ankle Int. 2000;21(5):413–9.

The first description of a non-anatomical repair by Watson-Jones, described complete transection of distal peroneus brevis and passage posterior to anterior through distal fibula and insertion onto talar neck. Short term results have been similar to anatomical repairs at around 80% success rate. However, abnormal ankle movements and excessive stiffness of the ankle and subtalar joint have led to a decline in its popularity. The Evans procedure is an alternative method of tenodesis by transecting peroneus brevis proximally, leaving its distal insertion and attaching it to the distal fibula. This again, stiffened the subtalar joint and led to residual anterior ankle instability. The function also deteriorated with time.

To address some of the issues of earlier reported non-anatomical reconstructions, the Chrisman-Snook reconstruction splits Peroneus Brevis proximally and passes a slip anterior to posterior distal fibula inserting on to calcaneus. This more closely approximates an anatomical repair without de-functioning the Peroneus brevis. Snook modified the Chrisman to include suturing of the end of tendon to anterior fibula, drill hole to calcaneus and gentle eversion rather than forced. Excellent results were reported in 38 of the 48 ankles with mean follow up of 10 years.

Snook GA, Chrisman OD, Wilson TC. Long-term results of the Chrisman-Snook operation for reconstruction of the lateral ligaments of the ankle. J Bone Joint Surg Am. 1985;67(1):1–7.

Comparative studies report similar short term results between anatomical and non-anatomical reconstructions. In addition, higher overall complications have been seen with non-anatomical repairs and long term studies indicate a decline in function, increased pain and stiffness. Some surgeons consider high impact sports men with instability as appropriate candidates for Chrisman-Snook repair given its increased resistance to inversion and relative hindfoot stiffness.

Krips R, van Dijk CN, Halasi PT, et al. *Long-term outcome of anatomical reconstruction versus tenodesis for the treatment of chronic anterolateral instability of the ankle joint: a multicenter study. Foot Ankle Int. 2001;22(5):415–21.*

There are currently no large long-term comparative studies comparing anatomical, non-anatomical and augmented repairs with synthetic grafts.

Osteochondral Lesion of the Ankle

The aetiology of non-traumatic osteochondral lesion of the ankle is unknown, but it may be related to a primary ischaemic event. Non-traumatic lesions can be familial. The majority of osteochondral lesions occur after a definite injury, but some have no clear history of injury. Most lesions occur on the talus, but about 10% occur on the tibial plafond, often as 'kissing lesions' with a talar defect. Only 50% of lesions are visible on plain radiographs.

Talar lesions usually occur in two distinct regions:

- Medial lesions constitute 70% of talar lesions. These lesions are deep and cup-shaped. They typically occur in the posterior half of the Talus. About 50% of cases have a history of injury.
- Lateral lesions constitute 30% of lesions and are almost always associated with injury. They often occur on the anterior third of the talar dome. These wafer-shaped superficial lesions are more likely to displace.

Classification

Osteochondral lesions were classified by Berndt and Harty in 1959 (Table 6.16) and by Hepple and colleagues in 1999 (Table 6.17). Cheng and colleagues developed the arthroscopic staging system shown in Table 6.18.

Table 6.16 Berndt and Harty classification of osteochondral lesion of the ankle

Stage	Description
1	Subchondral fracture
2	Partially detached fragment
3	Detached but undisplaced fragment
4	Displaced fragment

Table 6.17 Hepple and colleagues' classification of osteochondral lesion of the ankle

Stage	Description
1	Articular cartilage damage only
2	Cartilage injury with underlying fracture
2a	Cartilage injury with underlying fracture and edema
2b	Cartilage injury with underlying fracture but no edema
3	Detached (rim signal) but undisplaced fragment
4	Displaced fragment
5	Subchondral cyst formation

Table 6.18 Cheng and colleagues' arthroscopic staging system

Stage	Description	Stability
A	Smooth and intact, but soft or ballotable	Stable
B	Rough surface	Stable
C	Fibrillation/fissuring	Stable
D	Flap present or bone exposed	Unstable
E	Loose, undisplaced fragment	Unstable
F	Displaced fragment	Unstable

Berndt AL, Harty M. Transchondral fractures (osteochondritis dissecans) of the talus. J Bone Joint Surg Am. 1959;41-A:988–1020.

Hepple S, Winson IG, Glew D. Osteochondral lesions of the talus: a revised classification. Foot Ankle Int. 1999;20(12):789–793.

History and Examination

Most patients have an inversion injury to the lateral ligamentous complex. Patients typically present with chronic ankle pain along with intermittent swelling, locking, weakness, stiffness, instability and giving way.

Patients usually have tenderness in the joint. This can be localised, giving a clue as to the site of the lesion, or diffuse. Lateral lesions often have tenderness in the angle between the tibia and fibula, while medial lesions may have medial talar dome tenderness in plantar flexion. Anterolateral lesions may be tender when the anterolateral ankle joint is palpated with the joint in maximal plantar flexion, while tenderness behind the medial malleolus in dorsiflexion may indicate a posteromedial lesion. Occasionally a loose body may be palpable. There may be swelling or synovitis, and 30–50% of patients have ligament injuries. The anterior draw and talar tilt tests for instability may be positive.

Investigation

Plain films will show about half of all lesions and will also show other fractures, spurs and joint narrowing. Isotope bone scanning will show an area of increased activity at the site of an osteochondral lesion of the ankle, but has been largely superseded by MR and CT. MRI findings include areas of low signal intensity on T1-weighted images, which suggest sclerosis of the bed of the talus and indicate a chronic lesion. T2-weighted images reveal a rim that represents instability of the osteochondral fragment.

Management

Conservative management of osteochondral lesions of the talus should initially be attempted. This includes an initial period of immobilisation, followed by physical therapy.

Surgical treatment depends on a variety of factors, including patient characteristics (e.g., activity level, age, degenerative changes) and lesions (e.g., location, size, chronicity). Small symptomatic lesions are treated by loose-body removal, with or without stimulation of fibrocartilage growth (microfracture, curettage, abrasion or transarticular drilling). Larger lesions can be treated with fixation and bone grafting. More recently OATS, mosaicplasty and autologous chondrocyte implantation have been used successfully.

Outcomes of Surgery

Both curettage and curettage and drilling have high success rates. Curettage has a success rate of around 80%. The addition of drilling gives even better results.

Tol JL, Struijs PA, Bossuyt PM, Verhagen RA, van Dijk CN. Treatment strategies in osteochondral defects of the talar dome: a systematic review. Foot Ankle Int. 2000;21(2):119–26.

With regards to the maximal size of lesion that can be treated by arthroscopy and bone marrow stimulation, one study of 120 consecutive cases found a failure rate of 10.5% in lesions <150 mm^2 and an 80% failure rate in lesions >150 mm^2.

Lee KB, Bai LB, Chung JY, Seon JK. Arthroscopic microfracture for osteochondral lesions of the talus. Knee Surg Sports Traumatol Arthrosc. 2010;18(2):247–53.

Lesions that fail to settle or recur may be considered for further reconstructive surgery by bone and/or cartilage grafting. Osteochondral plug grafts can be harvested from the intercondylar notch of the femur or the non-weight-bearing surface of the talus. The success rate for this procedure is reportedly as high as 94%. However there is a concern regarding graft site morbidity of up to 50%. Autologous cultured chondrocyte grafts also give a high success rate. However, there is still a relative paucity of long term evidence. Current evidence contains low study numbers and variable outcomes. There needs to be an adequately powered randomised trial comparing cultured grafts to other established techniques before it can be adopted as routine practice.

Harris JD, Siston RA, Brophy RH, Lattermann C, Carey JL, Flanigan DC. Failures, re-operations, and complications after autologous chondrocyte implantation--a systematic review. Osteoarthritis Cartilage. 2011;19(7):779–91.

Lower-Limb Amputations

Most limb amputations are of the lower extremities. Foot and ankle amputations may be secondary to vascular compromise, trauma, tumour, infection or congenital deformity. Trauma is the most common cause in younger age groups and peripheral vascular disease in older patients.

Common amputations in the foot and ankle are Syme's, Boyd-Pirogoff, Boyd's, Lisfranc and Chopart amputations. All need adequate prosthetic foot and socket support because of the remaining short lever arm available.

A toe filler can be used for phalangeal and distal metatarsal amputations. Slightly proximal amputations such as toe disarticulation need a silicone boot.

Syme's Amputation

The most common indications for Syme's amputation are infection and limb deficiencies. A patent posterior tibial artery is needed for satisfactory healing of the flaps. Syme's amputation includes ankle disarticulation, removal of malleoli and anchoring the heel pad to the weight-bearing surface. The malleoli are resected flush with the joint and the fat pad is fixed to the residual bone.

Boyd-Pirogoff Amputation

Boyd's amputation provides a more solid stump because it preserves the function of the plantar heel pad. In this procedure, a portion of the calcaneus is left and fused to the tibia. The Boyd amputation can also be chosen for salvage after an unsuccessful Lisfranc or Chopart amputation.

Lisfranc Amputation

Lisfranc amputations are performed through all of the tarsometatarsal joints except the second, which should be osteotomised to preserve the stability of the medial cuneiform.

Chopart Amputation

Chopart amputation removes the fore- and mid-foot, saving the talus and calcaneus. This is an unstable amputation and is not performed for ischaemia. Chopart amputation can result in equinovarus deformity.

Transmetatarsal Amputation

Complete transmetatarsal amputations lead to a good functional result if the maximum length can be maintained to aid the terminal stance phase. Muscular balance between the dorsiflexors and plantarflexors of the foot is well conserved if a length of 3–4 cm can be kept. If necessary, the dorsal extensors can be sutured to the flexors, but only if the stumps do not have to be shortened by more than 1 cm.

The amputation levels of each metatarsal shaft should mimic the natural shape of the metatarsal bones. The amputation level should thus be more proximal laterally than medially, with a difference of 2 mm shorter beginning medially and going laterally between each stump. The recommended difference in remaining length of metatarsal stumps from medial to lateral is 2 mm between adjoining metatarsals. In order to avoid damage to the Lisfranc ligament, a minimum of 3 cm of the second metatarsal base should be maintained.

Toe and Ray Amputations

There is little disability from toe amputations. The big toe is amputated distal to insertion of the flexor hallucis brevis. The sesamoids must be stabilised, or they may potentially retract leading to uncovering of the metatarsal base.

Isolated second toe amputations are performed distal to metaphyseal flare of the proximal phalanx. This acts as a buttress and prevents the development of hallux valgus. Resections of one or more rays cause narrowing of the foot and late equinus deformity.

The first metatarsal ray may be amputated with only moderate loss of foot function.

Ankle and Foot Orthotics (AFO)

Foot and ankle orthoses can correct deformities, including distal deformities presenting from abnormal proximal joints. In addition, they transfer the weight proximally, augment muscle weakness and control motion.

The UCBL orthosis used for tibialis posterior insufficiency was introduced to control hindfoot valgus and midfoot pronation.

An AFO controls the joints of the foot and ankle and is a term used for a variety of designs. There are several different varieties:

- Posterior leaf-spring AFO—for patients requiring dorsiflexion assist for ground clearance in the swing phase.
- Solid ankle AFO—immobilises all the joints of the foot and ankle (e.g., in patients with paralysis or polio).
- Clamshell—an anterior shell is used to control the anterior portion of the leg (e.g., for pseudarthrosis of the tibia or fracture bracing).
- Floor-reaction AFO—used in patients with weak quadriceps and in those with spastic diplegia with tight gastrocnemius to improve crouch gait.
- Patellar tendon-bearing AFO—used to axially unload the foot; this is effective in treating diabetic and other neuropathic ulcers.

A Charcot restraint orthotic walker uses contact plastic technology. It is very effective in the treatment of Charcot foot.

Foot and Ankle Prosthesis

Commonly used designs for foot and ankle prostheses are the single-axis foot, solid ankle cushion heel and dynamic response foot.

The single-axis foot has an ankle hinge that provides dorsiflexion and plantar flexion. The dynamic-response foot additionally provides inversion and eversion, which are useful on uneven surfaces.

Further Reading

Alentorn-Geli E, Gil S, Bascuas I, et al. Correlation of dorsiflexion angle and plantar pressure following arthrodesis of the first metatarsophalangeal joint. Foot Ankle Int. 2013;34(4):504–11.

Alfredson H, Ohberg L, Forsgren S. Is vasculo-neural ingrowth the cause of pain in chronic Achilles tendinosis? An investigation using ultrasonography and colour Doppler, immunohistochemistry, and diagnostic injections. Knee Surg Sports Traumatol Arthrosc. 2003;11(5):334–8.

Armstrong DG, Lavery LA, Harkless LB. Validation of a diabetic wound classification system. The contribution of depth, infection, and ischemia to risk of amputation. Diabetes Care. 1998;21(5):855–9.

Baumhauer JF, Singh D, Glazebrook M, et al. Prospective, randomized, multi-centered clinical trial assessing safety and efficacy of a synthetic cartilage implant versus first metatarsophalangeal arthrodesis in advanced hallux Rigidus. Foot Ankle Int. 2016;37(5):457–69.

Berndt AL, Harty M. Transchondral fractures (osteochondritis dissecans) of the talus. J Bone Joint Surg Am. 1959;41-A:988–1020.

Boesen AP, Hansen R, Boesen MI, Malliaras P, Langberg H. Effect of high-volume injection, platelet-rich plasma, and sham treatment in chronic Midportion Achilles tendinopathy: a randomized double-blinded prospective study. Am J Sports Med. 2017;45(9):2034–43.

Bolland BJ, Sauve PS, Taylor GR. Rheumatoid forefoot reconstruction: first metatarsophalangeal joint fusion combined with Weil's metatarsal osteotomies of the lesser rays. J Foot Ankle Surg. 2008;47(2):80–8.
Bulstra GH, van Rheenen TA, Scholtes VA. Can we measure the heel bump? Radiographic evaluation of Haglund's deformity. J Foot Ankle Surg. 2015;54(3):338–40.
Carmont MR, Rees RJ, Blundell CM. Current concepts review: Freiberg's disease. Foot Ankle Int. 2009;30(2):167–76.
Chao KH, Lee CH, Lin LC. Surgery for symptomatic Freiberg's disease: extraarticular dorsal closing-wedge osteotomy in 13 patients followed for 2-4 years. Acta Orthop Scand. 1999;70(5):483–6.
Coester LM, Saltzman CL, Leupold J, Pontarelli W. Long-term results following ankle arthrodesis for post-traumatic arthritis. J Bone Joint Surg Am. 2001;83(2):219–28.
Cottino U, Collo G, Morino L, et al. Arthroscopic ankle arthrodesis: a review. Curr Rev. Musculoskelet Med. 2012;5(2):151–5.
Coughlin MJ. Treatment of bunionette deformity with longitudinal diaphyseal osteotomy with distal soft tissue repair. Foot Ankle. 1991;11(4):195–203.
Coughlin MJ. Hallux Rigidus: demographics, etiology and radiographic assessment. Foot and Ankle Int. 2003;24:731–4.
Coutts A, Kilmartin TE, Ellis MJ. The long-term patient focused outcomes of the Keller's arthroplasty for the treatment of hallux rigidus. Foot (Edinb). 2012;22(3):167–71.
Diaper R, Wong E, Metcalfe SA. The implications of biologic therapy for elective foot and ankle surgery in patients with rheumatoid arthritis. Foot. 2017;30:53–8.
Durlacher L. Corns, bunions, the diseases of nails and the general management of the feet. 1845:72.
Elmajee M, Shen Z, A'Court J, Pillai A. A systematic review of plantar plate repair in the management of lesser metatarsophalangeal joint instability. J Foot Ankle Surg. 2017;56(6):1244–8.
Erdil M, Bilsel K, Imren Y, et al. Metatarsal head resurfacing hemiarthroplasty in the treatment of advanced stage hallux rigidus: outcomes in the short-term. Acta Orthop Traumatol Turc. 2012;46(4):281–5.
Fuchs S, Sandmann C, Skwara A, Chylarecki C. Quality of life 20 years after arthrodesis of the ankle. A study of adjacent joints. J Bone Joint Surg Br. 2003;85(7):994–8.
Grennan DM, Gray J, Loudon J, Fear S. Methotrexate and early postoperative complications in patients with rheumatoid arthritis undergoing elective orthopaedic surgery. Ann Rheum Dis. 2001;60(3):214–7.
Haddad SL, Coetzee JC, Estok R, Fahrbach K, Banel D, Nalysnyk L. Intermediate and long-term outcomes of total ankle arthroplasty and ankle arthrodesis. A systematic review of the literature. J Bone Joint Surg Am. 2007;89(9):1899–905.
Harris E, Moroney P, Tourne Y. Arthrodesis of the first metatarsophalangeal joint-a biomechanical comparison of four fixation techniques. Foot Ankle Surg. 2017;23(4):268–74.
Harris JD, Siston RA, Brophy RH, Lattermann C, Carey JL, Flanigan DC. Failures, re-operations, and complications after autologous chondrocyte implantation--a systematic review. Osteoarthr Cartil. 2011;19(7):779–91.
Helal B, Gibb P. Freiberg's disease: a suggested pattern of management. Foot Ankle. 1987;8(2):94–102.
Hepple S, Winson IG, Glew D. Osteochondral lesions of the talus: a revised classification. Foot Ankle Int. 1999;20(12):789–93.
Jahss MH. The abnormal plantigrade foot. Orthop Rev. 1978;7:31–7.
Johnson KA, Strom DE. Tibialis posterior tendon dysfunction. Clin Orthop Relat Res. 1989;39:196–206.
Kang S, Thordarson DB, Charlton TP. Insertional Achilles tendinitis and Haglund's deformity. Foot Ankle Int. 2012;33(6):487–91.
Karlsson J, Eriksson BI, Bergsten T, Rudholm O, Sward L. Comparison of two anatomic reconstructions for chronic lateral instability of the ankle joint. Am J Sports Med. 1997;25(1):48–53.
Komenda GA, Ferkel RD. Arthroscopic findings associated with the unstable ankle. Foot Ankle Int. 1999;20(11):708–13.
Krips R, van Dijk CN, Halasi PT, et al. Long-term outcome of anatomical reconstruction versus tenodesis for the treatment of chronic anterolateral instability of the ankle joint: a multicenter study. Foot Ankle Int. 2001;22(5):415–21.
Kushioka J, Hirao M, Tsuboi H, et al. Modified scarf osteotomy with medial capsule interposition for hallux valgus in rheumatoid arthritis: a study of cases including severe first metatarsophalangeal joint destruction. J Bone Joint Surg Am. 2018;100(9):765–76.
Lee KB, Bai LB, Chung JY, Seon JK. Arthroscopic microfracture for osteochondral lesions of the talus. Knee Surg Sports Traumatol Arthrosc. 2010;18(2):247–53.
Lin MT, Chiang CF, Wu CH, Hsu HH, Tu YK. Meta-analysis comparing autologous blood-derived products (including platelet-rich plasma) injection versus placebo in patients with Achilles tendinopathy. Arthroscopy. 2018;34(6):1966–75.
Maffulli N, Longo UG, Spiezia F, Denaro V. Minimally invasive surgery for Achilles tendon pathologies. Open Access J Sports Med. 2010;1:95–103.
Mason LW, Tanaka H. The first tarsometatarsal joint and its association with hallux valgus. Bone Joint Res. 2012;1(6):99–103.
Maynou C, Szymanski C, Thiounn A. The adult cavus foot. EFORT Open Rev. 2017;2(5):221–9.
Monteagudo M, Maceira E, Garcia-Virto V, Canosa R. Chronic plantar fasciitis: plantar fasciotomy versus gastrocnemius recession. Int Orthop. 2013;37(9):1845–50.
Morgan S, Ng A, Clough T. The long-term outcome of silastic implant arthroplasty of the first metatarsophalangeal joint: a retrospective analysis of one hundred and eight feet. Int Orthop. 2012;36(9):1865–9.

Morton TG. A peculiar and painful affection of the fourth metatarso-phalangeal articulation. Am J Med Sci. 1876;71:37–45.

Myerson MS. Adult acquired flatfoot deformity: treatment of dysfunction of the posterior tibial tendon. Instr Course Lect. 1997;46:393–405.

Myerson MS, Komenda GA. Results of hallux varus correction using an extensor hallucis brevis tenodesis. Foot Ankle Int. 1996;17(1):21–7.

Naraghi R, Bremner A, Slack-Smith L, Bryant A. The relationship between foot posture index, ankle equinus, body mass index and intermetatarsal neuroma. J Foot Ankle Res. 2016;9:46.

Osti L, Del Buono A, Maffulli N. Arthroscopic debridement of the ankle for mild to moderate osteoarthritis: a midterm follow-up study in former professional soccer players. J Orthop Surg Res. 2016;11:37.

Paavola M, Orava S, Leppilahti J, Kannus P, Jarvinen M. Chronic Achilles tendon overuse injury: complications after surgical treatment. An analysis of 432 consecutive patients. Am J Sports Med. 2000;28(1):77–82.

Pagenstert GVV, Hintermann B. Lateral ankle ligament reconstruction with free Plantaris tendon graft. Techniques in Foot and Ankle Surg. 2005;4(2):104–12.

Pagenstert G, Knupp M, Valderrabano V, Hintermann B. Realignment surgery for valgus ankle osteoarthritis. Oper Orthop Traumatol. 2009;21(1):77–87.

Paley D, Lamm BM, Purohit RM, Specht SC. Distraction arthroplasty of the ankle--how far can you stretch the indications? Foot Ankle Clin. 2008;13(3):471–84.

Paterson R, Cohen B, Taylor D, Bourne A, Black J. Reconstruction of the lateral ligaments of the ankle using semi-tendinosis graft. Foot Ankle Int. 2000;21(5):413–9.

Pedersen E, Pinsker E, Younger AS, et al. Outcome of total ankle arthroplasty in patients with rheumatoid arthritis and noninflammatory arthritis. A multicenter cohort study comparing clinical outcome and safety. J Bone Joint Surg Am. 2014;96(21):1768–75.

Polzer H, Polzer S, Brumann M, Mutschler W, Regauer M. Hallux rigidus: joint preserving alternatives to arthrodesis–a review of the literature. World J Orthop. 2014;5(1):6–13.

Rompe JD, Furia J, Maffulli N. Eccentric loading versus eccentric loading plus shock-wave treatment for midportion achilles tendinopathy: a randomized controlled trial. Am J Sports Med. 2009;37(3):463–70.

Roukis TS. The need for surgical revision after isolated cheilectomy for hallux rigidus: a systematic review. J Foot Ankle Surg. 2010;49(5):465–70.

Roukis TS. Nonunion after arthrodesis of the first metatarsal-phalangeal joint: a systematic review. J Foot Ankle Surg. 2011;50(6):710–3.

Sackley C, Disler PB, Turner-Stokes L, Wade DT, Brittle N, Hoppitt T. Rehabilitation interventions for foot drop in neuromuscular disease. Cochrane Database Syst Rev. 2009;3:CD003908.

Saltzman CL, Mann RA, Ahrens JE, et al. Prospective controlled trial of STAR total ankle replacement versus ankle fusion: initial results. Foot Ankle Int. 2009;30(7):579–96.

Salvioli S, Guidi M, Marcotulli G. The effectiveness of conservative, non-pharmacological treatment, of plantar heel pain: a systematic review with meta-analysis. Foot (Edinb). 2017;33:57–67.

Schuh R, Hofstaetter J, Krismer M, Bevoni R, Windhager R, Trnka HJ. Total ankle arthroplasty versus ankle arthrodesis. Comparison of sports, recreational activities and functional outcome. Int Orthop. 2012;36(6):1207–14.

Shibata T, Tada K, Hashizume C. The results of arthrodesis of the ankle for leprotic neuroarthropathy. J Bone Joint Surg Am. 1990;72(5):749–56.

Silfverskiold N. Reduction of the uncrossed two-joints muscles of the leg to one-joint muscles in spastic conditions. Acta Chir Scand. 1924;56:315–30.

Snook GA, Chrisman OD, Wilson TC. Long-term results of the Chrisman-Snook operation for reconstruction of the lateral ligaments of the ankle. J Bone Joint Surg Am. 1985;67(1):1–7.

Sreekumar R, Gray J, Kay P, Grennan DM. Methotrexate and post operative complications in patients with rheumatoid arthritis undergoing elective orthopaedic surgery--a ten year follow-up. Acta Orthop Belg. 2011;77(6):823–6.

Tol JL, Struijs PA, Bossuyt PM, Verhagen RA, van Dijk CN. Treatment strategies in osteochondral defects of the talar dome: a systematic review. Foot Ankle Int. 2000;21(2):119–26.

Wagner FW Jr. The diabetic foot. Orthopedics. 1987;10(1):163–72.

Wilson F, Walshe M, O'Dwyer T, Bennett K, Mockler D, Bleakley C. Exercise, orthoses and splinting for treating Achilles tendinopathy: a systematic review with meta-analysis. Br J Sports Med. 2018;52(24):1564–74.

Wood PL, Karski MT, Watmough P. Total ankle replacement: the results of 100 mobility total ankle replacements. J Bone Joint Surg Br. 2010;92(7):958–62.

Wu KK. Morton's interdigital neuroma: a clinical review of its etiology, treatment, and results. J Foot Ankle Surg. 1996;35(2):112–9.

Hand

7

Julia Street and Sanjeev Agarwal

Extensor Tendon Injury

The dorsum of the wrist and hand contains 12 main extensor/abductor tendons that run in 6 dorsal compartments under the extensor retinaculum. These are illustrated in Fig. 7.1. The tendons are abductor pollicis longus (APL) and extensor pollicis brevis (EPB) in the first compartment; extensor carpi radialis longus (ECRL) and extensor carpi radialis brevis (ECRB) in the second compartment; extensor pollicis longus (EPL) in the third compartment; extensor digitorum (ED) and extensor indices (EI) in the fourth compartment; extensor digiti minimi (EDM) in the fifth compartment; and extensor carpi ulnaris (ECU) in the sixth compartment.

The location of an extensor tendon injury is described in zones in relation to the wrist and finger joints (Table 7.2). The zones for the thumb are defined differently to zones in the fingers with T I being IP joint, T II is proximal phalanx, T III is thumb MCPJ, T IV is thumb metacarpal and T V is carpal region (Fig. 7.2).

Extensor tendons derive vascularity from three sources (Table 7.1).

Extensor tendons are susceptible to injury as they are thin structures and have a superficial location. The most commonly injured digit is the middle finger and the most frequently injured zone is Zone VI.

The anatomy of the dorsal expansion is illustrated in Fig. 7.3. The lateral bands normally help in DIPJ extension. The triangular ligament prevents lateral bands from volar subluxation.

Diagnostic Pitfalls

Two factors should be considered when examining an extensor tendon injury:

The extensor digitorum communis tendons are also cross-connected to their adjacent neighbours by tendon slips called juncturae tendinum. An injury that divides an extensor tendon proximal to these juncturae will still allow active extension of the affected finger from an adjacent extensor tendon pulling through the juncturae.

A proximal interphalangeal joint (PIPJ) can still be actively extended via the lateral bands even if the central slip is completely divided. This can be differentiated by performing Elson's test (see below).

Extensor Tendon Repair

Indications for extensor tendon repair are–

1. Tendon laceration >50%.

J. Street
Wales Orthopaedic Program, Cardiff, UK
e-mail: juliastreet@doctors.org.uk

S. Agarwal (✉)
University Hospital of Wales, Consultant Orthopaedic Surgeon, Cardiff, UK

S. Agarwal (ed.), *Current Orthopaedic Practice*, https://doi.org/10.1007/978-3-030-78529-1_7

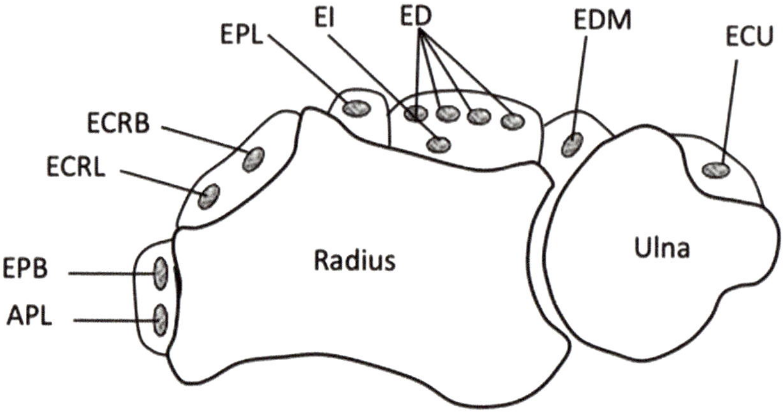

Fig. 7.1 Extensor compartments of the wrist

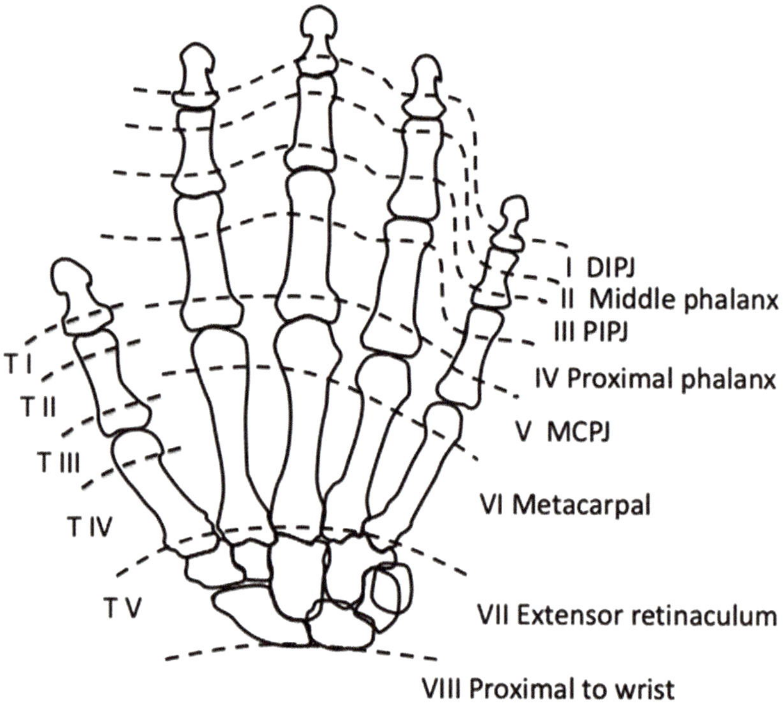

Fig. 7.2 Zones of extensor tendon injury

Table 7.1 Vascular supply to extensor tendons

Proximal to the dorsal retinaculum	Muscular arteries
Under the dorsal retinaculum	Synovial diffusion and mesotendon
Distal to the dorsal retinaculum	Arterial branches from the paratenon

Table 7.2 Leddy and Packer classification of FDP avulsion (Zone 1 injury)

Type I	The tendon end retracts into the palm	Vascularity of tendon impaired. Repair within 10 days
Type II	The tendon end retracts to the level of the PIPJ and rests against the A3 pulley	Intact vincula prevent further retraction. Repair within 6 weeks
Type III	Avulsion of a large bony fragment; A4 and A5 pulleys prevent retraction	Repair within 6 weeks

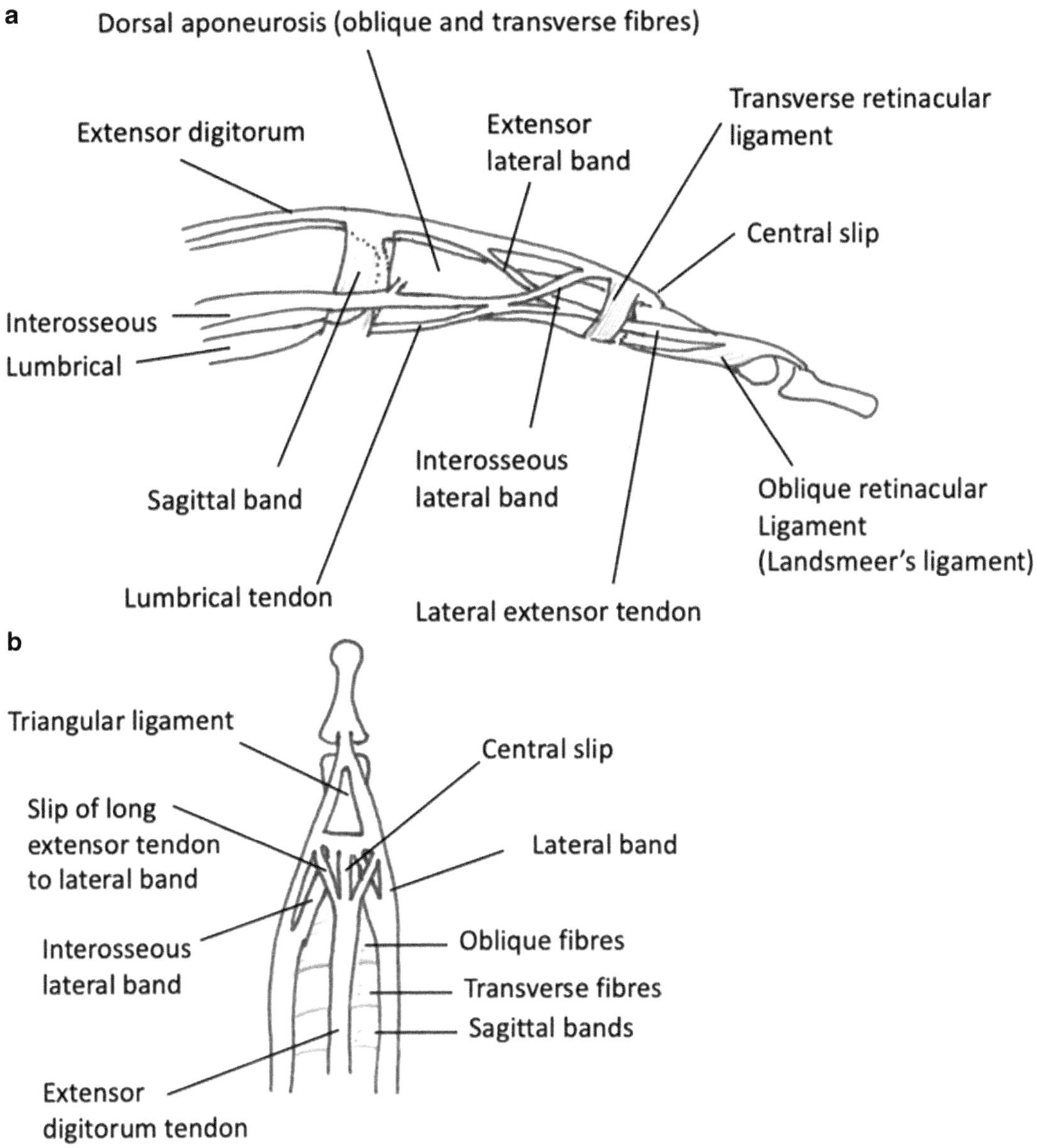

Fig. 7.3 (**a** and **b**): Anatomy of the extensor attachment on the dorsal aspect

2. Tendon laceration <50% with significantly decreased strength compared with contralateral finger.
3. Tendon laceration associated with significant overlying skin loss, joint space penetration, or bony fracture.

The method of repair differs according to the zone of the tendon injury.

Proximal to the middle of the proximal phalanx (zones IV–VII), the tendon is oval or cylindrical. A multistrand (4–6) 4/0 non-absorbable grasping or locking core suture can be used. This can be supplemented by a circumferential 6/0 monofilament suture.

Distal to the middle of the proximal phalanx (zone II and IV), the central slip is flattened. The lateral bands and their common tendon to the distal phalanx are also flattened and ribbon-like. A non-absorbable 4/0 or 5/0 suture is used as a continuous running suture. The joint must be immobilised for 4 weeks postoperatively either with transarticular wire or splint.

Repair tips to consider are as follows:

- Lacerations to the extensor digitorum communis tendons (especially distal to the juncturae tendinum) cause minimal retraction.
- Lacerations to the extensor pollicis longus tendons proximal to the metacarpophalangeal joint (MCPJ) are likely to cause retraction to Lister's tubercle. A separate incision at that level is often needed to retrieve the proximal tendon.
- A round-bodied non-cutting needle should be used, otherwise the needle will slice the tendon and possibly the core sutures.

Post-Operative

Historically immobilisation has been the mainstay of therapy following extensor tendon injuries as the repair site is protected from excessive motion which could threaten the repair.

CY Ng. Rehabilitation Regimens Following Surgical Repair of Extensor Tendon Injuries of the Hand—A Systematic Review of Controlled Trials. J Hand Microsurg. 2012:4(2);65–73. Early mobilisation regimens (active and passive) achieved quicker recovery of motion than static immobilisation in the post-operative treatment of extensor tendon injuries in zones IV—VI.

Management of Closed Tendon Avulsions

Mallet Finger (Zone 1)

Mallet finger is an avulsion of the extensor digitorum longus from the base of distal phalanx. This can be either pure tendinous avulsion, or with a bone fragment. The injury is caused by forced flexion of the extended DIP and results in loss of active DIP extension.

The management of mallet finger is summarised in Fig. 7.4.

A single dorsal distal phalanx avulsion fracture without subluxation can be ignored, irrespective of its size. Treatment is the same as with no fracture: continuous hyperextension splinting

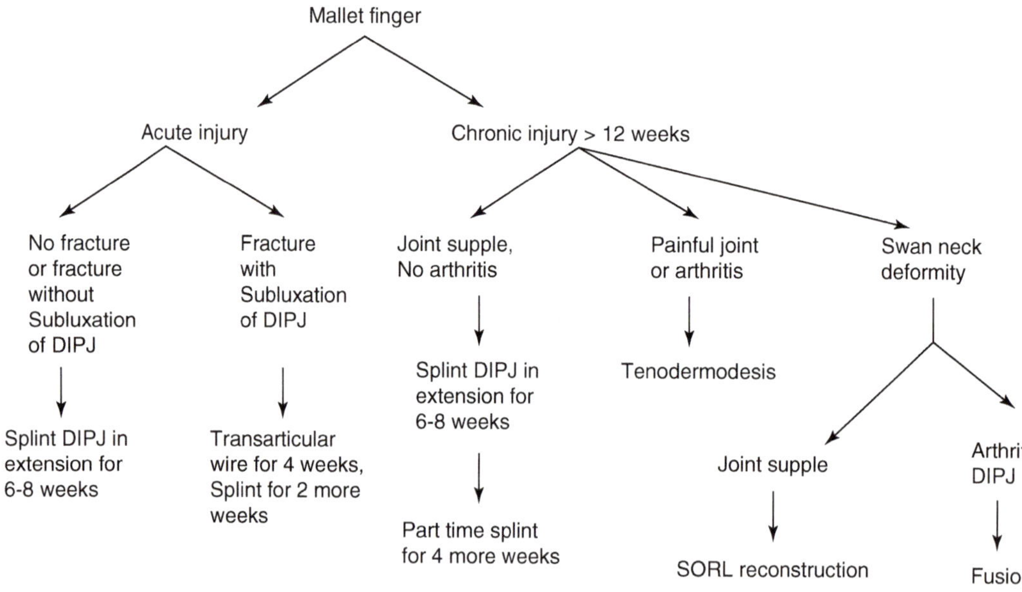

Fig. 7.4 Management of mallet finger

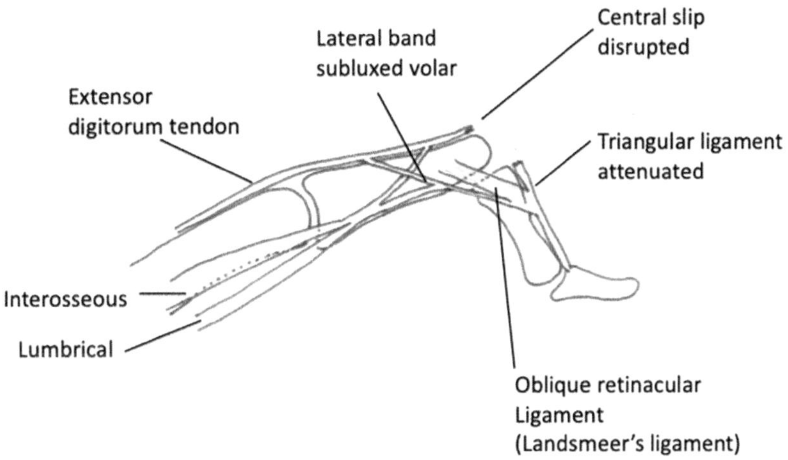

Fig. 7.5 Pathology of Boutonniere deformity

for 6–8 weeks. An X-ray must be taken in the splint. If the distal phalanx is subluxed in a palmar direction then the DIPJ is reduced in extension and held with a transarticular wire for 4 weeks and then a splint for a further 2 weeks.

Tenodermodesis is excision of a 3–4 mm elliptical wedge of skin, scar tissue and dorsal capsule of the DIPJ. The wound is closed in one layer and a transarticular K wire is used to maintain DIPJ extension.

Swan neck deformity in late presentations can be managed by Fowler's tenotomy or Spiral Oblique Retinacular Ligament (SORL) reconstruction. Fowler's procedure is tenotomy of the central slip, which can lead to a boutonniere deformity. SORL reconstruction has good results.

Boutonniere Deformity (Zone III)

The Boutonniere deformity (French for 'button hole') is described as a flexion deformity of the PIPJ and hyperextension of the DIPJ. It is rare for an acute central slip avulsion to present with a classic Boutonniere deformity. The deformity tends to develop in the weeks and months following injury. Rheumatoid patients may have central slip rupture following capsular distension. Pseudo-boutonniere deformity is flexion contracture of the PIPJ without DIPJ hyperextension.

The components of Boutonniere deformity are disruption of the central slip, attenuation of the triangular ligament and palmar migration of the lateral bands (Fig. 7.5).

In the acute setting a central slip avulsion can be diagnosed by tenderness over the central slip insertion. Palmar dislocation (diagnosed clinically or radiologically) of the PIPJ will be evident. The central slip has to detach for palmar subluxation.

The Elson test is done by holding the PIPJ at 90 degrees. Resistance is applied to prevent PIPJ extension by holding the middle phalanx. If the central slip is intact the lateral bands are not recruited and the DIPJ remains floppy. If the central slip is detached the DIPJ firmly extends.

The Zancolli test is done with the PIPJ extended. If flexion of the DIP is not possible, it correlates with poor outcome.

Treatment

The treatment plan is outlined in Fig. 7.6. Splintage for acute deformities should allow active DIPJ flexion.

For chronic deformity, the lateral bands are mobilised at the time of reconstruction. A variety of reconstructive options have been proposed including tenotomy of the tendon distal to triangular ligament; repositioning of lateral bands dorsally (Salvi); centralization of lateral bands with release of extrinsic and interosseous tendons (Littler); FDS to reconstruct central slip (Stack);

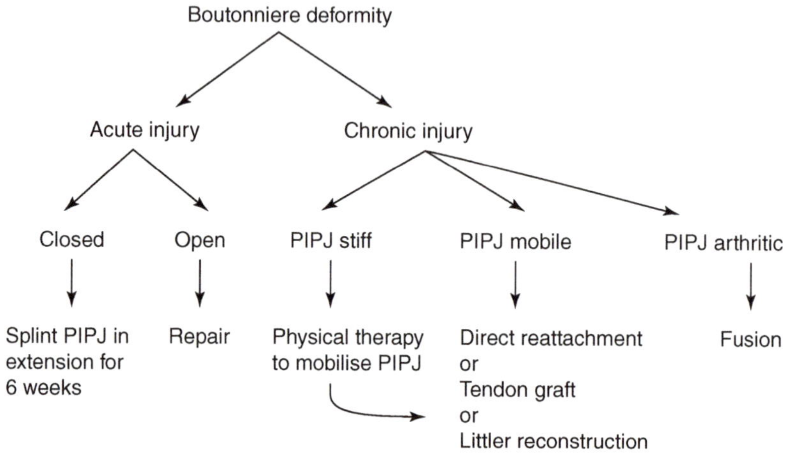

Fig. 7.6 Management of Boutonniere deformity

use of palmaris longus graft to reconstruct central slip (Hou); and the use of lateral band of one side to reconstruct the central slip (Matev).

Extension of the PIP should not be gained at the cost of losing flexion.

Fight Bite Injuries

These injuries are sustained when an individual punches another individual, and a tooth penetrates the skin, and often the sagittal band too. Such injuries can be associated with extensor tendon injury. Common site is the dorsum of index or middle finger MCPJ.

The position of the structures on the dorsum of the hand changes from flexion to extension (Fig. 7.7). With relative movement between the extensor tendon and joint capsule from flexion to extension, the path of contamination is not directly evident and a formal washout is needed in the operation theatre.

The human oral cavity houses a range of microorganisms and these can lead to infection in the wound. Common organisms are *staphylococcus aureus* and *streptococcus viridans*. *Eikenella corrodens* is a gram negative anaerobe, and a common organism in fight bite infections.

Radiographs are helpful to check for fractures or any foreign body.

Management is by intravenous antibiotics (augmentin), urgent exploration, and washout. The wound is left open for drainage.

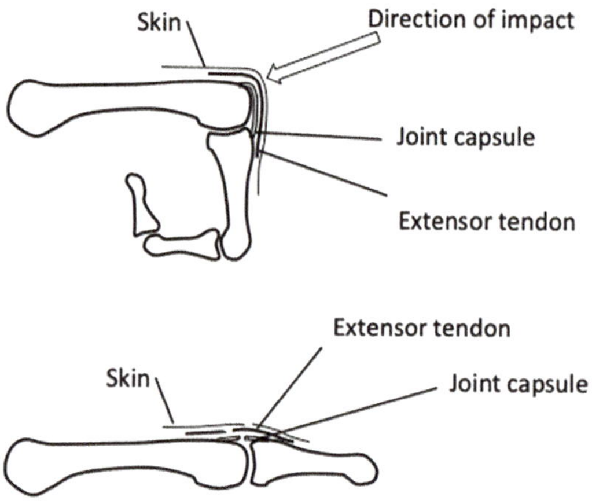

Fig. 7.7 Fight bite injuries

At surgery the finger should be assessed for an extensor tendon injury, traumatic MCPJ arthrotomy, metacarpal head or neck fracture, MCPJ chondral injury and any retained foreign body.

Extensor Pollicis Longus (EPL) Rupture

This specific tendon rupture can occur following conservative management of an undisplaced distal radial fracture. It usually occurs 3 weeks to 3 months following the injury.

This is treated with an EIP to EPL tendon transfer. A transverse incision is made over metacarpal head of index finger to harvest the extensor indicis tendon. A second incision is made to connect the distal stump of EPL to the harvested indicis tendon (Fig. 7.8). If the rupture of EPL is distal, a further incision is made to locate the stump and the indicis tendon is tunnelled to the repair site. Adequate tension should be restored.

Flexor Tendon Injuries

Flexor Tendon Nutrition

The vascular supply to the flexor tendons mainly comes from the vincula on the dorsal surface of the tendons. The digital artery gives off splits into four transverse branches along its course. Two branches are for the profundus tendon and two for the superficialis tendon (Fig. 7.9). The vascular supply is from the dorsal surface of the tendon.

Both tendons have avascular segments over the proximal phalanx and the flexor digitorum profundus (FDP) has an additional avascular segment over the middle phalanx.

Synovial fluid diffusion is another mechanism for tendon nutrition. When the digit is flexed and extended, a pumping mechanism known as imbibition moves the fluid into tendon interstices through rigid conduits on the surface.

Flexor Tendon Healing

Tendon healing occurs through the action of fibroblasts. There is an intrinsic and extrinsic healing process. Extrinsic healing leads to more adhesion formation.

Tendon healing has three phases.

The inflammatory phase extends to 3 to 5 days after repair. In this phase, the strength of repair depends on the strength of the sutures and minimally on the fibrin clot.

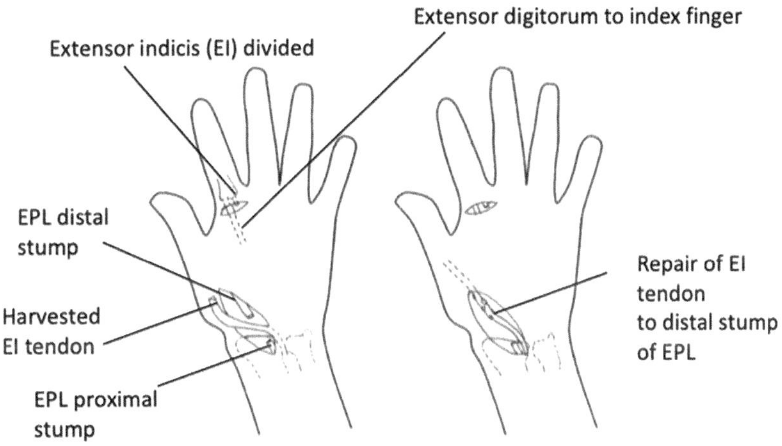

Fig. 7.8 Transfer of extensor indicis (EI) to EPL

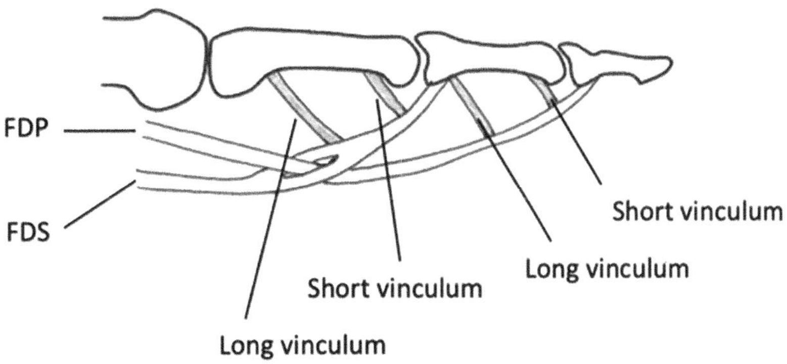

Fig. 7.9 Vascular supply for flexor tendons

The fibroblastic or collagen-producing phase begins on day 5 and lasts for 3 to 6 weeks. The fibroblasts proliferate, collagen is produced and new capillaries form. The tendon loses strength in the first 5–21 days.

The third phase is remodeling or maturation phase and lasts for 6 to 9 months. The collagen fibres become longitudinally oriented and stronger.

Biomechanics

Five annular (A1–A5) and three cruciate pulleys (C1–C3) prevent bowstringing of the tendon on flexion (Fig. 7.10).

A1, A3, A5 overlie the MCPJ, PIPJ and DIPJ, respectively. A2 and A4 arise from the periosteum of the proximal and middle phalanx, and are critical for mechanical function. A2 is almost 2 cm long and almost 50% can be resected without compromising function. Cruciate pulleys are thin and collapse to allow annular pulleys to approximate each other during digital flexion.

Zones of Injury

The location of a flexor tendon injury is described in zones (Fig. 7.11).

Clinical Features

The resting posture of the hand and the digital cascade is observed. Loss of finger flexion may be evident in flexor tendon injury.

For the FDP, flexion at DIPJ is checked keeping PIPJ stabilised in extension. For FDS, the patient is asked to flex at the PIPJ of the finger keeping other three fingers stabilised in extension. Keeping other fingers in extension will neutralise FDP. A flail DIP joint of the finger being examined indicates FDS is acting to flex the

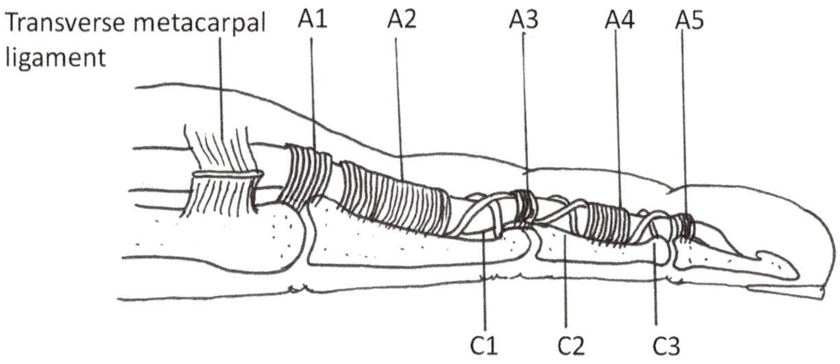

Fig. 7.10 Pulleys of the flexor tendon of the finger

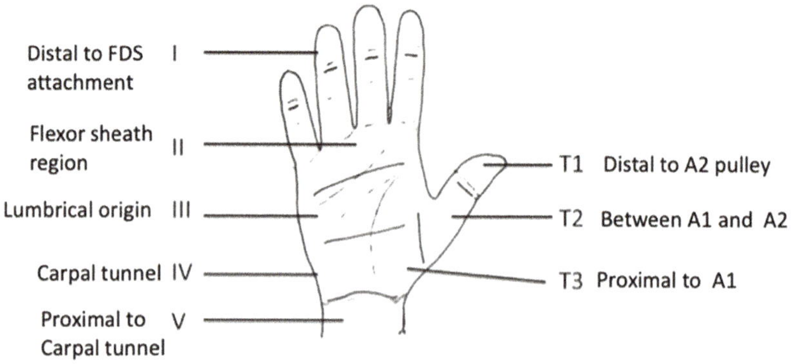

Fig. 7.11 Zones of flexor tendon injury

PIPJ. If the DIPJ is flexing, it implies the FDP is being recruited as the FDS is non-functional.

Principles of Flexor Tendon Repair

Repair is not an emergency and delayed primary repair has better results. Repair should not be delayed more than 3 weeks.

It is better to repair both the flexor digitorum superficialis (FDS) and FDP if both are cut. Badly contaminated wounds or wounds with skin loss should not be sutured primarily. Associated fractures should be stably fixed and primary repair performed. If there is concern regarding infection, repair should be delayed for a few days.

Wound Extension

Adequate exposure is needed to assess the extent of the injury, retrieve the tendons and perform the repair. The most common incision is a 'zigzag' or Brunner incision (Fig. 7.12).

Retrieval of Tendon Ends

Tendon ends retract and need to be retrieved with minimal damage to the tendon. Retrieval methods may be—proximal to distal milking of the tendon; reverse Esmarch bandage; skin hook to pull the tendon if the end is visible in the sheath; or an infant catheter to railroad the tendon through. A proximal incision is made and an infant catheter is passed from the distal wound through the sheath and retrieved from the proximal wound. The tendon is sutured to the catheter and the catheter is then pulled distally.

Once retrieved, the tendon can be transfixed through a pulley using a hypodermic needle.

Suture Methods for Repair

The strength of repair is proportional to the number of strands crossing the repair site. Various methods for core suture have been described (Fig. 7.13).

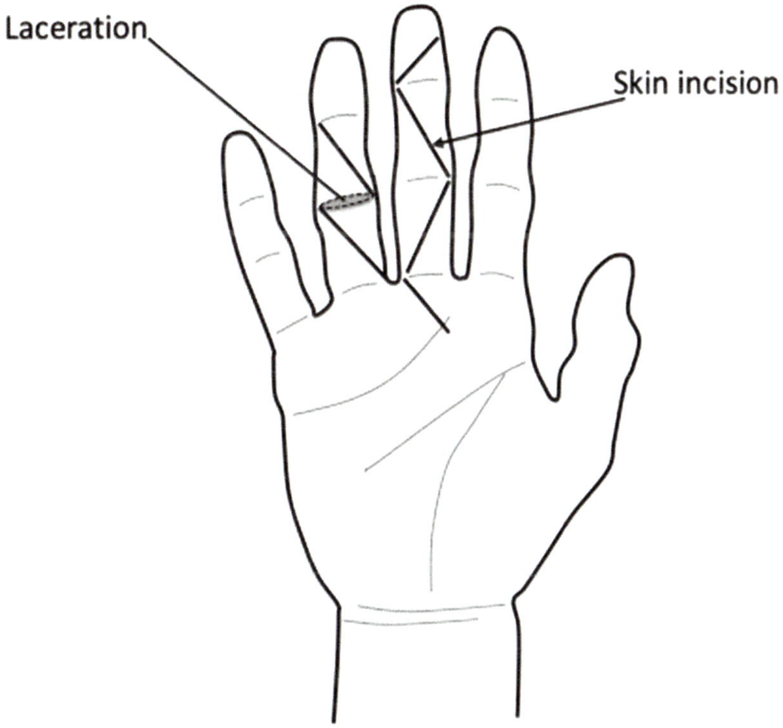

Fig. 7.12 Incision for flexor tendon repair

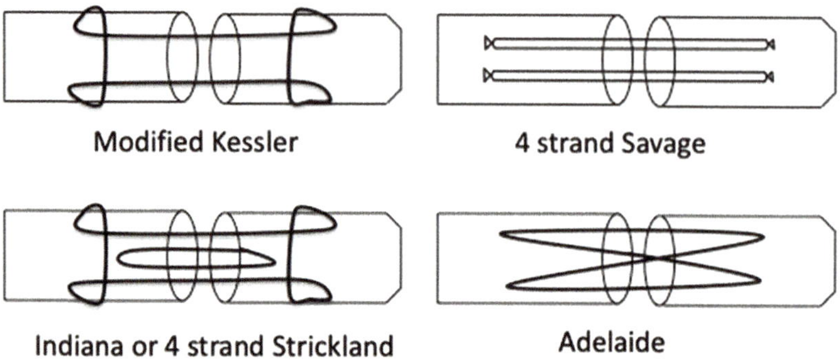

Fig. 7.13 Common methods of tendon repair

Repair

Core suture (4 or 6 strands) with a 4–0 braided polyester suture is most commonly used with a non-cutting needle. It is used as a grasping suture, which can be locked at the grasping site (Savage or Adelaide repair) or unlocked (Kessler). Anchor points, or 'purchase' on the tendon should be 10 mm from the ends of the cut tendon. This refers to the transverse segment of the suture.

All strands should be kept under a similar tension and knots should be located outside the repair site if possible. If a repair fails, it is usually at the knots. Partial lacerations of less than 60% do not need a core suture.

Peripheral epitendinous suture enhances the strength of repair by 10–50% and reduces gaps. A 6–0 monofilament suture is used with a non-cutting needle.

There is no definite advantage to repairing the tendon sheath, although it may improve synovial nutrition and act as a barrier to external adhesions. However, it may also cause narrowing and restrict gliding.

The A2 and A4 pulleys must be preserved as a minimum. If the repair is likely to catch on the pulley entrance, pulleys may be vented (partially divided) facing the repair.

Avulsion of the Flexor Digitorum Profundus Tendon: Zone 1 Injury

Avulsion of the FDP tendon usually occurs in athletes—known as 'rugger jersey finger'. The tendon avulses as the object being grasped (e.g., an opponent's shirt) is pulled out of the hand. The forced extension thus occurs during maximal contraction of the FDP. The ring finger is most commonly affected.

Classification of avulsion of the FDP tendon is based on the level of proximal retraction (Table 7.2).

In zone I injuries, only the FDP is divided or avulsed. The A5 pulley may have to be opened to find the distal stump. If the distal stump is too short (<1 cm), reattachment is performed directly to the bone. The osteoperiosteal flap is elevated and parallel oblique holes are drilled with a 1.2 mm K-wire through the distal phalanx, exiting through the nail. A straight needle 3–0 suture is placed in the proximal tendon end and pulled out through the bone holes. The suture is then tied over a button on top of the nail.

Zone II–V Repair

Zone II–V repair involves standard repair of the FDS and FDP tendons, preserving (as a minimum) the A2 and A4 pulleys if at the zone II level. A four strand repair with epitendinous suture is used for both tendons, and this will allow early mobilisation.

Zone 3 has better results compared to zone 2 given the absence of pulleys in this region. Lumbricals arise from FDP in zone 3.

Postoperative Management

Light dressings should be applied to the fingers. A dorsal slab is applied with the wrist in neutral and MCPJs are flexed at 45 degrees. The fingers are not bandaged to the slab to allow unresisted accidental flexion in the perioperative period.

Physical therapy should start within 3 days of repair. There are a number of different therapy regimens, of which the Belfast regimen is one. The principles are early active and passive motion protected by a dorsal finger and wrist extension block splint. Early motion leads to rapid healing, fewer adhesions and improved excursion. In tendon repairs that are mobilised early there is increased DNA content, collagen production and remodeling.

Small JO, Brennen MD, Colville J. Early active mobilisation following flexor tendon repair in zone 2. J Hand Surg Br 1989;14(4):383–91. 138 flexor tendon injuries treated with mobilisation within 48 hours. Excellent or good active range of movement in 77% patients. 9.4% had failed repair requiring secondary repair.

Complications

Rupture requires prompts re-exploration and repair. Typically, this happens at day 10 (6–12 days) as this is when the tendon ends soften, and the strength of the repair is entirely dependent on the sutures used and their hold in tendon tissue.

Joint contractures require splintage and physiotherapy.

Adhesions can form and if there is no improvement for several months, tenolysis is considered. In some series, almost half the patients may require tenolysis.

Quadriga effect is characterised by an active flexion lag in fingers adjacent to a digit with a previously repaired FDP tendon. This is due to shortening of the repaired flexor tendon. Release of the tight FDP may be needed.

Lumbrical plus finger occurs following a lax FDP tendon repair. While making a fist, the injured finger does not flex as much as normal fingers, and tends to stick out.

Finger Tip Injuries

The principles of managing finger tip injuries are.

- Preservation of sensation.
- Preservation of length.
- Provision of durable cover.
- Minimisation of hypersensitivity.
- Rapid return to work

Improper treatment may result in stiffness & long-term functional loss of the affected digits.

Length preservation is advisable in the thumb but is not always necessary in the fingers.

Digital-Tip Amputations with Skin or Pulp Loss Only

In situations with skin or pulp loss only, primary closure is advisable if sutures can be placed without much tension. Alternatively, non-adherent dressings are used and can be changed periodically.

Digital-Tip Amputations with Exposed Bone

Skeletal shortening and primary closure is the preferred treatment for digital-tip amputations with exposed bone. The nail bed should not be pulled distally to cover the distal phalanx. Instead, the nail bed is cut back to the level of bone loss so that it does not curve over the end of the bone, thus avoiding formation of a 'hook nail'.

Skin Flaps

The use of skin flaps to cover exposed bone is associated with a significant complication rate and is of questionable benefit. It is considered to preserve length when bone is exposed. A number of skin-flap methods that can be used to cover exposed bone in digital-tip amputations (Table 7.3).

Complications

The possible complications are.

Hypersensitivity. This can be addressed with a desensitisation program when the wound has healed.

Table 7.3 Methods of skin flap cover for digital-tip amputations

Skin-flap method	Description
Atasoy–Kleinert volar V-Y flap (5 mm advancement)	Better for volar distal–dorsal proximal oblique injuries Cut full-thickness skin only. The base of the triangle is sutured to the cut end of the nail bed, and the rest is closed as a 'Y'
Volar advancement flap (15 mm advancement)	The volar skin is advanced on the neurovascular pedicle
Cross-finger pedicle flap	The flap can be based distally, proximally, laterally or medially A full-thickness flap is raised off the extensor tendons. It is reflected over and sutured to the palmar defect on three sides. The fourth side is closed in the second stage The donor site is covered with a full-thickness skin graft The pedicle is detached at 2 weeks
Thenar flap	Can be used for the tips of index and long fingers Usually reserved for children; there is a risk of finger stiffness in adults

Stiffness is managed by hand therapy.

Decreased sensation. Advancement flaps and conservatively treated pulp loss often retain good sensation. Full-thickness skin grafting will usually provide only protective sensation.

Cold intolerance can develop in all finger tip injuries. In most patients it resolves after 2–3 years.

Flap failure can be due to either inadequate arterial or venous flow.

Nail deformity like a hook nail or nail spike.

Structure of the Nail

The structure of the nail is illustrated in Fig. 7.14. The germinal matrix gives rise to the nail plate while the sterile matrix helps increase the thickness of the nail plate. The lunula is the junction of germinal matrix and sterile matrix. The eponychium is the distal end of the proximal nail fold. Hyponychium is at the junction of the skin and distal nail bed. Paronychium is the lateral nail fold.

Nail Bed Injury

Nail bed injuries are common. The nail plate is removed, wound washed out and the sterile matrix repaired with 6–0 absorbable suture. The nail plate is repositioned. A flat nail bed repair reduces nail plate deformities.

Small subungual hematomas can be managed nonoperatively. Large hematomas are managed by trephining with a needle, or removal of nail plate, repair of nail bed and repositioning of nail plate.

Hand Infections

Hand infections are common and poor management can result in severe disability, including stiffness, contractures and possibly even amputation. Many organisms have been implicated and commonly include *staphylococcus aureus* and *streptococcus* species.

Paronychia (Infection of the Nail Fold)

If there is no obvious collection of pus then paronychia can be managed initially with oral antibiotics. A collection on one side of the nail fold is managed by incising along the margin of the nail bed (Fig. 7.15). A collection going across either side of the nail is again managed by incision. If there is also a suspicion of pus under the nail, the nail should be removed.

Felon (Infection of the Distal Phalanx Pulp)

The pulp of a digit contains multiple fibrous septa as well as multiple sensory nerve endings. As a result, even a small amount of pus in a septal compartment (even if not obvious) can cause pressure and significant pain. Increased pressure in the pulp caused by the accumulation of pus can cause pulp necrosis or osteomyelitis.

Pus is drained either through a lateral incision dorsal to the neurovascular structures (avoiding

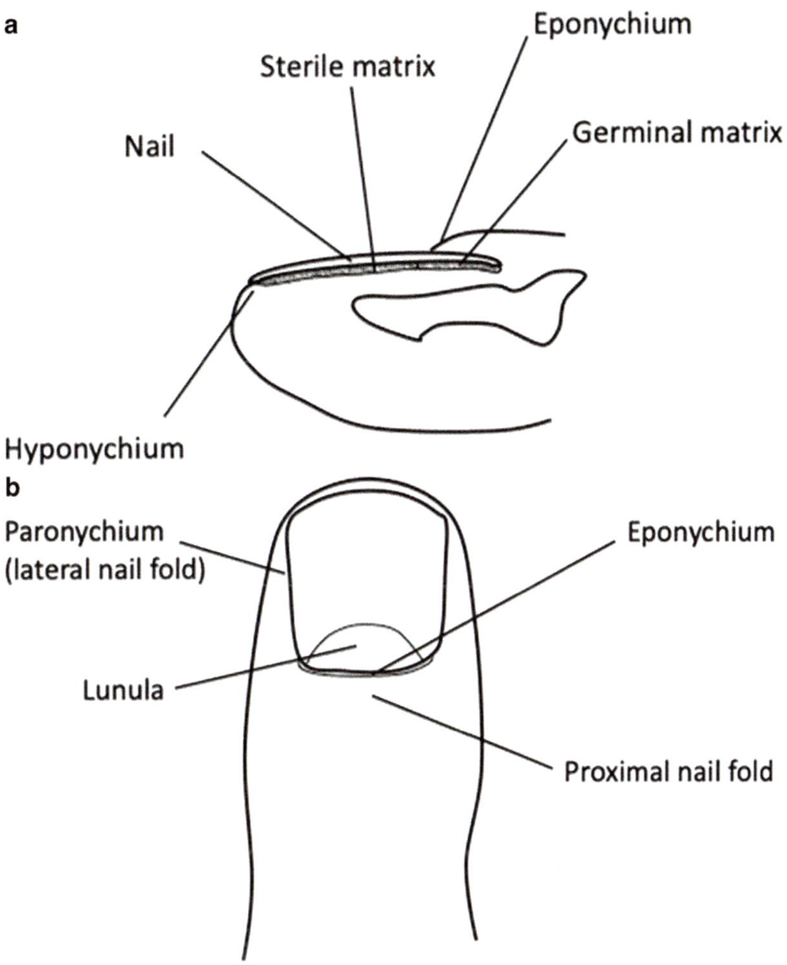

Fig. 7.14 (**a** and **b**): Structure of the nail

the sides involved in pinch) or with a volar longitudinal incision (Fig. 7.16). Early infection with mild pain and a soft pulp can initially be treated with antibiotics.

Collar Stud Abscess

Collar stud abscess is a web-space infection proximal to the superficial transverse metacarpal ligament. The palmar aspect is often the initiating site. Pus can track dorsally to form an abscess above and below the ligament. The palmar aspect of the abscess can spread to the deep palmar space. Drainage is through a dorsal and a palmar longitudinal incision (Fig. 7.17). The webs should not be incised.

Deep Fascial Space Infections

Deep fascial space infections are usually the result of a penetrating injury. The deep palmar space lies deep to the flexor tendons (Figs. 7.18 and 7.19). In the hand it is divided into three spaces separated by septa: the thenar space, the midpalmar space and the hypothenar space. In the forearm, the space is known as Parona's space and lies between the flexor tendons in the distal third of the forearm and the pronator quadratus.

Infections of the deep palmar space present with pain and tenderness over the space involved, swelling (often more noticeable on the dorsum of the hand) and restriction of finger movement.

Drainage of the midpalmar space is through a longitudinal incision in line with the middle finger from the distal palmar crease in a proximal direction. Thenar space infections can be drained through an incision on the dorsum parallel to first dorsal interosseous, or the volar aspect along the thenar crease (Fig. 7.20). Parona's space is drained through an incision on the volar aspect of the forearm ulnar to the midaxial line.

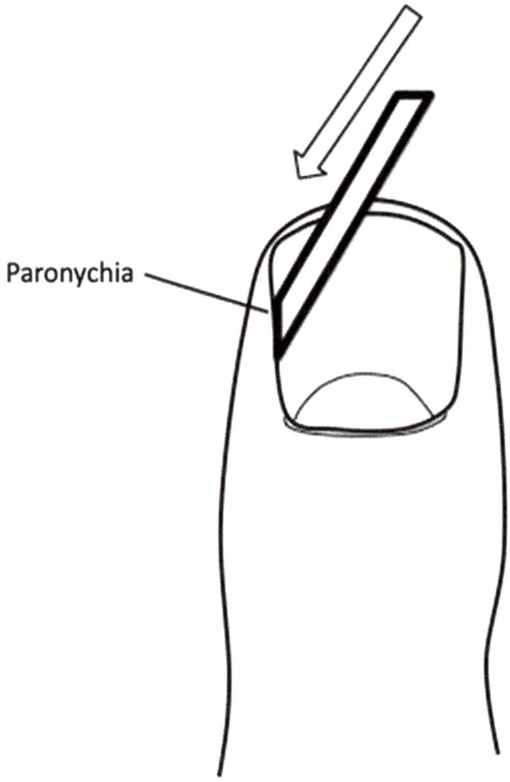

Fig. 7.15 Incision for paronychia

Flexor Sheath Infection

Flexor sheath infections are usually the result of a penetrating injury. Haematogenous or contiguous spread has been described as well. Untreated, they can cause destruction of the gliding mechanism and tendon necrosis.

Diagnosis

Kanavel in 1905 described four diagnostic signs:

- Flexed position of the finger.
- Symmetric enlargement of the whole finger.
- Excessive tenderness along the course of the sheath.
- Pain on passive extension of finger.

Treatment

The mainstay of treatment is operative drainage, intravenous antibiotics, rest and splint in the Edinburgh position. Early presentations can be treated with antibiotics alone.

Open drainage is through an oblique palmar incision centred on the DIPJ flexion crease. The synovium is incised between the A4 and A5 pulleys. A counterincision is made in the palm proximal border of the A1 pulley (Fig. 7.21). The tenosynovium is excised, leaving the annular pulleys intact. A small canula is passed proximally

Fig. 7.16 Incision for draining felon

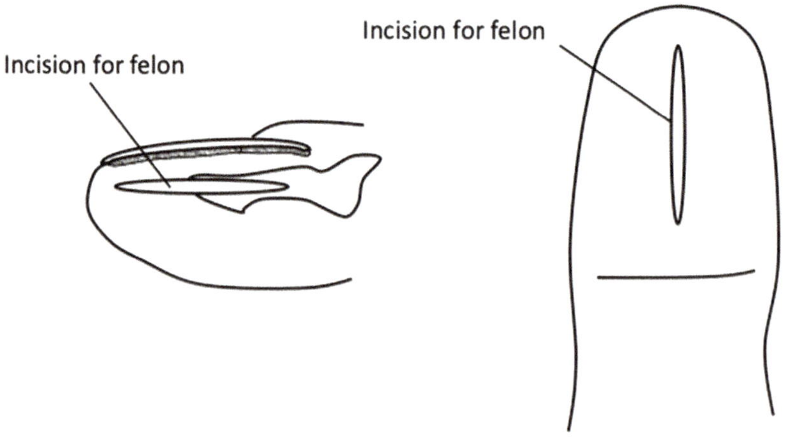

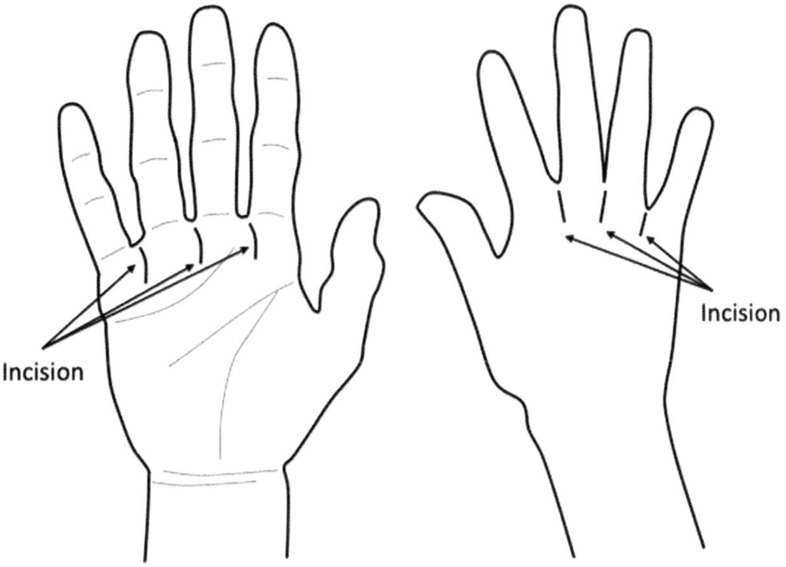

Fig. 7.17 Incision for draining collar stud abscess

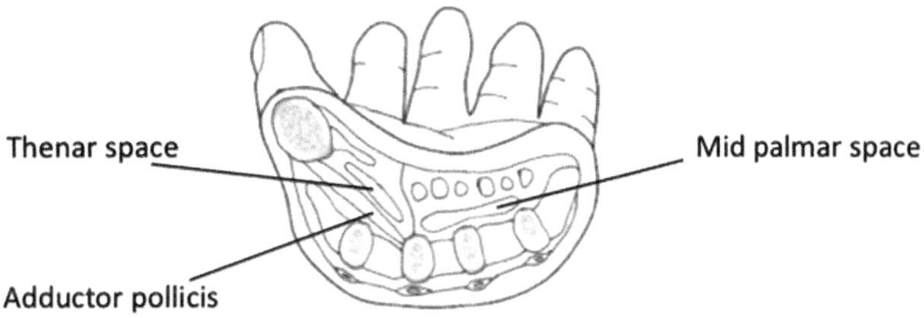

Fig. 7.18 The thenar and midpalmar space in cross section

into the sheath, which is irrigated with saline to ensure easy continuous flow. Free drainage should be ensured during irrigation. The surgeon should keep feeling how soft the finger is, if it starts to feel swollen and tense then no further irrigation should be performed.

A shiny tendon is visualised at both proximal and distal incisions and the finger is allowed to freely flex during irrigation. The flexor sheath of the thumb and small finger may communicate with the bursa of the wrist (Fig. 7.19), in which case the sheath may have to be opened proximal to the wrist flexor crease. This was classically the horse shoe abscess, although rarely seen in modern practice.

Stiffness of the wrist is a complication and hand therapy is needed.

Septic Arthritis of the Interphalangeal or Metacarpophalangeal Joints

Infections of the interphalangeal joints and MCPJs are usually the result of direct penetration. Contiguous spread can occur, but is much less common. Infections in the joint can lead to destruction of the articular cartilage and stiffness.

Diagnosis

Movement of the joint is painful and local swelling and tenderness is present. Aspiration of the joint fluid may help in the diagnosis.

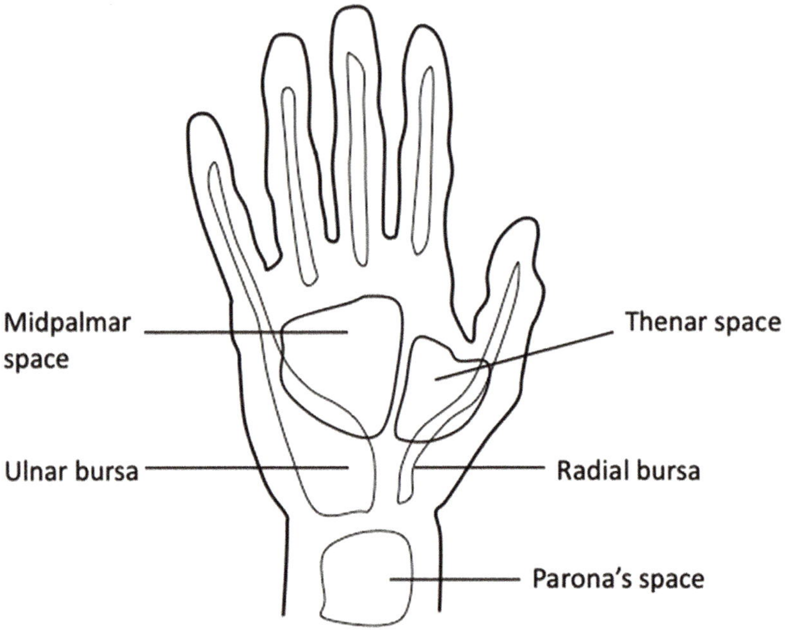

Fig. 7.19 The thenar and midpalmar space in relation to the flexor sheaths

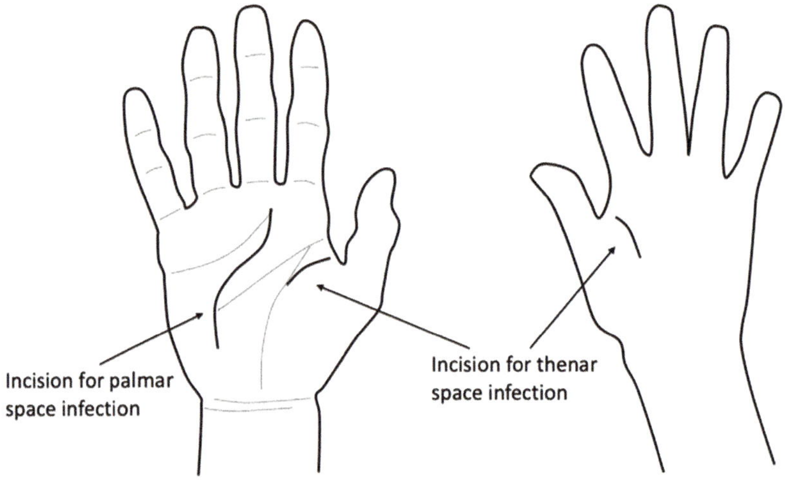

Fig. 7.20 Incisions for thenar and palmar space infections

Treatment

Washout of the joint is performed on an urgent basis. Approaches to finger joint washout are as follows–.

For MCPJ, access is through a longitudinal split in the extensor digitorum communis tendon. It should not go through the sagittal bands.

For PIPJ, the approach is between the central slip and the lateral band.

For DIPJ, the surgical approach is either (or both) sides of the terminal extensor tendon.

Carpal Tunnel Syndrome

Carpal tunnel syndrome is compression neuropathy of the median nerve in the carpal tunnel. It is the commonest compression neuropathy in the upper limb. In most instances it is idiopathic.

Other causes include trauma (distal radius fracture), rheumatoid arthritis, mucopolysaccharidosis, hypothyroidism, pregnancy, diabetes and systemic lupus erythematosus.

Anatomy

The carpal tunnel is bounded dorsally by the arch of carpal bones. The transverse carpal ligament is 3 cm long and completes the tunnel. The transverse carpal ligament inserts into the hamate and triquetrum on the ulnar side and the scaphoid and trapezium on the radial side (Fig. 7.22).

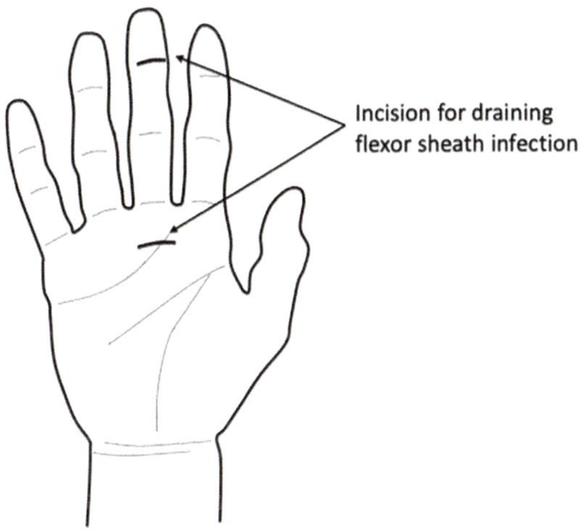

Fig. 7.21 Incision for draining flexor sheath infection

The contents of the carpal tunnel are the median nerve, the four FDS tendons, the four FDP tendons and the flexor pollicis longus. A total of 10 major longitudinal structures pass through the tunnel.

At the distal edge of the retinaculum the median nerve divides into six branches—one recurrent motor branch, three proper digital nerves and two common digital nerves.

The palmar cutaneous branch (Fig. 7.23) arises from the median nerve, 5 cm proximal to the wrist flexion crease from the radiopalmar aspect. It travels along with the nerve for 1.5–2.5 cm and then lies between the flexor carpi radialis (FCR) and the palmaris longus (PL). It emerges through the fascia 0.8 cm proximal to the wrist flexion crease and divides into ulnar and radial branches. Ulnar branches may be found in superficial tissue when doing a carpal tunnel release.

Certain variations in the median nerve may be encountered. There can be a high division separated by a persistent median artery or aberrant muscle. Also, the recurrent motor branch passes through or around the distal edge of the flexor retinaculum and can be extraligamentous (50–90%), subligamentous (30%) or transligamentous (25%). It can also arise from the ulnar border of the median nerve and lie on top of the transverse carpal ligament (Fig. 7.24). Patients with rarer variations of the recurrent motor branch often have a large palmaris brevis muscle.

Fig. 7.22 Contents of the carpal tunnel

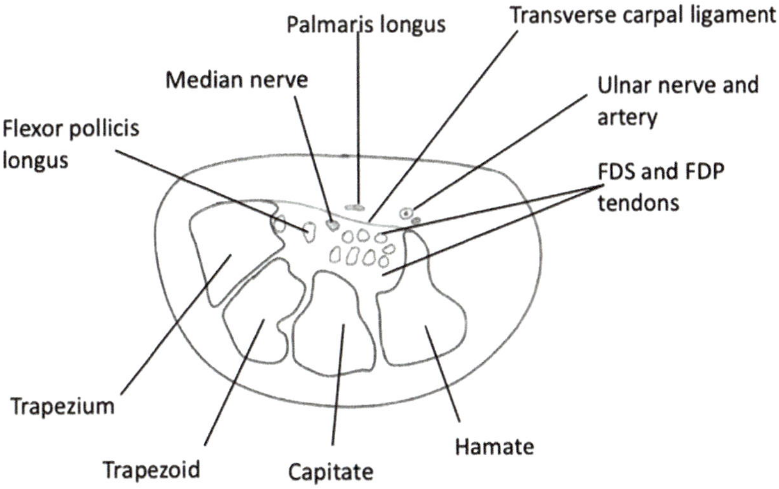

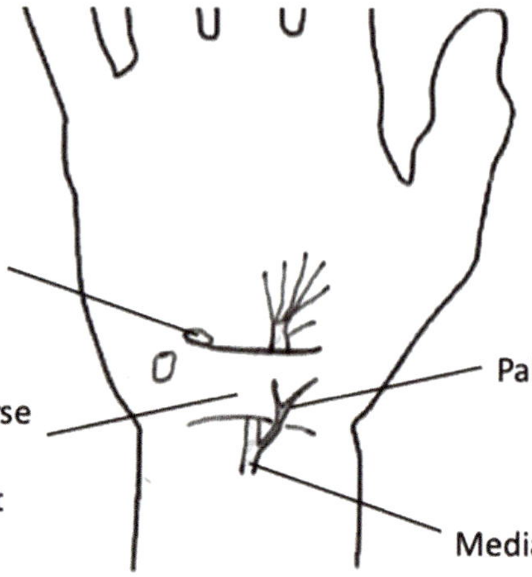

Fig. 7.23 Palmar cutaneous branch of median nerve

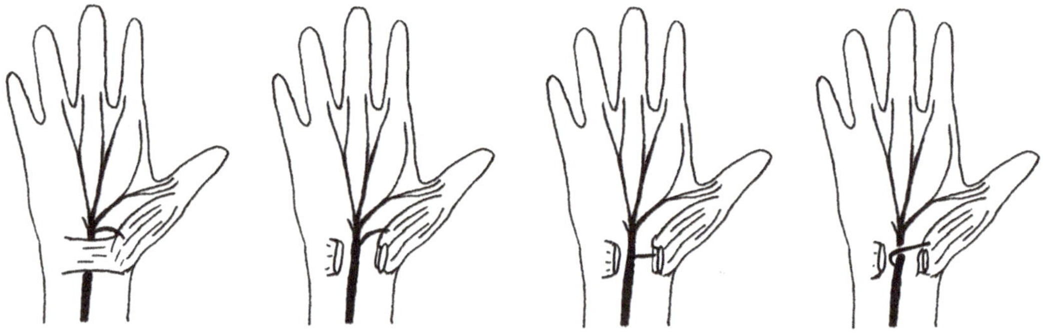

Fig. 7.24 Variations in the recurrent motor branch of median nerve

Symptoms

Patients present with pain and paraesthesia in the median nerve distribution in the digits. Symptoms are typically worse at night and may develop with activities involving gripping as the lumbricals are pulled into the tunnel. The palmar cutaneous branch is spared as it travels superficial to the carpal tunnel.

Signs

Phalen's wrist flexion is performed by holding the wrist in flexion for 60 seconds and checking for reproduction of paraesthesia.

Direct compression of the nerve (Durkan test) and Tinel's nerve percussion test are also useful tests.

Semmes Weinstein monofilament testing can be helpful to detect early signs of nerve dysfunction.

Thenar atrophy is present in late presentations.

Nerve Conduction Studies

Carpal tunnel syndrome is a clinical diagnosis and nerve conduction studies are only usually required where the diagnosis is uncertain. A negative result does not exclude carpal tunnel syndrome if the classic symptoms and signs are present.

Abnormal findings are—distal motor latencies greater than 4.5 ms; distal sensory latencies greater than 3.5 ms; and asymmetry of conduction between two hands of greater than 1 ms for motor and 0.5 ms for sensory conduction.

Electromyography of the thenar muscles is useful to look for signs of denervation.

Differential Diagnosis

Differential diagnoses are cervical nerve root compression, spinal cord lesions or peripheral nerve disorders.

Non-operative Treatment

Where symptoms at night predominate as a result of wrist flexion when sleeping, night splinting can be very effective. The splint prevents wrist flexion.

A permanent cure is rare following a steroid injection into the carpal tunnel. It is therefore used to confirm a diagnosis in equivocal cases or to provide temporary symptom relief.

Operative Treatment

Release of carpal tunnel can be performed through open surgery or arthroscopically. It is indicated for daytime symptoms and when splinting fails.

With open surgery, there is 96% patient satisfaction and 84% of patients return to their previous job.

With arthroscopic surgery, a general anaesthetic is needed, visualisation is often poor and there is an increased risk of iatrogenic nerve injury.

Ferdinand RD, Maclean JG. Endoscopic versus open carpal tunnel release in bilateral carpal tunnel syndrome. A prospective randomised blinded assessment. J Bone Joint Surg Br 2002;84(3):375–9. In 25 patients with bilateral carpal tunnel, the researchers performed one open and one endoscopic release. There was no difference in strength, relief or satisfaction between the two hands.

Open Release Technique

This technique is most commonly performed under local anaesthesia. The incision (approximately 3 cm long) is in line with the radial border of the ring finger (Fig. 7.25). It extends from the distal wrist crease to Kaplan's line. It is not necessary to cross the wrist crease with the skin incision. The transverse carpal ligament extends more proximal to the wrist crease and must be divided.

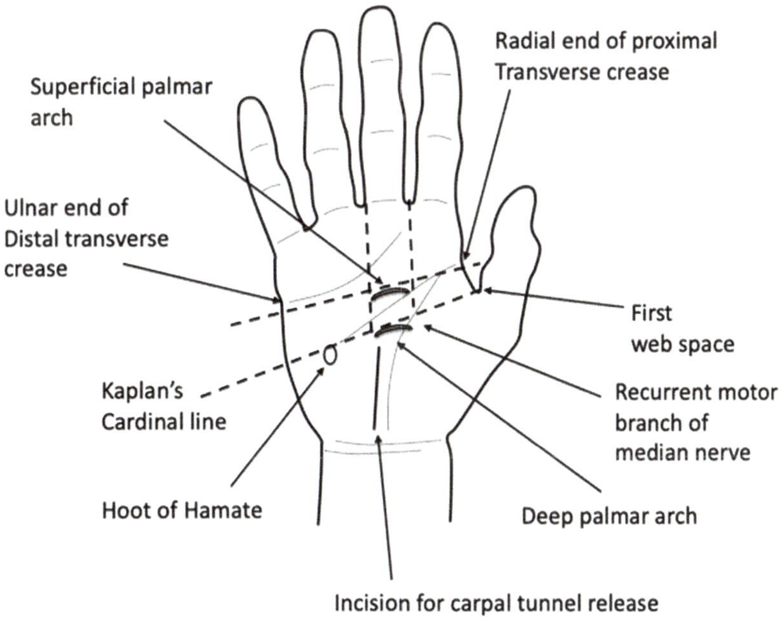

Fig. 7.25 Landmarks and incision for carpal tunnel release

Kaplan's cardinal line is drawn from the apex of the thumb–index web to the hook of hamate. The deep palmar arch lies under this line deep to the flexor tendons. The intersection of the line with the long finger flexed marks the recurrent motor branch. The superficial palmar arch is located between this line and the proximal palmar crease.

If ulna nerve symptoms are present there is no need to release Guyon's canal, as it enlarges itself following release of the transverse carpal ligament. Neurolysis of the medial nerve is not necessary.

Grip strength returns after 3 months and pinch strength returns after 6 weeks following open carpal tunnel decompression.

Bowstringing is not a problem as there is some repair of the flexor retinaculum with time.

Chronic Wrist Pain

Causes of chronic painful wrist can be classified according to the site of symptoms (Table 7.4).

Ganglion

Ganglia are the most common benign masses in the hand and wrist. They often arise from the synovial lining of the carpal joints or the tendon sheaths. The dorsal scapholunate ligament is the most common site of origin. The volar ganglia are related to the FCR tendon.

Table 7.4 Causes of chronic wrist pain according to the site of pain

Site	Causes
Radial-sided pain	de Quervain's tenosynovitis Intersection syndrome Trapeziometacarpal joint osteoarthritis Scaphoid non-unions and scaphoid non-union advance collapse Scaphotrapeziotrapezoid osteoarthritis Ganglion
Central pain	Scapholunate dissociation and scapholunate advanced collapse Kienbock's disease Intra-osseous ganglion Ganglion
Ulnar pain	Distal radioulnar joint instability, malalignment or osteoarthritis Triangular fibrocartilage tear Pisotriquetral osteoarthritis Hamate hook fracture ECU tendinitis

Clinically, ganglia appear as firm, fluctuant swellings, which may be mildly tender on palpation and can demonstrate transillumination. There is no specific initiating event and these swellings may have been present for a long time before treatment is sought. A sensation of aching or tiredness may sometimes be experienced.

Aspiration of the swelling reveals a gelatinous fluid. Aspiration with or without a steroid injection is associated with a high recurrence risk. Surgical excision under general anaesthetic and tourniquet control has the highest cure rate of approximately 95%. Excision involves removal of the stalk of the ganglion as well as a small part of the capsule of the joint from which it arises.

Patients should be warned about the risk of recurrence of the ganglion, which can be up to 30% following excision.

Carpal Instability

Carpal instability can be described by its pattern and can include dissociative, non-dissociative, adaptive or complex (Fig. 7.26).

Dissociative instability occurs within a carpal row. Example of this could be scaphoid fracture or scapholunate dissociation.

Scapholunate ligament injury can lead to dorsal intercalated segmental instability (DISI). In this the lunate is extended and scaphoid flexed.

Lunotriquetral ligament injury leads to volar intercalated segmental instability (VISI). The lunate is flexed and scaphoid is extended.

Non-dissociative carpal instability occurs between carpal rows—for instance midcarpal or radiocarpal instability. Carpal instability complex refers to instability within and between the carpal rows—like perilunate dislocation. Adaptive carpal instability is carpal malalignment secondary to distal radius malunion.

Gilula's arcs have been described on standard PA wrist radiographs (Fig. 7.27). Disruption of the arc may be present in carpal instability. Loss of carpal height is another sign (Fig. 7.28).

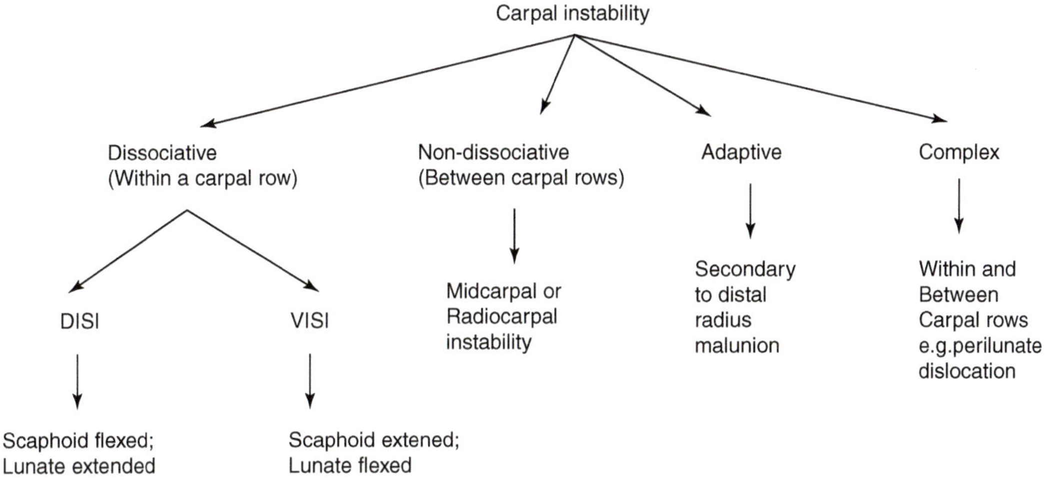

Fig. 7.26 Types of carpal instability

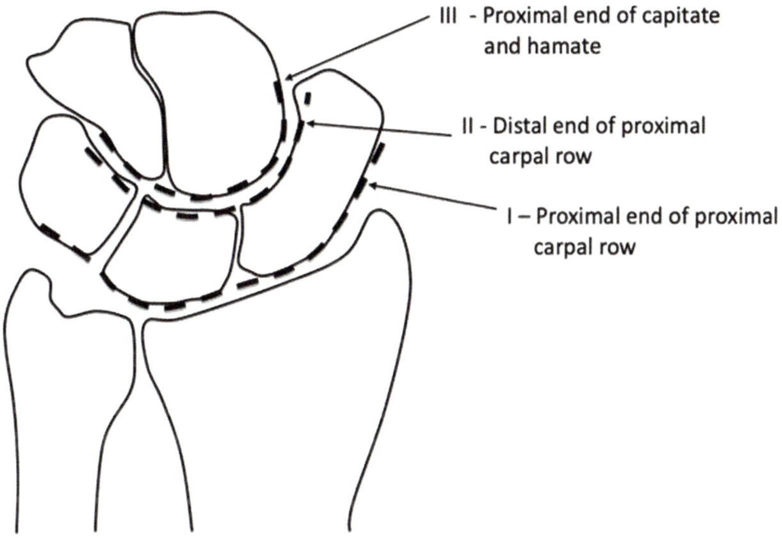

Fig. 7.27 Gilula's arcs on wrist radiographs

Normal ratio between height of carpus and length of third metacarpal is 0.54.

Scapholunate Ligament Instability

Scapholunate instability is the commonest presentation leading to DISI. Patients present with pain on the dorsum or dorsolateral aspect of the wrist. There may be a click, stiffness or weakness on movement. Tenderness is over the scapholunate interval. Watson scaphoid shift test and scaphoid ballotment test are checked.

The scapholunate angle is greater than 70 degrees (Figs. 7.29 and 7.30). The scapholunate interval is greater than 3 mm. Clenched fist radiograph may pick up subtle widening of the scapholunate interval.

Acute injury is managed with open ligament repair and wire stabilisation.

For chronic injuries (>6 weeks old), ligament reconstruction (modified Brunelli) can be performed if the joint is reducible and there is no arthritis. In the low-demand patient, a dorsal capsulodesis or equivalent procedure is adequate. For irreducible malalignment, scaphotrapezio-

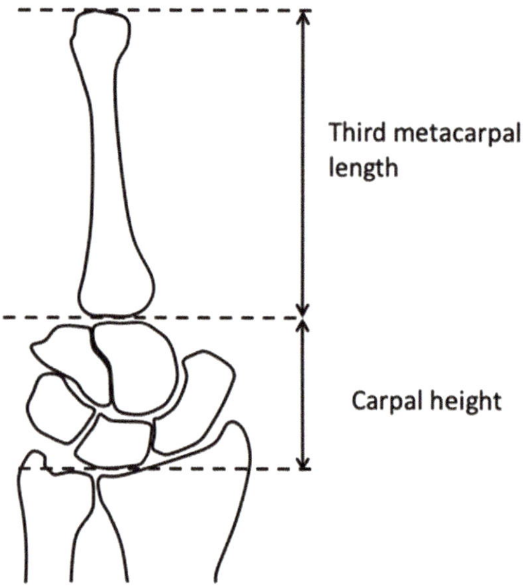

Fig. 7.28 Assessment of carpal height

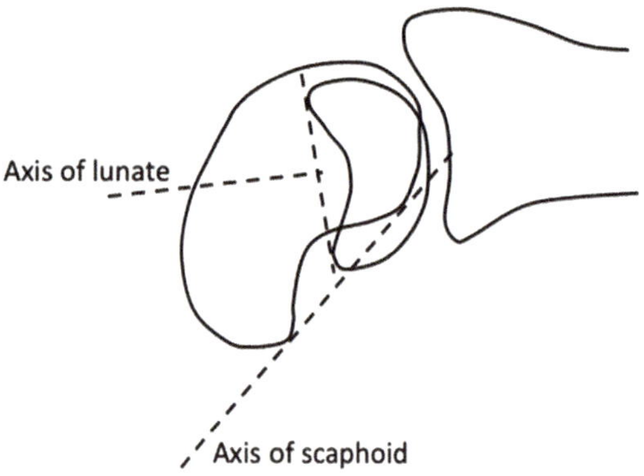

Fig. 7.29 The axis of lunate is perpendicular to the 2 distal points on the lateral view. The axis of scaphoid is drawn along the 2 proximal points on the proximal and distal pole

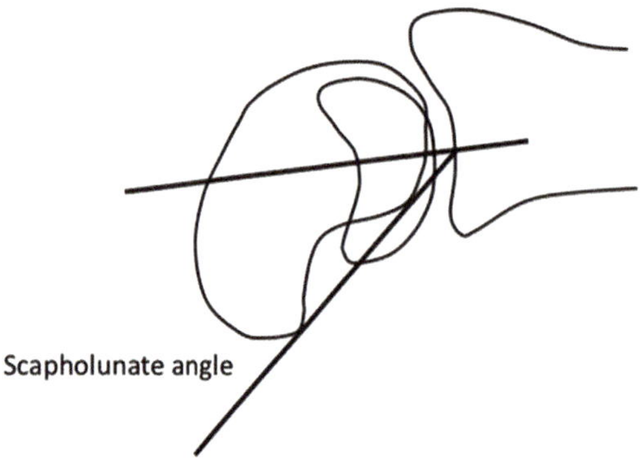

Fig. 7.30 Measurement of scapholunate angle

trapezoid (STT) fusion can be an option. Advanced arthritis can be managed with proximal row carpectomy or four corner fusion. Untreated injuries may progress to SLAC (Scapholunate advanced collapse) wrist.

Lunotriquetral instability causes ulnar sided pain and a positive lunotriquetral shear test. This is managed by repair in the acute phase. Lunotriquetral fusion is indicated in the chronic phase.

Acute perilunate dislocation is managed by acute reduction and repair of the ligaments through a dorsal approach along with K wire stabilisation of the proximal row. Operative intervention is needed and can be planned within a few days if the dislocation is reduced acutely.

Kienbock's Disease

Kienbock's disease is avascular necrosis and collapse of the lunate. The aetiology is unknown but it may be related to a single traumatic episode, or recurrent microtrauma events. It is associated with negative ulnar variance.

Clinical Features

Patients can be asymptomatic or can present with dorsal pain, weakness and/or stiffness of the wrist.

Imaging

Kienbock's disease is investigated with both radiographs and MRI. The radiological classification by Lichtman is given in Table 7.5.

From *Lichtman DM, Lesley NE, Simmons SP. The Classification and Treatment of Kienbock's Disease: The State of the Art and a Look at the Future. The Journal of Hand Surgery (European Volume, 2010)35E:7:549–54.*

Treatment

Treatment is conservative for most patients, but when this fails there are various surgical options.

Table 7.5 Lichtman classification and treatment options

Stage	Description	Treatment options
I	Normal architecture and density of the lunate on plain radiographs, with the possible exception of a linear or compressive fracture.	Immobilisation and anti inflammatory medication
II	Density changes, lytic and sclerotic, in the lunate on plain radiographs, but the size, shape and anatomic relationship of the bones are not altered.	Joint levelling procedure in patients with ulna minus Radial wedge osteotomy Revascularisation procedures
IIIA IIIB	Lunate sclerosis and loss of height in the absence of changes in carpal alignment. Carpal collapse with fixed scaphoid palmar flexion.	III A—Same as II For IIIB—STT fusion or proximal row carpectomy or scaphocapitate fusion
IV	Lunate collapse with radiocarpal or midcarpal degenerative arthritis.	Proximal row carpectomy or wrist fusion.

These are detailed in Table 7.5. Joint leveling can be radial shortening or ulnar lengthening.

Congenital Anomalies of the Hand and Upper Limb

Frantz and O'Rahilly (1966) proposed a classification system for congenital upper limb deficiencies that includes four types (Fig. 7.31). In terminal deficiencies, the limb distal to the abnormality is absent. Intercalary defects have a normal limb proximal and distal to the defect. In transverse defects, the abnormality affects the whole cross section of the limb. In paraxial defects, the missing part is either preaxial or postaxial.

This has been expanded by Swanson, Barsky and Entin to seven categories:

- Type 1—failure of formation of parts.
- Type 2—failure of differentiation.
- Type 3—duplication.
- Type 4—overgrowth.
- Type 5—undergrowth.
- Type 6—congenital constriction-band syndrome.
- Type 7—generalised skeletal abnormalities.

Swanson AB, Barsky AJ, Entin MA. Classification of limb malformations on the basis of embryological failures. Surg Clin North Am 1968;48(5):1169–79.

Radial Hemimelia

Radial hemimelia is the congenital absence of all or part of the radius and the associated deficiency of radial carpal bones. Classification is shown in Fig. 7.32.

Associated conditions include VATER (vertebrae, anal malformations, trachea, oesophagus anomalies and renal) syndrome, cardiovascular anomalies and Fanconi syndrome, and anomalies of the gastrointestinal and genitourinary tracts. Holt Oram syndrome is associated with cardiac abnormalities.

Treatment considerations include addressing the associated conditions which may have an impact on any planned surgical intervention for the upper limb deformities. In mild cases, stretching and manipulation may suffice. In more severe cases, the ulna can be centralised and fused to the wrist bones. Pollicisation of the index finger helps to provide opposition, replacing the thumb.

Ulnar Hemimelia

Ulnar hemimelia is partial or complete absence of the ulna. Ulnar longitudinal deficiencies are not as common as radial sided deficiencies.

Classification is shown in Fig. 7.33.

Treatment initially involves stretching and splinting, with forearm lengthening and osteotomies as surgical options.

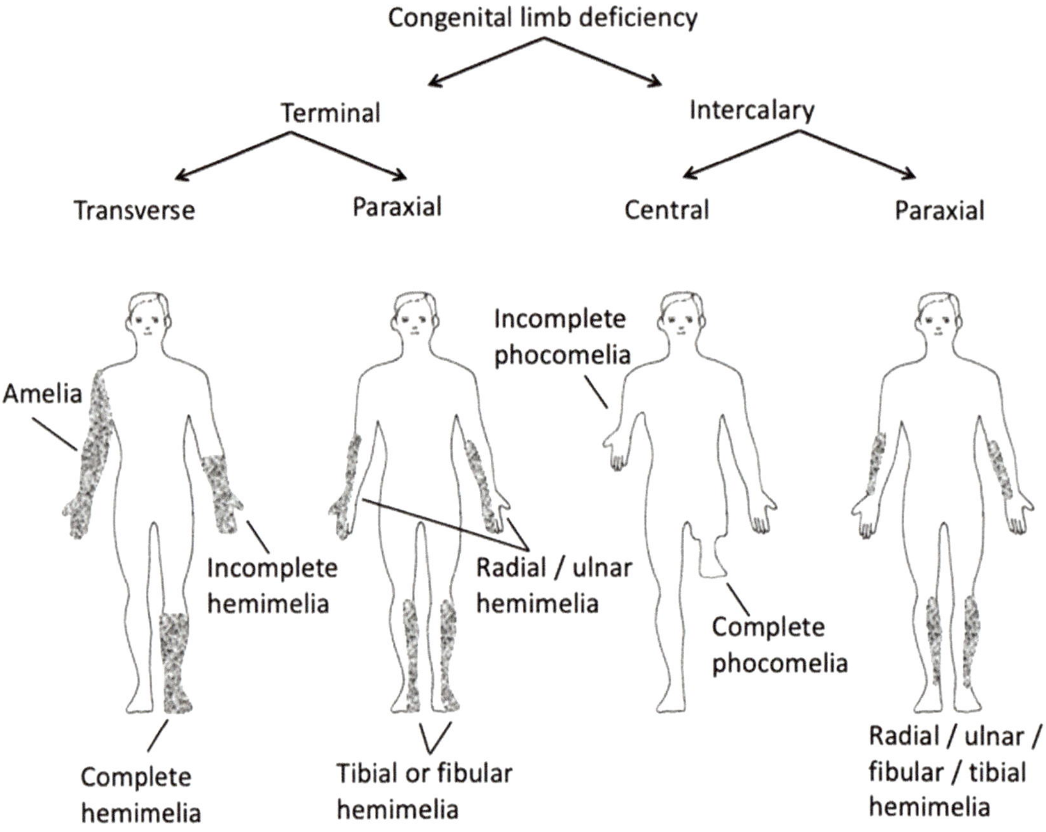

Fig. 7.31 Frantz and O'Rahilly classification and examples

Fig. 7.32 Classification of radial club hand

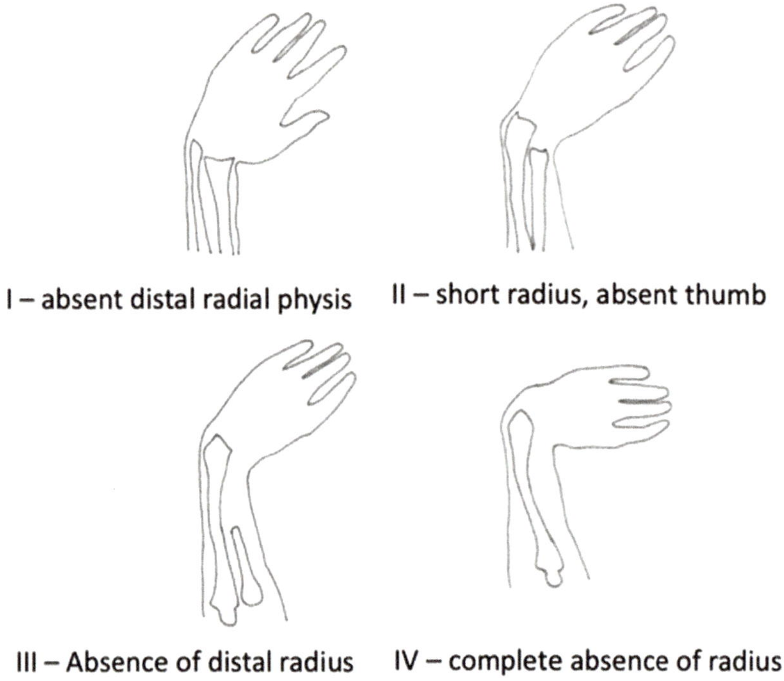

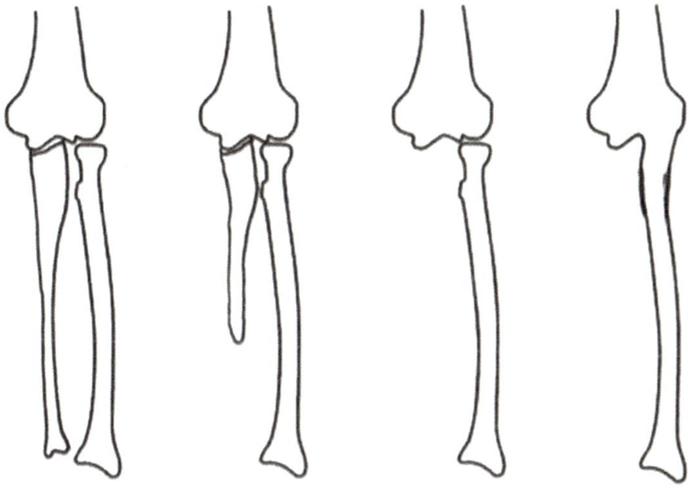

Fig. 7.33 Ulnar club hand

Madelung Deformity

This is a congenital condition caused by disruption of the ulnar volar physis of the distal radius causing growth arrest. It often manifests in adolescence when the distal radius demonstrates excessive radial inclination & volar tilt. Treatment depends on the age of the individual and the level of symptoms, particularly pain.

Cleft Hand

A cleft hand is the central absence of one or more digits and fusion of the other digits. It may be bilateral. The genetic transmission is autosomal dominant. If surgery is undertaken it must be individualised to the patient, as there are many variations and components to these abnormalities.

Syndactyly

Syndactyly is the most common congenital anomaly of the hand. It is partial or complete fusion of two or more digits. Simple syndactyly involves only the skin, while complex syndactyly involves the bones.

Polydactyly

Polydactyly is the presence of supernumerary digits. The accessory digit may be simple soft tissue, or may have a more complex structure with bones and tendons. Rarely, a metacarpal may be present.

Duplication of the Thumb

Duplication of the thumb is a common anomaly. It may be associated with cardiac abnormalities or Fanconi syndrome. The Wassel classification describes thumb duplication (Fig. 7.34).

Type 4 is the commonest. Triphalangism is similar to type 4, but with an extra phalanx at the end of one distal phalanx.

Hypoplasia of the Thumb

Thumb hypoplasia has been classified by Blouth (Fig. 7.35).

Surgical treatment depends on CMCJ presence and/or stability.

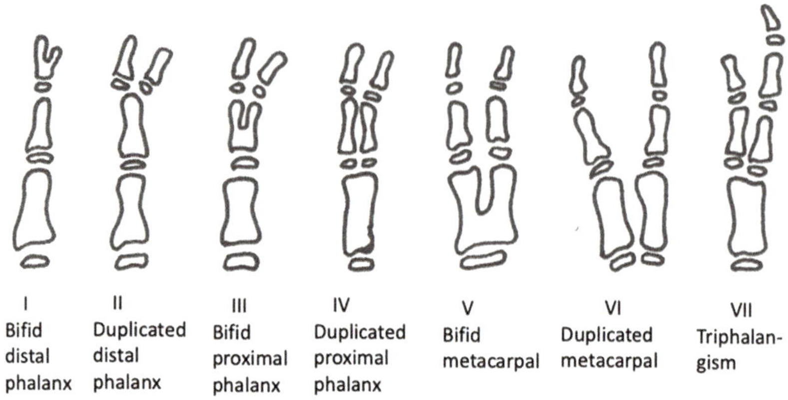

Fig. 7.34 Wassel classification

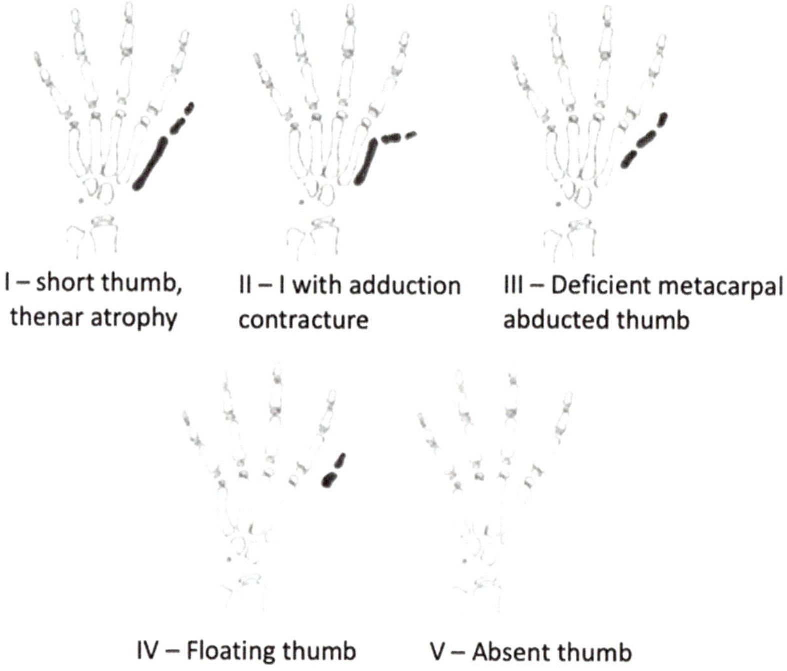

Fig. 7.35 Classification of thumb hypoplasia

Clinodactyly

Clinodactyly is deviation of the little finger laterally. It can be caused by a trapezoidal middle phalanx.

Camptodactyly

Camptodactyly is deviation of the digit in the sagittal plane. Flexion contracture of the little finger is the most common manifestation.

Kirner's deformity is incurling of the DIPJ of the little finger in prepubertal girls.

Macrodactyly

Macrodactyly is enlargement of one or more digits. Treatment can be observation or reduction in size or amputation.

Congenital Trigger Thumb

The underlying cause of congenital trigger thumb is stenosis of the A1 pulley. A third of cases resolve spontaneously by the age of 1 year, and those that do not are managed by surgical release between the ages of 18 months and 3 years.

Dupuytren's Contracture

Dupuytren's contracture was first described by Baron Guillaume Dupuytren (1777–1835).

The palmar fascia is a three-dimensional system of fine ligamentous structures. It forms a framework of guiding channels for the longitudinal structures. It also anchors the skin, allowing the hand to grip and rotate an object without the skin moving. In Dupuytren's contracture this flattened fibrous network thickens to form nodules and then cords. Contraction of these cords results in flexion deformities of the fingers.

Pathology

The proliferation phase is characterised by immature fibroblasts and myofibroblasts in whorl-like patterns. Growth factors, including interleukin 1 and platelet-derived growth factor, are produced by platelets and macrophages—IL-1, PDGF etc.

Once formed, cellular tissue responds to mechanical transduction. Fibroblasts respond to chemical signals and growth factors as well as to mechanical stimuli.

Etiology

The cause is largely unknown. Dupuytren's contracture is not related to alcohol intake, smoking, trauma or occupation. There is a possible correlation with diabetes or epilepsy medication. There is a genetic element, but only up to 20% of patients have a family history.

Several factors that may indicate an increasingly severe disease, known as Dupuytren's diathesis, with a more rapid progression:

- Young age (<40 yr).
- The presence of similar disease process at other sites—for example plantar fibromatosis (Ledderhose disease).
- A positive family history.
- Bilateral disease.

Anatomy

The palmar fascia can be considered to have three groups of fibres—Longitudinal, transverse and vertical.

The longitudinal system has four distinct bands from the palmaris longus tendon or flexor retinaculum to the four fingers (Fig. 7.36).

Beyond the transverse fibres, the fascia divides into three layers distally (Table 7.6).

The transverse component of the palmar fascia are the superficial (known as natatory ligament) and deep transverse metacarpal ligaments. Additionally, the transverse fibres of the fascia are a separate band of about 2 cm width and are known as fibres of Skoog. Fibres of the natatory ligament form the apex of the web and blend into the lateral digital sheet. The Grayson's and Cleland's ligaments are illustrated in Figs. 7.37 and 7.38.

The vertical component comprises fibres from the dermis to the flexor sheaths and metacarpals.

The patterns of cord contraction are as follows:

- Central cord—follows layer 1. Passes distally and attaches to the base of the middle phalanx.
- Lateral cord—runs from the natatory ligament to the lateral digital sheath.
- Spiral cord—formed from the pretendinous band, spiral band, Grayson's ligament and the lateral digital sheet.

The neurovascular bundle is fixed in the midpalm under the palmar fascia and at the base of the middle phalanx by Grayson's ligament. Between these two points the neurovascular bundle can be displaced.

Clinical Features

The presenting features are palpable nodules and cords. Patients present with progressive

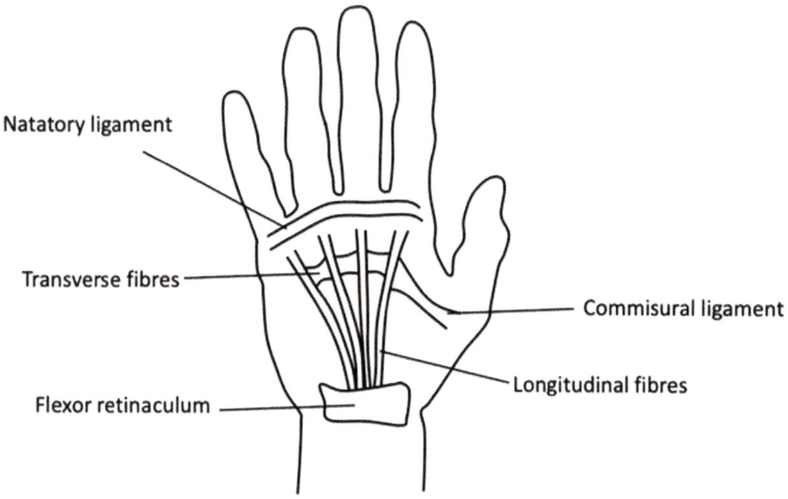

Fig. 7.36 Longitudinal fibres of palmar fascia

Table 7.6 Layers of the palmar fascia

Layer	Description
1	The superficial layer Inserts into the skin of the palm between distal palmar crease and proximal digital crease
2	The spiral band of Gosset on either side of the flexor tendon—Deep to the neurovascular bundle and join the– The lateral digital sheet The pretendinous band The natatory ligament Cleland's ligaments—Dorsal to the neurovascular bundle Grayson's ligaments—Palmar to the neurovascular bundle
3	The deepest layer Passes deep on either side of the metacarpophalangeal joint and attach to metacarpal bone and proximal phalanx

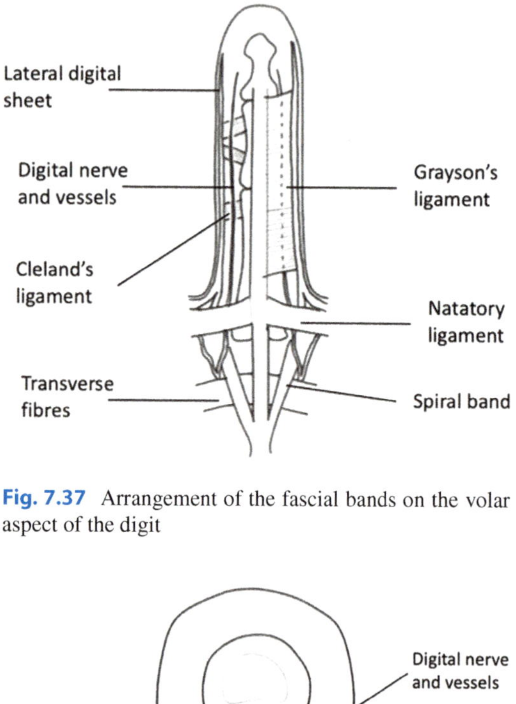

Fig. 7.37 Arrangement of the fascial bands on the volar aspect of the digit

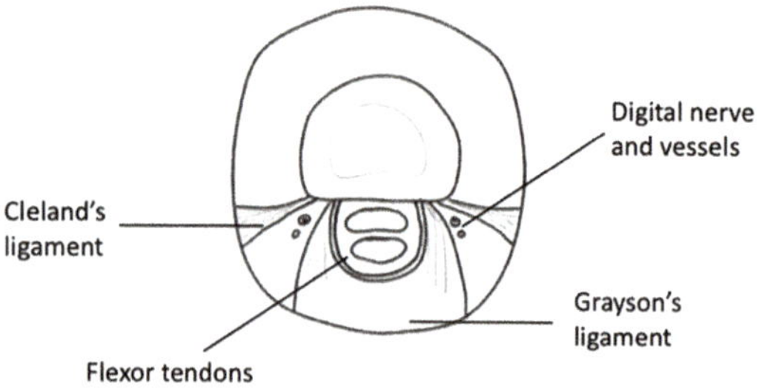

Fig. 7.38 The Cleland's and Grayson's ligament

flexion contractures of MCPJ and PIPJ. There may be pitting of the palmar skin. Finger, thumb and first web space contractures are present. Commonly the ring and little finger are affected.

Dupuytren's disease may be associated with fibromatoses elsewhere:

- Plantar fibromatosis (Ledderhose disease).
- Garrod's knuckle pads (circumscribed dermal nodules or plaques on the dorsal aspect of the PIPJs or MCPJs).
- Peyronie's disease of the penis.

The underlying cause and associated features are elicited in the history. The degree of flexion contracture of each digit and joint should be recorded. The table-top test of Hueston is performed by placing the palm prone on the table. Flexion of the interphalangeal joints will be evident.

Nodules can be painful when they initially form, but the pain decreases as they mature and therefore they rarely need excision. The table-top test of Hueston is a useful test. If the patient cannot place the palm flat on the table because of contractures then surgery is considered. Flexion contractures of >30° at the MCPJ and >15° PIPJ are considered indications for surgical treatment.

The aim of treatment is to release contractures by cutting or excising the diseased tissue. Releasing the associated joint contractures is also necessary in severe cases.

MCPJ contracture can be corrected regardless of duration, but PIPJ contracture is more difficult to correct.

Conservative Treatment

There are conservative measures that can be utilised in the treatment of Dupuytren's disease. Steroid injections may reduce the bulk of diseased tissue, but will not slow down the disease progression. *Clostridium histolyticum* (e.g. Xiapex) is licensed for use in some areas. This works by cleaving the collagen in the cords, allowing for a finger manipulation at 24 to 48 hours, which then tears the Dupuytren's cord. Radiotherapy can also be used to breakdown the pathological cords, but this does require multiple doses and is also only available in certain regions.

Needle Fasciotomy

This is a percutaneous technique performed using a hypodermic needle. It is most suited for well-defined cords causing MCPJ contractures, but the indications have been extended to include cords around the PIPJ. Complication rates are higher. It can be a good treatment method for patients who are not suitable or willing to undergo surgery, as it can be performed in the outpatient clinic.

Surgical Treatment

Standard Limited Fasciectomy

All involved fascia are removed by progressive longitudinal dissection. A longitudinal incision is made. The skin deficiency from the contracture is addressed using a Z-plasty, which brings skin from the sides of the finger to the palmar side and lengthens the scar. The limbs of the 'Z' need to be the same length (Fig. 7.39). If a Z plasty with angles of 60° is used then the wound can be lengthened by 75%.

Dermofasciectomy

Dermofasciectomy involves the removal of a section of skin and fascia. It is usually reserved for patients with poorly mobile skin and recurrence. A full-thickness skin graft, usually harvested from the antecubital fossa, is used to cover the defect. This helps prevent recurrence as the disease does not reoccur under a graft.

Segmental Fasciectomy

Small, spaced out incisions are made along the cord. A 1 cm section of cord is removed through each incision.

Skin Defects

Skin defects that remain in the palm after the deformity has been corrected can be left open to

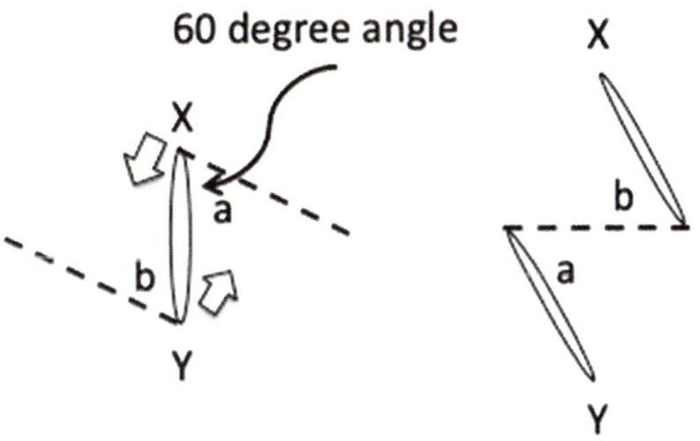

Fig. 7.39 Principle of Z-plasty

heal by secondary intention (open-palm technique) or grafted.

Joint Contractures

Residual PIPJ contracture may remain after Dupuytren's cord has been removed. The accessory collateral ligaments are released first, followed by the volar plate if necessary. More structures released corresponds to higher risk of postoperative stiffness.

Complications

The possible complications are–.

Injury to digital nerves is rare.

Injury to the digital artery—this may lead to ischaemic flaps and require reconstruction.

Wound healing problems including haematoma, infection and ischaemia.

Reflex sympathetic dystrophy.

Finger stiffness.

Postoperative Rehabilitation

Good therapy is the key to a successful outcome. If it is felt necessary, the hand can be splinted with the MCPJ flexed and PIPJ extended for 2–3 days. If a skin graft is used, a splint is applied for 10 days. A splint is continued in between periods of exercise, and night splintage continues for months. Early movement is encouraged.

Recurrence

There is a reported recurrence rate of 50% within 5–10 years. It is difficult to compare recurrence rates between the different techniques as there are many confounding variables.

Surgery for recurrent disease is made difficult by the presence of scar tissue. Other problems can include an altered anatomy, existing injury to the neurovascular structures, a non-compliant patient and unrealistic patient expectations. If the PIPJ cannot be straightened, consider PIPJ fusion. Amputation is not indicated, unless requested.

Hand Osteoarthritis

Before the age of 65 years, osteoarthritis of the hand is more common in men; after 65 years, it is more common in women. The most common joints involved are the DIPJ and PIPJ, and the carpometacarpal joint of the thumb.

Distal Interphalangeal Joint Arthritis

Clinical Features

Clinical features include Heberden's nodes and osteophytes. Deformity of the DIPJ may be present in severe arthritis.

Mucous cysts are ganglia arising from the DIPJ, often with an associated underlying osteophyte. These may cause nail deformity secondary to pressure on the germinal matrix. Mucous cysts can be treated by excising the base of the ganglion and the underlying osteophyte.

Treatment

Arthrodesis using wires or a Herbert screw can be considered for patients with significant malalignment or pain.

Proximal Interphalangeal Joint Arthritis

Clinical Features

Patients present with pain, deformity and stiffness due to osteophytes and soft tissue fibrosis.

Treatment

Treatment is conservative in the majority of cases.

The aim of surgery is pain relief. It is not usually possible to improve the range of movement.

Arthrodesis is the best way of permanently relieving pain at the cost of losing movement. Tension-band wire techniques, compression screws or plates are all accepted methods.

Arthroplasty is joint replacement surgery. All modern implants have yet to demonstrate good short- to medium-term implant survival. In most cases, range of movement is not improved.

Arthrodesis should be performed on the index and middle fingers. This gives a permanent reliable solution and allows a good stable pinch. Arthroplasty can be performed on the ring and small fingers to maintain range of movement for grip.

Metacarpophalangeal Joint Arthritis

The symptoms of arthritis in MCPJ are usually well tolerated. It is worth noting that isolated MCPJ arthritis can be associated with haemachromatosis.

If conservative treatment fails, arthrodesis or excision arthroplasty are poorly tolerated. Joint replacement is a much more reliable option in the MCPJ than in the PIPJ. Unlike in rheumatoid arthritis, the MCPJ in osteoarthritis is stable. Therefore, an unconstrained surface replacement arthroplasty can relieve pain and maintain range of movement and pinch stability.

Trapeziometacarpal Joint Arthritis

Clinical Features

Clinical features of trapeziometacarpal joint (TMCJ) arthritis are pain with use or movement of the thumb, pain on gripping and local deformity. There is tenderness over the capsule of the TMCJ.

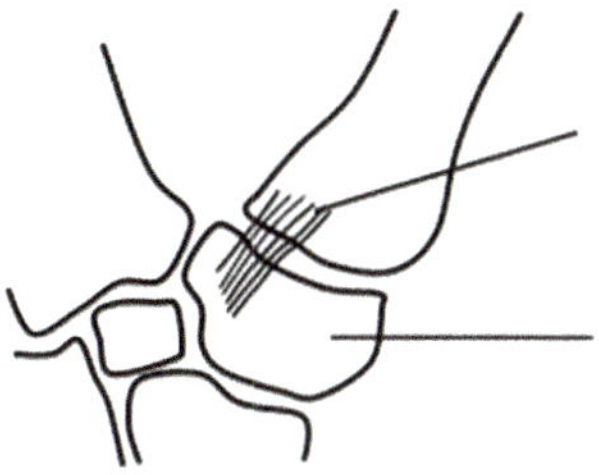

Fig. 7.40 The volar beak ligament

There are three main ligamentous stabilisers, of which the beak ligament or the palmar oblique ligament is key for stability (Fig. 7.40). The other two ligaments are the dorsal and lateral ligaments. Degeneration of the beak ligament can lead to joint instability.

Prominence of the subluxed metacarpal base on the radial aspect of the joint is known as the shoulder sign. Pain on axial loading and flexion extension can be assessed with the crank test, while pain on axial load and rotation can be assessed with the grind test.

Differential Diagnosis

Other conditions that can cause pain in the local area are thumb MCP arthritis, de Quervain's tenosynovitis, radiocarpal arthritis, Scaphoid nonunion, Kienbock's disease.

Imaging

Anteroposterior, lateral and oblique X-rays should be obtained. An anteroposterior stress view is achieved by pressing together the tips of the radial aspects of both thumbs. This is useful if testing for laxity.

Staging

The Eaton and Littler system is used to stage TMCJ arthritis (Fig. 7.41). However, it does not always correspond well with clinical symptoms.

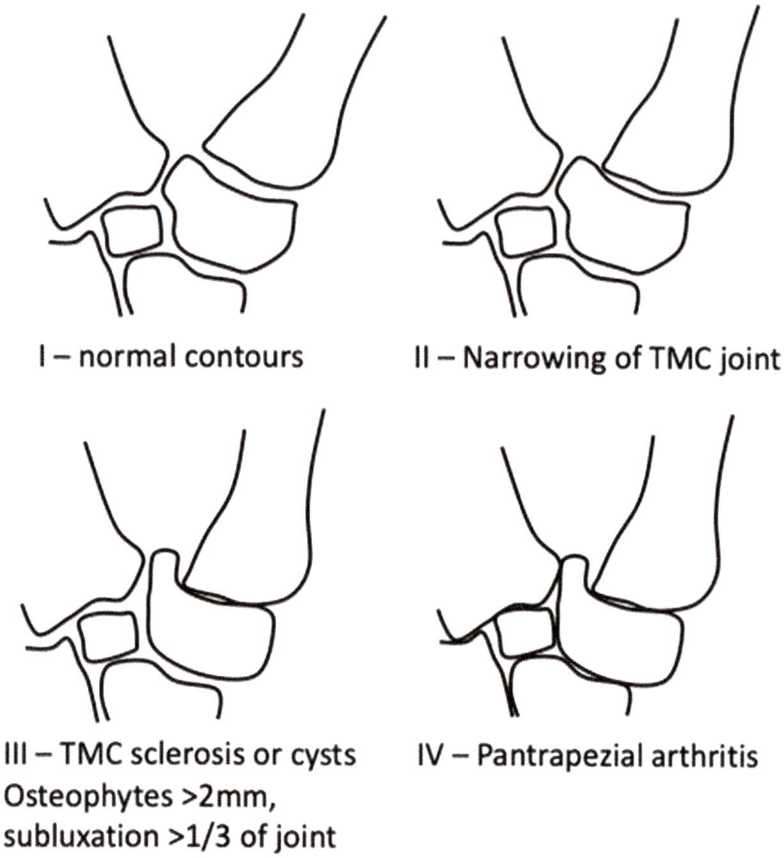

Fig. 7.41 TMCJ arthritis staging

Treatment

Treatment is based on clinical symptoms and not radiographic findings. Conservative treatment with appropriate splinting should be used first. Steroid injections can help confirm an uncertain diagnosis and offer temporary relief.

Stage 1 TMCJ arthritis is managed by carpometacarpal joint arthroscopy and thermal shrinkage of the palmar beak ligament and capsule. If symptoms return with time, the procedure can be repeated or a more permanent palmar beak ligament reconstruction (with split FCR) performed (Eaton Littler).

Stages 2, 3 and 4 are managed by salvage surgery. A number of options are available (Table 7.7).

Trapeziectomy

A dorsal or modified Wagner approach is used (Fig. 7.42). There is risk of damage to superficial radial nerve and radial artery.

Wrist Osteoarthritis

Scaphotrapeziotrapezoid Arthritis

Patients present with a painful wrist. Non-operative measures are adopted in early disease. The main surgical treatment is scaphotrapeziotrapezoid fusion. However, there is progressive TMC or radioscaphoid arthritis in 33% of patients. There is also a relatively high non-union

Table 7.7 Salvage surgery options for trapeziometacarpal joint arthritis

Surgery	Description
Trapeziometacarpal arthrodesis (for stages 2 and 3)	Good results, but may lead to wear of the scaphotrapeziotrapezoid joint Suitable for young and high-demand patients
Abduction extension osteotomy	Designed to offload the palmar surface of the joint Can be considered for high-demand young adults with early disease The failure rate is about 20%
Excisional arthroplasty (trapeziectomy)	Good pain relief Weakness in grip and pinch as a result of the operation is rarely noticed by the patient
Excision, ligament reconstruction and interposition—Flexor carpi radialis/joint capsule (LRTI)	The additional first metacarpal stabilisation or interposition procedures have yet to be proven superior to excision of the trapezium alone *Davis T, Brady O, Barton NJ, Lunn PJ, burke ED. Trapeziectomy alone, with tendon interposition or with ligament reconstruction? Journal of hand surgery (Br).1997; 22B (6) 689–694.*
Trapezial/metacarpal implants	Equivocal/poor results High early failure rate

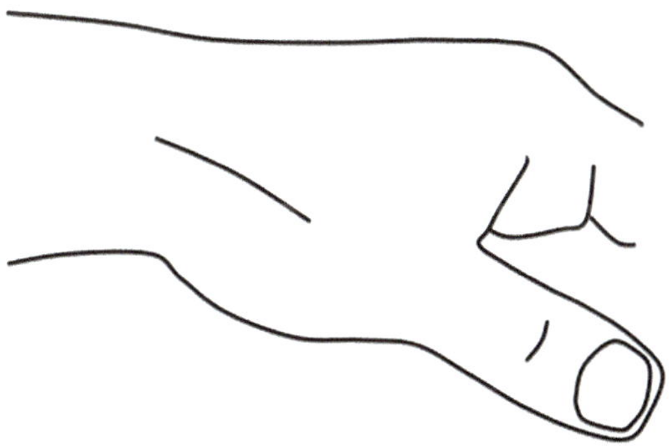

Fig. 7.42 Incision for trapeziectomy

rate. Alternatives to scaphotrapeziotrapezoid fusion are trapezium excision or excision of the distal pole of the scaphoid, with or without interposition arthroplasty.

Radiocarpal Arthritis

The underlying cause of radiocarpal arthritis may be secondary to a distal radius fracture, scaphoid fracture, radiocarpal dislocation or scapholunate ligament insufficiency.

Once conservative treatment fails arthrodesis is the treatment of choice (Table 7.8). Partial arthrodesis will preserve some wrist movement.

Scapholunate/Scaphoid Non-union Advanced Collapse

Scapholunate advanced collapse (SLAC) and scaphoid non-union advanced collapse (SNAC) follow untreated scapholunate ligament injury and non-union of a scaphoid fracture respectively.

Treatment depends on the stage of the disease and the status of the proximal capitate & radiolunate joint (which is often spared).

Surgical options include:

- Scaphoid excision and four-corner fusion.
- Proximal row carpectomy (remove scaphoid, lunate and triquetrum) with radial styloidectomy (contraindicated in presence of capitolunate arthritis).
- Wrist fusion.

Table 7.8 Treatment based on location of arthritis

Location	Treatment
Radiolunate	Radiolunate arthrodesis
Radioscapholunate	Radioscapholunate arthrodesis plus excision of the distal third of the scaphoid (to unlock the midcarpal joint)
Radiolunate and midcarpal	Total wrist fusion Wrist replacement arthroplasty Low-demand patients only

Rheumatoid Hand

Pathology

Rheumatoid arthritis is a chronic, systemic inflammatory disorder that principally attacks the joints. The pathological features are synovial proliferation and destructive pannus formation. This leads to cartilage, ligament and tendon destruction; and bone erosion.

Principles of Surgery

The principles are:

- Maximise medical treatment before considering surgery.
- Assess the timing and the natural course of the disease.
- Surgery should be performed before fixed joint contractures.
- Proximal joints should be operated on before the distal joints.
- Do not combine mobilisation procedures (arthroplasty) with stabilisation procedures (arthrodesis).

Extensor Tendons

Patients may present with extensor tenosynovitis and tendon ruptures. There is fraying of tendons, rupture, formation of nodules and pseudotendon. Rupture of extensor tendons due to erosion over the distal ulna is known as Vaughn–Jackson lesion.

Causes of inability to extend the fingers are–

- Tendon rupture.
- Subluxation of the extensor carpi ulnaris tendon.
- MCPJ dislocation.
- Posterior interosseous nerve (PIN) palsy.
- Tender nodules.

Differentiation Between Rupture and Subluxation

If tendons have ruptured then the patient is unable to hold the MCPJs in extension. If subluxed, when the MCPJ is extended passively the tendon returns to its normal position & the patient can then maintain the extended position.

Rupture Versus Palsy

In a PIN palsy (e.g. at radial neck) the fingers will extend when the wrist is flexed because of the tenodesis effect. However, this will not occur if the tendons have ruptured as the tenodesis effect is then lost.

Management of extensor tendon problems in the rheumatoid hand is shown in Table 7.9.

Flexor Tendons

Rupture of the flexor pollicis longus is known as Mannerfelt syndrome. This tendon ruptures due to erosion or an osteophyte on the scaphoid and

Table 7.9 Management of extensor tendon problems in the rheumatoid hand

Problem	Treatment
Rupture of little finger extensor	Distal end of ruptured tendon attached to ring finger extensor tendon
Rupture of ring and little finger extensors	Combine little and ring extensors and transfer extensor indicis proprius to both
Rupture of small, ring and middle finger extensors	Combine little and ring extensors and transfer extensor indicis proprius to both Suture middle finger extensor to index finger
Rupture of all four extensor digitorum tendons	Tendon graft or ring finger flexor digitorum superficialis transfer
Rupture of extensor pollicis longus	Extensor indicis to extensor pollicis longus transfer

synovitis. It is treated with a tendon bridge graft or a two-stage flexor graft.

Flexor tenosynovitis causes pain, triggering and tendon rupture. Steroid injection can be initially attempted, then a tenosynovectomy if the condition fails to respond.

Wrist

The problems in rheumatoid wrists include carpal supination, carpal ulnar subluxation, synovitis, joint destruction and distal radio ulnar joint pain.

Carpal supination is due to rupture of the dorsal radiocarpal ligaments, which leads to the ulna head becoming prominent.

In carpal ulnar subluxation, the carpus migrates down the radial slope secondary to erosive changes.

Synovitis involves the distal radioulnar and radiocarpal joints. A synovectomy can be considered for pain and removal of destructive tissue.

For joint destruction and pain, wrist arthrodesis or replacement can be considered.

Distal radioulnar joint pain—consider synovectomy with or without ulnar head excision. A Sauvé–Kapandji procedure is an option in young patients with a preserved ulnar head. This allows the ulna head to support the carpus. A Darrach's procedure is another option, where the distal ulna is resected.

Metacarpophalangeal Joint

Palmar dislocation and ulnar deviation of the proximal phalanges is caused by.

- Synovitis predominantly on the radial side, weakening the radial collateral ligament.
- Weakening of the radial sagittal band.
- Ulna subluxation of the extensor tendons.
- Normal pinch forces against the radial side of the fingers.

Synovitis is managed by synovectomy with or without extensor realignment.

Joint destruction and pain can be managed by implant arthroplasty with a silicone implant such as Swanson's, together with extensor tendon realignment.

Interphalangeal Joint

Swan-Neck Deformity

Swan-neck deformity is predominantly caused by PIPJ synovitis with attenuation of the volar plate and collateral ligaments, allowing hyperextension. In addition, patients may have intrinsic tightness.

A DIPJ mallet can be the initiating problem, due to extensor tendon rupture, with the PIPJ being susceptible to hyperextension because of an attenuated volar plate.

Pathology can also originate at the wrist—with carpal collapse causing relaxation of the extrinsics, which can then be overpowered by the intrinsics, causing MCPJ flexion & PIPJ extension.

Treatment varies depending on the type of deformity (Table 7.10).

Boutonniere Deformity

Boutonniere deformity is caused by synovitis at the PIPJ. This attenuates the extensor mechanism and elongates the central slip. The lateral bands then start to migrate towards the volar.

Again, treatment varies depending on the stage of deformity (Table 7.11).

Thumb

Problems associated with the thumb include swan-neck and Boutonniere deformities, as well as MCPJ pain (Table 7.12). Like in the digits,

Table 7.10 Treatment of swan-neck deformity

Type	Description	Treatment
I	Good passive motion at the PIPJ and no pain	A figure of eight splint to prevent hyperextension Tendon procedures (e.g., lateral band transfer) should be used to statically prevent extension
II	A positive result for the intrinsic test MCPJ extension limits PIP flexion	As for type I, plus intrinsic release
III	Loss of PIPJ motion without PIPJ destruction on X-ray	PIPJ manipulation with a temporary wire, with or without intrinsic release Once mobile, treatment is as for type I
IV	Limited PIPJ motion and joint destruction	Arthrodesis for the index and middle fingers Implant arthroplasty for the little and ring fingers

MCPJ metacarpophalangeal joint; *PIPJ* proximal interphalangeal joint

Table 7.11 Treatment of Boutonniere deformity

Stage	Description	Treatment
I	Pre-boutonniere deformity Normal PIPJ movement, but may have decreased DIP movement	Splint or synovectomy
II	Passively correctable PIPJ flexion of 30	Synovectomy and central slip repair or reconstruction using lateral bands
III	Fixed PIPJ contracture	Arthrodesis or arthroplasty
IV	Contracture >70	Arthrodesis

DIPJ distal interphalangeal joint; *PIPJ* proximal interphalangeal joint

treatment depends on whether the deformity is fixed or flexible.

Tendon transfers for Peripheral Nerve Dysfunction

Before tendon transfers can take place, certain prerequisites must be met (Table 7.13).

Table 7.12 Treatment of problems of the rheumatoid thumb

Problem	Description	Treatment
Swan-neck deformity	Interphalangeal joint flexed, MCPJ extended, CMC joint flexed	If originating from carpometacarpal joint degeneration and adducted first metacarpal—Trapeziectomy If originating from the MCPJ—MCPJ arthrodesis
Boutonniere deformity	IPJ extended, MCPJ flexed, carpometacarpal joint extended or normal	If comfortable and mobile—Divide the extensor pollicis longus distally and transfer to the proximal phalanx
MCPJ pain	–	Arthrodesis

MCPJ metacarpophalangeal joint; *IPJ* Interphalangeal joint

Table 7.13 Prerequisites for tendon transfers

Category	Prerequisites
Joints	Good preoperative range of motion
Donor muscle/tendon	Good power (5/5 MRC grade) Sufficient excursion for satisfactory function Preferably synergistic Preferably has a straight line of pull Under voluntary control with independent action Expendable
Patient	Motivation and mental capacity to re-train

There are many different types of tendon transfers. Those below mention some of the accepted transfers for the conditions described.

Low Median Nerve Palsy

Problem

Loss of thumb abduction and opposition. Thumb abduction and opposition are frequently retained after an isolated median nerve injury because of innervation by the ulnar nerve. Even with marked thenar muscle wasting, adequate abduction and opposition is possible.

Treatment

Treatment depends on the presence of the PL.

If the PL is present, a Camitz transfer is performed. This transfer restores palmar abduction. When abducted, the flexor pollicis longus can then oppose the thumb.

A strip of palmar fascia is dissected in continuity with the PL tendon. This effectively extends the length of the tendon. This is passed subcutaneously and attached to the abductor pollicis brevis insertion. Release of the carpal tunnel is performed.

If the PL is absent, donor tendons choice is extensor indices proprius, FDS to ring or long fingers or abductor digiti minimi (Huber transfer).

High Median Nerve Palsy

Problems are loss of forearm pronation; flexion of wrist, index finger, middle finger and thumb; and thumb opposition.

Treatment

Treatment is summarized in Table 7.14.

Low Ulnar Nerve Palsy

Problem is loss of intrinsic muscles and loss of thumb to index finger pinch.

Treatment

- Static clawing—MCPJ volar plate advancement.
- Dynamic clawing—the FDS of the long finger tendon is split to attach A2 pulleys to all fingers (Table 7.15).

Table 7.14 Tendon transfers for high median nerve palsy

Function needed	Common method
Thumb IPJ flexion	Brachioradialis to FPL
Opposition	EIP
Index & middle finger flexion	ECRL to the index finger FDP

High Ulnar Nerve Palsy

Problem

Loss of flexor carpi ulnaris and FDP to ring and little fingers.

Treatment

Treatment is similar to that for low ulna nerve palsy, with suturing of the FDP tendon of the little and ring fingers to that of the middle finger.

Radial Nerve Palsy

In low radial nerve palsy, the extensor carpi radialis longus, extensor carpi radialis brevis and brachioradialis are spared. The available muscles are the wrist flexors: flexor carpi ulnaris, FCR, FDS, PL and pronator teres (Table 7.16).

In a high radial nerve palsy, there is loss of wrist extension in addition to the dysfunction in low radial nerve palsy. Pronator teres transfer can be used for regaining active wrist extension.

Complications

Some patients develop adhesions which need treatment with intensive hand therapy with or without tenolysis.

Table 7.15 Tendon transfers for low ulnar nerve palsy

Function needed	Common method
Thumb adduction	ECRB, brachioradialis or ring finger FDS
Index finger abduction	Accessory slip of the APL

Table 7.16 Tendon transfers for low radial nerve palsy

Function needed	Common method
Wrist extension (extensor carpi radialis brevis)	Pronator teres
Finger extension	Flexor carpi ulnaris
Thumb extension	Palmaris longus
Thumb abduction	Palmaris longus

Procedures for the Paralytic Hand

Trying to improve hand function for patients who have cerebral palsy or suffered a stroke is complex. The surgical options depend on the following and are assessed on an individual patient basis:

- Extent of motor involvement.
- Degree of spasticity.
- Extent of contracture.
- Voluntary control of the muscles.
- Mental capacity to maximise function following surgery.

In principle, the following treatment options can be used:

- Muscles with high resting tone or spasticity can be lengthened to weaken them.
- Tendons can be transferred if there is a degree of motor control.
- An improved functional position of the hand can be achieved with arthrodesis.

In most cases the condition is too severe for a useful tendon transfer. Most often, a mixture of tendon lengthening/division, joint releases and arthrodesis can improve function and personal care.

Replantation

Unsurprisingly, trauma is the most common cause for upper extremity replantation.

Indications

The factors that influence the decision for replantation are shown in Table 7.17.

Management

All patients must be managed rauma is the most common cause for upper extremity replantation in accordance with Advanced Trauma and Life Support (ATLS) principles.

Table 7.17 Factors influencing replantation

Factor	Implications for replantation
Level of injury	Replantation is considered for: • amputation of the thumb • multiple-digit amputations • amputation through the palm, wrist and distal forearm Single-digit amputation is a controversial indication (unless in a child) Results are variable with amputation through the proximal forearm, elbow and arm
Age	Increasing age is a negative factor. Outcomes worsen with age
General medical condition	Cardiac disease and diabetes reduce the success rate
Ischaemic time	Cold ischaemia of 12 hours and warm ischaemia of 6 hours are the upper limit for proximal amputations These limits can be doubled for digit amputations
Injury mechanism	Avulsion and crush are negative factors

The amputated part is wrapped with moist gauze, placed in a bag, and then that bag is placed in a bag of ice for transfer.

Reattachment

The order of reattachment is flexible, but in general:

- Obtain skeletal stability.
- Tendons.
- Arteries.
- Veins.
- Nerves.

The needs for prophylactic fasciotomies should be considered.

Post- Replantation

Patients with successful digit replantations commonly complain of stiffness, cold intolerance and poor sensibility. As a result, the patient often excludes the digit from use following a single finger replantation.

Hand Transplants

The UK Hand Transplant Programme is based in Leeds. To date, 72 upper limb and hand transplants have been performed. 18 transplants have survived past 5 years and 7 of 8 transplants have survived to 10 years.

Outcomes are greatly dependent on the individual. Several patients have experienced osteomyelitis or skin necrosis. Most patients had protective sensation, but poor localisation.

Most patients were hospitalised for several months. Prolonged immunosuppression is required. Better outcomes are associated with younger patients and more distal injuries.

References

From http://www.handtransplantuk.com/index.php/information-for-professionals/outcomes (accessed 01/02/2019)

de Quervain's Disease

This is a stenosing tenosynovitis of the first dorsal extensor compartment (containing APL and EPB). It is seen predominantly in women aged 30 to 50 years, and is noted to affect post-partum women.

Clinical Features

It presents with dorsoradial wrist pain, exacerbated by thumb movement. This is shown in Finkelstein's test, where folding the thumb into the palm and ulnar deviation of wrist reproduce the pain.

Treatment

Treatment involves rest, steroid injection into the first extensor compartment and surgical release. Conservative measures are less likely to be successful if the APL and EPB tendons have more than one tendon sheath. When releasing the first extensor compartment care must be taken to assess for multiple tendon sheaths, as well as to avoid injuring the sensory branch of radial nerve.

Further Reading

Ferdinand RD, Maclean JG. Endoscopic versus open carpal tunnel release in bilateral carpal tunnel syndrome. A prospective randomised blinded assessment. J Bone Joint Surg Br. 2002;84(3):375–9.

Lichtman DM, Lesley NE, Simmons SP. The classification and treatment of Kienbock's disease: the state of the art and a look at the future. J Hand Surg Am (European Volume. 2010;35E(7):549–54.

Ng CY. Rehabilitation regimens following surgical repair of extensor tendon injuries of the hand—a systematic review of controlled trials. J Hand Microsurg. 2012;4(2):65–73.

Small JO, Brennen MD, Colville J. Early active mobilisation following flexor tendon repair in zone 2. J Hand Surg Br. 1989;14(4):383–91.

Swanson AB, Barsky AJ, Entin MA. Classification of limb malformations on the basis of embryological failures. Surg Clin North Am. 1968;48(5):1169–79.

Bone and Soft Tissue Tumours

8

Robert Ashford and Randeep S. Aujla

Assessment of Tumours

Assessment of patients with any potential bone or soft tissue tumour should include a full history (particularly including previous malignancies and family history), a detailed clinical examination (including the breasts or prostate) and appropriate imaging.

Blood tests are helpful to rule out infection, although raised inflammatory markers (ESR/CRP) may be present in certain tumours, such as Ewing's sarcoma.

Plain radiographs are the initial investigation of choice for bone tumours and potential imaging studies are detailed in Table 8.1.

After local and systemic staging (Table 8.1), a biopsy should be undertaken either at, or following discussion with the regional sarcoma unit.

MRI scans are used to assess the extent of the lesion within the bone and any soft tissue extension. Whole body MRI is utilized for certain subtypes of soft tissue sarcoma e.g. myxoid liposarcoma. CT scans of the chest are highly sensitive compared to plain radiographs in detection of lung metastasis. Isotope bone scans are useful to detect other distant lesions and may show a primary lesion. Bone scans should be done prior to biopsy to avoid a false positive result. PET-CT can be used for detection of occult metastases.

R. Ashford (✉)
East Midlands Sarcoma Service and Leicester Cancer Research Centre, University Hospital of Leicester, Leicester, UK

University Hospital of Leicester, Leicester, UK
e-mail: robert.ashford@uhl-tr.nhs.uk

R. S. Aujla
University Hospital of Leicester, Leicester, UK

Biopsy and Staging of Tumours

Biopsy for bone and soft tissue tumours should be performed by, or in consultation with, the surgeon who will be definitively resecting the tumour and who is therefore familiar with the surgical approach that will be utilised for that resection.

Indications for Biopsy

The following features are indications for biopsy:

- Solitary bone lesions with aggressive features (presumed bone sarcoma)
- New bone lesions with no or distant history of cancer
- Soft tissue lesions with concerning features (e.g. large, deep to fascia, painful and growing) or radiological concerning features.
- When an accurate diagnosis cannot be made on imaging or when the lesion appears aggressive on imaging.

S. Agarwal (ed.), *Current Orthopaedic Practice*, https://doi.org/10.1007/978-3-030-78529-1_8

Table 8.1 Plan for evaluating bone and soft tissue tumours

Staging	Primary bone tumour	Soft tissue sarcoma	Skeletal metastasis
Local	Plain radiograph Whole bone MRI	Plain radiograph Ultrasound Lesion MRI	Plain radiograph (including joint above and joint below)
Systemic	Chest X-ray Chest CT Isotope bone scan or PET-CT	Chest X-ray Chest ± abdomen/pelvis CT PET-CT Whole Body MRI (for certain pathologies)	Chest and abdomen CT[a] Isotope bone scan[a]

[a]Where appropriate
CT computed tomography, *MRI* magnetic resonance imaging, *PET-CT* positron emission tomography-CT, *WBMRI* Whole Body MRI

Biopsy is not needed for the following:

- Non-ossifying fibromas.
- Unicameral bone cysts.
- Osteochondroma/exostoses.
- Enchondromata.
- Ganglia.
- Fatty tumours that completely suppress on magnetic resonance imaging (MRI) (e.g., lipoma, atypical lipomatous tumours, low-grade liposarcomas)—these should be marginally excised.

Types of Biopsy

1. *Closed/Core needle biopsy*
   Core needle biopsy (CNB) is utilised by most sarcoma services worldwide, in most cases under radiological guidance. Typically a Tru-Cut type needle is used for soft tissue lesions and a Jamshidi type for bone lesions (Fig. 8.1).
   CNBs are used for bone lesions with large soft tissue extensions and soft tissue tumours. The advantages and disadvantages of CNB are shown in Table 8.2.
2. *Open biopsy*
   The advantages and disadvantages of open biopsy are shown in Table 8.3.
   There are different types of open biopsy: incisional (a small area of tissue is taken from the lesion); excisional (the lesion is removed in its entirety and sent as a sample);

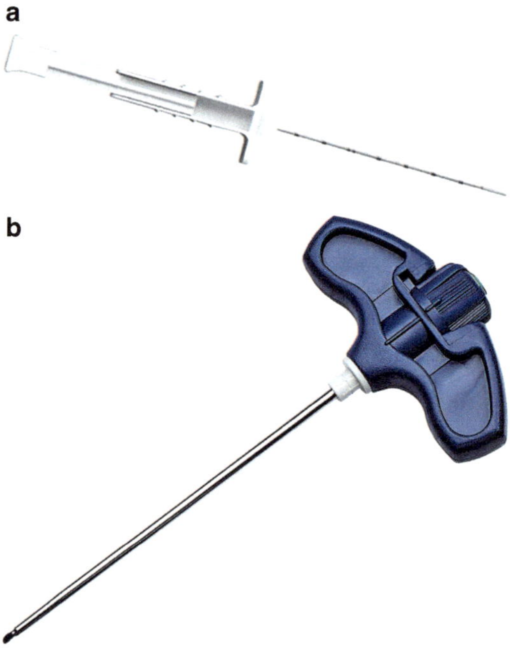

Fig. 8.1 (**a**) Trucut type biopsy needle (**b**) Jamshidi type biopsy needle

Table 8.2 Advantages and disadvantages of core needle biopsy compared with to open biopsy

Advantages	Disadvantages
Local anaesthetic Less invasive (may need image guidance) Less contamination Useful in spine and pelvis	Small sample size—insufficient/unrepresentative tissue Diagnostic accuracy is 85% (better at tumour centres) Needle tract has to be excised *en bloc* with main mass resection

Table 8.3 Advantages and disadvantages of open biopsy compared with core needle biopsy

Advantages	Disadvantages
Better/large sample size Diagnostic accuracy is 96% (better in tumour centres)	More time and expense—needs an operating theatre Risk of pathological fracture, infection or haematoma Biopsy tract must be excised *en bloc* with definitive surgery Higher risk of contamination

and primary wide excision (where the entire lesion is excised along with a cuff of normal tissue).

In incisional biopsies, all tissue touched or manipulated, including sutures and drain sites at definitive resection, is considered contaminated and should therefore be excised *en bloc* at definitive resection.

Incisional biopsy may be indicated for several types of lesions:

- Larger than 3–4 cm.
- Distal to the elbow and ankles, even for small lesions.
- Close to major vessels and nerves.
- Non-diagnostic CNB

It can also be useful for lesions in the axilla, groin, antecubital and popliteal fossae, hand and foot (difficult sites).

The advantages and disadvantages of excisional and primary wide excision methods are shown in Table 8.4.

A fine needle biopsy (FNB)/fine needle aspiration cytology (FNAC) is used in some centres using a 22–23 G needle. The smears are used for cytological diagnosis and the diagnostic accuracy is 80–90%. It is not compatible with immunohistochemical studies.

Surgical Technique for Open Biopsy

These principles apply for biopsies of both bone and soft tissue tumours.

Table 8.4 Advantages and disadvantages of incisional, excisional and primary wide excision biopsy

Type of biopsy	Advantages	Disadvantages
Incisional	Allows tissue diagnosis prior to planning definitive surgery Can avoid larger surgery if benign	Tumour seeding—tract will need to be excised at final surgery Further procedure may be needed
Excisional	Large sample size Serves as treatment (if benign or intermediate tumour)	Extensive contamination if the tumour proves aggressive and a wide margin is not achieved Nerve or vascular contamination can result in need for amputation
Primary wide excision	Single operation (particularly if high index of suspicion of malignancy in relatively medically unfit patient)	Lesion may not be malignant (therefore over treated) Negates role of neoadjuvant chemotherapy (inability to assess response)

Incision

A tourniquet can be used, with elevation rather than exsanguination and deflation prior to closure. Meticulous haemostasis should then be secured. A longitudinal incision is used with short oblique segments when crossing joint creases. The planned incision for definitive resection for the limb salvage should be marked and utilised in part. The most direct approach is used, going directly through the compartment, not in between compartments. Flaps should not be raised. Dissection should not be in between muscle planes. To prevent contamination, vessels, nerves or tendons should not be exposed (Neurovascular structures should be avoided).

Biopsy

A peripheral soft tissue sample is obtained. The Codman's triangle is to be avoided for biopsy, as periosteal new bone can be misdiagnosed as tumour. A round window (3.5 mm drill bit) is made in the bone if necessary—a core biopsy can then be taken through this hole. A frozen section is helpful to confirm that the tissue is representative. A culture sample is obtained before administering antibiotics—biopsies should always be sent for histology and microbiology.

A frozen section should be utilised for all patients being biopsied under general anaesthesia. The accuracy of frozen section for diagnosis is approximately 80%, but is less reliable for cartilage and fatty lesions. The primary role of the frozen section is to ensure representative tissue has been obtained. The representative tissue should allow definitive histopathological analysis.

Closure

Meticulous haemostasis is mandatory. If a drain is necessary, it should exit through the same compartment and in line with (and at one end of) the longitudinal incision. This is performed with a view to excise the drain tract at any further resection. Closure is performed in layers. A light pressure dressing is applied.

Mankin HJ, Lange TA, Spanier SS. The hazards of biopsy in patients with malignant primary bone and soft-tissue tumours. J Bone Joint Surg Am 1982;64:1121–7. Open Biopsy had a 20% inaccuracy rate when performed in a referring centre. The complication rate was higher when biopsy was performed by non-tumour surgeons.

Mankin HJ, Mankin CJ, Simon MA. The hazards of the biopsy, revisited. Members of the Musculoskeletal Tumor Society. J Bone Joint Surg Am 1996;78:656–63. The authors found no improvement from the 1982 study.

Pollock RC, Stalley PD. Biopsy of musculoskeletal tumours—beware. ANZ J Surg 2004;74:516–9. Definitive treatment was hindered by a badly performed open biopsy in 38% of patients biopsied by the referring surgeon. In 25%, treatment had to be changed either to a more radical procedure than would originally have been necessary or to palliative rather than curative intent.

Ashford RU, McCarthy SW, Scolyer RA, et al. Surgical biopsy with intra-operative frozen section. An accurate and cost-effective method for diagnosis of musculoskeletal sarcomas. J Bone Joint Surg Br 2006;88:1207–11. Accuracy was 99% and there were no inadequate biopsies. Surgical biopsy with intra-operative frozen section was 38% more expensive than CT-guided biopsy.

Staging of Malignant Bone Tumours

MSTS Staging (Enneking's) is based on three factors:

- Grade of tumour—low grade (G1) or high grade (G2).
- Anatomic site—intra-compartmental, confined to bone, (T1) or extra-compartmental, spread outside the bone including the periosteum, (T2).
- Metastasis—no distant metastasis (M0) or presence of distant metastasis (M1).

These three factors determine the staging (Table 8.5).

Classification of Benign Tumours

Benign bone tumours are classified into latent, active and aggressive, based on Enneking's classification (Table 8.6).

Enneking WF. A staging system of musculoskeletal neoplasms. Clin Orthop Relat Res 1986;204:9–24.

Table 8.5 Staging of malignant bone tumours

Stage	Grade	Site	Metastasis
IA	G1	T1	M0
IB	G1	T2	M0
IIA	G2	T1	M0
IIB	G2	T2	M0
III	Any grade	Any site	M1

Table 8.6 Classification of benign bone tumours

Type	Characteristics	Tumour type
Latent	Well-defined margin Grows slowly then stops Remains static/heals	Non-ossifying fibroma Chondroma Eosinophilic granuloma Osteoid osteoma
Active	Progressive growth Limited by natural barriers Recurs	Aneurysmal bone cyst Osteoblastoma Chondroblastoma
Aggressive	Aggressive growth, not limited by natural barriers Grows from bone to soft tissues	Giant cell tumour

Key Points for Biopsy and Staging of Tumours

- Biopsy of a tumour should be conducted by the centre who will be performing definitive treatment, or at least after discussion with them.
- Core needle biopsies are less invasive, can be performed under local anaesthetic and can access areas that can cause morbidity with open technique.
- Open biopsies provide a better diagnostic accuracy due to ease of accessing a representative sample.

In this chapter, bone neoplasms will be considered under

A. Benign cartilaginous tumours
B. Benign osteoblastic tumours
C. Benign cystic lesions
D. Benign locally aggressive tumours
E. Malignant primary bone tumours
F. Soft tissue sarcomas
G. Skeletal metastasis

A. Benign Cartilaginous Tumours

Benign cartilaginous tumours include osteochondroma, chondroma, chondroblastoma and chondromyxoid fibromas (CMFs).

Osteochondroma (Exostosis)

Osteochondroma is the most common benign bone lesion. It is a cartilage-capped projection on the external surface of bones. Lesions can be solitary or multiple. Solitary osteochondroma is a different pathological entity to multiple osteochondroma (multiple hereditary exostoses or MHE).

Etiology

The etiology of osteochondroma is linked to mutations in the Exostosin-1 *(EXT1) and Exostosin-2 (EXT2)* genes. 44–66% of multiple osteochondroma families show EXT1 linkage. The underlying histological process is of abnormal growth of cartilage.

MHE is associated with bone deformities and bone growth abnormalities and occurs with an incidence of 1:50,000. It is autosomal dominant in 70% of patients and sporadic mutation in 30% of patients.

Clinical Features

Patients most commonly present with osteochondromata in the second decade of life, and the male to female ratio is 2:1. The actual incidence of osteochondroma in the general population is unknown as they can often be asymptomatic and impalpable.

Osteochondromas are seen as bony prominences at the metaphyseal ends of long bones—usually around the knee, although the pelvis and scapula are also commonly involved. They can occur in any bone.

MHE can interfere with joint movements and lead to flexion deformities (Fig. 8.2). Clinical features include abnormal bone growth, leg-length inequalities, forearm bowing and valgus knees and ankles.

The risk of malignant transformation is about 1% in solitary osteochondromas and increases to 10% in MHE. Malignant transformation never occurs before skeletal maturity. Increasing size, onset of pain and an increase of more than 1 cm in the thickness of the cartilage cap indicate possible malignant transformation. Malignant transformation is usually to a low-grade

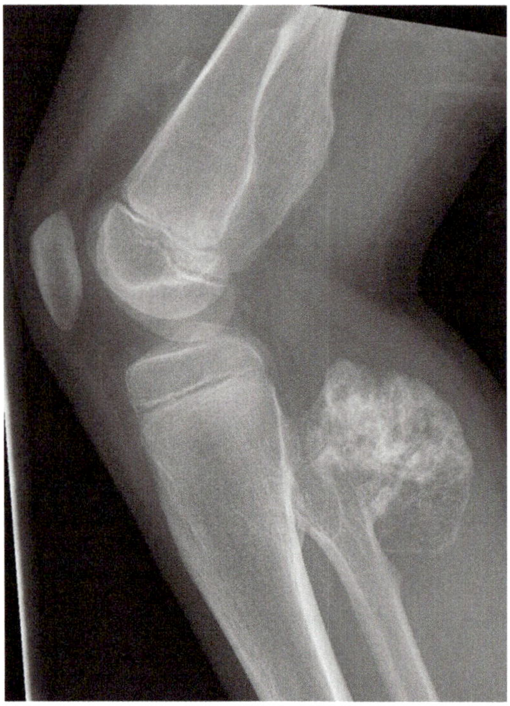

Fig. 8.2 Multiple Hereditary Exostoses in an 8 year old boy. The fibular exostosis required excision due to pressure effects and interference with knee movements

chondrosarcoma with a local recurrence rate of less than 2%.

Staals EL, Bacchini P, Mercuri M, Bertoni F. Dedifferentiated chondrosarcomas arising in preexisting osteochondromas. J Bone Joint Surg Am 2007;89:987–93. Dedifferentiated chondrosarcomas from osteochondroma were extremely rare, but were associated with a poor prognosis.

Imaging

On radiographs, the osteochondroma can be a pedunculated or sessile outgrowth from the metaphyseal region. The direction of growth of the pedunculated lesion is away from the adjoining joint. The cortex of the osteochondroma is always contiguous with the normal cortex and adjacent medullary cavity.

There is a hyaline cartilage cap on the bony prominence, the thickness of which decreases with skeletal maturity. This can usually readily be demonstrated on ultrasound. An increase in the thickness of the cartilage cap indicates possible malignant transformation.

Malghem J, Vande Berg B, Noël H, Maldague B. Benign osteochondromas and exostotic chondrosarcomas: evaluation of cartilage cap thickness by ultrasound. Skeletal Radiol 1992;21:33–7. Ultrasound is accurate for assessing cartilage cap thickness.

Management

The removal of a benign osteochondroma may be indicated for functional limitation of the adjoining joint, formation of painful bursa overlying the growth, neurological or vascular pressure symptoms, fracture or rarely cosmetic concerns.

Osteochondromas should be investigated if there is pain or growth after skeletal maturity. Recurrence after excision raises suspicion of malignancy. The risk of malignancy is 5–25%.

Porter DE, Lonie L, Fraser M, et al. Severity of disease and risk of malignant change in hereditary multiple exostoses. A genotype–phenotype study. J Bone Joint Surg Br 2004;86:1041–6. The presence of an EXT1 mutation indicated significantly worse disease. The lifetime sarcoma risk was 3%.

Chondromata

Chondromata are common cartilaginous tumours, second only to osteochondromata in prevalence. Broadly, chondromata can be divided into two groups: enchondroma, which occur within the bone; and periosteal chondroma, which occur on the bone surface.

Enchondroma

Patients usually present with enchondroma in the second decade of life, however they are often incidental findings. Enchondroma commonly involve the small bones of the hand; other sites include the long bones, pelvis and scapula. Long bone lesions are located in the metaphysis and diaphysis.

The tumour is usually asymptomatic, although local swelling due to bone expansion is sometimes evident. Pain, when it occurs, is commonly due to a pathological fracture, which can draw attention to the presence of an enchondroma. If the lesion is painful without pathological fracture, chondrosarcomatous dedifferentiation should be considered.

Imaging shows an intraosseous radiolucent lesion with a varying amount of mineralisation and calcification (Fig. 8.3). The edges are rounded and well defined. The cortex is well preserved in long bones, while in small bones there can be cortical thinning and expansion. There is a high MRI signal on T2 and a low MRI signal on T1.

Histologically, the tumour is composed of well-differentiated mature hyaline cartilage cells. It can be difficult to distinguish between enchondroma, atypical cartilaginous tumour (ACT) and low-grade chondrosarcoma.

Periosteal Chondroma

Periosteal chondroma is an often painful tumour on the bone surface. It is rare and usually occurs in adolescents or young adults.

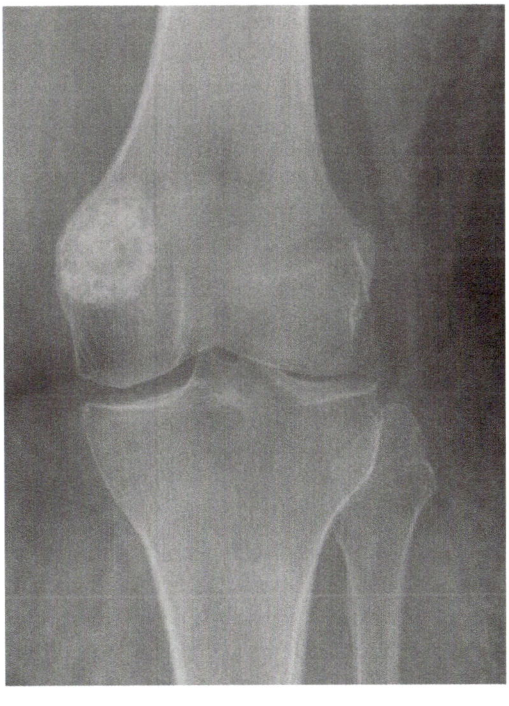

Fig. 8.3 Calcified enchondroma in a 74 year old woman. This was an incidental finding

The pathological appearance is similar to that of enchondroma. The tumour is usually smaller than 5 cm in diameter. A mass lies on the bone surface, with scalloping of the underlying cortex and a dense sclerotic rim.

Multiple Chondromata

Conditions resulting in multiple chondromata are much rarer than MHE.

- Ollier disease—caused by an error in osseous development. It is characterised by multiple intraosseous and subperiosteal cartilage tumours. The development of bone destruction or soft tissue masses suggests malignant transformation. The risk of secondary malignancy is 10–25% and the malignancy risk is 25%.
- Maffucci syndrome—a congenital condition characterised by the same skeletal lesions as Ollier disease plus soft tissue haemangiomas. Calcified phleboliths are a feature on radiographs. The risk of secondary malignancy is 15–56% and the malignancy risk is reported to be 100%.

Management of Chondromata

Benign asymptomatic chondromas can be simply followed-up with regular radiographs. In the presence of a pathologic fracture, the fracture should be allowed to heal with non-operative measures and the lesion can be treated with curettage and bone grafting if needed. Alternatively, the fracture can be stabilised internally along with curettage and bone grafting of the lesion primarily.

Chondroblastoma

Chondroblastomas are small cartilaginous tumours in the epiphysis of long bones, appearing as well-demarcated lytic lesions. They account for less than 1% of all primary bone tumours.

Clinical Features

Patients usually present with chondroblastoma in the second decade of life, and the male to female ratio is 3:2. The knee is a common site, while other sites include the proximal femur and proximal humerus. Patients present with local pain and restricted movement. Pain has often been present for many months.

Imaging

The neoplasm appears as a lytic lesion in the center of the epiphysis. Aggressive tumours may sometimes extend to the metaphysis or the soft tissues. Mineralisation is present in approximately 50% of lesions. MRI scans demonstrate 'vigorous' oedema surrounding the lesion.

Pathology

The tumour is composed of round or polyhedral cells with large nuclei. Mitotic figures can be present but are never atypical. Multinucleated giant cells may be present. Pericellular chicken-wire-like calcifications are pathognomonic of chondroblastoma and stain positively for S100.

Management

Management of the majority of chondroblastomas is with curettage and bone grafting. Local recurrence occurs in up to 15% of patients. Recurrent chondroblastoma is likely to be malignant and is best managed by *en bloc* resection.

Chondromyxoid Fibroma (CMF)

Clinical Features

CMF is the least common benign bone tumour of chondrogenic origin. The male to female ratio is 2:1. CMF shows a predilection for the tibia, the small bones of the feet and the ilium. There are two peaks of incidence: one in the first and second decades of life, and a second at ages 50–70 years. Risk of malignant transformation is small (<2%).

Imaging

The main features are well-circumscribed, round or oval osteolytic lesions with an eccentric metaphyseal location. The cortex is frequently eroded. With MRI scanning, there is a low signal on T1 sequences of the lesion and a high signal on T2.

Pathology

Histologically, the lesion is lobulated and well demarcated from the surrounding bone. The lesion is hypocellular centrally and hypercellular peripherally. Spindle cells are present in an abundant myxoid matrix.

Management

Treatment of CMF is by curettage with bone grafting if necessary. Adjuvants, such as cement, liquid nitrogen and phenol, should be considered. Local recurrence is less than 5%. *En bloc* resection with appropriate reconstruction may be necessary for extensive lesions.

Rahimi A, Beabout JW, Ivins JC, Dahlin DC. Chondromyxoid fibroma: a clinicopathologic study of 76 cases. Cancer 1972;30:726–36. CMF was aggressive locally and distinguishable from chondrosarcoma on imaging. It will recur if not treated properly.

Key Points for Benign Cartilaginous Tumours

- Osteochondroma is the most common benign bone lesion and can be associated with conditions leading to multiple osteochondromata (MHE, Ollier disease, Maffucci syndrome).
- Chondroblastomas appear as lytic lesions in the epiphysis of long bones and are usually treated with curettage and bone grafting.
- Chondromyxoid fibromas are benign and usually have an eccentric metaphyseal location.

B. Benign Osteoblastic Tumours

Osteoid Osteoma

Osteoid osteoma is a benign bone neoplasm.

Clinical Features

The common age of presentation is 4–25 years and the male to female ratio is 2:1. The main presenting symptom is pain. The pain can be severe, is often worse at night and is typically relieved by non-steroidal anti-inflammatory drugs (NSAIDs). The common sites of osteoid osteoma are the diaphysis and metaphysis in the long bones.

Lesions in the spine involve the posterior elements and the resulting pain leads to a non–structural, painful, concave scoliosis on the side of the lesion.

Imaging
The radiographic appearance is of a small lytic lesion with surrounding cortical sclerosis with a central nidus. A fine-cut CT scan is the best imaging modality to demonstrate the nidus and plan treatment.

Pathology
The pain in osteoid osteoma is related to a high level of local prostaglandins, and hence is effectively alleviated by NSAIDs.

The nidus is composed of immature osteoid trabeculae and mineralised matrix, with blood vessels and a fibrovascular stroma. The nidus is surrounded by dense sclerotic bone.

Management
The management options for osteoid osteoma include the following:

- CT-guided radiofrequency/laser ablation.
- Intralesional resection with the use of a burr or adjuvants such as phenol.
- Resection of the nidus.

CT-guided radiofrequency/laser ablation is usually the first-line "surgical" treatment and is particularly useful for lesions that are difficult to access surgically. It is minimally invasive, but the procedure often has to be performed under general/regional anaesthesia. There is a risk of injury to nearby nerves and soft tissues, and histological diagnosis can be difficult due to the limited amount of tissue obtained. However, radiofrequency ablation has successfully been used in spinal osteoid osteomata. Recurrence rate (10–15%) is higher than with surgical excision.

Surgery can be utilised for easily accessible lesions as it provides tissue for histological diagnosis and is also associated with a low rate of recurrence (5–10%).

Hoffmann RT, Jakobs TF, Kubisch CH, et al. Radiofrequency ablation in the treatment of osteoid osteoma—5-year experience. Eur J Radiol 2010;73:374–9. Biopsy was possible in 50% of patients. Thirty-eight of 39 patients successfully treated. One patient developed an infection and there was one broken needle.

Cribb GL, Goude WH, Cool P, et al. Percutaneous radiofrequency thermocoagulation of osteoid osteomas: factors affecting therapeutic outcome. Skeletal Radiology 2005;34(11):702–6. Recurrence rate 16%. No complications recorded in 45 cases.

Osteoblastoma

Osteoblastoma is a benign bone neoplasm.

Clinical Features
Patients usually present with osteoblastoma in the second and third decades of life. Males are more often affected than females.

The posterior element of the spine is the most common site of osteoblastoma, although any bone can be involved. The metaphysis is the preferred location in long bones.

Neurological symptoms may arise from pressure or pathologic fracture. Osteoblastoma in the spine can cause painful scoliosis.

Imaging
The lesions are either mixed lytic and blastic or predominantly lytic.

A CT scan is the ideal imaging method to assess the size and location of the neoplasm. The presence of mineralisation within the lesion helps to differentiate it from an aneurysmal bone cyst (ABC).

An MRI scan may reveal oedema in the surrounding tissues and bone, known as 'flare phenomenon'. This can raise suspicion of malignancy.

Pathology
Osteoblastomas are histologically similar to osteoid osteoma but have increased size. They are predominantly lytic with a fibrovascular stroma. There is less surrounding sclerosis than in osteoid osteomata. Immature osteoid trabeculae and

giant cells are seen. It has a more organized structure than osteoid osteomata.

Management

Surgical excision (intralesional curettage or en-bloc resection) is the treatment of choice to achieve the lowest recurrence rate. If the location of the tumour precludes wide excision then curettage and treatment with adjuvants (e.g., phenol) or cryosurgery is an option. Bone grafting is often required and prophylactic fixation should be considered for larger lesions.

Key Points for Benign Osteoblastic Tumours

- Osteoid osteoma and osteoblastoma are benign lesions of bone.
- They usually present in the second or third decades of life.
- Pain is the main symptom, and is characteristically relieved by the use of NSAIDs.
- Radiologically, lytic lesions are surrounded by sclerotic bone with a central nidus.
- Radiofrequency ablation or surgery are the treatment modalities.

C. Benign Cystic Lesions

Unicameral (Simple) Bone Cyst

Clinical Features

Patients present with unicameral bone cysts (UBC) in the first two decades of life. The male to female ratio is 2:1.

The majority of UBCs are asymptomatic, although some patients can present with pain, pathological fracture or swelling.

UBCs are usually located in the metaepiphyseal areas and most frequently involve the proximal humerus (60–70%), proximal femur (15%), and proximal tibia (5%).

Imaging

On imaging there is a central lucency within the medullary cavity, with a narrow zone of transition. A fallen fragment sign may be seen in pathological fractures. With MRI, the lesion is very bright on T2 sequences and there is a low signal on T1.

Pathology

The pathological features are of a unilocular cyst with clear fluid, a thin fibrous wall, dilated vessels and scattered lymphocytes.

Management

Management is usually observation. If a pathological fracture occurs then it should be allowed to heal. In the event of recurrence, curettage and adjuvants can be considered. Injections of steroid, bone marrow or calcitonin have been tried to stimulate healing with variable results. Healing of the UBC may be stimulated by fracture.

If there is an expanding lesion in weight-bearing bone, curettage and bone grafting is the treatment of choice.

Aneurysmal Bone Cyst (ABC)

Clinical Features

ABCs are benign cystic lesions of bone that expand the cortex. They can be primary (arising *de novo*—translocation TRE17/USP6) or secondary (as a result of cystic change in a giant cell tumour [GCT] or chondroblastoma); approximately 30% are secondary. The male to female ratio is 1:1.

The symptoms are usually pain and swelling. Occasionally a pathological fracture is the presenting feature.

Imaging

ABCs are typically expansile, lytic lesions, eccentrically located in the medullary cavity of long bones. They can arise in the cortex or periosteum and can cross joints.

MRI of expansile ABCs often reveals multiple fluid levels.

Pathology

At surgery the feature is typically a 'hole containing blood' but 5% manifest in the solid form.

Histologically ABCs are cavernous spaces with walls that lack any endothelial cell lining.

Differential Diagnosis

The differential diagnosis of ABC includes GCT (however secondary ABC can occur in GCTs) and Telangiectatic osteosarcoma.

Management

The treatment of ABC depends on the location. Most lesions are treated with intralesional curettage, with or without bone grafting or cementation. Recurrence occurs in 10–20% of patients and is reduced by adjuvants. Expendable bones can be excised. Embolisation should be considered for large and pelvic lesions. The concept of curopsy (percutaneous limited curettage at time of biopsy) has been shown to resolve ABCs in 81% of patients. There is some evidence for injection of ABC with bone marrow or doxycycline but this can only be considered experimental at this stage.

Marcove RC, Sheth DS, Takemoto S, Healey JH. The treatment of aneurysmal bone cyst. Clin Orthop Relat Res 1995;311:157–63. With curettage alone, the authors reported 59% recurrence. Curettage plus cryosurgery resulted in an 82% rate of cure, rising to 96% with a second treatment.

Reddy KIA, Sinnaeve F, Gaston CL, Grimer RJ, Carter SR. Aneurysmal Bone Cysts: Do simple treatments work? Clin Orthop Relat Res 2014;472:1901–10.

Key Points for Benign Cystic Lesions

- Unicameral bone cysts appear in the young and are often an incidental finding. Usually found in the meta-epiphyseal region. Observation is the treatment of choice.
- Aneurysmal bone cysts (ABC) are primary in 70% of cases.
- Secondary ABC can occur due to giant cell tumours or chondroblastoma.
- ABCs classically have multiple fluid levels on MRI.

D. Benign Locally Aggressive Tumours

Giant Cell Tumour (Osteoclastoma)

A GCT is a mesenchymal tumour. The cell of origin is a mononuclear stromal cell that produces type I and II collagen. Most GCTs are benign and the risk of local recurrence is 20–50%. Malignant transformation occurs in 10% of recurrent GCTs. Pulmonary metastasis can occur in 1–4%.

Clinical Features

Almost half of GCTs occur around the knee. Other common sites are the distal radius, proximal humerus and pelvis. GCTs are typically epiphyseal and have an eccentric location in the bone. Patients usually present in the second to fourth decade of life, and the male to female ratio is 1.5:1.

Clinically, GCT presents with local swelling, warmth and pain unrelated to weight bearing. Pathologic fracture occurs in up to 15% of cases.

Imaging

Epiphyseal location of a lucent lesion in a patient between 20 and 40 years of age should raise the possibility of a Giant Cell tumour (Fig. 8.4).

With CT, the density is 20–70 HU. CT is useful for evaluating the intraosseous extent of the tumour. With MRI, GCTs are typified by a high signal in T2-weighted images. They demonstrate high contrast enhancement. MRI is useful to detect extension of the tumour into the bone marrow and soft tissues. Secondary ABC formation can often occur in GCT.

Pathology

GCTs arise from undifferentiated mesenchymal cells in the bone marrow. The giant cells are derived from fusion of mononuclear stromal cells or nuclear division. They are approximately 60 μ (microns) in size and the nuclei are arranged centrally. The giant cells stain positively for tartrate-resistant acid phosphatase (TRAP) and have receptors for calcitonin.

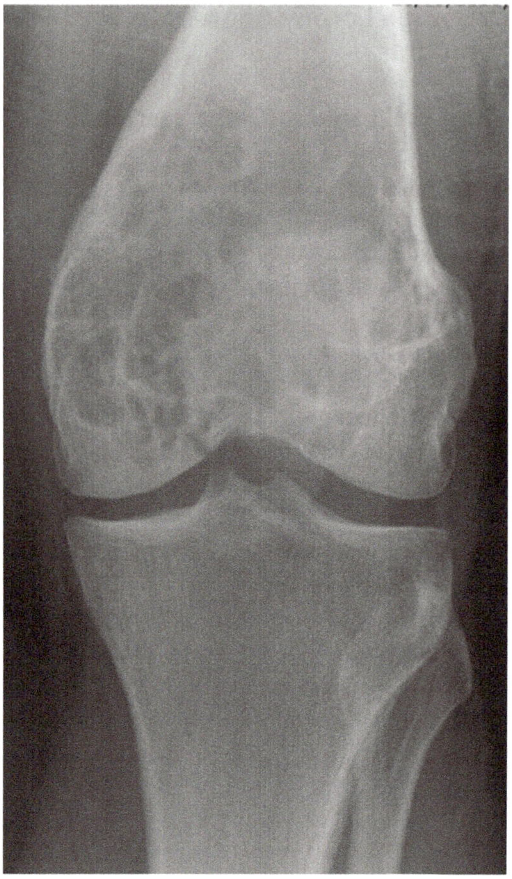

Fig. 8.4 Giant Cell tumour of distal femur in a 36 year old patient

Mononuclear stromal cells have two cell lines:

- Round cells—non-neoplastic and express TRAP.
- Spindle-shaped neoplastic cells—produce type I and II collagen and alkaline phosphatase, and have receptors for parathyroid hormone. These cells are genetically unstable and have high expression of p53. They secrete macrophage colony-stimulating factor, interferon-γ, and tumour necrosis factor-α.

Round cells and giant cells are the reactive components of the tumour, while spindle cells represent the neoplastic component.

Histology

Confirmatory needle biopsy should usually be obtained prior to definitive management.

Immunohistochemical staining can be used to assess the relationship between the rate of proliferation and recurrence. Overexpression of the *p53* and *MYC* oncogenes is seen in tumours metastasising to the lung.

Differential Diagnosis

Differential diagnosis of GCT includes

- ABC.
- Brown tumour of hyperparathyroidism (need to check serum PTH at diagnosis).
- Giant cell reparative granuloma (rare).
- Non-ossifying fibroma (rare).
- Giant-cell-rich osteosarcoma (rare).

Grading

GCTs are graded using the Enneking and Campanacci staging system (Table 8.7).

Campanacci M et al. Giant cell tumours of bone. J Bone Joint Surg Am 1987;69(1);106–14.

GCTs can occasionally be polyostotic, which can either be simultaneous or metachronous with an interval of many years. Malignancy can occur and can either be primary and sarcomatous from

Table 8.7 Giant cell tumour grading with the Enneking and Campanacci staging system

Grade	Activity, nature	Description
I	Benign, latent	Well-marginated border of a thin rim of mature bone Cortex is intact and not deformed
II	Benign, active	Relatively well defined margins but no radiopaque rim Moderately expanded cortex
III	Aggressive	Tumour with fuzzy borders suggesting rapid and possibly permeative growth Cortical breach and a soft tissue component Often cause a pathological fracture

the onset or secondary due to malignant transformation of a recurrent tumour.

Rarely, GCT can occur in a benign metastasising form, with nodules in the lung. This is believed to be due to embolisation. Lung metastases may be present at the first presentation of the tumour or a few years later. CT lung staging should be performed for all recurrent GCTs.

Benign GCT

Simple curettage can have a recurrence rate of 20–50%. This is decreased with the use of adjuvants and when performed in a specialist centre.

For benign tumours, wide local excision (*en bloc* resection) is associated with a recurrence rate 7%. This usually requires resection of the articular surface and reconstruction with an endoprosthetic replacement or allograft.

The relative indications for *en bloc* resection and reconstruction are as follows:

- Extensive grade 3 tumour with no remaining mechanically supportive bone.
- Repeated recurrences.
- Displaced intra-articular fracture.
- Distal radial site.
- Articular collapse after previous curettage.
- Involvement of 50% of the distal femur (a relative indication).

Radiotherapy has been occasionally utilised for GCT in the pelvis, vertebra or inoperable sites. The form is 40–60 Gy using a linear accelerator and super-voltage therapy. Local control is achieved in 85–90% of patients. The risk of radiation-induced sarcoma is 0–8%.

The distal radius is the third most common site for GCT and reconstruction is challenging. Options include ulnocarpal arthrodesis or replacing the bone defect with a vascularised or non-vascularised fibular graft.

Feigenberg SJ, Marcus RB Jr, Zlotecki RA, et al. Radiation therapy for giant cell tumours of bone. Clin Orthop Relat Res 2003;411:207–16. From 26 tumours, 20 were controlled locally. One patient developed a radiation-induced sarcoma.

Recurrent GCT

Several factors influence recurrence:

- Original tumour stage. Recurrence rate in Stage 1 is 7%; stage 2 is 20%; and stage 3 is 41%.
- Adequacy of primary treatment (surgical margin, aggressiveness of curettage).
- Adjuvant agents.
- Tumour behaviour.

Pathologic fracture does not increase the risk of recurrence. Recurrent GCT can be managed with wide excision or repeat curettage with adjuvants.

Adjuvants help to reduce recurrence. These include high-speed burr, liquid nitrogen, polymethyl methacrylate (PMMA), phenol and alcohol. Bone cement (PMMA) is useful because it is inexpensive and helps detect recurrence. Excellent results noted in 85% of cases. Liquid nitrogen is also very effective and has been associated with a 7.9% recurrence rate. The use of a dental burr to remove tumour tissue has been found to reduce recurrence rates to 12%. Denosumab can be used in unresectable or advanced GCT and has been shown to change tumour composition, reduce bony destruction and lead to clinical improvement. Optimum duration of treatment is currently unknown and cessation of treatment can result in reactivation of disease.

Malawer MM, Bickels J, Meller I, et al. Cryosurgery in the treatment of giant cell tumor. A long-term follow-up study. Clin Orthop Relat Res 1999;359:176–88.

Blackley HR, Wunder JS, Davis AM, et al. Treatment of giant-cell tumors of long bones with curettage and bone-grafting. J Bone Joint Surg Am 1999;81:811–20.

Balke M, Hardes J, Denosumab: a breakthrough in treatment of giant-cell tumour of bone. Lancet Oncol. 2010;11:218–19.

Malignant GCT

Malignant GCT has a mortality rate of 15–20%. Lung lesions should usually be excised (if significant co-morbidities, can be treated with radiotherapy.)

Campanacci M, Baldini N, Boriani S, Sudanese A. Giant-cell tumor of bone. J Bone Joint Surg Am 1987;69:106–14. In nearly 300 patients, 74% had grade 2 GCT and 22% grade 3. Nine percent presented with a pathological fracture. The local recurrence rates were 27% for intralesional procedures, 8% for marginal procedures and 0% for wide excision.

Szendröi M. Giant-cell tumour of bone. J Bone Joint Surg Br 2004;86:5–12.

Zhen W, Yaotian H, Songjian L, et al. Giant-cell tumour of bone. The long-term results of treatment by curettage and bone graft. J Bone Joint Surg Br 2004;86:212–6. This study looked at 92 patients with a 5- to 11-year follow-up. The patients were treated with 50% zinc chloride for 5 min and auto- or allograft bone grafting. The recurrence rate was 13%, and 93% achieved at least good function. Patients underwent wide excision of soft tissues if the lesion perforated through the cortex.

Prosser GH, Baloch KG, Tillman RM, et al. Does curettage without adjuvant therapy provide low recurrence rates in giant-cell tumors of bone? Clin Orthop Relat Res 2005;435:211–8. The local recurrence rate of GCTs confined to bone (Campanacci grades 1 and 2) was only 7%, compared with 29% in tumours with extraosseous extension (Campanacci grade 3).

E. Malignant Primary Bone Tumours

Primary bone tumours (PBTs) are rare and account for only 0.2% of all malignant tumours. Approximately 380 people were diagnosed with bone sarcomas annually in England between 1979 and 2007.

Management of malignant PBTs is at supra-regional centres and through specialist MDTs. In England these are at Stanmore, Birmingham, Oswestry, Oxford and Newcastle.

Osteosarcoma

Osteosarcoma is a malignant bone tumour characterised by spindle cells and the production of osteoid matrix. It is the most common primary malignant bone tumour (excluding haematological bone marrow cancers such as multiple myeloma).

Epidemiology

Osteosarcoma has a bimodal distribution. It is most common in the second decade of life and in men (M:F 2:1). Adults in the fifth to sixth decades of life may develop osteosarcoma in association with Paget's disease (with a 1% incidence of malignant transformation). Ionising radiation also predisposes to osteosarcoma.

Hereditary retinoblastoma and Li–Fraumeni syndrome are linked to the development of osteosarcoma. *c-MYC* and c-*FOS* proto-oncogenes are overexpressed in the disease.

Clinical Features

Osteosarcoma tumours are usually metaphyseal and the symptoms are principally related to fast bone growth. The most common sites are the distal femur, proximal tibia and proximal humerus. Half of osteosarcomas occur around the knee as it is the area of most active bone growth.

The most common presenting symptoms are pain (85%) and a tender swelling. Pain at rest and at night is commensurate with the diagnosis. Occasionally, a patient will have a pathologic fracture.

In up to 20% of patients, the disease has metastasized, usually to the lungs, at the time of presentation. Less common sites of metastasis include bone, kidneys, lymph nodes, brain and pleura. The presence of metastasis at initial presentation is a very poor prognostic sign.

Widhe B, Widhe T. Initial symptoms and clinical features in osteosarcoma and Ewing sarcoma. J Bone Joint Surg Am 2000;82:667–74. Strain-related pain was reported in 85% of patients with osteosarcoma and 64% of those with Ewing sarcoma. Night pain was experienced by 21% and 19%, respectively, and 39% and 34% had a mass. Symptoms developed at 9 weeks with osteosarcoma and at 19 weeks with Ewing sarcoma.

Imaging

Radiographs typically show a metaphyseal lesion with bone destruction (Figs. 8.5 and 8.6). Soft tissue calcification may be visible and is described as having a 'star-burst' appearance. The periosteum is elevated at the periphery of the lesion due to rapid growth, and laying down of bone under the elevated periosteum is known as Codman's triangle. There is little endosteal bone formation and the transition zone is wide.

A CT scan of the chest is useful to look for lung metastases. A 99-Tc bone scan or PET-CT is used to identify other lesions or bone metastasis, as well as the extent of the lesion in the affected bone.

MRI of the whole bone is undertaken to evaluate the extent of the tumour and skip lesions—both in the soft tissues and the medullary canal. The relationship of the tumour to the local neurovascular structures is of particular importance when it comes to surgery.

Pathology

Transformed osteoblasts are the malignant cells that produce the osteoid matrix. Pleomorphism and anaplasia are seen.

Laboratory Studies

Alkaline phosphatase and lactic dehydrogenase (LDH) levels can be raised and are poor prognostic signs.

Types of Osteosarcomas

Types of osteosarcomas are summarised in Table 8.8.

Management

Surgery and chemotherapy are the mainstays of treatment. Chemotherapy is usually given pre- and post-operatively as discussed in more detail below.

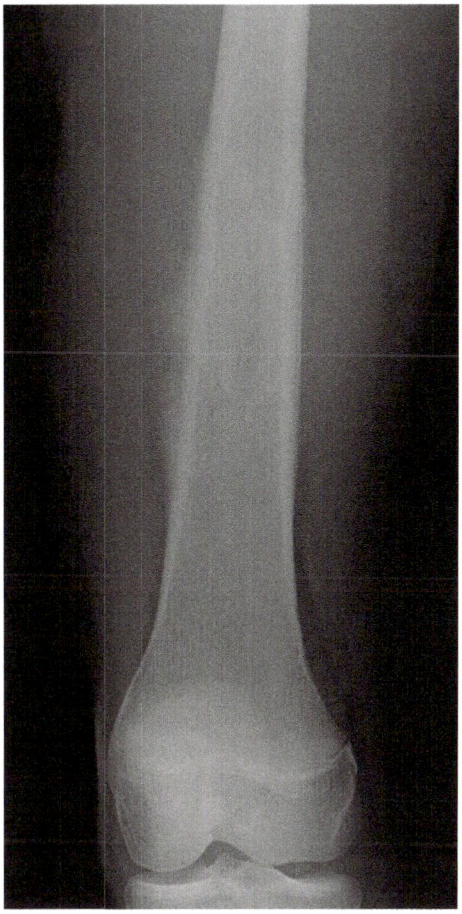

Fig. 8.5 An osteosarcoma in distal femoral metaphysis. Note the cortical destruction, soft tissue extension and the Codman's triangle

Surgical resection should have a negative margin (wide excision), and this is an important factor determining local recurrence. The inability to achieve wide margins at resection is a contraindication to limb salvage. Other relative contraindications include very young patients, distal limb tumours and, historically, pathologic fractures. Recent studies have however found that pathologic fractures can be salvageable as long as the fracture haematoma is resected *en bloc* with the primary tumour.

Following resection, reconstructive options include endo-prosthesis (mega-prosthesis), allograft or allograft–prosthesis composites (Table 8.9). Novel reconstructions such as extra-

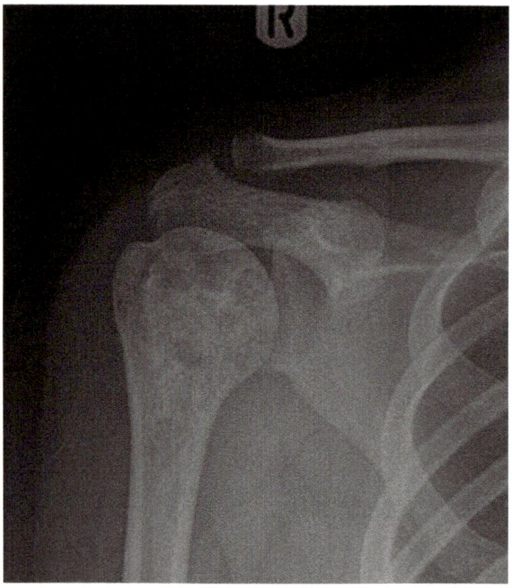

Fig. 8.6 Plain radiograph of a mixed lytic and sclerotic ill defined lesion in the proximal humerus. Biopsy confirmed high grade chondroblastic osteosarcoma

Table 8.8 Types of osteosarcomas

Type	Percent	Description
Classic high-grade central	90%	As detailed in main text
Parosteal	4%	Low-grade. Common location is posterior surface of distal femur. Seen in older patients (third or fourth decade). Densely mineralized. Surgical resection has a high cure rate. Chemotherapy is not indicated
Telangiectactic	3.6%	High-grade. Vascular lesion with little osteoid formation. Radiographically similar to ABC. Chemotherapy response is usually good
Periosteal	1.5%	Moderate-grade. Common location is proximal tibia. Usually presents in second decade of life. Surgery and chemotherapy are usually indicated
Juxtacortical	Rare	High-grade. Arises from surface of bone rather than metaphysis.
Mutlifocal		Tumour at more than one site
Secondary		From Paget's disease or following radiotherapy. Poor prognosis.

corporeal irradiation and reimplantation supplemented by vascularised fibular grafting, rotationplasties, lengthening and bone transport procedures are sometimes utilised, dependent on pathology and location.

Jeys LM, Kulkarni A, Grimer RJ, et al. Endoprosthetic reconstruction for the treatment of musculoskeletal tumors of the appendicular skeleton and pelvis. J Bone Joint Surg Am 2008;90:1265–71. At 10 years, implant survival was 75% with mechanical failure as the endpoint and 58% with failure from any cause as the endpoint. The limb salvage rate was 84% at 20 years.

Sewell MD, Spiegelberg BG, Hanna SA, et al. Total femoral endoprosthetic replacement following excision of bone tumours. J Bone Joint Surg Br 2009;91:1513–20. This study looked at 33 patients with a mean age of 31 years. Total femoral endoprosthetic replacement resulted in no cases of aseptic loosening and no recurrence.

Resection options for the upper extremities include intra- and extra-articular resection. Tikhoff–Linberg resection is a limb-sparing procedure for tumours around the proximal humerus and shoulder girdle. Reconstruction can involve the implantation of a prosthesis to maintain arm length.

Resection of tumours around the knee follows similar principles and a range of reconstruction prostheses are available. A consideration in young people is to use an expandable prosthesis that makes up for growth of the limb. Repeated procedures may be required to lengthen the prosthesis. An implant that is expandable (magnetically), without surgical intervention may be used.

Van Nes rotationplasty is a procedure in which a knee tumour is excised and reconstructed with the tibial segment arthrodesed to the distal femur and the ankle rotated 180° to function as the knee joint. Extensive patient counselling and information is imperative prior to planning this procedure. Good function is achievable, but the procedure is still unacceptable to many patients (and parents), who will often choose endoprosthetic replacement ahead of rotationplasty, particularly in the United Kingdom.

Table 8.9 Relative advantages and disadvantages of allograft reconstruction and endoprosthesis

Reconstruction	Advantages	Disadvantages
Endoprosthetic replacement (EPR)	Durable Easily available Stable (immediately) Immediate mobilisation	Soft tissue reconstruction is required and may be difficult/unsatisfactory. Loosening[a] Mechanical failure[a] Infection[b]
Allograft	Reattachment of soft tissues Maintains joint anatomy with restoration of tendons and ligaments	High infection rate Graft failure and fracture are possible Chemotherapy and radiotherapy interfere with host–graft union Resorption of graft Availability dependent

[a]Loosening and mechanical failure are late disadvantages and better survival is being seen with improved technology, including the use of rotating-hinge knee prostheses and hydroxyapatite coating of collars
[b]Surface coatings to reduce biofilm formation and infection

Chemotherapy

The development of effective chemotherapy regimens has improved the survival of patients with osteogenic sarcoma. Chemotherapy is usually given as part of a multinational trial—for this tumour type, the main group currently recruiting patients for trials is the European and American Osteosarcoma Study Group (EURAMOS).

Induction (preoperative) chemotherapy is used to improve chances of limb salvage and reduce tumour size, although there is a lack of evidence for this practice. The main role is to eradicate the disease from distant sites.

In EURAMOS-1, induction chemotherapy is with the combination of cisplatin, doxorubicin and methotrexate (CDM). This has shown to produce a survival benefit and locally control the disease. After surgery, patients are randomised based on their response rate to induction chemotherapy. Good responders (>90% tumour kill) are randomised to CDM with or without interferon-α. Poor responders (>10% viable tumour) receive CDM with or without ifosfamide and etoposide.

Recent advances in chemotherapy treatment include the use of Mifamurtide, an immune macrophage stimulant. It is authorized to use in patients aged 2–30 with high-grade non-metastatic osteosarcoma after macroscopic complete surgical resection. It has been shown to improve survival from 71 to 78% when used in conjunction with chemotherapy.

Grimer RJ, Taminiau AM, Cannon SR; Surgical Subcommittee of the European Osteosarcoma Intergroup. Surgical outcomes in osteosarcoma. J Bone Joint Surg Br 2002;84:395–400. In this study of 202 patients following surgery, the survival rates were 57% at 5 years and 54% at 10 years. The local recurrence rate was 8%, and all local occurrences were in patients undergoing limb salvage surgery using endoprosthetic replacements (there were no local recurrences in amputations). Local recurrences did not occur when the necrosis rate was over 90%.

Davis AM, Bell RS, Goodwin PJ. Prognostic factors in osteosarcoma: a critical review. J Clin Oncol 1994;12:423–31.

McDonald DJ, Capanna R, Gherlinzoni F, et al. Influence of chemotherapy on perioperative complications in limb salvage surgery for bone tumours. Cancer 1990;65:1509–16. In this study of 304 patients, the incidence of complications was 25.2% (29/115) for no chemotherapy, 32.8% (20/61) for adjuvant chemotherapy and 55.4% (71/128) for neoadjuvant chemotherapy.

Bielack SS, Smeland S, Whelan JS, et al. Methotrexate, Doxorubicin, and Cisplatin (MAP) plus maintenance pegylated Interferon Alfa-2b versus MAP alone in patients with resectable high-grade osteosarcoma and good histologic response to preoperative MAP: First results of the EURAMOS-1 good response randomized controlled trial. J Clin Oncol 2015;33(20):2279–87.

Prognostic Indicators

The following factors are indicators of poor prognosis:

- Metastases at initial presentation.
- Large tumours.
- Skip lesions—separate foci within the same bone.
- Tumours of the axial skeleton and more proximally located tumours.
- Poor response to chemotherapy (<95% necrosis).
- Pathological fracture.
- Elevated LDH and ALP levels.

Ewing's Sarcoma

Ewing's sarcoma is the second most common malignant bone tumour. Ewing's sarcoma is part of the family of Ewing's Family of Tumours (EFT), which also includes extraosseous Ewing's tumour and peripheral primitive neuro ectodermal tumour. The incidence is 0.6 per one million and the male to female ratio is 1.6:1.

Etiology

The gene associated with the development of Ewing's sarcoma is *EWS*, which is responsible for triggering changes in fibroblasts. The translocation t(11;22) is present in 90% of patients with Ewing's sarcoma. This results in fusion of EWS to FLI1 (Fig. 8.7).

Clinical Features

The bones commonly involved in Ewing's sarcoma are the femur, tibia, humerus, fibula, pelvis, ribs, scapula, clavicle and spine. The location within the bone is usually diaphyseal.

The common presenting features are pain (90%) and swelling (70%) in the involved extremity. There may be a history of incidental trauma. Tumours involving the spine may present with neurological disturbance. Pathological fractures are the presenting feature in 5–10% of patients.

Systemic signs may be present, including fever, weight loss and malaise. However, an absence of these symptoms is not an indicator of benign disease.

Laboratory Studies

There can be elevated white blood cell count and erythrocyte sedimentation rate and normochromic normocytic anaemia.

LDH and alkaline phosphatase levels may be elevated. The rise and fall in LDH levels correlate with tumour progression or response to chemotherapy, respectively. A raised LDH level is a poor prognostic indicator at presentation.

Imaging

The lesion is usually diaphyseal and may extend to the metaphysis (Fig. 8.8). In plain radiographs, the pattern of bone destruction is permeative and is accompanied by cortical changes. The appearance is described as 'onion skin' due to the lamel-

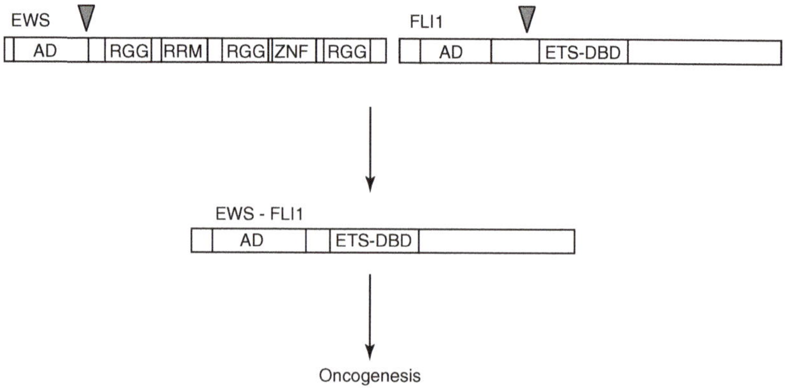

Fig. 8.7 EWS-FLI1 fusion seen in Ewing's sarcoma

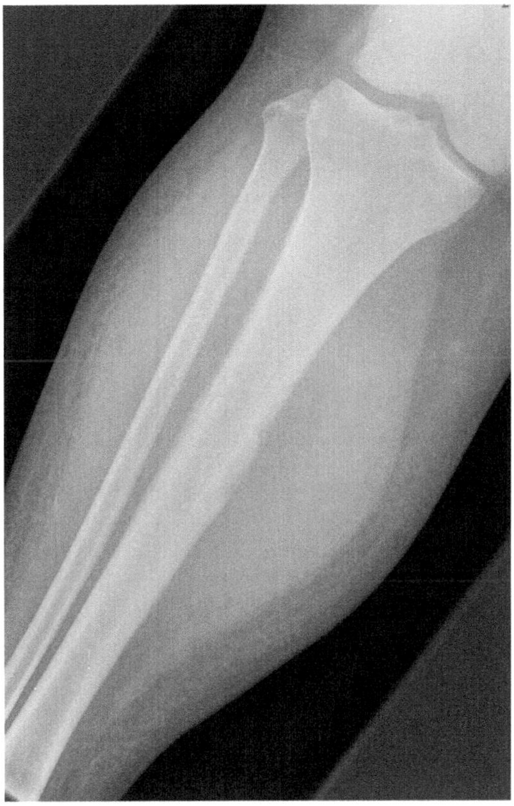

Fig. 8.8 Ewing's tumour of tibial diaphysis. The cortical destrction is poorly defined with a wide zone of transition

lated appearance and Codman's triangle may be seen due to rapid growth of the lesion.

MRI is used to demonstrate the soft tissue component; intramedullary extent and presence of skip lesions.

Metastasis is commonly to the lungs, but also to other sites in the skeleton. This can be detected early on bone scan or PET-CT scan.

Histology

Sheets of closely packed small, round, blue cells with large nuclei are evident on microscopy. The presence of glycogen makes them stain positive with periodic acid–Schiff staining.

Management

Chemotherapy is the first line of treatment for Ewing's sarcoma. Systemic control is usually achieved by induction chemotherapy, which is almost always part of a clinical trial (currently Euro-EWINGS 2012). Euro-EWINGS 2012 is aiming to randomise two induction chemotherapy regimes (VIDE; vincristine/ifosfamide/doxorubicin/etoposide vs. alternative VDC (vincristine/doxorubicin/cyclophosphamide) and IE (ifosfamide/etoposide). A second randomization occurs for further consolidation regimes dependent on presence of pulmonary metastasis, presence of regional disease and good or poor risk factors.

Radiation is effective for local control and is preferable to surgery in some anatomic sites. The recurrence rate is 10% and there is a risk of development of secondary neoplasm. Radiation can also cause growth arrest in the immature skeleton, avascular necrosis in the femoral head, joint contracture, muscle atrophy and pathological fracture. However for pelvic tumours radiotherapy may offer an advantage functionally with similar outcomes for local control.

Surgery is used after induction chemotherapy to achieve local control of the disease and is followed by adjuvant chemotherapy. If adequate margins can be achieved, local recurrence is reduced. Surgery has the advantages of preserving function and avoiding some of the complications of radiation therapy. Radiation may be needed after surgery if there is a possibility of residual tumour tissue.

Prognostic Indicators

The following factors are indicators of poor prognosis in Ewing's sarcoma:

- Large volume tumours (>200 mL).
- More than one bone metastasis site.
- Bone marrow metastasis
- Lung metastasis
- Older age at presentation (>14 vs. <14).

Ladenstein R, Potschger U, Le Deley MC et al. Primary disseminated multifocal Ewing sarcoma: results of the Euro-EWING 99 trial. J Clin Oncol 2010;28(20):3284–91.

Chondrosarcoma

Chondrosarcoma is the third most common primary bone tumour and has varying malignant potential. Even within the same tumour mass, different areas may have different degrees of malignancy.

Two-thirds of chondrosarcomas occur in the trunk, or proximal humerus and or femur. The genetic translocation t(9;22) is present in 25% of tumours.

Several factors are associated with a higher rate of malignancy:

- Larger tumour.
- Older patient.
- Persistent or night pain.
- Multiple lesions (Maffucci's syndrome, Ollier's disease or hereditary multiple exostoses).
- Lesions within the bone.
- Centrally placed tumours.
- Increased uptake on bone scan.
- Local recurrence.

Clinical Features

Most chondrosarcomas present as a slowly growing mass. Pain may indicate possible malignant growth. Pathologic fractures can be present with enostotic lesions.

Imaging

The soft tissue calcification seen in chondrosarcoma is typically described as having a 'popcorn-ball' appearance (Fig. 8.9). There is a thick cap of cartilage and the presence of a soft tissue mass indicates malignancy. Bone destruction is often evident.

Classification

Chondrosarcoma is classified using the following categories:

- Grade:
  - ½—ACT: Atypical cartilaginous tumour.
  - 1—low.
  - 2—medium/intermediate.
  - 3—high.

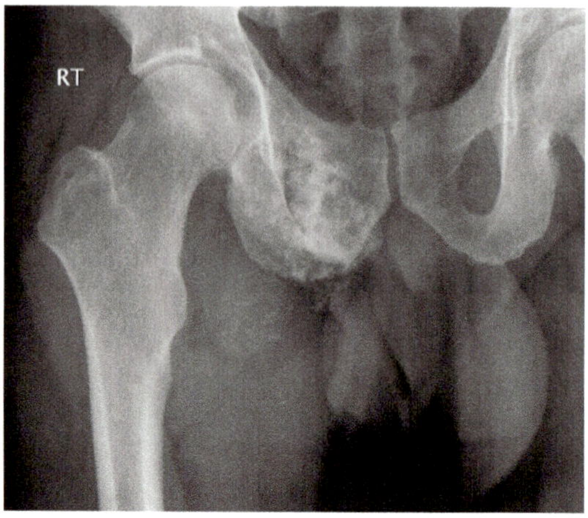

Fig. 8.9 Chondrosarcoma of pelvis. Note the calcification and soft tissue extension

- Primary or secondary.
- Central or peripheral.
- Histological subtype:
  - Clear cell.
  - Mesenchymal.
  - Chondrosarcoma of soft parts.
  - Dedifferentiated.

Management

For grade ½ or 1 lesions, curettage plus cementation is usually appropriate—careful histological examination is necessary to ensure the tumour is not more aggressive.

The mainstay of treatment of grade 2 and 3 lesions is wide surgical excision. The adequacy of the margin can be planned depending on the site of the lesion. Reconstructive options after surgery are typically endoprostheses but also allografts and allograft–prosthesis composites.

These are usually resistant to chemotherapy and radiotherapy, but these modalities are employed where there is a dedifferentiated tumour, which has a very poor prognosis.

Patients should be followed up regularly for the development of local recurrence and metastasis in the lung. If a solitary lesion is detected, surgical excision after staging isusually the accepted treatment.

Daly PJ, Sim FH, Wold LE. Dedifferentiated chondrosarcoma of bone. Orthopedics 1989;12:763–7. Patients had a 5-year survival rate of 10%.

Barnes R, Catto M. Chondrosarcoma of bone. J Bone Joint Surg Br 1966;48:729–64.

Dahlin DC, Beabout JW. Dedifferentiation of low-grade chondrosarcomas. Cancer 1971;28:461–6. Ten percent of low-grade chondrosarcomas had areas of dedifferentiation. These patients rapidly deteriorated.

Giuffreda AY et al. Chondrosarcoma in the Unites States (1973–2003): An analysis of 2890 cases from the SEER database. J Bone Joint Surg am 2009;91(5):1063–72. Current treatment protocols have not improved survival in Chondrosarcoma over the last 30 years.

Key Points for Malignant Primary Bone Tumours

- Osteosarcoma has a bimodal age distribution. It can occur secondarily due to Paget's disease and ionising radiation. Radiologically a "starburst" appearance is seen.
- Osteosarcoma is treated with surgery plus chemotherapy.
- Ewings sarcoma occurs in the young presenting with pain and swelling in a limb. Lung metastasis is common.
- Chondrosarcoma commonly occur in the trunk or proximal humerus/femur. Radiologically a "popcorn-ball" appearance is seen

F. Soft Tissue Sarcomas

Incidence

The incidence of soft tissue sarcomas (STS's) is 45 per one million of the population and it accounts for <1% of all malignancies. There were approximately 3300 cases reported in 2010 in the UK, and 46% of these occur in the lower extremities.

Clinical Features

Concerning features are:

- Size larger than 4 cm.
- A painful lump.
- Growing lesion.
- Lesion located beneath the deep fascia.

The presence of all four characteristics carries a high risk of malignancy. Recurrent lesions can also be suggestive of a malignant process. Approximately 20% of STS's are small and superficial.

Pathology

There are many subtypes of soft tissue sarcomas based on tissue of origin.

The common subtypes are:

- Liposarcoma (fat):
  - Myxoid liposarcoma.
  - Pleomorphic liposarcoma.
- Leiomyosarcoma (smooth muscle).
- Rhabdomyosarcoma (skeletal muscle):
  - Embryonal (two-thirds of patients)—ages 10–20 years (alveolar, botyroid or spindle-cell).
  - Pleomorphic (one-third)—ages 50–70 years.
- Synovial sarcoma
- Malignant peripheral nerve sheath tumour (neural tissue).
- Undifferentiated Pleomorphic sarcoma (High grade sarcoma not otherwise specified (HGSNOS)—tissue type of origin not identifiable)

Pathogenesis

Several different factors contribute to the pathogenesis of soft tissue sarcomas (Table 8.10).

The genetic factors associated with soft tissue sarcomas are shown in Table 8.11.

Post-irradiation Sarcoma

The criteria for post-irradiation sarcoma have been defined by Cahan *et al.* and later modified by Arlen et al.:

- The sarcoma developed in an irradiated field.
- Histological confirmation.
- Latency of 3 years or more.
- The region bearing the tumour was normal prior to irradiation.

It has subsequently been suggested that a latency period of even 6 months is sufficient to affirm diagnosis.

Cahan WG et al. Sarcoma arising in irradiated bone. Cancer 1:3;1948.

Arlen M et al. Radiation induced sarcoma of bone. Cancer 28:1087;1971.

Gladdy RA, Qin LX et al. Do radiation-associated soft tissue sarcomas have the same prognosis as sporadic soft tissue sarcomas? J Clin Oncol 2010;28(12):2064.

Table 8.10 Pathogenesis of soft tissue sarcomas

Environmental factors	– Trauma (anecdotal) or implants (surgical) – Chemicals (asbestos, phenoxyacetic acid herbicides, vinyl chloride) – Radiation
Oncogenic viruses	– Epstein–Barr virus in smooth muscle tumours of patients positive for HIV – Human herpes virus 8 in Kaposi's sarcoma
Immunologic factors	– Immunodeficiency/therapeutic immunosuppression associated with leiomyosarcomas – Acquired regional immunodeficiency associated with angiosarcomas in lymphoedema
Genetic factors	– Bilateral retinoblastoma is associated with secondary sarcoma (germline deletion of *RB1* locus on chromosome 13) – Li–Fraumeni syndrome (germline deletion of *p53* locus) results in familial rhabdomyosarcoma

Management

For most soft tissue sarcomas, combined modality treatment of surgery and radiotherapy is the treatment of choice. For lower grade STSs, surgical excision with clear surgical margins is the treatment of choice for local control. The definition of an acceptable margin is debated but in the UK a microscopically clear margin is essential. Planned marginal resection is sometimes used (e.g. in elderly patients when major nerve resection would otherwise be needed). In some situations amputation may be the most appropriate treatment option to gain local control and potential cure. Unplanned positive margins should ideally undergo re-resection after morbidity and co-morbidity has been taken into consideration.

Pre- and post-operative radiotherapy is used for large (>5 cm), deep and intermediate/high-grade tumours or where margins are suboptimal. Induction (pre-operative) radiotherapy is more commonly used despite increased complications following surgery because of the reduced toxicity to uninvolved tissues.

Proton therapy is considered in defined indications which may include spinal or paraspinal STS's.

Chemotherapy is reserved for treatment where the disease is metastatic. Typically it comprises doxorubicin and ifosfamide.

Table 8.11 Genetic factors associated with soft tissue sarcomas

Genetic factor	Sarcoma	Gene	Chromosome
Neurofibromatosis type 1	Malignant peripheral nerve sheath tumour	*NF1*	17q11.2
Retinoblastoma	Soft tissue sarcoma or osteosarcoma	*RB1*	13q14
Li–Fraumeni	Soft tissue sarcoma or osteosarcoma	*TP53*	17p13
Gardner	Fibrosarcoma or desmoid tumours	*APC*	5q21
Werner	Soft tissue sarcoma	*WRN*	8p12
Gorlin	Fibrosarcoma or rhabdomyosarcoma	*PTC*	9q22.3
Tuberous sclerosis	Rhabdomyosarcoma	*TSC1*, *TSC2*	9q34 16p13.3

APC adenomatous polyposis coli, *NF-1* neurofibromin 1, *PTC* phenylthiocarbamide, *RB1* retinoblastoma 1, *TSC* tuberous sclerosis, *TP53* tumour protein p53, *WRN* Werner syndrome

Tunn PU, Kettelhack C, Dürr HR. Standardized approach to the treatment of adult soft tissue sarcoma of the extremities. Recent Results Cancer Res 2009;179:211–28.

Khatri VP, Goodnight JE Jr. Extremity soft tissue sarcoma: controversial management issues. Surg Oncol 2005;14:1–9.

Cribb GL, Loo SC, Dickinson I. Limb salvage for soft tissue sarcomas of the foot and ankle. J Bone Joint Surg Br 2010; 92(3): 424–9. 27 patients managed by limb salvage. Synovial sarcoma was the commonest histological diagnosis. Successful in 26 out of 27. Two had local recurrence.

Albertsmeier M, Rauch A, Roeder F, Hasenhütl S, Pratschke S, Kirschneck M, Gronchi A, Jebsen NL, Cassier PA, Sargos P, Belka C. Annals of surgical oncology. 2018;25(3):754–67. External beam radiation therapy for resectable soft tissue sarcoma: a systematic review and meta-analysis.

O'Sullican B, Davis AM et al. Preoperative versus postoperative radiotherapy in soft-tissue sarcoma of the limbs: a randomised trial. The Lancet 2002;359(9325):2235–41. Wound complications in 35% (pre-operative) and 17% (post-operative) patients.

Issels RD, Lindner LH, Verweij J, Wessalowski R, Reichardt P, Wust P, Ghadjar P, Hohenberger P, Angele M, Salat C, Vujaskovic Z. Effect of neoadjuvant chemotherapy plus regional hyperthermia on long-term outcomes among patients with localized high-risk soft tissue sarcoma: the EORTC 62961-ESHO 95 randomized clinical trial. JAMA oncology. 2018 Apr 1;4(4):483–92.

Key Points for Soft Tissue Sarcomas

- Any patient with a soft tissue mass increasing in size, size >4 cm or painful should be referred for imaging/specialist review.
- Ultrasound scan by a musculoskeletal radiologist should be considered the first-line investigation. MRI ± guided core biopsy as needed.
- Imaging of the chest should be performed prior to radical treatment.
- Surgery is the standard treatment commonly with pre- or post-operative radiotherapy.

G. Skeletal Metastasis

The skeleton is the third most common site for metastasis, after the lungs and liver. Skeletal metastases are much more common than primary bone tumours. In the USA, 1.2 million new cases of skeletal metastases are diagnosed each year compared with 2700 primary bone tumours.

Metastasis Sites

The common sites for skeletal metastasis are the spine, sacrum, pelvis, ribs, femur and humerus (Fig. 8.10). Metastases distal to the elbow and knee are uncommon apart from those associated with lung cancer.

Cortical metastases are less common, but can be detected early on plain films. The appearance is of punched-out lesions known as 'cookie-cutter' metastasis. These lesions again are generally from the lung and the most common site is the femur.

Tumours Metastasising to Bone

Any malignant tumour can metastasise to bone. The breast (22%), prostate (32%), lung, kidney (16%) and thyroid directly drain to the vertebral venous system. Less common causes include gastric and colorectal carcinoma, melanoma and neurogenic tumours. Neuroblastoma and leukaemia can cause bone metastases in children.

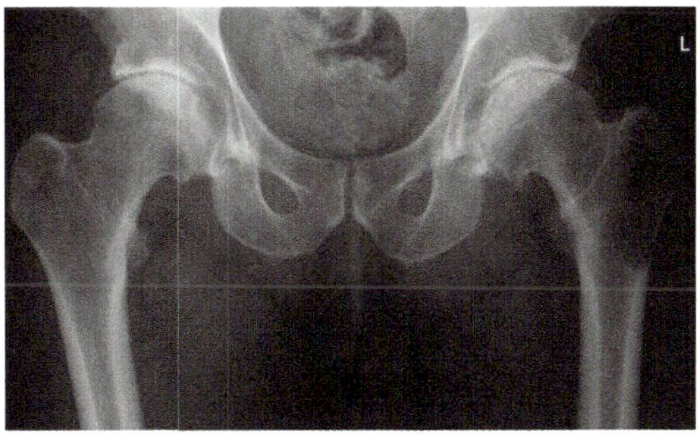

Fig. 8.10 Metastasis from a melanoma into the left proximal femur

Evaluation of a patient presenting with an unknown primary tumour should include focus on identifying the primary tumour sites. Lung and prostate tumours can often spread to bone and present as a metastasis with an unknown primary lesion. Melanoma and colorectal cancer are less common. In lymphoma and leukaemias, bone metastasis may be the first presentation.

A detailed multi-faceted investigation of patients presenting with skeletal metastases from cancer of an unknown primary origin is probably unnecessary. A CT scan of the chest, abdomen and pelvis, an isotope bone scan and a biopsy of the most accessible lesion will usually give sufficient diagnostic and prognostic information on most tumours.

Pathology

Bone destruction is most often through activation of osteoclasts by the tumour cells. The pathological steps are shown in Fig. 8.11.

Several mechanisms are involved in osteoclast-mediated bone resorption:

- Increased osteoclasts binding to bone.
- Stimulation of osteoclastic bone resorption.
- Increased osteoclast formation from precursors and increased osteoclast survival.

Type I collagen is a chemotactic factor for tumour cells in bone.

Clinical Features

Skeletal metastases may be incidentally identified on radiographs, although this is relatively uncommon. Usually a radiograph will have been performed for pain, which may have been misinterpreted as pain from osteoarthritis. The features of skeletal metastases typically are

- Pain—usually at night and progressive. The pain may be localised to the lytic area. Pain on mobilisation with femoral or tibial metastases often indicates an impeding pathological fracture as may activity-related pain with upper limb metastasis.
- Swelling—this is generally a late sign and tumours are often identified before they get to this stage. Swelling signifies soft tissue extension or a pathological fracture with haematoma.
- Neurological dysfunction—sometimes seen with vertebral tumours.

In a solitary lesion, the diagnosis should be confirmed before treatment is undertaken. Patients aged over 40 years may have primary bone tumours and the management of these is fundamentally different to that of metastases. Inadvertent management of these as a metastasis can compromise survival and may render what was previously treatable, unsalvageable (Table 8.12).

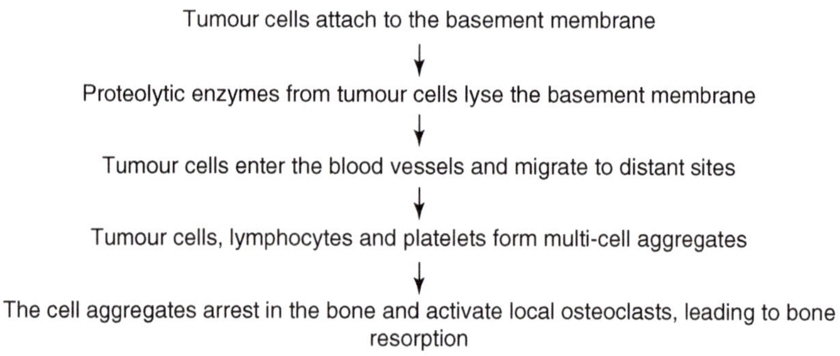

Fig. 8.11 The pathological process of osteoclast activation in skeletal metastasis

Table 8.12 Differential diagnosis of lytic lesions in patients aged over 40 years

Lesion	Differential diagnosis
Benign	Paget's disease of bone Hyperparathyroidism (Brown's tumour)
Primary malignancy	Haematological malignancy—myeloma, lymphoma Chondrosarcoma Spindle cell sarcoma Secondary osteosarcoma

Evaluation

Radiographs (Whole of Involved Bone and Chest)

Radiographs of the lesion and the whole bone (joint above and below) are taken in two planes (the anteroposterior and lateral views). Approximately 30–50% of the mineral content of the bone has to be lost before the lesions are apparent on radiographs.

Lytic lesions are common in renal cell and thyroid metastasis. Other tumours may produce varied appearances. Prostate cancer is typically sclerotic, while breast cancer is usually lytic or mixed in appearance. Lung cancer produces a lytic or permeative, moth-eaten appearance. Myeloma produces punched-out lesions with no surrounding sclerosis.

The risk of pathologic fracture is usually determined by plain radiographs (although there is increasing evidence for the role of CT). It is necessary to visualise the whole bone for further metastases prior to planning stabilisation.

A chest radiograph is taken to check for lung metastases (or a primary cancer), which can indicate poor prognosis.

Radiographs can also help to assess response to treatment, as evidenced by increased sclerosis, reduced size or lesion disappearance.

Cross Sectional Imaging

A CT scan of the chest, abdomen and pelvis is useful for spinal and pelvic lesions where plain radiographs may not provide sufficient information. CT scans are also necessary for staging of the primary disease and planning appropriate surgery.

Isotope Bone Scan

A Tc 99 isotope bone scan indicates 'hot' areas with increased blood flow and increased bone turnover. It is useful for determining singularity versus multiplicity of a lesion. A bone scan may be positive before the lesion is evident on radiographs. It also helps to assess the response to treatment.

In myeloma, a Tc 99 bone scan is often negative because of low bone turnover. Renal cell carcinoma may give a false-negative bone scan because of its highly aggressive nature, with little or no reactive bone.

Widespread metastasis can lead to a high level of diffuse uptake in the skeleton while inhibiting uptake in the kidneys and bladder, which are normally visible on the bone scan. The appearance of the entire skeleton as 'hot' is known as a superscan.

Plain radiographs should be obtained of any areas with increased uptake.

Magnetic Resonance Imaging

MRI is extremely sensitive for the detection of bony metastatic disease. Because of the high water content in metastases, they usually appear dark on T1 and bright on T2 imaging.

T1 imaging is more sensitive for detection and the low-signal (dark) metastases show up well against the background of high-signal (bright) marrow fat. Short tau inversion recovery (STIR) sequences are useful to detect metastases on T2 as the fat signal is suppressed. Sclerotic metastases are dark on T1 and T2. Ideally, T1 should be combined with T2 or STIR sequences to detect metastases.

For spinal metastases, MRI can detect cord compression and soft tissue extension. MRI is less sensitive for differentiating acute fractures from metastases, but is able to differentiate old fractures from metastases.

MRI is a good modality for detecting and staging primary breast tumours, which may be undetected by clinical examination and mammography (PET-CT is also a good investigation here).

MRI is not a good screening tool because of its cost and because only a part of the skeleton can be assessed at any one time. Whole-body scans are expensive and time consuming, although scanners are improving in quality and scanning is becoming cheaper. Whole body MRI is being increasingly utilized for myeloma. The use of 99Tc bone scan is decreasing because of the advances in alternative imaging.

PET-CT (Positron Emission Tomography—Computed Tomography)

PET-CT uses the 18F-fluorodeoxyglucose tracer and helps to detect occult primary tumours (particularly in the head and neck area) and differentiate scar tissue from recurrent disease. There may be a role for this imaging modality in cancers of unknown primary origin and surveillance for sarcoma recurrence.

Yanagawa T, Shinozaki T, Iizuka Y, et al. Role of 2-deoxy-2-[F-18] fluoro-d-glucose positron emission tomography in the management of bone and soft-tissue metastases. J Bone Joint Surg Br 2010;92:419–23. In this study, PET-CT scanning was not helpful in evaluating occult primary lesions in patients with bone metastasis.

Blood Tests

A full blood count and electrolyte levels should be taken for all patients. Positive findings often include anaemia or a low platelet count.

Serum electrophoresis often demonstrates features consistent with myeloma and there is often an elevated sedimentation rate (>100 mm/h). Serum free lights chains should be performed to rule out multiple myeloma.

Serum calcium, phosphate and liver function tests should be performed. Alkaline phosphatase can be elevated and is a poor prognostic indicator.

The prostate-specific antigen (PSA) level is useful in screening for prostate cancer. This should be evaluated in light of PSA density (the rise in the PSA level in relation to the size of the gland on ultrasound) and PSA velocity (the rate of rise of PSA over a period of time).

Carcinoembryonic antigen levels are often elevated in gastrointestinal or hepatocellular carcinoma. These are helpful in monitoring response to treatment, but are not useful as diagnostic tests. This is the same for many other tumour markers.

Needle Biopsy ± Imaging Guidance

Multiple specimens should be obtained and may be checked for representative tissue by frozen section. Biopsies are ideally obtained from areas of bone destruction. Reactive bone, which may not have tumour cells, and the centre of the lesion, which may be largely necrotic tissue, should be avoided. Biopsies should be sent for microbiology as well as histology.

Indications for Biopsy

There are several indications for taking a biopsy of a lesion suspected of being a bone malignancy.

- A patient with a known primary malignancy but no known metastases who develops a first bony lesion.
- A patient with a known malignancy who presents with a pathological fracture.
- A patient with a history of long stable malignancy (e.g., breast, renal, prostate cancer) who was considered cured, but develops a new bony lesion.
- A previously healthy patient who presents with new multiple bony lesions indicative of disseminated metastatic disease of unknown origin.
- A healthy patient who presents with a pathological fracture suspected of being metastatic in origin.
- To assess for phenotypic changes between primary tumour and metastases.

Salai M. Surgical biopsy of bone metastases. In: Jasmin C, Coleman RE, Coia LR, et al. (eds) Textbook of Bone Metastases. Wiley: Chichester,2005:123–31.

Preparation for Surgery

Surgery for skeletal metastases is rarely an emergency (excluding spinal cord compression). Patients should be medically optimised and ideally operated on from a planned list within normal working hours. A number of measures should be undertaken prior to performing surgery:

- Check or perform cervical spine radiographs/CT if symptomatic—metastases can lead to instability.
- Correct hypercalcaemia (see below).
- Correct electrolyte imbalance (rehydration and correction).
- Consider preoperative embolisation, especially for renal or thyroid tumours and multiple myeloma. Surgery should be undertaken soon after embolisation (within 24 h) prior to formation of a collateral circulation.
- Check the white blood cell count and avoid surgery if the patient is neutropenic after chemotherapy or radiotherapy.
- Correct anaemia and thrombocytopenia and any other haematological or biochemical abnormalities.

Prediction of Fracture Possibility

The prediction of pathologic fractures in skeletal metastasis is based on Mirels' scoring system (Table 8.13).

Mirels H. Metastatic disease in long bones: a proposed scoring system for diagnosing impending pathologic fractures. Clin Orthop Relat Res 1989;249:256–64. Patients with a score of 8 had a 15% risk of fracture, while those with a score of 9 had a 33% risk. Hence, impending fracture is indicated by a score of 9 or more.

Capanna R, Campanacci DA. The treatment of metastases in the appendicular skeleton. J Bone Joint Surg Br 2001;83:471–81. Patients with fracture had a mean score of was 10, while those without fracture had a mean score of 7.

Mirels' scoring system is a guide and the decision to prophylactically stabilise a possible fracture should be based on the characteristics of the individual lesion and the patient.

A CT scan and rigidity analysis are research tools that may help in predicting the risk of an impending fracture.

Table 8.13 Mirels' scoring system for pathologic fractures

	Score		
	1	2	3
Site	Upper limb	Lower limb	Peritrochanteric
Pain	Mild	Moderate	On weight bearing
Lesion type	Blastic	Mixed	Lytic
Relation to bone diameter	<1/3	1/3–2/3	>2/3

Prognosis

The prognosis is worse with the following:

- Site:
  - Extraosseous/visceral metastasis.
  - Metastasis below the lumbosacral junction.
- Duration:
  - A short interval from the diagnosis of the primary tumour to metastasis.
  - Metastasis at presentation.
- Pathology:
  - Non-small-cell lung cancer.
  - Cancer of unknown primary origin.
- Laboratory results and imaging:
  - Hypercalcemia
  - Elevated alkaline phosphatase levels
  - Lytic lesions

Survival following skeletal metastases is variable and generally ranges from 6 months to 4 or more years (Table 8.14).

The revised Tokuhashi score has been devised to predict survival following spinal metastasis (Table 8.15).

Tokuhashi Y, Matsuzaki H, Oda H, Oshima M, Ryu J. A revised scoring system for preoperative evaluation of metastatic spine tumor prognosis. Spine 2005;30:2186–2191.

Table 8.14 Type of cancer and 5-year survival after metastasis

Type of Cancer	% of cases that metastasize after 5 years	5-year Survival after metastasis (%)
Prostate	24.5	6
Lung	12.4	1
Renal	8.4	5
Breast	6.0	13
GI	3.2	3

Table 8.15 Revised Tokuhashi Score

Characteristic	Group	Score
Performance status	Poor (10–40%)	0
	Moderate (50–70%)	1
	Good (80–100%)	2
Number of extraspinal bone metastases	>2	0
	1–2	1
	0	2
Number of metastases in the vertebral body	>2	0
	2	1
	1	2
Metastases to the major internal organs	Unremovable	0
	Removable	1
	None	2
Primary site of cancer	Lung, osteosarcoma, stomach, bladder, esophagus, pancreas	0
	Liver, gallbladder, unidentified	2
	Other	2
	Kidneys, uterus	3
	Rectum	4
	Thyroid, breast, prostate, carcinoid tumour	5
Neurological status	Frankel A/B	0
	Frankel C/D	1
	Frankel E	2

Prognosis from score; 0–8 (less than 6 months); 9–11 (6–12 months); 12–15 (>12 months)

Clinical Evaluation of the Unknown Primary Tumour

A clinical evaluation should be performed to identify the unknown primary tumour (Table 8.16).

Table 8.16 Clinical features of primary tumours

Primary tumour	Clinical features
Lung	History of smoking or exposure to asbestos Cough, haemoptysis Bronchial breathing, consolidation, pulmonary effusion Clubbing
Breast	Breast lumps, enlarged axillary lymph nodes
Prostate	Symptoms of prostate enlargement—Hesitancy, frequency, dysuria Rectal examination for enlargement or mass
Renal	Haematuria Palpable mass, flank pain
Thyroid	Swelling of enlargement of the thyroid gland
Colorectal	Altered bowel habits, blood with faeces
Melanoma	History of pigmented or non-pigmented lesions with a recent increase in size, asymmetric shape, change in colour, itching or bleeding

Non-Surgical Treatment of Bone Metastasis

Non-surgical treatment aims to achieve local or systemic control of the tumour, or both.

Radiotherapy

Once the bone has been surgically stabilised, postoperative radiotherapy is essential to control tumour growth. Radiotherapy can be given once the surgical incision is healed, usually 2–3 weeks after surgery. In the event of a bony procedure, the whole bone should be irradiated (an intramedullary nail will disseminate the tumour throughout the bone).

There is increasing evidence that a palliative single dose of radiotherapy is as effective as multiple doses.

Endocrine Therapy

Endocrine therapy is the treatment of choice for hormone-receptor-positive breast cancer. Cancer cells that express oestrogen and progesterone receptors are more susceptible to endocrine therapy. Luteinising hormone-releasing hormone (LHRH) agonists are frequently prescribed to premenopausal women and tamoxifen is prescribed to postmenopausal women.

Prostate cancers can respond to endocrine therapy in the form of LHRH agonists and antiandrogens.

Radioisotopes

The increased uptake of radioisotopes by tumour cells allows the use of radioisotopes to control metastases. Commonly used isotopes include ^{131}I for metastatic thyroid carcinoma, ^{131}I MIBG (mono-iodo benzylguanidine) for neuroblastoma and ^{89}Sr for osteoblastic prostate and breast metastasis.

Management of Bone Pain

The causes of bone pain in metastasis have been postulated to include the following:

- Increased intraosseous pressure.
- Periosteal stretching.
- Local inflammation and release of mediators that activate pain receptors.
- Impending fracture.

The treatment of bone pain is based on the WHO analgesic ladder. Patients with mild to moderate pain are managed with NSAIDs. Weak opioids can be added to NSAIDs in a fixed-dose combination if pain is not controlled. Severe pain requires opioid analgesia. The dosage of opioid analgesia is determined by the response to the drug and the susceptibility to adverse effects.

Fentanyl patches can be considered where pain is not controlled by oral analgesia. Bisphosphonates can also be useful for metastatic bone pain.

Treatment of Hypercalcemia

Hypercalcemia causes nausea, vomiting, dehydration, polyuria, polydipsia, confusion and, in severe cases, coma.

Several mechanisms contribute to hypercalcemia:

- Paraneoplastic production of parathyroid hormone-related peptide.
- Local osteolytic hypercalcemia due to bone resorption.
- Reduced renal elimination.

Initial management of hypercalcemia is by rehydration to restore intravascular volume, followed by intravenous bisphosphonate therapy. It can take 3–5 days to restore calcium ions Ca^{2+} levels to normal. Long-term management is normally aimed at controlling the neoplastic process. Hypercalcaemia is a poor prognostic indictor.

Surgical Treatment of Bone Metastasis

The BOOS BOA guidelines for management of metastatic disease provide a framework for surgical management of metastatic bone disease.

http://www.boos.org.uk/wp-content/uploads/2016/03/BOOS-MBD-2016-BOA.pdf

The prerequisites for surgery to treat skeletal metastases are

- A single operation can be performed with a reconstruction that will not fail in the patient's lifetime.
- Stabilisation of the whole bone.
- The operation will enable immediate weight-bearing.
- The recovery time from surgery is not longer than the probable life expectancy.

With improved survival rates, more aggressive treatment strategies (e.g., endoprosthetic replacement) are becoming necessary to restore quality of life.

Katagiri H, Takahashi M, Wakai K, et al. Prognostic factors and a scoring system for patients with skeletal metastasis. J Bone Joint Surg Br 2005;87:698–703. This study identified five significant prognostic factors for survival: the site of the primary lesion, performance status, the presence of visceral or cerebral metastases, previous chemotherapy and multiple skeletal metastases. The prognostic score was calculated by totaling the scores for individual factors. Patients with a prognostic score of six or more had a survival rate of 31% at 6 months and 11% at 1 year. By contrast, patients with a prognostic score of two or less had survival rates of 98% and 89%, respectively.

Pelvic Metastasis

A thorough preoperative evaluation is performed to assess the extent of the lesions and integrity of the remaining bone. Percutaneous options such as cementoplasty may be appropriate and should be considered. The surgical options include reconstruction using cemented hip replacement with augmentation of the acetabular bone defects using cup-cage reconstruction. Extensive disease may not be amenable to surgical treatment.

Harrington described a reconstruction technique of the pelvis using threaded pins inserted into the intact hemipelvis to transfer load. This requires an extensile exposure and is technically demanding. Tillman described a modified version through a percutaneous approach augmented by a cemented hip arthroplasty.

Harrington KD. The management of acetabular insufficiency secondary to metastatic malignant disease. J Bone Joint Surg Am 1981;63:653–64.

Tillman RM, Myers GJ, Abudu AT, et al. The three-pin modified 'Harrington' procedure for advanced metastatic destruction of the acetabulum. J Bone Joint Surg Br 2008;90:84–7. In this study of 19 patients, there were no deep infections, dislocations or nerve or major vessel injuries.

Femoral Neck Pathologic Fracture

Plain radiographs of the entire femur and acetabulum are necessary to identify occult lesions. A Tc 99 isotope bone scan or MRI scan can be undertaken to detect any radiologically occult lesions. Preoperative embolisation is typically employed for renal metastasis unless the metastasis is being excised *en bloc*.

Arthroplasty is the treatment of choice for femoral neck fractures due to the high risk of failure of fixation implants.

Long-stem cemented implants should be used and the tip of the stem should bypass the most distal lesion by twice the bone diameter. Long stems are preferable even if there are no identifiable lesions distally because of the possibility of lesion development at a later stage.

Acetabular involvement requires appropriate reconstruction. If possible a cemented acetabulum is preferable, as a cementless socket can have impaired bone ingrowth if radiation is required following surgery.

Peritrochanteric Fractures

The treatment method chosen should be expected to function beyond the life expectancy of the patient.

A sliding hip screw is inappropriate for the management of intertrochanteric metastatic fractures because of the following:

- There is a high risk of failure because of the nature of the device.
- A sliding hip screw does not address any distal defects.

- Non-union and cut out are major problems.
- Postoperative irradiation can lead to a stress riser at the distal end of the implant.
- Disease progression will result in failure of the reconstruction.

Cephalomedullary nails can be used and should be long, stabilising the entire femur to avoid the risk of fracture at the tip of the nail, which is a problem with the short version of the nail locked in the diaphysis.

Total hip replacement can be a conventional cemented design or with calcar replacement type designs that supports the deficient medial wall. The greater trochanter and abductor attachments are important for hip stability and should be preserved if possible. If the greater trochanter is involved, conversion to a proximal femoral replacement may be needed. Arthroplasty for metastatic disease is palliative; therefore, even if the greater trochanter is involved, it can be preserved and residual disease irradiated.

Cemented stems are preferred to achieve primary stability in bone. Ingrowth is unreliable due to pathologic bone and the radiation requirement. The exothermic reaction by which bone cement cures will also potentially kill tumour cells.

The arthroplasty can be technically difficult and has a higher risk of infection and dislocation than primary hip arthroplasty. Consideration should be given to larger-diameter heads to reduce the dislocation rate. Dual-mobility components can be used to improve stability if extensive soft tissue loss is found.

Subtrochanteric Fractures

Mechanisms for internal fixation include an intramedullary implant and proximal femoral replacement.

Dependent on pathology and disease load, intramedullary fixation is the preferred treatment, if possible. It avoids the risk of implant failure associated with extramedullary implants (there is no place for sliding hip screws because of the risk of disease progression or implant failure) and the risk of instability associated with proximal femoral replacement endoprostheses.

Second-generation (reconstruction-type) nails provide secure fixation proximally in the femoral head using two screws and distal interlocking.

The mode of failure is generally by screw cut-out from the femoral head. This can be caused by involvement of the head in the disease process, disease progression or inappropriate positioning of the implant (technical error).

Third-generation nails (long intramedullary hip screw/Gamma nails) have a single large proximal-locking screw as well as distal locking. Failure is less frequent.

Proximal femoral replacement is useful in the event of fixation failure, disease progression or extensive disease involving the entire proximal femur. The surgery is more extensive compared to internal fixation, with greater blood loss and an increased risk of infection (particularly if the patient is on chemotherapy). Stability can be a concern and reattachment of the abductors to the prosthesis or vastus lateralis may provide some support. Because this is a palliative procedure, preserving the greater trochanter and its soft tissue attachment will improve stability, as will the use of unipolar heads (hemiarthroplasty), bipolar heads and dual-mobility cups.

Chandrasekar CR, Grimer RJ, Carter SR, et al. Modular endoprosthetic replacement for tumours of the proximal femur. J Bone Joint Surg Br 2009;91;108–12.

Ashford RU, Hanna SA, Park DH et al. Proximal femoral replacements for metastatic bone disease: financial implications for sarcoma units. Int Orthop 2010;34(5):709–13.

Proximal Humerus Metastasis

Certain lesions can be treated with curettage and cement augmented fixation. Involvement of the head and neck requires hemiarthroplasty. A long stem may be needed to achieve distal fixation. The tuberosities (if salvageable) or the rotator cuff can be reattached to the prosthesis.

Using an allograft–prosthesis composite can help the reattachment of the host rotator cuff to the soft tissue on the allograft. Allograft is uncommonly used in the United Kingdom.

Humerus Diaphysis

Options for reconstruction include an intramedullary nail with or without cement augmentation, or diaphyseal replacement. The latter allow excision of the tumour. They also provide good axial and rotational stability, but reduced function.

Spencer SJ, Holt G, Clarke JV, et al. Locked intramedullary nailing of symptomatic metastases in the humerus. J Bone Joint Surg Br 2010;92:142–5. Thirty-five patients had a mean postoperative survival of 7.1 months. There were no failures of fixation and no reoperations.

Distal Humerus Metastasis

There are two surgical reconstructive options:

- Double plating with cement augmentation. The plates are placed in different planes for maximum mechanical advantage and the defect is curetted and filled with cement.
- Excision of the lesion and endoprosthetic distal humeral replacement.

Spinal Metastasis

The aim of management of spinal metastases is to alleviate pain, restore stability and prevent the compression of neural elements. Detailed review of spinal metastatic disease is beyond the scope of this chapter.

NICE guidelines (CG75) for metastatic spinal cord compression (MSCC) are well established and includes

- Treatment within cancer networks with availability of MRI within 24 h of suspected diagnosis.
- An MSCC coordinator who can coordinate the care pathway.
- Analgesia (including bisphosphonates in myeloma, prostate or breast cancer).
- Radiotherapy for non-mechanical pain.
- Consideration of vertebroplasty, kyphoplasty and surgery.
- Corticosteroids (loading dose of 16 mg dexamethasone then 16 mg once daily).
- Mechanical and chemical thromboprophylaxis.
- Pressure ulcer prevention.
- Bladder and bowel continence management.

Diagnostic surgical procedures include open or percutaneous biopsy to establish a tissue diagnosis. Percutaneous biopsy can be performed under fluoroscopy, CT or MRI guidance.

Malignant spinal cord compression is often best treated with radiotherapy, but surgical treatment is more appropriate in some cases. The indications for radiotherapy are

- No spinal instability.
- Radiosensitive tumour.
- Stable or slowly progressive neurology.
- Multilevel disease.
- Surgery is precluded by the general condition.
- Poor prognosis.
- Postoperative adjuvant treatment.

It is possible to deliver radiotherapy to the posterior vertebral body. Supplemental dexamethasone should be administered and the course of radiotherapy should be short (24 Gy in 6 fractions or 30 Gy in 10 fractions).

The indications for surgical treatment of malignant spinal cord compression are -.

- Spinal instability evidenced by pathological fracture, progressive deformity and/or neurological deficit.
- Clinically significant neurological compression, especially by bone.
- The tumour is insensitive to radiotherapy, chemotherapy or hormonal manipulation.

Surgical stabilisation is indicated where there is impending instability. The Denis three-column concept has been extended to include a left and right division in each column, making a total of six columns. Involvement of three or four columns out of six is an indication for stabilisation. Those with involvement of five or six columns will often require anterior and posterior stabilisation.

For the dorsal and lumbar spine, the anterior approach is preferred as the disease commonly involves the body of the vertebrae. The posterior approach can be used for isolated posterior disease (which is quite rare) or in conjunction with the anterior approach when the disease extends to more than two vertebral levels.

The anterior approach is also best for lower cervical spine disease. The upper cervical spine may require posterior stabilisation with or without anterior reconstruction.

Preoperative embolisation should be utilised for renal cell metastases and considered for myeloma in view of high vascularity to reduce blood loss during surgery.

Fürstenberg CH, Wiedenhöfer B, Gerner HJ, Putz C. The effect of early surgical treatment on recovery in patients with metastatic compression of the spinal cord. J Bone Joint Surg Br 2009;91:240–4. In 35 patients with incomplete cord compression, those who underwent decompression within 48 h had better neurologic outcomes than those with compression delayed for more than 48 h.

Further Reading

Albertsmeier M, Rauch A, Roeder F, Hasenhütl S, Pratschke S, Kirschneck M, Gronchi A, Jebsen NL, Cassier PA, Sargos P. Belka C. Ann Surg Oncol. 2018;25(3):754–67.

Arlen M, et al. Radiation induced sarcoma of bone. Cancer. 1971;28:1087.

Ashford RU, McCarthy SW, Scolyer RA, et al. Surgical biopsy with intra-operative frozen section. An accurate and cost-effective method for diagnosis of musculoskeletal sarcomas. J Bone Joint Surg Br. 2006;88:1207–11.

Ashford RU, Hanna SA, Park DH, et al. Proximal femoral replacements for metastatic bone disease: financial implications for sarcoma units. Int Orthop. 2010;34(5):709–13.

Balke M, Hardes J. Denosumab: a breakthrough in treatment of giant-cell tumour of bone. Lancet Oncol. 2010;11:218–9.

Barnes R, Catto M. Chondrosarcoma of bone. J Bone Joint Surg Br. 1966;48:729–64.

Bielack SS, Smeland S, Whelan JS, et al. Methotrexate, doxorubicin, and cisplatin (MAP) plus maintenance pegylated interferon alfa-2b versus MAP alone in patients with resectable high-grade osteosarcoma and good histologic response to preoperative MAP: first results of the EURAMOS-1 good response randomized controlled trial. J Clin Oncol. 2015;33(20):2279–87.

Blackley HR, Wunder JS, Davis AM, et al. Treatment of giant-cell tumors of long bones with curettage and bone-grafting. J Bone Joint Surg Am. 1999;81:811–20.

Cahan WG, et al. Sarcoma arising in irradiated bone. Cancer. 1948;1:3.

Campanacci M, et al. Giant cell tumours of bone. J Bone Joint Surg Am. 1987a;69(1):106–14.

Campanacci M, Baldini N, Boriani S, Sudanese A. Giant-cell tumor of bone. J Bone Joint Surg Am. 1987b;69:106–14.

Capanna R, Campanacci DA. The treatment of metastases in the appendicular skeleton. J Bone Joint Surg Br. 2001;83:471–81.

Chandrasekar CR, Grimer RJ, Carter SR, et al. Modular endoprosthetic replacement for tumours of the proximal femur. J Bone Joint Surg Br. 2009;91:108–12.

Cribb GL, Goude WH, Cool P, et al. Percutaneous radiofrequency thermocoagulation of osteoid osteomas: factors affecting therapeutic outcome. Skelet Radiol. 2005;34(11):702–6.

Cribb GL, Loo SC, Dickinson I. Limb salvage for soft tissue sarcomas of the foot and ankle. J Bone Joint Surg Br. 2010;92(3):424–9.

Dahlin DC, Beabout JW. Dedifferentiation of low-grade chondrosarcomas. Cancer. 1971;28:461–6.

Daly PJ, Sim FH, Wold LE. Dedifferentiated chondrosarcoma of bone. Orthopedics. 1989;12:763–7.

Davis AM, Bell RS, Goodwin PJ. Prognostic factors in osteosarcoma: a critical review. J Clin Oncol. 1994;12:423–31.

Enneking WF. A staging system of musculoskeletal neoplasms. Clin Orthop Relat Res. 1986;204:9–24.

Feigenberg SJ, Marcus RB Jr, Zlotecki RA, et al. Radiation therapy for giant cell tumours of bone. Clin Orthop Relat Res. 2003;411:207–16.

Fürstenberg CH, Wiedenhöfer B, Gerner HJ, Putz C. The effect of early surgical treatment on recovery in patients with metastatic compression of the spinal cord. J Bone Joint Surg Br. 2009;91:240–4.

Giuffreda AY, et al. Chondrosarcoma in the unites states (1973–2003): an analysis of 2890 cases from the SEER database. J Bone Joint Surg Am. 2009;91(5):1063–72.

Gladdy RA, Qin LX, et al. Do radiation-associated soft tissue sarcomas have the same prognosis as sporadic soft tissue sarcomas? J Clin Oncol. 2010;28(12):2064.

Grimer RJ, Taminiau AM, Cannon SR, Surgical Subcommittee of the European Osteosarcoma Intergroup. Surgical outcomes in osteosarcoma. J Bone Joint Surg Br. 2002;84:395–400.

Harrington KD. The management of acetabular insufficiency secondary to metastatic malignant disease. J Bone Joint Surg Am. 1981;63:653–64.

Hoffmann RT, Jakobs TF, Kubisch CH, et al. Radiofrequency ablation in the treatment of oste-

oid osteoma—5-year experience. Eur J Radiol. 2010;73:374–9.
Issels RD, Lindner LH, Verweij J, Wessalowski R, Reichardt P, Wust P, Ghadjar P, Hohenberger P, Angele M, Salat C, Vujaskovic Z. Effect of neoadjuvant chemotherapy plus regional hyperthermia on long-term outcomes among patients with localized high-risk soft tissue sarcoma: the EORTC 62961-ESHO 95 randomized clinical trial. JAMA Oncol. 2018;4(4):483–92.
Jeys LM, Kulkarni A, Grimer RJ, et al. Endoprosthetic reconstruction for the treatment of musculoskeletal tumors of the appendicular skeleton and pelvis. J Bone Joint Surg Am. 2008;90:1265–71.
Katagiri H, Takahashi M, Wakai K, et al. Prognostic factors and a scoring system for patients with skeletal metastasis. J Bone Joint Surg Br. 2005;87:698–703.
Khatri VP, Goodnight JE Jr. Extremity soft tissue sarcoma: controversial management issues. Surg Oncol. 2005;14:1–9.
Malawer MM, Bickels J, Meller I, et al. Cryosurgery in the treatment of giant cell tumor. A long-term follow-up study. Clin Orthop Relat Res. 1999;359:176–88.
Malghem J, Vande Berg B, Noël H, Maldague B. Benign osteochondromas and exostotic chondrosarcomas: evaluation of cartilage cap thickness by ultrasound. Skelet Radiol. 1992;21:33–7.
Mankin HJ, Lange TA, Spanier SS. The hazards of biopsy in patients with malignant primary bone and soft-tissue tumours. J Bone Joint Surg Am. 1982;64:1121–7.
Mankin HJ, Mankin CJ, Simon MA. The hazards of the biopsy, revisited. Members of the Musculoskeletal Tumor Society. J Bone Joint Surg Am. 1996;78:656–63.
Marcove RC, Sheth DS, Takemoto S, Healey JH. The treatment of aneurysmal bone cyst. Clin Orthop Relat Res. 1995;311:157–63.
McDonald DJ, Capanna R, Gherlinzoni F, et al. Influence of chemotherapy on perioperative complications in limb salvage surgery for bone tumours. Cancer. 1990;65:1509–16.
Mirels H. Metastatic disease in long bones: a proposed scoring system for diagnosing impending pathologic fractures. Clin Orthop Relat Res. 1989;249:256–64.
O'Sullican B, Davis AM, et al. Preoperative versus postoperative radiotherapy in soft-tissue sarcoma of the limbs: a randomised trial. Lancet. 2002;359(9325):2235–41.
Pollock RC, Stalley PD. Biopsy of musculoskeletal tumours—beware. ANZ J Surg. 2004;74:516–9.
Porter DE, Lonie L, Fraser M, et al. Severity of disease and risk of malignant change in hereditary multiple exostoses. A genotype–phenotype study. J Bone Joint Surg Br. 2004;86:1041–6.
Prosser GH, Baloch KG, Tillman RM, et al. Does curettage without adjuvant therapy provide low recurrence rates in giant-cell tumors of bone? Clin Orthop Relat Res. 2005;435:211–8.
Rahimi A, Beabout JW, Ivins JC, Dahlin DC. Chondromyxoid fibroma: a clinicopathologic study of 76 cases. Cancer. 1972;30:726–36.
Reddy KIA, Sinnaeve F, Gaston CL, Grimer RJ, Carter SR. Aneurysmal bone cysts: do simple treatments work? Clin Orthop Relat Res. 2014;472:1901–10.
Salai M. Surgical biopsy of bone metastases. In: Jasmin C, Coleman RE, Coia LR, et al., editors. Textbook of bone metastases. Wiley: Chichester; 2005. p. 123–31.
Sewell MD, Spiegelberg BG, Hanna SA, et al. Total femoral endoprosthetic replacement following excision of bone tumours. J Bone Joint Surg Br. 2009;91:1513–20.
Spencer SJ, Holt G, Clarke JV, et al. Locked intramedullary nailing of symptomatic metastases in the humerus. J Bone Joint Surg Br. 2010;92:142–5.
Staals EL, Bacchini P, Mercuri M, Bertoni F. Dedifferentiated chondrosarcomas arising in preexisting osteochondromas. J Bone Joint Surg Am. 2007;89:987–93.
Szendröi M. Giant-cell tumour of bone. J Bone Joint Surg Br. 2004;86:5–12.
Tillman RM, Myers GJ, Abudu AT, et al. The three-pin modified 'Harrington' procedure for advanced metastatic destruction of the acetabulum. J Bone Joint Surg Br. 2008;90:84–7.
Tokuhashi Y, Matsuzaki H, Oda H, Oshima M, Ryu J. A revised scoring system for preoperative evaluation of metastatic spine tumor prognosis. Spine. 2005;30:2186–91.
Tunn PU, Kettelhack C, Dürr HR. Standardized approach to the treatment of adult soft tissue sarcoma of the extremities. Recent Results Cancer Res. 2009;179:211–28.
Widhe B, Widhe T. Initial symptoms and clinical features in osteosarcoma and Ewing sarcoma. J Bone Joint Surg Am. 2000;82:667–74.
Yanagawa T, Shinozaki T, Iizuka Y, et al. Role of 2-deoxy-2-[F-18] fluoro-d-glucose positron emission tomography in the management of bone and soft-tissue metastases. J Bone Joint Surg Br. 2010;92:419–23.
Zhen W, Yaotian H, Songjian L, et al. Giant-cell tumour of bone. The long-term results of treatment by curettage and bone graft. J Bone Joint Surg Br. 2004;86:212–6.

Infections

9

Sanjeev Agarwal

Acute Osteomyelitis

Incidence

The incidence of acute osteomyelitis varies, but has been reported as 1 in 5000 per year in children, peaking in late summer. Boys are three times more prone to infection than girls. It generally involves rapidly growing bones, hence the predominance in children under the age of 5 years.

Pathogenesis

The common infecting organisms are summarized in Table 9.1.

Staph aureus is the commonest organism overall. *Haemophilus influenzae* is rare in countries following immunization programs. *Strep pneumoniae* can cause invasive disease progressing to bacteremia and meningitis. Community acquired MRSA (Methicillin Resistant *Staphylococcus aureus*) can be a possible causative organism.

Kingella kingae is a slow growing Gram negative coccobacillus is increasingly recognized as the causative pathogen in children under the age or 4 years. *Kingella* was first described by Elizabeth King in 1960s. The availability of better identification techniques indicated *K. kingae* may be the predominant organism for osteoarticular infections in children under the age of 4 years.

Table 9.1 Common infecting organisms in Acute haematogenous osteomyelitis

Age/patient group	Common infecting organism
Neonates	*Staph aureus* Group B *Strep* *Neisseria gonorrhoeae*
Children	*Staph aureus* Group A Strep Coliforms *Kingella kingae*
Adults	*Staph aureus*
Sickle cell disease	*Staph aureus* *Salmonella* *Strep pneumoniae*
Intravenous drug use/ puncture wounds	*Staph aureus* *Pseudomonas aeruginosa* *Candida*
Trauma/diabetes	Polymicrobial
Animal bite	*Pasturella multocida* *Eikenella corrodens*

Infections caused by *Kingella kingae* are more indolent and demonstrate a lesser inflammatory response compared to Staphylococcal infections.

The infection is commonly haematogenous. Several features of the metaphysis make it a common site of infection:

S. Agarwal (✉)
University Hospital of Wales, Consultant Orthopaedic Surgeon, Cardiff, UK

S. Agarwal (ed.), *Current Orthopaedic Practice*, https://doi.org/10.1007/978-3-030-78529-1_9

- The blood flow is slow, allowing bacteria to migrate through fenestrations in the capillary wall (Fig. 9.1).
- Deficient ability of endothelial cells to phagocytise particles in the metaphysis.
- Medullary vessels become thrombosed and white cells cannot reach the bacteria.

The initial phase is inflammatory with rising intraosseous pressure causing intense pain. Pus formation follows. In long bones, pus exits laterally and forms a subperiosteal abscess. Because of pressure the blood supply to the cortex is cut off, which can lead to the formation of sequestrum.

Intra-articular metaphysis is found in the proximal femur, proximal humerus, distal tibia and the radial neck. At these sites, the joint can become infected by contiguous spread from the metaphysis (Fig. 9.2).

In the later phase, after about 2 weeks, new bone formation takes place under the elevated periosteum. This new bone formed over the sequestrum is called involucrum.

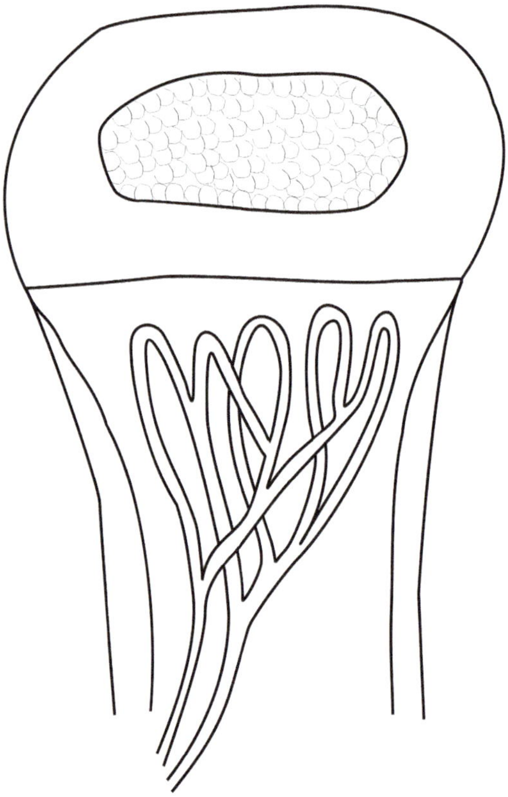

Fig. 9.1 Medullary vessels 'hairpin' loops

Clinical Features

Common site are around the knee or proximal humerus. Patients commonly present with pseudoparalysis (reluctance to use the extremity), pain, a limp and refusal to walk. Sympathetic effusion may be present in the adjoining joint. Acute infection is often associated with systemic signs.

Differential diagnosis includes septic arthritis, trauma, osteoid osteoma, acute lymphoblastic leukemia, Ewing's sarcoma, osteosarcoma, bone infarction in sickle cell disease, glycogen storage diseases and avascular necrosis.

Investigations

Blood Tests

The white cell count (WCC) is normal in 75% patients. The erythrocyte sedimentation rate (ESR) is elevated in 90%, but although it can be

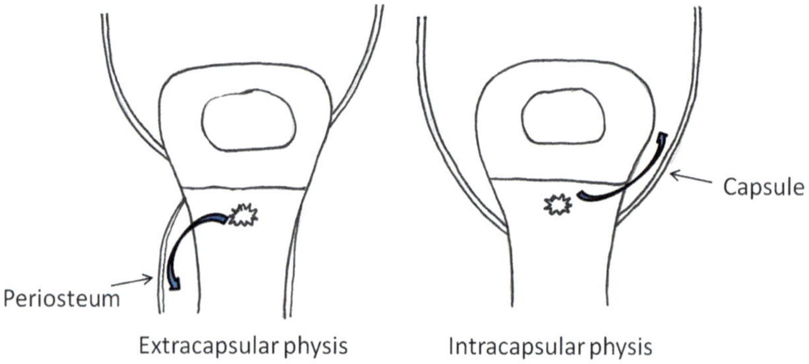

Fig. 9.2 Spread of infection in intraarticular physis

normal in patients with sickle cell disease, those undergoing steroid therapy and neonates. The ESR rises 3–5 days after the onset of infection and starts declining in 1–2 weeks.

The C-reactive protein level peaks in 2 days, and starts declining within 6 h of appropriate therapy. This is the most sensitive indicator of the course of infection and response to treatment.

Blood cultures are positive in 30–50% of patients.

Imaging

Radiographs within 3 days may show displacement of the muscle planes. In 7 days, the muscle planes are typically obliterated. Bone changes appear after 1–2 weeks.

A Tc99 bone scan has a high false-negative rate. It should be performed within 48 h of aspiration, otherwise false-positivity is high. Patients with cold bone scans may have more aggressive infection.

Other radioisotopes scans with increasing sensitivity and specificity are available. These include gallium 67, indium-111-labeled WBC, indium-111-labeled immunoglobulin and Tc-99 ciprofloxacin scans.

A computed tomography scan will show bone changes. This can help to differentiate osteomyelitis from chondroblastoma and osteoid osteoma.

Magnetic resonance imaging (MRI) can detect changes due to bone oedema within 3–5 days due to bone oedema. Gadolinium enhancement helps define areas of necrosis. MRI is a sensitive and commonly used investigation. In children under the age of 5 years, anesthetic may be needed for MR scan.

An ultrasound scan can be performed to detect subperiosteal abscesses ('sandwich appearance of periosteum'). Elevation of the periosteum by 2 mm is suggestive of an underlying infection.

Positron emission tomography scanning has nearly 99% sensitivity for the detection of bone infections.

Bone Marrow Aspiration

Bone marrow aspiration is performed to obtain material for Gram stain and culture. Ideally, blood culture and bone marrow aspiration should be done before antibiotic therapy, if possible.

If the patient has underlying chronic diseases then the aspirate should be tested for anaerobes, acid-fast bacilli and fungi should be tested.

Polymerase chain reaction can detect bacteria and help in determining the causative organism.

Treatment

The choice of antibiotic therapy depends on sensitivity. Empiric therapy can be started once samples have been obtained for bacteriological diagnosis. Commonly used antibiotics are oxacillin, cefazolin, clindamycin and vancomycin. Once the infecting organism has been identified, the choice of antibiotic therapy is based on the sensitivity.

Kingella kingae is generally sensitive to penicillins and aminoglycosides (like gentamicin). It is less sensitive to flucloxacillin and is often resistant to glycopeptides such as teicoplanin and vancomycin.

Bacteraemia may interfere with the absorption of oral agents. Duration of intravenous antibiotics is usually 3 days followed by 3–6 weeks of oral antibiotics based on microbiology advice.

Jagodzinski NA, Kanwar R, Graham K, Bache CE. Prospective Evaluation of a Shortened Regimen of Treatment for Acute Osteomyelitis and Septic Arthritis in Children. J Pediatr Orthop 2009;29(5):518–25. Prospective data on 70 children aged 2 weeks to 14 years. Staphylococcus was the only organism for osteomyelitis and Strep was more common in septic arthritis. 3 days of intravenous antibiotics followed by 3 weeks of oral antibiotics was sufficient for treatment. All patients returned to normal at 1 year follow up.

Indications for surgery include a lack of response to antibiotic therapy, subperiosteal abscess, intramedullary pus, sequestrum and secondary septic arthritis. Surgery is rarely needed. The local pus is drained, periosteum incised to check for subperiosteal collection, and drill holes made in the metaphysis to drain intraosseous pus.

Long-term sequelae are limb-length discrepancy, recurrent infection, joint deformity and gait abnormalities.

Brodie's Abscess

Brodie's abscess is subacute osteomyelitis in the metaphysis of long bones. It appears as a lytic area surrounded by sclerotic bone. As the infection is localised, systemic sepsis is rare. Local symptoms may be pain and limp. Recurrent flare-ups of infection from a Brodie's abscess are managed by debridement, curettage, and antibiotics. A preoperative image guided aspiration is helpful to establish the diagnosis and plan antibiotic therapy.

Chronic Osteomyelitis

Chronic osteomyelitis can be the result of persistent infection following acute osteomyelitis or local/haematogenous spread. Open fractures and postsurgery infection can lead to chronic osteomyelitis. Immune deficiency predisposes to chronic infection.

Three types of patients are identified on the basis on immune resistance (Cierney—Table 9.2).

Anatomically, chronic osteomyelitis can be of four types (Fig. 9.3).

Cierny G 3rd, Mader JT. Approach to adult osteomyelitis. Orthop Rev, 1987;16(4):259–70.

Sequestrum is dead bone surrounded by infected granulation tissue. This refers to areas of bone which have separated as part of the infective process. With time, periosteum may form new bone around the sequestrum, which is known as involucrum. Holes in the involucrum, called cloaca, allow the pus to drain through sinus tracts. Chronic osteomyelitis may or may not be associated with a sinus tract.

Table 9.2 Host types for chronic osteomyelitis

Host type	Characteristic
Type A	Normal immune response, non-smoker
Type B	Mild systemic disorders, or smoker
Type C	Major nutritional or systemic disorder

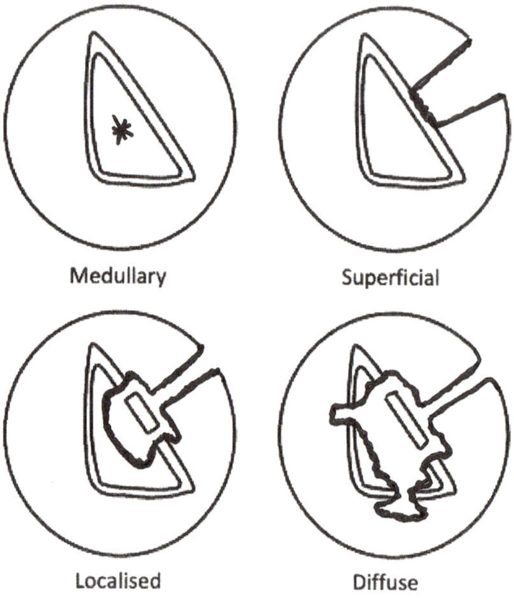

Fig. 9.3 Types of chronic osteomyelitis proposed by Cierny and Mader

Investigations

In addition to blood tests and radiographs, MRI scan will help determine soft tissue involvement, the presence of marrow edema and areas of pus collection.

Culture from the sinus tract is not helpful because it is colonised by a variety of bacteria. Deep cultures are more representative of the causative organism.

Tc-99 scan will show increased local uptake in all three phases. A white cell labeled Indium scan is highly specific for infections. A PET scan is considered most sensitive for diagnosis of osteomyelitis. PET scans are rarely needed.

Polymerase chain reaction techniques can aid diagnosis.

Treatment

Treatment is based on thorough debridement of all dead and infected tissue, appropriate antibiotics, obliteration of dead space and soft tissue cover. In the localised form of chronic osteomyelitis, local debridement may involve excising dead bone; the diffuse form is managed by *en bloc* resection of a segment of bone, with the defect managed by one of the techniques described below.

A flap cover is very useful to cover soft tissue defects and bring a greater blood supply to the local area. Open cancellous grafting (Papineau technique) is rarely used. Negative pressure dressings are helpful in wound healing.

Local antibiotic delivery can be achieved by gentamicin beads, or by using absorbable calcium sulphate preparations. Absorbable preparations can be used for a wide range of antibiotics and antifungal agents. These get absorbed completely and hence do not require removal at second stage, which is a problem when gentamicin beads are used.

McNally described a technique that was performed in two stages. The first stage was radical debridement with the use of gentamicin beads. The second stage, performed 3–6 weeks later, involved further debridement and bone grafting. The reported success rate was 92%.

McNally MA, Small JO, Tofighi HG, Mollan RA. Two stage management of chronic osteomyelitis of the long bones. The Belfast technique. J Bone Joint Surg Br 1993;75:375–80.

Another technique from Oswestry describes excision of sinus tracks, removal of internal fixation devices and double-ended reaming. An endoscope is passed into the canal to ensure bleeding bone surfaces. A closed suction irrigation tube is inserted, and removed at the end of treatment. Only one operation is planned, although some patients may require repeat debridement.

Caesar BC, Morgan-Jones R, Warren RE, et al. Closed double-lumen suction irrigation in the management of chronic diaphyseal osteomyelitis: long-term follow-up. J Bone Joint Surg Br 2009;91:1243–8. Oswestry technique. Thirty-five patients were managed by reaming, arthroscopic debridement of the medullary canal and closed double-lumen suction irrigation. Infection was cleared in 85%.

Vascularised bone grafts are indicated for long defects (>6 cm) and require close coordination between plastic and orthopaedic surgeons.

The Ilizarov method of corticotomy, bone transport and distraction histogenesis is helpful when a bone segment must be excised. Docking of the two ends can be performed acutely and then length regained by distraction, or the length can be maintained and a segment transported to fill the gap.

The Masquelet technique or Induced Membrane technique (IMT) is being used increasingly commonly for chronic infections. This is a two stage procedure. The first stage is radical debridement and removal of dead and infected bone, stabilisation of bone and insertion of cement spacer in the defect. The cement spacer induces formation of a hypervascular membrane. The second stage is undertaken after 6 weeks whereby the cement spacer is removed preserving the membrane, and autogenous cancellous graft placed in the membrane cavity.

Masquelet AC, Fitoussi F, Begue T, Muller GP. Reconstruction of the long bones by the induced membrane and spongy autograft. Annales de Chirurgie Plastique et Esthetique 2000;45(3):346–353.

Morelli I, Drago L, George DA, Gallazzi E, Scarponi S, Romanò CL. Masquelet Technique: Myth or Reality? A Systematic Review and Meta-Analysis. Injury 2016;47 Suppl 6:S68–S76. Meta-analysis of 17 papers. Union rate 89% and infection clearance achieved in 91%.

Septic Arthritis

Septic arthritis is acute bacterial infection of a joint.

The most common route of spread is haematogenous via the blood. Local spread, trauma or surgery may be responsible in some instances.

Infecting organism are commonly *Staphylococcus aureus* while *Kingella kingae* is increasingly recognized as the causative organism in children under the age of 4 years.

Clinical Features

Septic arthritis can present in any age group but is more common in boys aged less than 2 years. There may be a history of upper respiratory tract infection or local infection.

Common presenting symptoms include fever, local pain, swelling, tenderness and inability to bear weight.

Blood Parameters

An ESR of more than 40 mm/h and a WCC of greater than 12,000/mm^3 are suggestive of septic arthritis.

If three characteristics out of fever, inability to bear weight, raised ESR and raised WCC are present, there is a 93% chance of septic arthritis. If all four characteristics are present, the odds rise to 99.6%.

Imaging

X-ray features include joint-space widening, obliteration of normal fat planes and soft tissue swelling. In later stages, bone destruction may be evident.

A Tc-99 bone scan is useful in detecting multifocal lesions. In addition, in certain areas such as the foot, pelvis, hip, spine and scapula, clinical and radiological signs may not be readily evident and these can be evaluated with a Tc-99 scan/SPECT scan.

Computed tomography and MRI cannot differentiate infection from non-septic inflammation. Ultrasound is non-specific and operator dependant.

Aspiration

Joint aspiration can provide a definitive diagnosis and is the definitive test, if positive. Table 9.3 shows the tests performed on the fluid and indicators of infection.

Treatment

Septic arthritis is an emergency. The immediate management is resuscitation of the patient, ensuring adequate analgesia and hydration. Blood cultures should be sent for culture, and it is worth taking a sample for microbiology analysis prior to starting antibiotics. Open irrigation and debridement is undertaken and the joint closed over drains. In gonococcal arthritis, aspiration only may be sufficient.

Intravenous antibiotics, usually cephalosporins, are started pending culture results. Oxacillin and ceftriaxone are used in immunocompromised patients. The duration of antibiotic therapy is a debated issue, but in most cases it should continue for 6 weeks.

With early diagnosis and adequate treatment, a 90% cure rate can be expected. Ongoing infec-

Table 9.3 Tests performed on the joint aspiration fluid and indicators of infection

Test	Indicator of infection
Gram stain	Positive
Culture—aerobic, anaerobic	Positive Cultures are positive in 50–60% of patients
WCC count	WCC >50,000/mm^3 with >90% polymorphonuclear neutrophils
Synovial glucose test	Ratio of synovial fluid glucose to blood glucose of <0.5
Mucin clot test	Acetic acid is added to the fluid, and an appearance like curdled milk indicates infection In rheumatic fever, a mucin clot forms a rope-like appearance

tion and damage to the physis account for most of the disability following acute osteomyelitis. Damaged physis leads to deformity, shortening or sometimes compensatory overgrowth. A pathological fracture can occur through the infection site.

Alpha Defensin

There has been a lot of interest recently in alpha defensin for diagnosis of prosthetic joint infections. Alpha defensin is an antimicrobial peptide secreted by neutrophils. The alpha defensin kills the bacteria by incorporating into the cell membrane of the invading pathogen.

Alpha defensin is measured in the synovial fluid. There are other synovial fluid biomarkers like C reactive protein (CRP) and synovial leucocyte esterase (LE). Of these, alpha defensin displays the best sensitivity and specificity.

The laboratory assessment of alpha defensin is an ELISA (Enzyme Linked Immunosorbent Assay) and shows a very high predictive value in diagnosis of prosthetic joint infections.

Wyatt MC, Beswick AD, Kunutsor SK et al. The alpha-defensin immunoassay and leukocyte esterase colorimetric strip test for the diagnosis of periprosthetic infection: a systematic review and meta-analysis. J Bone Joint Surg Am 2016;98:992–1000. 100% sensitivity and 96% specificity of alpha defensin.

Lateral flow devices allow assessment of alpha defensin by the bedside or intraoperatively within 10 min. However, the alpha defensin lateral flow test (marketed as synovasure) is not as accurate as lab based tests.

Alpha defensin levels are not influenced by prior antibiotic therapy, which is a significant advantage over bacterial cultures done while patients are on antibiotics. However, these tests only confirm or rule out infection and do not provide a microbiological diagnosis.

Osteoarticular Tuberculosis

Tuberculosis of the skeletal system is caused by *Mycobacterium tuberculosis* and *M. bovis*. It is relatively common in the developing world. In developed countries, it is predominantly seen in those with compromised immune systems.

1.8 million people died from tuberculosis worldwide in 2015. 10% patients have extrapulmonary manifestations, of which 5% are in the skeletal system. HIV targets CD4 cells, and this results in a reduced cellular response to Mycobacterium. Patients with HIV may have increased incidence as well and increased reactivation of tuberculosis. HIV targets CD4 cells, and results in a reduced cellular response to Mycobacterium.

Primary tuberculosis presents as a pulmonary infection in children and often resolves. The primary focus lesion is subpleural and is known as a Ghon's focus. Reactivation of the primary tuberculosis, often related to a drop in immune resistance, leads to a more severe infection. The reactivation can be related to a drop in immune resistance. Haematogenous spread of the infection leads to involvement of the bones and joints.

Clinical Features

The features of post-primary tuberculosis include cough, haemoptysis, weight loss, night sweats and lymphadenopathy. The systemic signs depend on the system involved.

The onset of symptoms is insidious and presentation is often delayed. Weight loss is a common symptom.

Investigations

The ESR is markedly raised in tuberculosis, with minimal elevation in white cell count. Differential count shows relative lymphocytosis.

Microscopic identification of *Mycobacteria* is performed using Ziehl–Neelsen staining. The disease is paucibacterial, and AFB may not be seen in the microscopy. Tissue has a better yield for bacterial detection compared to pus.

Culture is done on Lowenstein–Jensen medium for 6 weeks. The histology is characterised by a delayed-type hypersensitivity picture, with tuberculoid granulomas, Langhan's giant cells, central caseating necrosis, abundant lymphocytes and epithelioid macrophages.

Polymerase Chain Reaction (PCR) is very helpful to detect genetic material of the bacilli and can give a result within 2 days. Specificity of PCR is between 80 and 90% and sensitivity is up to 95%. It also helps in detection of antibiotic resistance.

Treatment

The treatment of osteoarticular tuberculosis is mainly medical and is based on combination therapy with rifampicin, isoniazid, ethambutol and pyrazinamide. Resistant or recurrent tuberculosis requires second-line drugs.

WHO recommends an initial 2 months period of intense therapy using four drugs—Isoniazid, Ethambutol, Rifampicin and Pyrazinamide. This is followed by a continuation phase using Isoniazid and Rifampicin. The total duration of therapy is 9 months. In countries with high prevalence of tuberculosis, three drugs are used in the continuation phase—Rifampicin, isoniazid and ethambutol—for a period of 10–16 months.

Patients with HIV are treated with four drugs for 9 months or longer, depending on response to treatment.

Involvement of the hip or knee joint leads to joint destruction and arthroplasty is an option. Adequate debridement must be performed and the implant can be inserted as a single- or two-stage procedure. Antitubercular medication should be given both pre- and postoperatively to minimise the risk of recurrent infection.

Prevention of Surgical Site Infections

Surgical site infections account for substantial morbidity in the postoperative period. A range of practices have been proposed to minimise surgical site infection, and include patient-dependant aspects as well as factors related to the operation room environment and perioperative management. NICE (National Institute for Health and Care Excellence) has published guidelines for preventing surgical site infections in 2019.

An adequate nutrition status and control of concurrent infections is essential before elective procedures.

An impaired immunological response is associated with a higher risk of infection.

Local hair removal, if needed, should be performed using clippers and not razors. It should be performed just before the operation, preferably in the anaesthetic room.

The use of clean-air operation theatres with vertical laminar flow significantly reduces the risk of infection.

Chlorhexidine is more effective and longer lasting than iodine based antiseptics. Iodine antiseptics should be allowed to dry for maximal efficacy.

High-pressure pulse lavage can increase damage to soft tissues and increase the penetration of bacteria.

The use of drains has not been shown to make a difference to the infection rate or wound breakdown following elective surgery. Drains may increase the transfusion rate, but this can be offset by the use of reinfusion drains. Reinfusion drapes are contraindicated where the operation is done for infection.

Sutures are considered to be better than skin clips for wound closure.

The maintenance of normal glucose levels, normothermia and oxygenation reduces the risk of infection.

Occlusive dressing allows a hypoxic and acidic environment, which retards the growth of skin pathogens and improves healing.

Prophylactic Perioperative Antibiotics

Prophylactic antibiotics should be given prior to starting an operation involving a prosthesis. Antibiotics are not routinely used for uncomplicated, clean, non-prosthetic surgery.

For closed fractures and elective orthopaedic procedures, cefuroxime or cefazolin is considered to be effective against the common infective organisms (*Staph. aureus* and *Staph. epidermidis*). In some hospitals, the emergence of resistance has led to the use of co-amoxiclav(Augmentin), vancomycin or teicoplanin as the prophylactic antibiotics of choice.

Antibiotics should be given before surgery, at the time of start of anaesthesia. For operations lasting longer than the half life of the antibiotic, a second dose is administered.

Antibiotics are given for a maximum of 24 h postoperatively. A longer period of therapy does not reduce infection risk and may increase the risk of resistant organisms and systemic infections. Patients with open wounds or infections need antibiotics for longer periods.

Prosthetic infection management is discussed in Chap. 14.

Further Reading

Caesar BC, Morgan-Jones R, Warren RE, et al. Closed double-lumen suction irrigation in the management of chronic diaphyseal osteomyelitis: long-term follow-up. J Bone Joint Surg Br. 2009;91:1243–8.

Cierny G 3rd, Mader JT. Approach to adult osteomyelitis. Orthop Rev. 1987;16(4):259–70.

Jagodzinski NA, Kanwar R, Graham K, Bache CE. Prospective evaluation of a shortened regimen of treatment for acute osteomyelitis and septic arthritis in children. J Pediatr Orthop. 2009;29(5):518–25.

Masquelet AC, Fitoussi F, Begue T, Muller GP. Reconstruction of the long bones by the induced membrane and spongy autograft. Ann Chir Plast Esthet. 2000;45(3):346–53.

McNally MA, Small JO, Tofighi HG, Mollan RA. Two stage management of chronic osteomyelitis of the long bones. The Belfast technique. J Bone Joint Surg Br. 1993;75:375–80.

Morelli I, Drago L, George DA, Gallazzi E, Scarponi S, Romanò CL. Masquelet technique: myth or reality? A systematic review and meta-analysis. Injury. 2016;47(Suppl 6):S68–76.

Wyatt MC, Beswick AD, Kunutsor SK, et al. The alpha-defensin immunoassay and leukocyte esterase colorimetric strip test for the diagnosis of periprosthetic infection: a systematic review and meta-analysis. J Bone Joint Surg Am. 2016;98:992–1000.

Non-Union

10

Sanjeev Agarwal

Non-union

Non-union is defined as cessation of the normal biological healing process at the fracture site, with no progression of healing for at least 3 months. Non-unions require intervention for union to be achieved.

Delayed union is a delay in the healing of a fracture. There is some progression, but the rate of healing is less than expected for that site.

In view of the various factors that influence fracture healing, it is difficult to provide a standard fixed timescale to define non-union.

The rate of delayed and non-union varies with the site and type of injury. For instance in tibial fractures, the rate of non-union is around 2.5% and that of delayed union is about 5%. This will depend on a variety of injury and treatment related factors.

Causes

Causes of nonunion are summarized in Table 10.1.

Table 10.1 Contributory factors for nonunion

Patient factors	Injury factors	Surgical factors
Smoking Diabetes Steroid intake NSAIDs Rheumatoid arthritis Malnutrition—a serum albumin level of less than 3.4 g/dL and a lymphocyte count of less than $1500/mm^3$ is suggestive of a reduced nutrition level	Initial displacement of fragments Degree of comminution Degree of periosteal stripping Bone loss Local infection or open injuries Disruption of blood supply	Inadequate reduction Inadequate stabilisation Ongoing sepsis Distraction at fracture site Periosteal stripping

Types of Non-union

Radiologically, non-union can be of three types (LaVelle)—Table 10.2.

The distinction between these types is based on the vascularity of the bone ends. This can be determined with strontium 85 scanning.

Dror Paley has classified non-unions into type A (<1 cm bone loss) and type B (>1 cm bone loss). They can be further classified based on deformity and shortening (Fig. 10.1).

Mora R, Paley D. Nonunion of the long bones: diagnosis and treatment with compression distraction techniques. Springer 2006.

S. Agarwal (✉)
University Hospital of Wales, Consultant Orthopaedic Surgeon, Cardiff, UK

S. Agarwal (ed.), *Current Orthopaedic Practice*, https://doi.org/10.1007/978-3-030-78529-1_10

Table 10.2 Types of nonunion

Hypertrophic	Oligotrophic	Atrophic
Abundant callus	Inadequate callus	No callus
Adequate blood supply	Adequate blood supply	Inadequate blood supply
Insufficient stability	Due to lack of reduction or lack of contact	Deficient biology
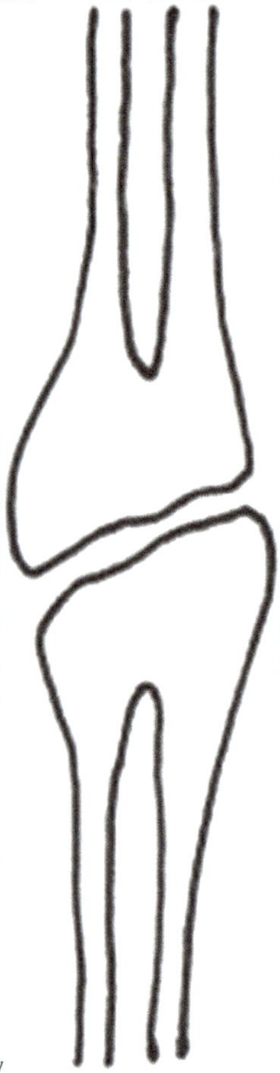	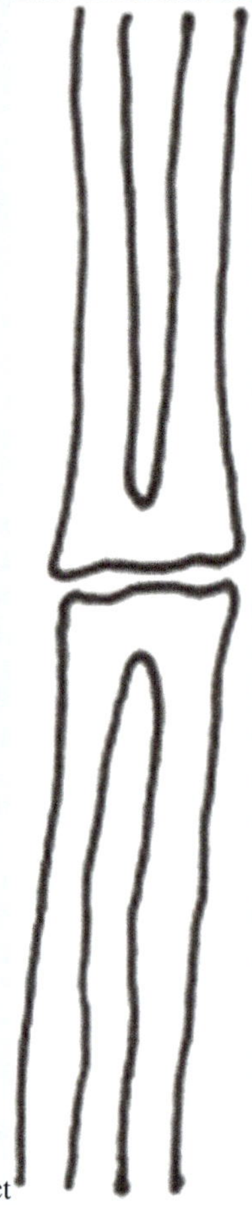	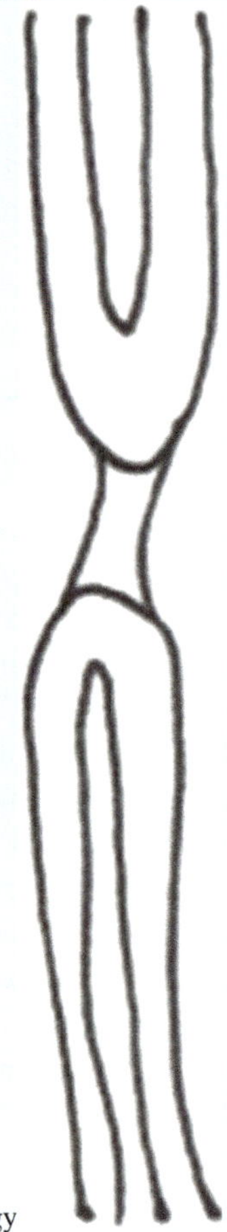

Diagnosis

Plain radiographs are the basis for the diagnosis of non-union. CT scans are very helpful for detecting a gap between the fragments if it is not obvious on plain films.

Ultrasound examination can reveal a discontinuity in the cortex, implying incomplete healing.

Management

Evaluation for the cause of non-union is an integral part of management. Bone loss, sepsis, malalignment and previous operations can affect planning of the treatment modality.

The principles of management are as follows:

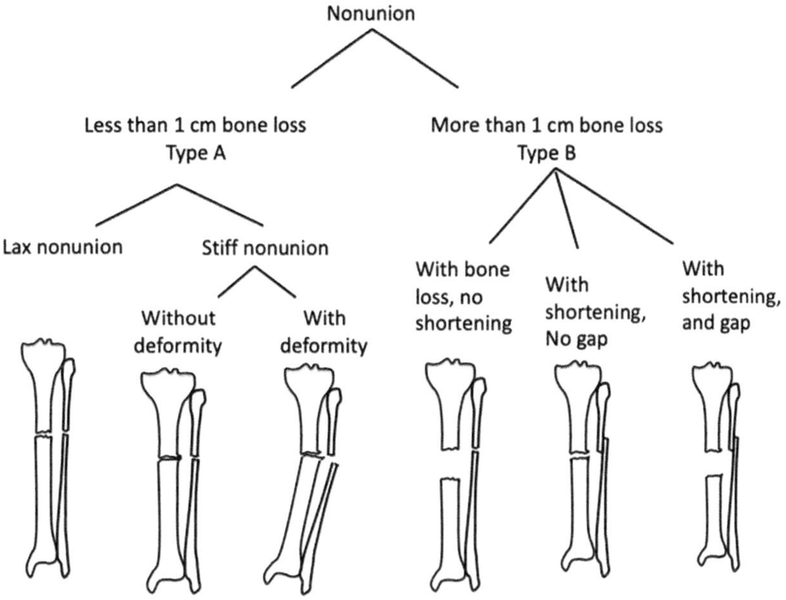

Fig. 10.1 Paley classification of nonunion

- Radical debridement to minimise the risk of sepsis.
- Adequate stability and contact between bone ends.
- Preservation of blood supply.
- Adequate soft tissue cover—either directly or flap cover.
- Bone grafting.
- Use of supplementary treatments to encourage healing like bone morphogenetic protein.
- Antibiotic therapy guided by culture results

Management of Tibial Delayed Union and Non-union

Intramedullary Nailing

An intramedullary nail is commonly used to treat tibial fractures. In the absence of sepsis, it is an effective method of treatment. In the presence of sepsis the use of nails is debatable, with some studies showing a higher risk of persistent infection with the use of nails in infected non-unions.

Reaming stimulates healing by generating an autogenous graft. In fractures managed with external fixation, removal of the fixator and insertion of a nail is an option, but carries a high risk of infection.

Dynamisation of the nail involves removal of the locking screws, which allows the fracture fragments to impact together. Hypertrophic non-union is considered suitable for dynamisation. The exact timing of dynamisation is not universally agreed. However, the value of dynamisation is debatable.

Court-Brown CM, Christie J, McQueen MM. Closed intramedullary tibial nailing. Its use in closed and type I open fractures. J Bone Joint Surg Br 1990;72:605–11. In this study involving 125 patients, all healed with closed intramedullary tibial nailing and no use of dynamisation. Forty-one percent of patients experienced knee pain and 26% had the nail removed.

The SPRINT trial was a prospective study of 1226 tibial fractures comparing reaming and non reamed technique. No conclusive superiority was demonstrated of either technique.

Investigators SPERINPTF. Randomized trial of reamed and unreamed intramedullary nailing of tibial shaft fractures. J Bone Joint Surg Am 2008;90:2567.

Exchange nailing involves removing the existing nail and replacing with a larger-diameter nail.

This provides greater stability and 'internal bone graft' in the form of reamings to the site of delayed union. There is no difference in statically locked versus dynamically locked exchange nails in terms of healing time. A fibular osteotomy for tibial exchange nails may enhance healing. It is an effective treatment for delayed union in the tibia.

Templeman D, Thomas M, Varecka T, Kyle R. Exchange reamed intramedullary nailing for delayed union and nonunion of the tibia. Clin Orthop Relat Res 1995;315:169–75. In this study involving 28 patients, 93% healed after exchange nailing and the rest healed after a second exchange nailing. The infection rate was 11%.

In view of the high risk of infection reported with exchange nailing, the reaming should be cultured and antibiotics given for 6 weeks if culture is positive.

Bone Grafting

A variety of bone grafts and substitutes have been used in the management of non-unions. The ideal graft is an autogenous cancellous graft, usually obtained from the iliac crest. Autogenous iliac crest graft provides osteogenic, osteoconductive and osteoinductive properties. Autograft carries no risk of disease transmission or rejection, but have limited availability and donor site morbidity.

Grafts can be onlay or inlay grafts. The recommended approach for the tibia is posterolateral, which is through less traumatised tissue compared with the anterolateral approach. The incision is medial to the fibular border and the dissection plane is along the interosseous membrane, lifting the deep posterior compartment from the tibia.

An alternative method of obtaining autograft is RIA—Reamer Irrigation, Aspiration. This is a method to ream the femur and collect the endosteal reaming for use as bone graft.

Compression Plate

Hypertrophic non-union can be managed with compression plating, which provides enough stability to allow healing. Atrophic non-union will require supplementary bone grafting. The disadvantages of using a compression plate include soft tissue damage, infection and the inability to bear weight until satisfactory union.

External Fixator

External fixators are commonly used for the management of open tibial fractures. Uniplanar fixation can be converted to an intramedullary nail within 1–2 weeks. Fixators applied for over 2 weeks have risk of pin site infection and this can lead to intramedullary infection when the fixator is exchanged to a nail.

In the presence of bone loss, circular fixators provide stability and allow bone regeneration through distraction histogenesis. Advantages are minimal trauma to the soft tissues, the ability to correct deformities and the ability to compress and regenerate bone. In addition, the patient can immediately bear weight. Disadvantages are pin-site infection, a prolonged period in a fixator, joint stiffness and the risk of damage to neurovascular structures.

The principle of doing a corticotomy along with circular fixators improves vascularity and encourages union.

Paley D. Treatment of tibial nonunion and bone loss with the Ilizarov technique. Instr Course Lect 1990;39:185–97.

Electrical Stimulation

Electrical stimulation has been shown to enhance fracture healing. Stimulation can be delivered by implantable devices, percutaneously or non-invasively.

In most studies, the reported healing rate for these methods is 75–90%. The implantable device allows weight bearing, while the other two methods involve a period of non-weight bearing. Implantable devices require surgery for implantation and removal.

The clinical efficacy of electrical stimulation in randomised controlled studies is debatable.

Sharrard WJ. A double-blind trial of pulsed electromagnetic fields for delayed union tibial fractures. J Bone Joint Surg Br 1990;72:347–55. Out of 45 patients with tibial shaft non-unions, 20 had electrical stimulation and 25 a dummy device. Significantly better healing was observed in patients with the functioning electrical stimulation device.

Goldstein C. Sprague S, Petrisor BA. Electrical stimulation for fracture healing. Current evidence. J Orthop Trauma 2010; 24 Suppl 1: S62–65. Four meta-analysis reviewed and concluded that evidence in support of electrical stimulation in nonunion is debatable.

Ultrasound

Low Intensity Pulsed Ultrasound (LIPUS) has been used to help healing in tibial fractures. Hypertrophic non-unions respond better to ultrasound than atrophic non-unions.

Griffin XL, Smith N, Parsons N, Costa ML. Ultrasound and shockwave treatment for acute fractures in adults. Cochrance Database Syst Rev 2012; 2: CD008579. Evidence insufficient to support routine use for acute fractures in clinical practice.

Bone Morphogenetic Protein

Recombinant human bone morphogenetic protein-7 (rhBMP-7) has been shown to be as effective as an autogenous graft in the treatment of tibial non-unions.

The rhBMP-7 is applied to an absorbable collagen sponge placed over the fracture site.

Friedlaender GE, Perry CR, Cole JD, et al. Osteogenic protein-1 (bone morphogenetic protein-7) in the treatment of tibial nonunions. J Bone Joint Surg Am 2001;83-A(Suppl. 1):S151–8. A total of 122 patients with established tibial non-unions were treated with a nail with rhBMP7 or a nail with autogenous graft. At 9 months, 81% of patients with BMP and 85% of patients with an autogenous graft showed healing.

Govender S, Csimma C, Genant HK, et al. Recombinant human bone morphogenetic protein-2 for treatment of open tibial fractures: a prospective, controlled, randomized study of four hundred and fifty patients. J Bone Joint Surg Am 2002;84-A:2123–34. Patients were divided into three groups: nail only; nail plus 0.75 mg/mL rhBMP2; and nail plus 1.5 mg/mL rhBMP2. The group with 1.5 mg/mL rhBMP2 underwent significantly fewer secondary interventions.

Management of Bone Loss

Open fractures with bone loss present a range of challenges to the treating surgeon. They are often associated with other injuries which may influence management of the orthopaedic injury. The management of limb injury requires input from other specialties—plastic surgery, vascular surgery, microbiology, intensive care as well as specialised physiotherapy and nursing care. The treatment may be complex, time consuming and throws up financial, social, psychological and functional challenges for the patients. Despite months of treatment and multiple procedures, the end result may be an amputation. The decision to amputate acutely versus attempting reconstruction has to be individualised based on patient factors, injury factors and surgeon factors.

The cause of bone loss can be extrusion at the time of injury, gun shot wounds, or following debridement of devascularised segment of bone.

Multiple assessment scores have been devised to help decision making e.g. Mangled Extremity Severity Score (MESS), Limb Salvage Index (LSI) and Hannover Fracture Scale-97 (HFS 97). The clinical usefulness of these scores is low.

Bosse MJ, MacKenzie EJ, Kellam JF, et al. A prospective evaluation of the clinical utility of the lower-extremity injury-severity scores. J Bone Joint Surg [Am] 2001; 83-A:3–14. Multicentre prospective study unable to establish usefulness of scoring systems.

The aim of treatment is surgical stabilisation, preservation of length and alignment, and to optimize function. Severe soft tissue injury, neurological compromise or warm ischemia time of over 6 h are poor prognostic signs. The extent of bone loss and its location—diaphyseal, metaphyseal or articular will influence decision making.

Keating JF, Simpson AHRW, Robinson CM. The management of fractures with bone loss. J Bone Joint Surg Br 2005; 87B: 142–150.

A common management plan for these injuries can be radical debridement, stabilisation of the fracture using a nail, closure of the wound within 48 h and secondary bone grafting, with or without exchange nailing.

Mitchell SE, Keating JF, Robinson CM. The treatment of open femoral fractures with bone loss. J Bone Joint Surg Br 2010;92(12):1678–84. 31 open femoral fractures with bone loss. Managed as above. Mean time to healing 51 weeks.

Nails confer multiple advantages—adequate stabilisation of fracture, maintaining length and rotation, allow access for soft tissue coverage, preserve periosteal blood supply, and cause minimal further soft tissue injury. The length of the bone can be judged by x-rays of the contralateral uninjured side. Nailing may not always be possible in forearm and humerus depending on location of the fracture. Plates provide good stability in situations where nails are not usable.

External ring fixators provide excellent stability with the ability to shorten the limb for wound closure and subsequent distraction to regain length. Fixators can be used for bone transport alongside a nail *in situ*. Fixators can be used in fractures close to the joint, where nails are not usable. Pin site infection, prolonged need for fixator, and joint stiffness are problems with external fixators. The advantage with external fixators is they can be used to acutely shorten the limb at the fracture site to allow soft tissue closure without needing a flap cover. At the same time, a corticotomy can be done at a different site in the bone to lengthen the bone while the fracture is healing and is stabilised with the fixator.

Free fibular grafts are an option for large defects. Advantages are availability of up to 20 cm segment of bone, which works like a structural autograft. Disadvantages are need for microvascular expertise, difference in diameter compared to femoral or tibial defects, nonunion at proximal or distal end, and prolonged need for restricted weight bearing. These can be more useful for upper limb defects.

In patients with extensive soft tissue injury and absence of plantar sensation, amputation is an option. The decision is based on patient factors, surgeon factors and injury factors as well as patient expectations.

MacKenzie EJ, Bosse MJ, Kellam JF, et al. Factors influencing the decision to amputate or reconstruct after high-energy lower extremity trauma. J Trauma 2002;52:641–9. The degree of bone loss was not a predictor for amputation. Plantar sensation and extent of soft tissue injury correlated with need for amputation.

Telescoping intramedullary nails may be an option to regain length in patients with bone loss. Experience with these has evolved from paediatric limb lengthening, and its application in trauma is limited at present.

Fresh allografts are useful for large articular defects in young patients. Joint replacement can be considered for older patients.

These are complex injuries and are best managed in specialist centres.

Further Reading

Bosse MJ, MacKenzie EJ, Kellam JF, et al. A prospective evaluation of the clinical utility of the lower-extremity injury-severity scores. J Bone Joint Surg Am. 2001;83-A:3–14.

Court-Brown CM, Christie J, McQueen MM. Closed intramedullary tibial nailing. Its use in closed and type I open fractures. J Bone Joint Surg Br. 1990;72: 605–11.

Friedlaender GE, Perry CR, Cole JD, et al. Osteogenic protein-1 (bone morphogenetic protein-7) in the treatment of tibial nonunions. J Bone Joint Surg Am. 2001;83-A(Suppl. 1):S151–8.

Goldstein C, Sprague S, Petrisor BA. Electrical stimulation for fracture healing. Current evidence. J Orthop Trauma. 2010;24(Suppl 1):S62–5.

Govender S, Csimma C, Genant HK, et al. Recombinant human bone morphogenetic protein-2 for treatment of open tibial fractures: a prospective, controlled, randomized study of four hundred and fifty patients. J Bone Joint Surg Am. 2002;84-A:2123–34.

Griffin XL, Smith N, Parsons N, Costa ML. Ultrasound and shockwave treatment for acute fractures in adults. Cochrance Database Syst Rev. 2012;2:CD008579.

Investigators SPERINPTF. Randomized trial of reamed and unreamed intramedullary nailing of tibial shaft fractures. J Bone Joint Surg Am. 2008;90:2567.

Keating JF, Simpson AHRW, Robinson CM. The management of fractures with bone loss. J Bone Joint Surg Br. 2005;87B:142–50.

MacKenzie EJ, Bosse MJ, Kellam JF, et al. Factors influencing the decision to amputate or reconstruct after high-energy lower extremity trauma. J Trauma. 2002;52:641–9.

Mitchell SE, Keating JF, Robinson CM. The treatment of open femoral fractures with bone loss. J Bone Joint Surg Br. 2010;92(12):1678–84.

Mora R, Paley D. Nonunion of the long bones: diagnosis and treatment with compression distraction techniques. Cham: Springer; 2006.

Paley D. Treatment of tibial nonunion and bone loss with the Ilizarov technique. Instr Course Lect. 1990;39:185–97.

Sharrard WJ. A double-blind trial of pulsed electromagnetic fields for delayed union tibial fractures. J Bone Joint Surg Br. 1990;72:347–55.

Templeman D, Thomas M, Varecka T, Kyle R. Exchange reamed intramedullary nailing for delayed union and nonunion of the tibia. Clin Orthop Relat Res. 1995;315:169–75.

Inflammatory Joint Disorders

11

Anurag Negi and Kaushik Rajamani

Rheumatoid Arthritis

Rheumatoid arthritis (RA) is a systemic autoimmune inflammatory arthritis. In United Kingdom the prevalence of RA in adults is 0.81% (females 1.16% and males 0.44%) with female to male ratio of 2.7. Around 1.5 men and 3.6 women per 10,000 people develop RA every year. The peak age of incidence in the UK for both men and women is the 70s, but people of all ages can develop the disease (Overview | Rheumatoid arthritis in adults: management | Guidance | NICE. https://www.nice.org.uk/guidance/ng100).

D. Symmons et al. The prevalence of rheumatoid arthritis in the United Kingdom: new estimates for a new century. Rheumatology 2002;41:793–800.

There is no known cause for RA. Environmental factors like smoking are important contributors. If not adequately treated, RA can lead to joint damage, severe disability, and premature mortality. Early diagnosis and treatment reduces joint damage and disability. There is an association with HLA DRb1 gene and twin studies show 30% identical twin and 5% non-identical twin concordance.

It is estimated that up to a third of RA patients will stop work within 2 years of diagnosis due to their disease. The total cost of RA in the UK, including indirect costs and work-related disability, has been estimated at around £2.4 billion per year (NICE 2018).

The American College of Rheumatology (ACR)/ European League Against Rheumatism (EULAR) 2010 Classification criteria for Rheumatoid Arthritis are summarized in Table 11.1 (Arthritis Rheum. 2010 Sep;62(9):2569–81. https://doi.org/10.1002/art.27584). The criteria are applicable to patients

Table 11.1 The ACR/ EULAR Classification criteria for RA

Criteria	Score
A. Joint Involvement	
1 large joint	0
2–10 large joints	1
1–3 small joints	2
4–10 small joints	3
>10 joints (at least 1 small joint)	5
B. Serology (at least 1 test result is needed for classification)	
Negative RF and negative ACPA	0
Low positive RF or Low-positive ACPA	2
High positive RF or high positive ACPA	3
C. Acute phase reactants (at least 1 test result is needed for classification)	
Normal CRP and normal ESR	0
Abnormal CRP or abnormal ESR	1
D. Duration of symptoms	
<6 weeks	0
≥6 weeks	1

MCP metacarpophalangeal joints, *MTP* metatarsophalangeal joint. *Anti CCP* anti cyclic citrullinated peptide antibody, *CRP* C Reactive Protein, *ESR* Erythrocyte Sedimentation Rate

A. Negi (✉) · K. Rajamani
University Hospital of Wales, Cardiff, UK
e-mail: krajamani@doctors.org.uk

S. Agarwal (ed.), *Current Orthopaedic Practice*, https://doi.org/10.1007/978-3-030-78529-1_11

with at least one swollen joint and no better explanation for synovitis. The maximum score is 10, and a score of 6 or over indicates Rheumatoid arthritis.

A large joint refers to shoulder, elbow, hip, knee or ankle. Joint involvement is any swollen or tender joint on examination. Negative serology refers to value less than or equal to ULN (Upper Limit of Normal); low positive is IU value >ULN but <3 × ULN; and high positive is >3 × ULN. If rheumatoid factor is only reported as negative or positive, a positive result should be scored as a low-positive. At least one acute phase reactants test result is needed for using criterion C. Duration of symptoms is patient's self-reported duration of pain, swelling, tenderness in the joints clinically involved at the time of assessment, regardless of treatment status.

Clinical Features

The main symptoms include joint pain and swelling, morning stiffness, myalgia, fatigue and tenosynovitis.

Typically RA is polyarticular with involvement of the small joints of the hands and feet. It tends to spare the distal inter-phalangeal joints although it can affect any synovial joint. Spinal involvement typically affects the atlanto-axial joint leading to instability. This is relevant for the anaesthetist and surgical team if the patient needs intubation for a surgical procedure. Deafness can result from involvement of the stapedius. Splenomegaly is part of Felty's syndrome. Sicca symptoms indicate dry eyes and mouth. Involvement of the cricoarytenoid cartilage can cause hoarseness. Joint swelling can cause symptoms of nerve entrapment like carpal tunnel syndrome.

Extraarticular manifestations are summarized in Fig. 11.1.

Other Presentations

Although the typical presentation of RA is acute onset symmetrical polyarthritis involving the small joints of the hands and feet, it can also present as oligoarticular arthritis, palindromic symptoms, and a polymyalgia rheumatica like illness. Palindromic onset indicates bursts of severe inflammation that may settle after a few days. Polymyalgic onset is with limb-girdle pain and stiffness.

Inflammation is a driver for atherosclerosis. Cardiovascular morbidity and mortality are significantly increased in patients with rheumatoid arthritis independent of the presence of the traditional cardiovascular risk factors. This is comparable in magnitude to the cardiovascular disease risk in type 2 Diabetes mellitus.

Peters MJL et al. Does rheumatoid arthritis equal diabetes mellitus as an independent risk

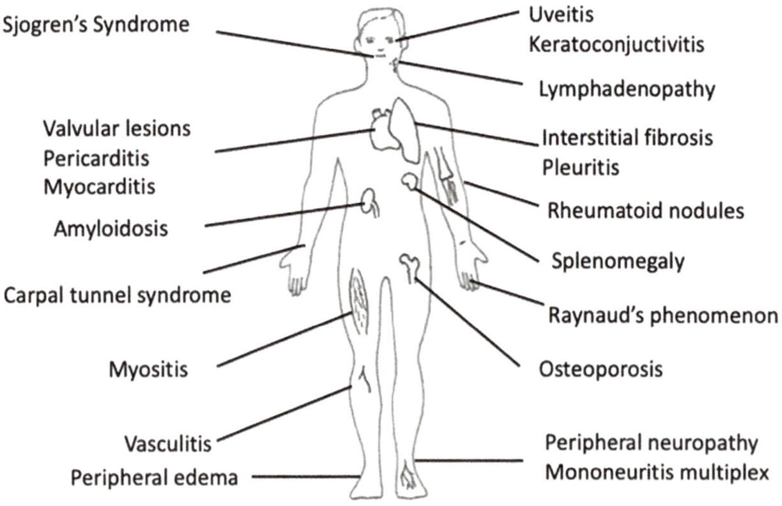

Fig. 11.1 Extraarticular manifestations of Rheumatoid arthritis

factor for cardiovascular disease? A prospective study. Arthritis Rheum 2009;61(11):1571–9.

European League against Rheumatism (EULAR) has published recommendations for cardiovascular disease risk management in patients with rheumatoid arthritis and other forms of inflammatory joint disorders.

Peters MJL et al. EULAR recommendations for cardiovascular disease risk management in patients with rheumatoid arthritis and other forms of inflammatory joint disorders: 2015/2016 update. Ann Rheum Dis. 2017;76(1):17–28.

Pathogenesis

The underlying process is characterised by synovitis, nodules and vasculitis. Histopathology of the involved synovium reveals an increase in the synovial lining layer, increased vascularity and an abundance of T and B lymphocytes, macrophages and activated cells of all types, with increased production of cytokines and their receptors. RF is an IgM antibody that antagonizes the Fc fragment of IgG. Histological changes are illustrated in Fig. 11.2.

Investigations

Periodic monitoring of FBC, ESR, CRP, renal & liver function helps to monitor disease activity and the toxicity of anti-rheumatoid drugs. Iron deficiency anemia may be present.

Rheumatoid factor (RF) and anti-CCP antibodies (ACPA) do not need to be repeated frequently and are not useful in assessing disease activity. These are not diagnostic in isolation and should only be requested in the right clinical context. RF has a sensitivity of 50% for the detection of RA and anti-CCP antibodies are 95% specific for diagnosis. Presence of RF and ACPA might indicate a more aggressive disease and a less favourable prognosis. Up to 4% of normal population may have positive rheumatoid factor, but no evidence of rheumatoid arthritis.

Other autoantibody tests: ANA, anti-Ds DNA and ENA screen can be present and are also useful in patients who have symptoms to suggest an overlapping syndrome e.g. RA and SLE.

Urinalysis for proteinuria is a useful screening for asymptomatic renal involvement. This can be

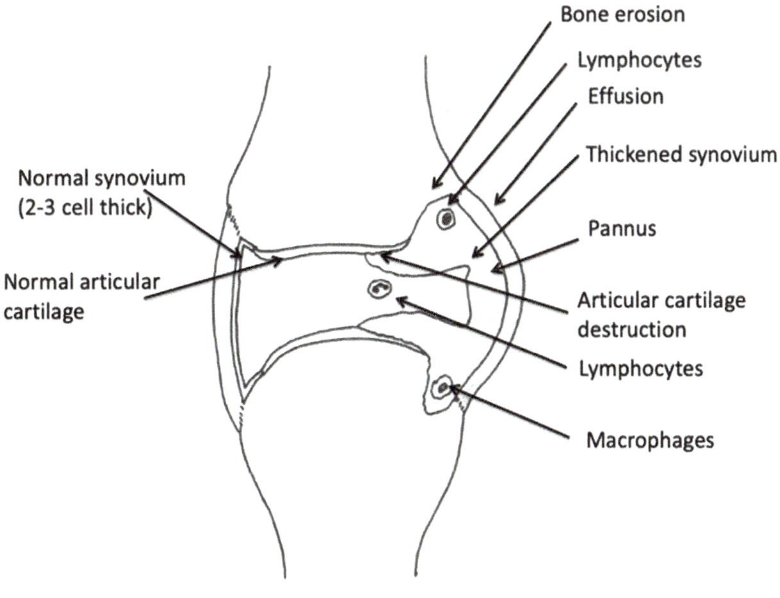

Fig. 11.2 Histological changes in inflammatory arthritis

easily done in clinic using a commercially available testing strip.

Imaging

X-rays are likely to be normal in early disease. Typical features in established disease include articular subluxation, peri-articular osteopenia and erosions.

Musculoskeletal ultrasound is a very useful tool in detecting early synovial & tenosynovial inflammation and erosions.

MR scan is useful for early detection of joint and tendon inflammation and joint damage. However, availability and cost may be factors in some healthcare systems.

Other useful investigations include chest x-ray (if respiratory symptoms and/or signs present; and before commencing treatment with Methotrexate), lung function test and CT scan of chest for patients with suspected interstitial lung disease.

Management

The modern management of rheumatoid arthritis aims to achieve disease remission or a state of low disease activity. There have been significant advances in the management of rheumatoid arthritis including the use of ultrasound for early diagnosis, early arthritis clinics and the development of targeted therapy in the form of biological agents.

Treat-to-Target Strategy This strategy aims to set a treatment target of complete remission (based on disease activity score—DAS) or low disease activity if remission cannot be achieved. This involves close monitoring with frequent clinic visits and adjusting the treatment to achieve the agreed target.

Education (NICE 2009, 2018) It is important to explain the risks and benefits of the treatments offered to patients with RA in simple language and to involve patients in decision making. Adults with RA who wish to know more about their disease and its management should be offered the opportunity to take part in existing educational activities, including self-management programmes.

Rheumatology specialist nurses play a key role in educating the patient about the disease and management. Patients should be encouraged to read the Arthritis research UK (ARUK) and 'Versus Arthritis' booklets on RA and medication. Local and national help groups provide very useful information and patients are encouraged to use their services.

Pain Relief NSAIDS and analgesics. It is recommended to use the lowest effective dose of NSAIDs for the shortest period needed.

Steroids These can be prescribed for oral or parenteral use including joint injections. Steroids are used for their quick onset of action and to bridge the treatment gap until the disease modifying anti-Rheumatic drug (DMARD) takes full effect. Long term steroid use carries the risk of adverse effects like osteoporosis and drug induced diabetes.

Disease Modifying Anti Rheumatic Drugs (DMARDs) Methotrexate, Sulphasalazine, Hydroxychloroquine and Leflunomide are all commonly used. The treatment is usually started with one or more DMARDs with or without corticosteroids. With the exception of hydroxychloroquine, all other DMARDs need regular blood monitoring. Patients on hydroxychloroquine need screening for retinopathy through the local ophthalmology service. Hydroxychloroquine-and-Chloroquine-Retinopathy-Monitoring-Guideline.pdf (rcophth.ac.uk). These agents do not have to be stopped perioperatively, as opposed to biologic agents (see Table 10.2).

Royal college of Ophthalmology guideline 2018 for Hydroxychloroquine and chloroquine retinopathy: recommendations on screening.

Biological Agents and Jak inhibitors Use of these agents in United Kingdom is subject to NICE criteria for their use (Table 11.2).

Table 11.2 Biologic agents for inflammatory arthritis

Drug	Target
Infliximab[a] Etanercept[a] Adalimumab[a] Certolizumab pegol Golimumab	Tumour Necrosis factor-α(TNFα)
Anakinra	Interleukin-1 (IL-1) not NICE approved
Tocilizumab (TCZ) Sarilumab	IL-6
Rituximab[a] (RTX)	Targets the B lymphocytes, CD20
Abatacept	CTLAIg Inhibits T cell activation by binding to CD80 and CD86 receptors on antigen presenting cells
Tofacitinib Baricitinib	Janus kinase

[a]These agents have a licensed biosimilar drug

MDT Approach All patients with RA should have access to Physiotherapy, Occupational therapy and podiatry.

Disease Activity Assessment In addition to the clinical assessment and patient reported severity, there are objective tools to assess disease activity of RA. Disease activity score (DAS28) is widely used and validated for use in RA patients.

This is a composite score based on the tender and swollen joint count (Joints included are all hand joints except the DIPJs, wrists, elbows, shoulders and the knees), Patient global (VAS 0–100), ESR or CRP.

Peri-operative Care British society for Rheumatology (BSR) recommends the following- The British Society for Rheumatology biologic DMARD safety guidelines in inflammatory arthritis—Executive summary *https://doi.org/10.1093/rheumatology/key207*

1. The potential benefit of preventing post-operative infections by stopping biologics (different surgical procedures pose different risks of infection and wound healing) should be balanced against the risk of a peri-operative flare in disease activity.
2. For most biologics (exceptions: RTX and TCZ), consideration should be given to planning surgery when at least one dosing interval has elapsed for that specific drug; for higher risk procedures consider stopping 3–5 half-lives before surgery (if this is longer than one dosing interval).
3. Biologics may be recommenced after surgery when there is good wound healing (typically around 14 days), all sutures and staples are out, and there is no evidence of infection.
4. For patients receiving RTX, treatment should ideally be stopped 3–6 months prior to elective surgery.
5. For patients receiving TCZ, i.v. TCZ should be stopped at least 4 weeks before surgery; s.c. TCZ should be stopped at least 2 weeks before surgery.

Spondyloarthritis

Spondyloarthritis (SpA) is a group of disorders characterised by inflammation of the axial skeleton, peripheral joints and entheses. Patients with SpA are often rheumatoid factor negative. Genetic factors are important and there is a strong association with human leukocyte antigen (HLA)-B27. Concordance rates among monozygotic (MZ) twins with AS range between 50 and 75% compared with 10–15% among dizygotic (DZ) twins.

The types of SpAs are shown in Fig. 11.3.

Epidemiology

The incidence is approximately 6.9–7.2 per 100,000 per year. The gender ratio is estimated at 2:1 to 3:1 (men to women) and the peak age of onset is 20–40 years. The gender ratio for nr AxSpA is reported as 1:1.

The prevalence of SpA varies according to the geographical region and with the background prevalence of HLA B27 in the local population (Table 11.3).

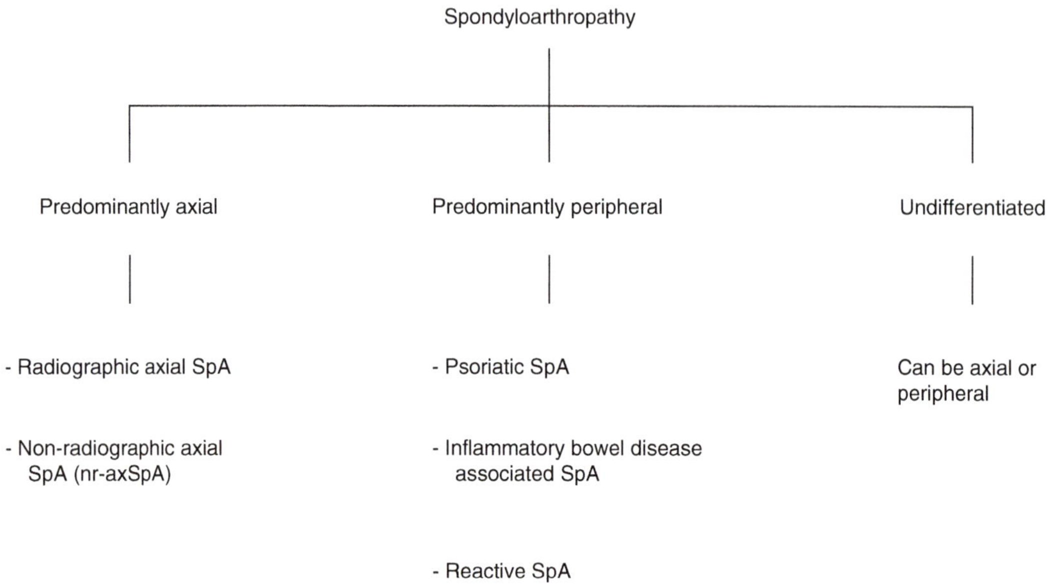

Fig. 11.3 Types of Spondyloarthritis (SpA)

Table 11.3 Geographical variation in prevalence of Spondyloarthritis (Ramirez et al. 2018)

	Lowest prevalence	Highest prevalence
Spondyloarthritis	0.20% in South-East Asia	1.61% in Northern Arctic
Ankylosing spondylitis	0.02% Sub Saharan Africa	0.35% in Northern Arctic
Psoriatic arthritis	0.01% in middle east	0.19% in Europe

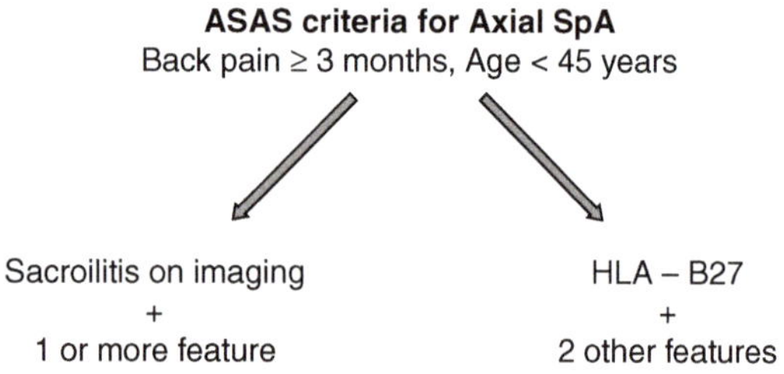

Fig. 11.4 Classification criteria for axial SpA

Carmen Stolwijk et al. Global Prevalence of Spondyloarthritis: A Systematic Review and Meta-Regression Analysis. Arthritis Care Res (Hoboken). 2016 Sep;68(9):1320–31. https://doi.org/10.1002/acr.22831.

Inflammatory back pain is a common symptom of axial SpA. For a diagnosis of 'inflammatory' back pain, four out of the following five criteria have to be present.

- Onset at age <40 years.
- Symptoms >3 months.
- Insidious onset.
- Early morning stiffness lasting for >60 min.
- Improvement of pain with exercise.

Assessment of Spondylo Arthritis international Society (ASAS) has developed classification criteria for use in clinical trials.

ASAS criteria for classification of Axial SpA are shown in Fig. 11.4.

The additional features are illustrated in Fig. 11.5.

Rudwaleit M et al. The development of Assessment of Spondylo Arthritis international Society classification criteria for axial spondyloarthritis (part II): validation and final selection. Ann Rheum Dis 2009;68:777–83.

ASAS classification criteria for peripheral SpA are illustrated in Fig. 11.6.

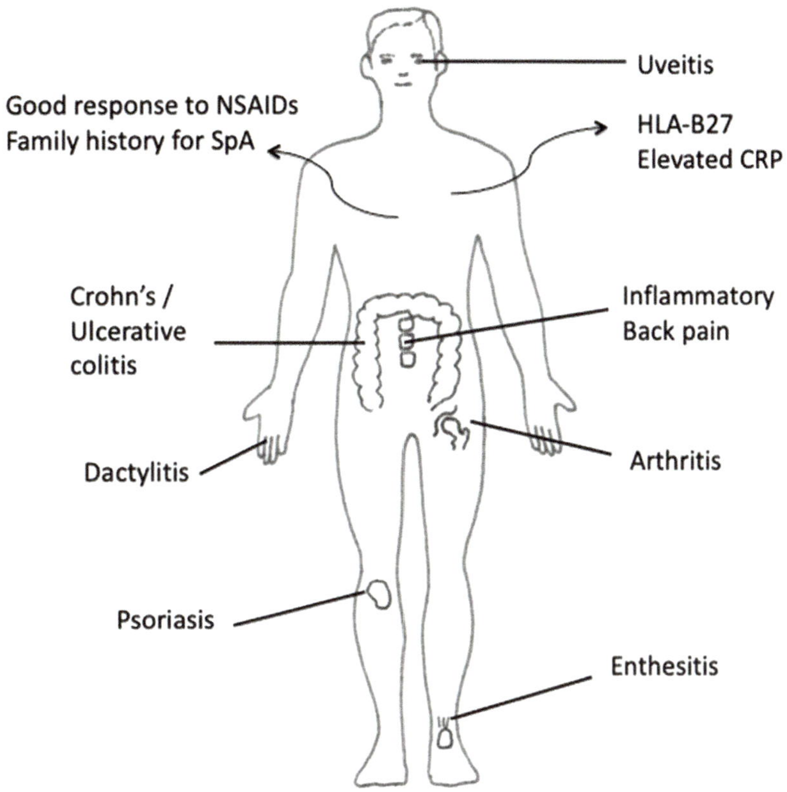

Fig. 11.5 SpA Features

Rudwaleit M et al. The Assessment of Spondylo Arthritis international Society classification criteria for peripheral spondyloarthritis and for spondyloarthritis in general. Ann Rheum Dis 2011;70:25–31.

Ankylosing Spondylitis

The modified New York criteria for Ankylosing Spondylitis (AS) are summarised in Table 11.4.

Definite Ankylosing spondylitis is considered if the radiologic criterion is associated with at least one clinical criterion.

Probable Ankylosing spondylitis is considered if.

(a) Three clinical criteria are present.
(b) The radiologic criterion is present without any signs or symptoms satisfying the clinical criteria. (Other causes of sacroiliitis should be considered).

One of the drawbacks of the modified New York criteria was the reliance on X-rays for the diagnosis. This can potentially delay diagnosis, as there can be a lag of up to 8 years between the onset of symptoms and the appearance of radiographic changes.

Clinical Features

Clinical features are summarized in Fig. 11.7.

Inflammatory low back pain and stiffness is a key feature, often located in the buttock region. Arthritis of peripheral joints, this is usually asymmetric, involves the large-joints and is oligoarticular.

Atlanto-axial subluxation and cauda equina syndrome may be seen in advanced disease. Extra-articular features are uveitis, aortic regurgitation and apical lung fibrosis.

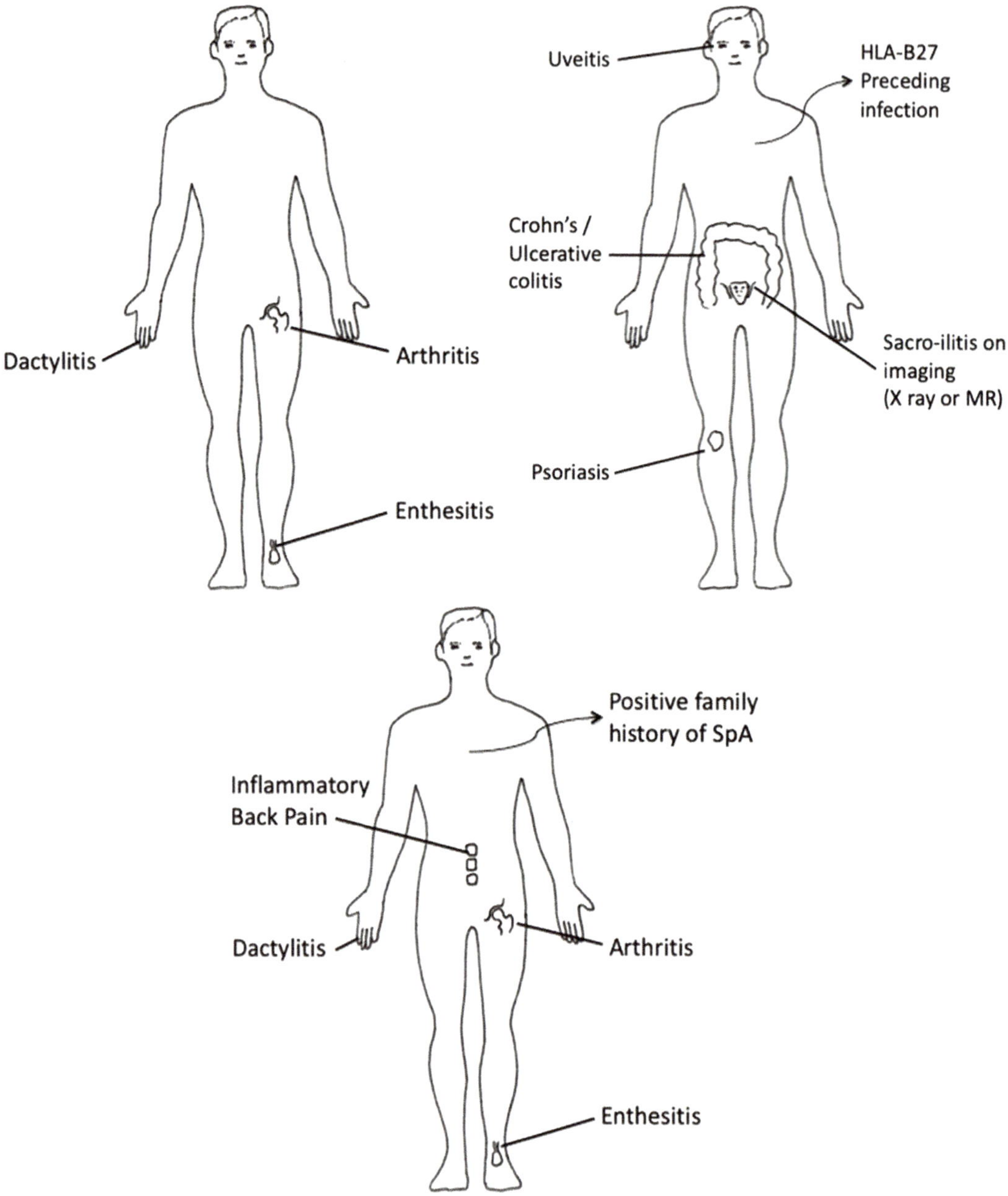

Fig. 11.6 Classification criteria for peripheral SpA

Investigations

The initial haematological investigations are similar to those for Rheumatoid arthritis. HLA B27 is useful for diagnosis.

Imaging

X-ray of the spine, sacroiliac joints and the symptomatic peripheral joint(s) are obtained. These may show erosions, sclerosis and squaring of vertebrae.

'Romanus' lesion is florid anterior spondylitis evident at the attachment of the annulus fibrosus to vertebral end plate. In the inflammatory phase, there is irregularity and erosion of the end plate. Post-inflammatory changes are 'shiny corners' which are sclerotic lesions at vertebral end plates. Syndesmophytes and enthesitis may be evident.

MRI is done using the Spondyloarthritis protocol including the STIR sequences.

Ultrasound is useful for assessment of subclinical synovitis in the peripheral joints and soft tissue inflammation (tenosynovitis and enthesitis).

Table 11.4 Modified New York criteria for Ankylosing Spondylitis

Clinical criteria	Low back pain and stiffness for >3 months which improves with exercise and is not relieved by rest
	Limited lumbar movements in both frontal and sagittal planes
	Reduced chest expansion relative to normal values corrected for age and sex
Radiological criteria	Bilateral sacroilitis grade ≥2 on X-ray
	Unilateral sacroilitis grade 3–4 on X-ray

Bone Density Scan (DXA)

According to one meta-analysis, the prevalence of osteoporosis and fractures in axial SpA varied from 11.7 to 34.4% and 11 to 24.6%, respectively. The authors concluded that alcohol intake, corticosteroid use, and low levels of 25-OH-vitamin D should be taken into account in osteoporosis assessment in patients with axial SpA.

Ramirez et al. Prevalence and risk factors for osteoporosis and fractures in axial spondyloarthritis: A systematic review and meta-analysis. Semin Arthritis and Rheum. 2018;48(1):44–52.

Assessment of Disease Activity

1. Visual Analogue Scale (VAS): A 10 point scale is used.
2. BASDAI (Bath Ankylosing Spondylitis Disease Activity Index): This is based on six questions relating to five symptoms of AS (Fig. 11.8). Each question is answered from a

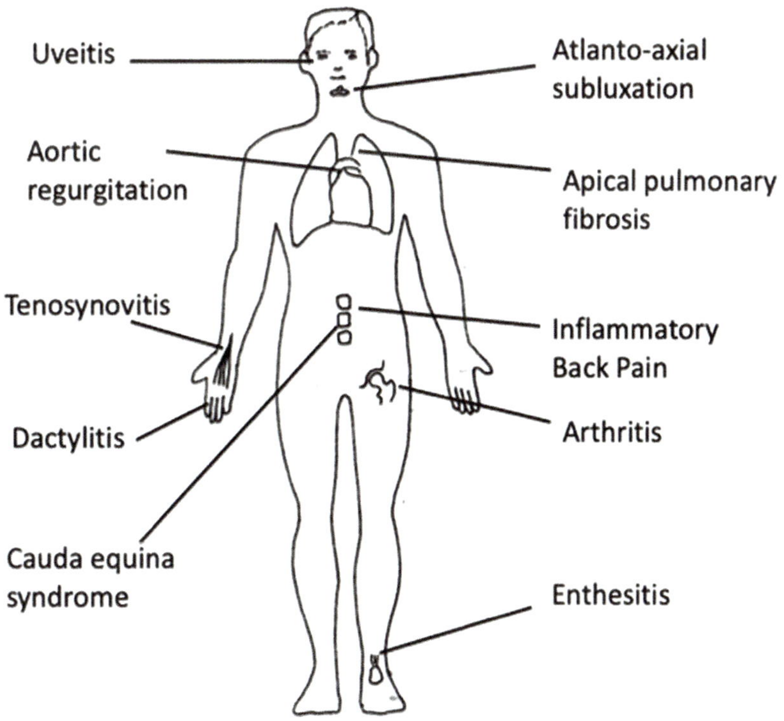

Fig. 11.7 Clinical features of Ankylosing spondylitis

The Bath Ankylosing Spondylitis Disease Activity Index (BASDAI)

Please place a mark on each line below to indicate your answer to each question relating to **the past week**

1. How would you describe the overall level of **fatigue/tiredness** you have experienced?

   NONE ____ VERY SEVERE

2. How would you describe the overall level of AS **neck, back or hip pain** you have had?

   NONE ____ VERY SEVERE

3. How would you describe the overall level of pain/swelling in joints other than **neck, back, hips** you have had?

   NONE ____ VERY SEVERE

4. How would you describe the overall level of **discomfort** you have had from any areas tender to touch or pressure?

   NONE ____ VERY SEVERE

5. How would you describe the overall level of **morning stiffness** you have had **from the time you wake up?**

   NONE ____ VERY SEVERE

6. How long does your morning stiffness last from the time you wake up?

   ____

   0 hrs ½ 1 1½ 2 or more hours

Fig. 11.8 BASDAI for assessment of disease severity for Ankylosing Spondylitis

scale of 0 (minimal problem) to 10 (maximal problem).
3. ASDAS: considers both the patient perceived symptoms and the acute phase reactants.

The mean of 5 and 6 is calculated. The total of 1 to 4 is added to mean of 5 and 6 (total out of 50). The total divided by 5 is the BASDAI score.

Management

All patients with axial SpA should have multidisciplinary care involving rheumatologist, specialist nurse and the allied health specialist.

NSAIDs, both conventional (e.g., Naproxen and Diclofenac) and the cyclo-oxygenase-2 selective Inhibitors (e.g., Etoricoxib) are effective and are the first line of management. DMARDs (e.g. Methotrexate and sulphasalazine) are effective for peripheral disease.

Corticosteroids are useful as they have a quick onset of action. These can be prescribed as oral tables or as intravenous, intramuscular, intra-articular or a soft tissue injection, depending on the clinical situation.

Patient education including advice on smoking cessation is important.

Kaut et al. Axial Spondyloarthritis and Cigarette Smoking. Open Rheumatol J. 2017;11:53–61.

Biological therapy is a major advance in the therapeutics of inflammatory arthritis. In UK the use of biological agents is subject to fulfilment of the NICE criteria:

1. Confirmed diagnosis of AS. Failed response to NSAID therapy (full dose for 3 months) and
2. Active disease defined by
   a. Back pain visual analogue score 4 or more on 2 separate occasions 12 weeks apart.
   b. BASDAI (Bath Ankylosing spondylitis disease activity score) of 4 or more on 2 separate occasions 12 weeks apart.

Drugs Approved for Axial SpA in the UK

TNF inhibitors: Adalimumab, certolizumab pegol, etanercept, golimumab, and infliximab, Secukinumb (IL-17A inhibitor).

NICE recommends that response to biological treatment should be assessed 12 weeks after the start of treatment. Treatment should only be continued if there is clear evidence of response, defined as:

1. A reduction in the Bath Ankylosing Spondylitis Disease Activity Index (BASDAI) score to 50% of the pre-treatment value or by 2 or more units; and.
2. A reduction in the spinal pain visual analogue scale (VAS) by 2 cm or more.

Surgical Treatment

Surgical treatment is for end stage joint disease like hip osteoarthritis and spinal surgery for severe pain, deformity and neural involvement. Perioperative care in patients on biological agents is same as mentioned in the rheumatoid arthritis section.

Psoriatic Arthritis

Psoriatic arthritis (PsA) can have varied presentations, including a predominantly axial arthritis and a rheumatoid arthritis like presentation. Prevalence is between 7% and 26% in patients with Psoriasis. Prevalence in UK is estimated to be 0.1% to 0.3% of the total population.

It can occur at any age but in most common presentation is between 30 and 50 years of age. Unlike RA the sex ratio in PsA is equal. Skin lesions predate the onset of PsA in the majority of patients. Severity of skin psoriasis, nail dystrophy, scalp, inter-gluteal, or perianal lesions, family history of psoriasis or PsA confer a higher risk of developing PsA.

Kristine Busse et al. Which psoriasis patients develop psoriatic arthritis? Psoriasis Forum. 2010;16(4):17–25.

Moll and Wright Classification of PsA

The classification describes five subtypes (Table 11.5).

These sub-types are not mutually exclusive and may evolve with time.

Other musculoskeletal features include dactylitis, enthesitis and tenosynovitis. Extra-articular features include psoriasis affecting the skin, scalp and the nails.

Ocular inflammation may be present.

Classification Criteria for PsA (CASPAR)

These were developed to facilitate further research.

To meet the CASPAR (ClASsification criteria for Psoriatic ARthritis) criteria, a patient must have inflammatory articular disease (joint, spine, or entheseal) with three points from the following five categories (Table 11.6).

The CASPAR criteria have specificity of 98.7% and sensitivity of 91.4%. Current psoriasis is assigned a score of 2; all other features are assigned a score of 1.

Laboratory Investigations

These are not diagnostic. Raised ESR, CRP and anaemia of chronic disease are useful to assess disease activity and monitor response to treatment. RF and anti-CCP can be present in a small proportion of patients.

Table 11.5 Moll and Wright classification of psoriatic arthritis

Arthritis with predominant distal interphalangeal joint involvement
Arthritis mutilans
Asymmetric oligoarticular arthritis
Symmetric polyarthritis-indistinguishable from RA
Predominant spondylitis

Table 11.6 CASPAR classification for psoriatic arthritis

1. Evidence of current psoriasis, a personal history of psoriasis, or a family history of psoriasis.
   Current psoriasis is defined as psoriatic skin or scalp disease present on the day of examination, as judged by a rheumatologist or dermatologist. A personal history of psoriasis is defined as a history of psoriasis that may be obtained from a patient, family physician, dermatologist, rheumatologist, or other qualified health care provider
   A family history of psoriasis is defined as a history of psoriasis in a first- or second-degree relative according to patient report
2. Typical psoriatic nail dystrophy including onycholysis, pitting, and hyperkeratosis observed on current physical examination
3. A negative test result for the presence of rheumatoid factor
4. Either current dactylitis, defined as swelling of an entire digit, or a history of dactylitis recorded by a rheumatologist
5. Radiographic evidence of juxtaarticular new bone formation, appearing as ill-defined ossification near joint margins (but excluding osteophyte formation) on plain radiographs of the hand or foot

Imaging

The radiological changes predominantly affect the interphalangeal joints, in the hands as opposed to the metacarpophalangeal joints. Asymmetric joint involvement is common, and sometimes a symmetric polyarthropathy picture is evident.

The main feature is periostitis with proliferative new bone formation. Thickened cortices can be seen along the shafts of the digital bones. Bone proliferation leads to 'fuzzy appearance' around the joint. The joints may be subluxed.

Marginal bone erosions may occur, causing 'pencil-in-cup' appearance in advanced disease (Fig. 11.9). 'Pencil in cup' deformity is common but is not pathognomonic of PsA.

Ultrasound and MRI scan are more sensitive than x-rays in picking up early erosions and presence of enthesitis and tenosynovitis. 'Sausage digits' are swollen digits due to underlying tenosynovitis and synovitis.

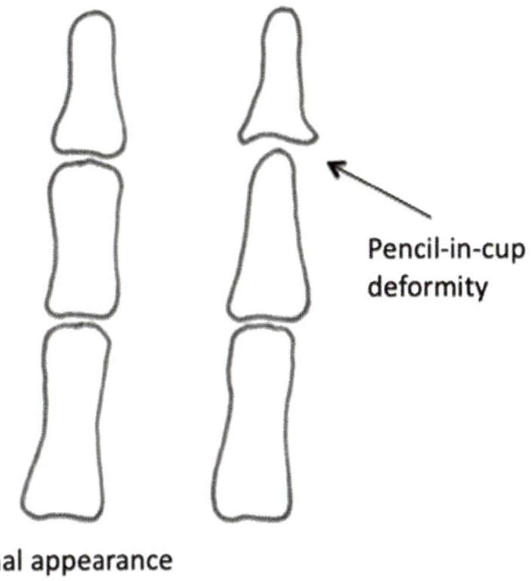

Fig. 11.9 Pencil in cup deformity

Arthritis mutilans is a particularly severe form with marked bone resorption causing severe joint deformity. This can lead to 'telescoping fingers'.

Management

NSAIDs are prescribed for musculoskeletal pain and stiffness and treating mild PsA.

Corticosteroids are used to manage active disease as mentioned in RA, however they should be used with caution as corticosteroid use can make skin psoriasis to worsen including evolution to a more severe form.

Non-biological disease modifying anti Rheumatic drugs (DMARDs) like Sulphasalazine, Methotrexate, Leflunomide and Cyclosporine.

As mentioned in the RA section, these drugs need careful blood monitoring.

Biological and Other Drugs

The anti-TNF- α agents (Infliximab, Etanercept, Certolizumb, Golilumab and adalimumab), Ustekinumab (anti-IL12 and 23 inhibitor), Apremilast (inhibitor of phosphodiesterase 4 (PDE4)), Secukinumab & Ixekizumab (IL-17 A antagonist) and Tofacitinib (Janus Kinase inhibitor) are licensed and approved for PsA by NICE in the UK. The use of these drugs in UK is subject to fulfilling the NICE criteria. Some of these drugs are also available as biosimilars of the originator drug.

PsARC (Psoriatic Arthritis Response Criteria) is a useful tool to monitor response to treatment.

Inflammatory Bowel Disease-Associated Spondyloarthritis

Up to 60% of patients with AS have inflammation on ileocolonoscopy and up to 25% of patients with Crohn's disease have inflammatory arthritis.

Investigation and management of the disease is similar to the other spondyloarthritides and is done in association with the gastroenterologist.

Reactive Arthritis

Reactive arthritis is inflammatory arthritis triggered by a stimulus away from the site of the joint inflammation. Most often this trigger is an infection. Gut (e.g., *Salmonella*), airway (*Streptococcus)* and genitourinary infections (e.g., *Chlamydia*) are common triggers. The joint inflammation may be accompanied by inflammation of the eye (conjunctivitis), rash, urethritis, diarrhoea and mouth ulcers. The triad of joint inflammation, urethritis and eye inflammation is termed Reiter's syndrome. The skin may also be involved, with scaly patches on the genitalia or the sole of the foot (keratoderma blennorrhagica).

The joints involved are usually the lower limbs (knees, ankles or toes), but upper limb joints and the spine may also be involved. As in other spondyloarthritis, the tendons (e.g., Achilles) may be involved.

Management

The underlying infection is treated. Symptom control is through NSAIDs and appropriate analgesia. Steroids can be injected locally into the joint or administered systemically. DMARDs like Sulphasalazine are needed for more refractory cases. Majority of patients with reactive arthritis achieve remission.

Undifferentiated Spondyloarthritis

Undifferentiated spondyloarthritis is where the symptoms and signs do not match a specific disease pattern. Some of these patients will eventually develop a classic pattern like ankylosing spondylitis. Treatment is largely directed at controlling symptoms and inflammation.

Juvenile Idiopathic Arthritis (JIA)

Juvenile idiopathic arthritis is a group of disorders characterized by arthritis persisting for at least 6 weeks with onset before the age of 16 years and other causes have been excluded.

International League of Associations for Rheumatology (ILAR) classification of juvenile idiopathic arthritis describes seven types.

1. Systemic-onset JIA: Systemic arthritis is diagnosed if there is arthritis in 1 or more joints with, or preceded by, fever of at least 2 weeks' duration. Signs or symptoms must have been documented daily for at least 3 days and accompanied by 1 or more of the following: evanescent rash, generalised lymphadenopathy, hepato/splenomegaly, serositis. (Exclusions are A, B, C, and D from the exclusion list below.)
2. Persistent or extended oligoarthritis: Oligoarthritis is diagnosed if there is arthritis affecting 1 to 4 joints during the first 6 months. Persistent oligoarthritis affects up to 4 joints throughout the course of the disease, and extended oligoarthritis affects more than 4 joints after the first 6 months of disease. (Exclusions are A, B, C, D, and E from the exclusion list below.)
3. RF-negative polyarthritis: Polyarthritis (RF-negative) is diagnosed if there is rheumatoid factor (RF)-negative arthritis affecting 5 or more joints during the first 6 months of disease. (Exclusions are A, B, C, D, and E from the exclusion list below.)
4. RF–positive polyarthritis: Polyarthritis (RF-positive) is diagnosed if there is RF-positive arthritis affecting 5 or more joints during the first 6 months of disease. Two or more RF tests (taken at least 3 months apart) are positive during the first 6 months of disease. (Exclusions are A, B, C, and E from the exclusion list below.)
5. Psoriatic JIA: Psoriatic arthritis is diagnosed if there is arthritis and psoriasis, or arthritis and at least 2 of the following: dactylitis, nail pitting, onycholysis, and/or family history of psoriasis (in a first-degree relative). (Exclusions are B, C, D, and E from the exclusion list below.)
6. Enthesitis-related arthritis: Enthesitis-related arthritis is diagnosed if there is arthritis and/or enthesitis with at least 2 of the following: presence or history of sacroiliac joint tenderness with or without inflammatory lumbosacral pain; presence of HLA B27 antigen; onset of arthritis in a male over 6 years of age; acute (symptomatic) anterior uveitis; history of ankylosing spondylitis, enthesitis-related arthritis, sacroiliitis with inflammatory bowel disease, Reiter's syndrome, or acute anterior uveitis in a first-degree relative. (Exclusions are A, D, and E from the exclusion list below.)
7. Undifferentiated: Undifferentiated arthritis is diagnosed if there is arthritis that does not fulfil criteria in any of the above categories or that fulfils criteria for 2 or more of the above categories.

Exclusions

A. Psoriasis or history of psoriasis in patients or first-degree relatives.

B. Arthritis in HLA B27 positive males beginning after the age of 6 years.
C. Ankylosing spondylitis, enthesitis-related arthritis, sacroiliitis with inflammatory bowel disease, Reiter's syndrome, acute anterior uveitis, or history of 1 of these disorders in first-degree relatives.
D. Presence of IgM rheumatoid factor on at least 2 occasions at least 3 months apart.
E. Presence of systemic JIA in patients.

The incidence is reported to be between 2 and 23/100,000 children younger than 16 years and prevalence is 16–140/100,000. Oligoarthritis is the most common subtype. Overall, girls are more commonly affected. ANA is the commonest autoantibody present in JIA. It is most commonly seen in oligoarthritis and is an independent risk factor for uveitis.

Laboratory Investigations

These are not diagnostic and are mainly done to rule out other causes like infections. ANA, RF and HLA B27 should be checked in JIA patients, this helps in further categorization. ESR and CRP levels might help in differentiating an inflammatory cause from non-inflammatory disorders.

Imaging

X-rays are not helpful in early disease. Musculoskeletal ultrasound and MRI are very useful diagnostic tools and also for assessing response to therapy.

Management

The multidisciplinary team approach is essential. The main emphasis of management is to help the child regain normal levels of physical and social activities. This is accomplished with the use of physical therapy, pain management and social support.

Pharmacotherapy

This includes NSAIDs and DMARDS like methotrexate, sulphasalazine and leflunomide. Biological drugs like adalimumab, etanercept, abatacept and tocilizumab have been approved for use in polyarthritis JIA. Anakinra, canakinumab, golimumab are licensed for use in some forms of JIA.

Intra-articular or systemic corticosteroids may be of help.

Surgical Intervention

The advances in the medical management have reduced the need for orthopedic surgery in JIA patients. Synovectomy and arthroplasty are occasionally required. Surgeons should liaise closely with the paediatric rheumatologist especially in children who are on immunosuppressive therapy.

Connective Tissue Diseases

Although they may cause considerable musculoskeletal pain (polyarthralgia), these conditions are rarely the primary reason for orthopaedic intervention.

Sjögren's Syndrome

Described in 1933 by the Swedish ophthalmologist Henrik Sjögren, this syndrome is probably the most common of the connective tissue diseases. It may occur as a primary disorder or secondary to other rheumatic diseases, especially rheumatoid arthritis. It is characterised by dry eyes and mouth, caused by inflammation and damage to tear and salivary glands (sicca symptoms), as well as polyarthralgia, muscular aching and fatigue. The salivary glands may become visibly swollen. Rare sequelae include peripheral neuropathy and lung fibrosis. The risk of non-Hodgkin's B-cell lymphoma is increased in patients with the syndrome. It occurs mostly in women between the ages of 40 and 60 years, with a 1:10 male to female ratio. Viruses (e.g., Epstein–Barr virus, retroviruses) may trigger the syndrome in genetically susceptible people.

ANA, anti-Ro and anti-La antibodies are present in some patients. Babies of women with the syndrome are at an increased the risk of congenital heart block if mother has Anti-Ro antibodies.

Management may require a multispecialty approach including a rheumatologist, ophthalmologist and dentist. Artificial saliva and tear preparations are used for sicca symptoms. Pilocarpine may be used for recalcitrant dry mouth. Musculoskeletal and systemic involvement requires symptomatic treatment and use of corticosteroids, hydroxychloroquine or more potent immunosuppressants.

Systemic Lupus Erythematosus (SLE, Lupus)

SLE is a diverse condition, varying in organ involvement and severity. It mainly affects young women, particularly black African and Caribbean. The main symptoms of Lupus include, a facial rash typically in the malar distribution, photosensitivity to UV light, joint pain, fatigue, alopecia and Raynaud's phenomenon. Patients may also experience fever, weight loss, lymphadenopathy and mouth ulcers.

In severe cases patients develop organ threatening disease including acute renal failure due to glomerulonephritis, serositis, cardiomyopathy, anaemia, thrombocytopenia, bone marrow suppression, neuropathy and CNS involvement.

Patients are at a significantly increased risk of cardiovascular disease and thrombosis may occur, particularly if anti-phospholipid antibodies are present.

Majority of patients with SLE are positive for the antinuclear antibody. Anti double-stranded DNA antibody is more specific for SLE and its levels may correlate with disease activity. Anti-Ro antibodies can be present and overlapping features with Sjögren's syndrome are more likely in these patients. A low complement level (C3 or C4) might indicate SLE activity.

Treatment: Corticosteroids, Hydroxychloroquine and other immunosuppressive medications (including Azathioprine, Methotrexate, Mycophenolate mofetil, Cyclophosphamide and rituximab) are used alone or in combination depending on the disease severity.

Avascular bone necrosis can occur as a manifestation of SLE or any other autoimmune connective tissue disease as well as a complication of corticosteroid use. Surgical intervention for arthroplasty is needed if disease activity causes joint damage.

Scleroderma

The term 'scleroderma' means hard skin, but the condition may affect the connective tissues surrounding the joints, blood vessels and internal organs. It is uncommon and affects women more than men. It usually begins between the ages of 25 and 50 years. It can occur as localised (termed 'morphoea'), limited, or systemic disease. The latter affecting the blood vessels, joints, internal organs including gut, lungs, heart, kidneys and muscles.

Raynaud's phenomenon can be very severe. Severe case of scleroderma can result in digital ischemia and acro-osteolysis. Advanced disease can result in cutaneous calcinosis, pulmonary fibrosis, pulmonary arterial hypertension, accelerated atherosclerosis and renal failure.

Antinuclear antibodies may be positive. Blood pressure, renal & pulmonary function and cardiovascular assessment are essential part of disease monitoring.

Individual manifestations are treated with targeted therapies (e.g., angiotensin-converting enzyme inhibitors in hypertension). Evidence for agents with an overall benefit in controlling the disease remains poor, although specific aspects of scleroderma are being treated more effectively. Mycophenolate mofetil may have a role in improving skin disease. Cyclophosphamide is used for active pulmonary fibrosis; vasodilators are used for vasculopathy (iloprost, Bosentan, sildenafil).

Steroids should be used with caution in scleroderma.

Surgical intervention might be required for debridement of large calcinosis, correction of digital flexion deformities or for indications unrelated to scleroderma. The presence of thickened skin and poor blood supply raises the concern regarding wound healing. However, one study concluded that surgery performed electively in systemic sclerosis is not linked to difficulty with wound healing. Even larger operations, such as wrist arthrodesis or wrist replacement, can be performed safely. The authors commented that for cases with established skin ulcers and digital ischemia several procedures may be necessary to achieve skin healing.

Tägil M et al. Wound healing after hand surgery in patients with systemic sclerosis—a retrospective analysis of 41 operations in 19 patients . J Hand Surg Eur Vol. 2007;32(3):316–9.

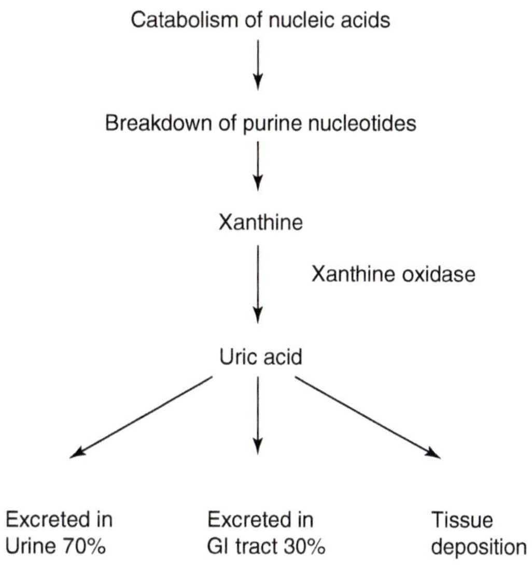

Fig. 11.10 Formation of uric acid in the body

Dietary risk factors are beverages sweetened with high fructose corn syrup, seafood, beer (with or without alcohol), spirits and high protein diet especially red meat.

Gout

Gout is the most common inflammatory arthritis in the western hemisphere. Epidemiological studies show an increase in Gout prevalence across the world and in both sexes. The prevalence in UK rose from 1.5% in 1997 to 2.49% in 2012.

Kuo CF et al. Rising burden of gout in the UK but continuing suboptimal management: a nationwide population study. Ann Rheum Dis 2015; 74: 661–7.

This has partly been attributed to diet and behavioral changes.

Men are more commonly affected and it is uncommon in premenopausal women.

The risk factors for hyperuricemia include male gender, CKD and metabolic syndrome, diuretics, low dose aspirin, ethambutol, cyclosporin and tacrolimus. Xanthine oxidase converts Xanthine to Uric acid (Fig. 11.10).

Pathophysiology of Gout

A simplistic explanation is a state of hyperuricemia due to increased production or reduced excretion or both. When serum uric acid levels reach a saturation point, microcrystals of uric acid form in joint and soft tissues (Fig. 11.11). This is followed by larger aggregates and micro shedding in the joint, triggering an inflammatory response. Crystal formation is facilitated in peripheral (cooler) joints. Repeated trauma to first MTP joint provides a nidus for crystal formation.

Advances in Pathophysiology of Gout

The two important developments are identification of genes encoding for uric acid transport (URAT1) and their interaction with environmental factors; and secondly, discovery of NLRP3 inflammosome

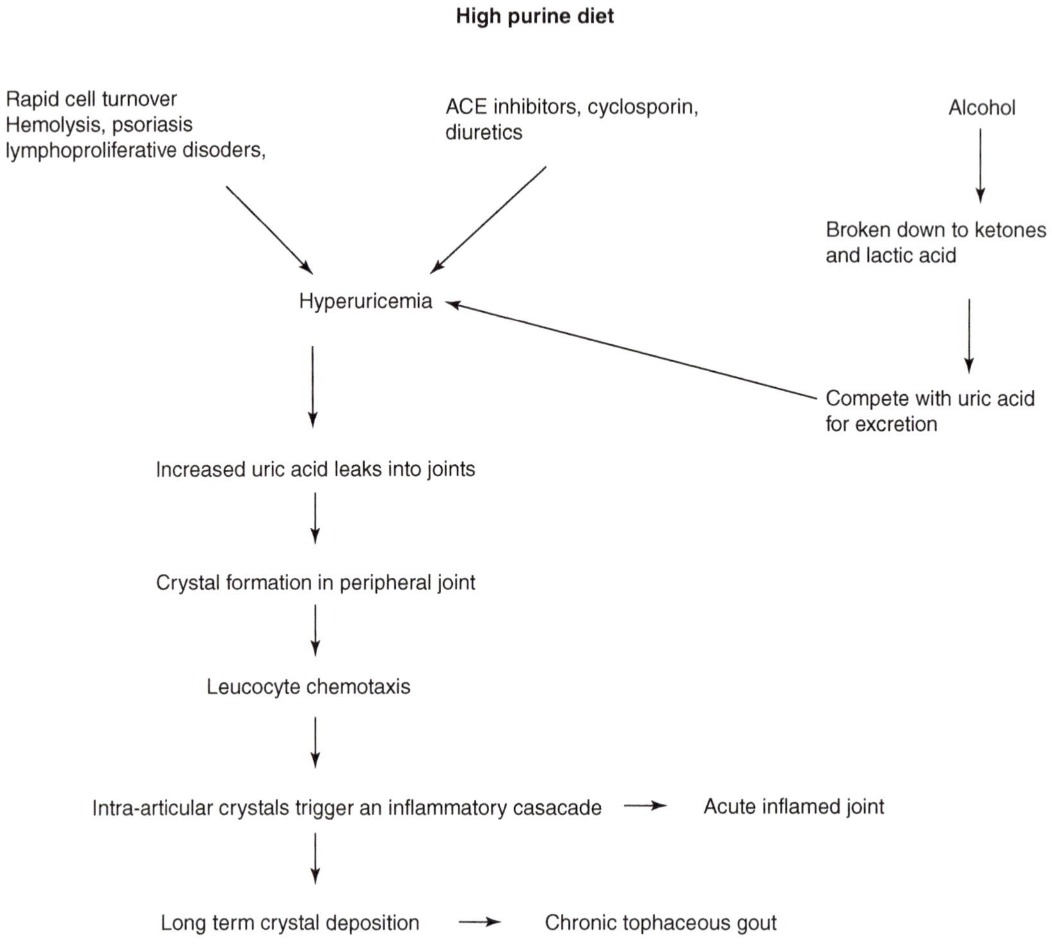

Fig. 11.11 Pathophysiology of gout

and role of IL-1. These advances have led way in identifying new therapeutic targets for Gout.

Clinical Features

Acute gout presents as sudden, severe joint pain and swelling. Typically described in the first MTPJ, but can also present as monoarthritis of another joint or as a polyarticular presentation. This phase usually last days to weeks followed by a period of calm until the conditions are right for another acute episode. The acute phase may be clinically indistinguishable from acute septic arthritic.

The period between the acute attacks is called the intercritical phase. Eventually some patients develop chronic tophaceous Gout. Tophi (tophus) are seen as subcutaneous chalky deposits. These can grow in size and can cause mechanical symptoms.

Laboratory Investigations

Routine bloods tests including serum uric acid are not diagnostic. Serum uric acid levels can be normal in acute gout. Monitoring serum uric acid is important for adjusting the dose of urate lowering therapy. ESR and CRP are useful in assessing disease activity and response to therapy during acute attacks.

The only diagnostic test for gout is demonstration of monosodium urate crystals in synovial fluid or a tophus. These appear as needle shaped crystals and demonstrate negative birefringence under polarized light.

Patients presenting with acute, red, swollen painful knee joint where septic arthritis is being considered should routinely have aspiration and examination of fluid under microscope for crystals in addition to investigations for infection.

X-rays changes are only seen in established disease. These show soft tissue deposits, secondary OA changes and bony erosions typically in juxta-articular location.

Application of ultrasound (USS) is a recent development and can detect changes much earlier, including synovitis and crystal deposition in the articular cartilage described as a "double contour sign", which is considered typical for gout.

DECT (Dual Energy Computerised Tomography) is a technique using two different energy x-ray beams. This allows differentiation between uric acid deposits and other chemical deposits like calcium. Both USS and DECT need greater standardization and are not routinely used for gout in clinical practice at present.

Management

Education about the mechanism of gout, lifestyle modification and dietary advice should be offered to all patients. Literature on gout including dietary advise is available in print and online on arthritis research UK (now called versus arthritis) website.

Acute Gout

NSAIDs, colchicine and corticosteroids are all used to control inflammation. Dose adjustment and caution is required in patients with renal impairment and other co-morbidity like congestive heart failure. Use of Proton pump inhibitors are normally advised alongside NSAIDs.

Newer Agents

These all target IL1 and include Anakinra, Rilonacept and Canakinumab. None have been approved by NICE. Canakinumab has been approved by FDA in USA and by the European medicines agency (EMEA).

Additionally, medication like diuretics which are known to cause hyperuricaemia should be reduced in dose, or changed.

Management of Hyperuricaemia

BSR recommends that urate-lowering therapy (ULT) should be discussed and offered to all patients who have a diagnosis of gout. ULT should particularly be advised in patients with the following: recurring attacks (⩾2 attacks in 12 months); presence of tophi; chronic gouty arthritis; joint damage due to gout; renal impairment (eGFR < 60 ml/min); a history of urolithiasis; ongoing diuretic therapy use; primary gout starting at a young age.

Xanthine Oxidase (XO) Inhibitors

Allopurinol starting at 50–100 mg/day and increasing the dose by 100 mg every 4 weeks up to 900 mg/day aiming for a serum urate of 360 μmol/l (European recommendation) or 300 μmol/l (British recommendation), dose adjustment is required in renal impairment.

Febuxostat

This is a more potent XO inhibitor. In UK, NICE recommends using Febuxostat if patients are unresponsive to or cannot take allopurinol. It has better safety profile in CKD but use in patients with ischaemic heart disease or congestive heart failure is not recommended.

Uricosuric Agents

These include sulfinpyrazone, probenecid and benzbromarone. The latter was removed from some countries due to a rare risk of hepatotoxicity. In UK benzbromarone is available on a named patient basis.

Lesinurad is new drug targeting URAT1 and reducing uric acid reabsorption in the kidneys. The FDA and EMEA have approved it for use in combination with a Xanthine oxidase inhibitor.

Pegloticase (Uricase)

Uricase is the enzyme that converts uric acid to allantoin, which is more easily excreted. Lack of this enzyme in humans and higher primates makes them more susceptible to hyperuricemia and Gout.

Pegloticase is a recombinant mammalian uricase. NICE does not approve its use for gout in UK. BSR advises use in severe refractory cases. Use is contraindicated in patients with G6PD deficiency. Uricase is immunogenic and is associated with development of uricase antibodies and drug reactions.

Calcium Pyrophosphate Deposition Disease (Pseudogout)

Calcium pyrophosphate dihydrate (CPPD) deposition disease is a common but under recognised condition. It mostly occurs in older adults.

Pseudogout refers to the clinical syndrome of acute arthritis triggered by CPPD.

Chondrocalcinosis refers to the radiographic evidence of calcification in hyaline and/or fibrocartilage. Not all patients with chondrocalcinosis will develop an acute inflammatory arthritis.

Underlying OA is not uncommon in this group of patients. While most cases are sporadic, CPPD deposition disease can be associated with hyperparathyroidism, hemochromatosis, hypophosphataemia, Wilson's disease and hypomagnesemia. The knee is the most commonly affected joint in pseudogout. Wrist involvement is also common. It mostly presents as a monoarthritis but polyarticular involvement is well recognised when it can be confused with Rheumatoid arthritis.

The joint aspirate can be blood tinged and microscopy shows CPPD crystals, which confirms the diagnosis. Often no trigger is identified, but an injury, post operative state and intercurrent illness can all trigger an attack.

'Crowned dens syndrome' is a description of CPPD deposition around the Dens (odontoid process). This can cause neck pain, meningism, restricted cervical spine movements and even cervical cord compression.

Diagnosis of pseudogout is by microscopic analysis of joint fluid, which shows rhombus-shaped, positively birefringent crystals. Plain X-rays show chondrocalcinosis.

Intra-articular corticosteroid injection, systemic corticosteroids, NSAIDs and colchicine are all useful in treating acute attacks. EULAR recommends that for chronic CPP crystal inflammatory arthritis, the pharmacological options in order of preference are oral NSAIDs (plus gastroprotective treatment if indicated) and/or colchicine (0.5–1.0 mg daily) and low-dose corticosteroid. Methotrexate & hydroxychloroquine can be used for more resistant cases.

Further Reading

Busse K, et al. Which psoriasis patients develop psoriatic arthritis? Psoriasis Forum. 2010;16(4):17–25.

Kaut IK, et al. Axial Spondyloarthritis and Cigarette Smoking. Open Rheumatol J. 2017;11:53–61.

Kuo CF, et al. Rising burden of gout in the UK but continuing suboptimal management: a nationwide population study. Ann Rheum Dis. 2015;74:661–7.

Peters MJL, et al. Does rheumatoid arthritis equal diabetes mellitus as an independent risk factor for cardiovascular disease? A prospective study. Arthritis Rheum. 2009;61(11):1571–9.

Peters MJL, et al. EULAR recommendations for cardiovascular disease risk management in patients with rheumatoid arthritis and other forms of inflammatory joint disorders: 2015/2016 update. Ann Rheum Dis. 2017;76(1):17–28.

Ramirez J, et al. Prevalence and risk factors for osteoporosis and fractures in axial spondyloarthritis: a systematic review and meta-analysis. Semin Arthritis Rheum. 2018;48(1:44–52.

Rudwaleit M, et al. The development of Assessment of Spondylo Arthritis international Society classification criteria for axial spondyloarthritis (part II): validation and final selection. Ann Rheum Dis. 2009;68:777–83.

Rudwaleit M, et al. The Assessment of Spondylo Arthritis international Society classification criteria for peripheral spondyloarthritis and for spondyloarthritis in general. Ann Rheum Dis. 2011;70:25–31.

Symmons D, et al. The prevalence of rheumatoid arthritis in the United Kingdom: new estimates for a new century. Rheumatology. 2002;41:793–800.

Tägil M, et al. Wound healing after hand surgery in patients with systemic sclerosis—a retrospective analysis of 41 operations in 19 patients. J Hand Surg Eur Vol. 2007;32(3):316–9.

Arthrodesis and Amputation

12

Sanjeev Agarwal

Hip Arthrodesis

Hip arthrodesis (fusion) has been carried out for over 100 years for infections, arthritis and hip dysplasia. The operation is increasingly rare, largely due to advances in hip replacement techniques, materials and results.

Hip fusion arthrodesis can be achieved by intra-articular or extra-articular techniques, or a combination of the two.

Internal fixation to achieve union was first proposed by Watson Jones and Charnley.

Morris JB. Charnley compression arthrodesis of the hip. J Bone Joint Surg Br 1966;48(2):260–79.

In modern practice hip fusion is a rare operation, although it may be indicated in young men with advanced arthritis who are involved in heavy labour. A normal lumbar spine, contralateral hip and ipsilateral knee are prerequisites. Arthrodesis produces further shortening, hence any existing shortening will be accentuated. Active sepsis is a contraindication.

The recommended position for hip fusion is 30° of flexion, 0°–5° of adduction and 0°–15° of external rotation. Abduction will lead to a lurch and internal rotation will cause tripping from the opposite limb while walking. Flexion allows ability to sit in a chair, but excess flexion will worsen the shortening. Movements of the lumbar spine compensate for lack of flexion and extension at the hip.

Assessment of patients should cover muscle wasting, ongoing infection, true shortening of the limb, neurological deficit and the position of the limb. Thomas test is essential to assess flexion deformity at the hip.

Various techniques have been described for hip fusion:

- Debridement of the joint and fixation with transacetabular cancellous screws. A subtrochanteric osteotomy can be performed at the same time.
- Application of a cobra plate to the lateral aspect of the femur, fixed to the outer surface of the ilium. A greater trochanter osteotomy is performed to elevate the abductors to preserve abductor function (Fig. 12.1). After plate fixation (Fig. 12.2) the greater trochanter is reattached to the femur over the plate (Fig. 12.3). Preservation of abductors does not influence the arthrodesis but may be relevant if a future conversion procedure to a hip replacement is planned. The distal end of the plate may act as a stress riser due to the long lever arm for forces in the absence of a mobile hip joint.
- Fixation after fusion is performed with a dynamic compression screw and supplemented by cancellous screws.

S. Agarwal (✉)
University Hospital of Wales, Consultant Orthopaedic Surgeon, Cardiff, UK

S. Agarwal (ed.), *Current Orthopaedic Practice*, https://doi.org/10.1007/978-3-030-78529-1_12

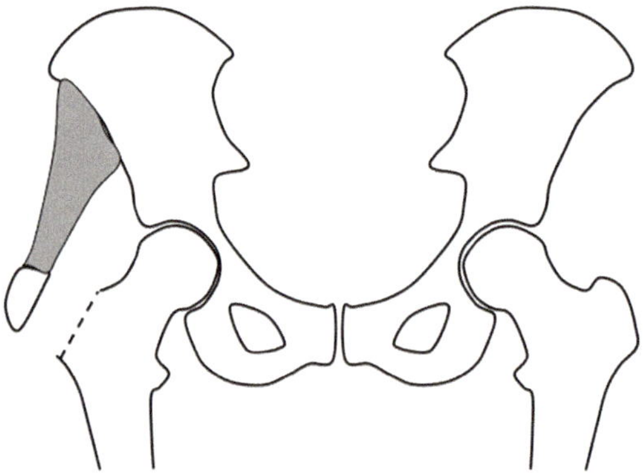

Fig. 12.1 Trochanteric osteotomy for hip arthrodesis

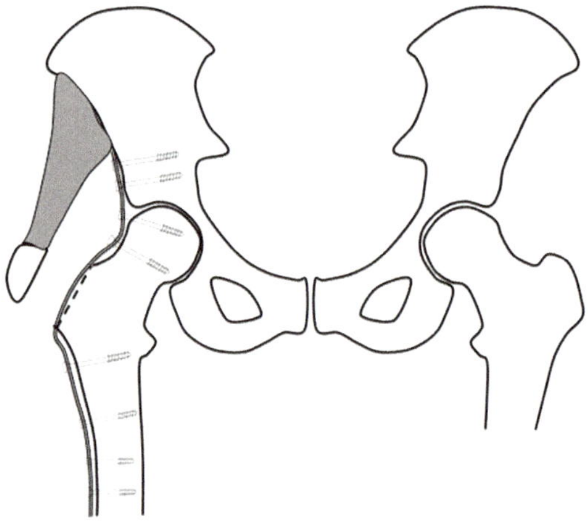

Fig. 12.2 Fixation of hip using a contoured plate

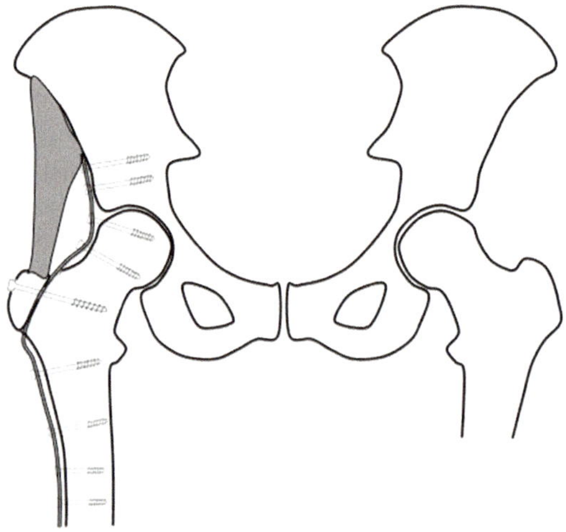

Fig. 12.3 Reattachment of the trochanter over the plate

In the long term, 50% patients may suffer from low back pain, 40% may have ipsilateral knee pain and 20% may have contralateral hip pain. Presence of these symptoms, or difficulty in managing daily activities, are indications for conversion of hip fusion to arthroplasty.

Conversion of hip fusion to total hip arthroplasty is associated with a high risk of complications, including infection, recurrent dislocation and poor mobility. A preoperative MR scan is helpful to determine the condition of the abductors and CT scan to assess bone stock and templating. Ongoing infection should be ruled out.

Technical problems are difficult approach due to lack of mobility, scarring, altered anatomy, lack of normal landmarks and existing metalwork. The neck has to be divided in situ and reaming of the acetabulum is done to place the component. Intraoperative radiographs help placement at the correct level and orientation of acetabulum. Abnormal proximal femoral anatomy may make femoral component fixation difficult. Capsular and soft tissue release is needed because of extensive contracture and scarring. Poor abductor function increases risk of dislocation and dual mobility or constrained acetabular component should be considered. Prophylaxis for heterotopic ossification is recommended.

Total knee arthroplasty for knee pain after hip fusion should be performed after conversion of the fusion to hip arthroplasty. Knee replacement below a hip fusion has a poor outcome.

Aderinto J, Lulu OB, Backstein DJ, Safir O, Gross AE. Functional results and complications following conversion of hip fusion to total hip replacement. J Bone Joint Surg Br 2012;94(11) Suppl A. 18 hip fusions converted to total hip replacement. Mean 5 year follow up. Two hips revised and two had injury to peroneal component of sciatic nerve.

Knee Arthrodesis

With the reliability and success of knee arthroplasty, knee fusion is an increasingly rare operation. Historically, the indications included gross instability, tuberculosis of the knee, pyogenic infection and neuropathic joints. These were also sometimes performed in young patients with arthritic knees who were involved in heavy manual work.

Most of these situations are now managed by knee arthroplasty. Failed knee arthroplasty with extensive bone loss or recurrent infection is now the most common indication for knee arthrodesis. Other indications include a grossly unstable knee in a young patient, failed extensor mechanism or a neuropathic joint.

A successful knee fusion alleviates pain, but imposes significant limitations in mobility and the ability to perform activities of daily living. A preoperative trial using a long leg cast for 2–3 weeks is sometimes recommended to emphasise the limitations following knee fusion.

A relatively normal contralateral limb is essential to allow optimum mobility after knee fusion. Contralateral knee pathology and ipsilateral hip or ankle disease are contraindications to this procedure.

The recommended position for knee fusion is 10°–15° of flexion and physiological valgus (3°–5°). A stiff fully extended knee will necessitate a circumduction of the limb while walking. Flexion allows the patient to clear the ground without circumduction. However, in situations with bone loss and shortening, fusion in extension is acceptable.

Several techniques have been proposed to achieve fusion such as external fixators, compression plate and intramedullary nail.

External Fixators

External fixators were effectively used by Sir John Charnley, achieving 98.5% union using a pin above and below the knee connected to clamps on either side. The indications in his patients were osteoarthritis, rheumatoid arthritis and tuberculosis. Problems included pin-site infections and difficulty in mobilising.

Charnley J, Lowe HG. A study of the end results of compression arthrodesis of the knee. J Bone Joint Surg Br 1958;40(4):633–5.

More recently, ring fixators have been used to stabilise fusions. Extensive bone loss results in shortening, and compressing with a fixator accentuates the problem. However, ring fixators can be used in conjunction with debridement in patients with ongoing sepsis. It is possible to adjust the alignment postoperatively with external fixators.

Compression Plates

Compression plates can be used when the knee is opened for debridement, using the same exposure for stabilising the fusion with one or two plates. Two plates at right angles or a medial and lateral plate can be used. The plates should be staggered to avoid a stress riser at the end of the plate. Wound closure can be difficult due to the added bulk of the plates. Weight bearing is restricted until the fusion is solid.

Intramedullary Nails

Intramedullary nails provide reliable fixation without the problems associated with external fixation. They allow debridement and nail insertion, with early weight bearing.

The nails can be a long antegrade intramedullary nail, or comprise a separate femoral and tibial nail connected at the level of the knee joint. Long intramedullary nails can be locked proximally and distally for added stability. The nail has a fixed diameter throughout, and as the femoral canal is wider than the tibial canal, the nail is relatively narrow in the femoral segment. Using separate femoral and tibial nails has the advantage of using different diameters for the two segments, but the disadvantage of difficult removal, if required. Removal in this situation requires opening a window in the bone at the fusion site and disarticulating the nail. Articulated nails can be cemented which allows a high local dose of antibiotics mixed with the cement.

MacDonald JH, Agarwal S, Lorei MP, Johanson NA, Freiberg AA. Knee arthrodesis. J Am Acad Orthop Surg 2006;14(3):154–63.

Razii N, Abbas AM, Kakar R, Agarwal S, Morgan-Jones R. Knee arthrodesis using a long intramedullary nail as limb salvage for complex periprosthetic infections. Eur J Orthop Surg Traumatol 2016;26(8):907–14.

Ankle Arthrodesis

Ankle fusion provides pain relief and allows mobility in end stage ankle arthritis. The common indications for ankle fusion include post-traumatic arthritis, rheumatoid arthritis, chronic infections, neuromuscular conditions, tumours around the ankle and failed ankle replacement. Restriction of hind foot movement after ankle fusion makes walking on uneven surfaces difficult. An ankle fusion will cause additional force on the adjacent joints of the foot, leading to degenerative changes in due course.

The recommended position for ankle fusion is 0° of flexion, 0°–5° of valgus and 5°–10° of external rotation. A plantar flexed position of 10° is preferred in patients with cerebral palsy.

The surgical technique should allow thick skin flaps, a large cancellous surface for contact, rigid internal fixation and optimum alignment. The approach can be anterior through the sheath of tibialis anterior, transmalleolar, transfibular or posterior. The joint surfaces are debrided and fixation can be with an external fixator, cancellous screws or intramedullary rod.

Arthroscopic ankle fusion is increasingly popular as it creates minimal soft tissue disruption and better cosmesis. The technique is useful in patients with minimal deformity. Success rates of over 80% have been reported in most series.

In patients with severe deformity an open technique is the gold standard at present, but success has been reported with arthroscopic techniques as well.

Smith R, Wood PL. Arthrodesis of the ankle in the presence of a large deformity in the coronal plane. J Bone Joint Surg Br 2007;89:615–9. The researchers performed open fusion using compression screws in a consecutive series of 23 patients (25 ankles). Primary union was achieved in 24 ankles.

Gougoulias NE, Agathangelidis FG, Parsons SW. Arthroscopic ankle arthrodesis. Foot Ankle Int 2007;28:695–706. Arthroscopic ankle arthrodesis was performed in 30 ankles with more than 15° deformity. A good outcome was reported in 80% of the ankles.

Postoperatively, a cast is used for 3 months with the first 6 weeks being non weight bearing and the second 6 weeks allowing partial weight bearing thorough the cast. Full weight bearing can commence once bony union is evident, usually at 3 months stage.

Shoulder Arthrodesis

Shoulder arthrodesis has been used for over 100 years for the management of chronic shoulder infections. Extra-articular fusion was initially proposed to reduce the risk of infection, and Charnley devised an external fixator with pins in the proximal humerus and the acromion to achieve compression.

The success of shoulder arthroplasty and stabilisation procedures has led to a reduction in arthrodesis procedures. The current indications for arthrodesis are paralytic disorders, brachial plexus injury, massive cuff tears, tumours around the shoulder and failed shoulder arthroplasty.

Chronic infections in the shoulder can be managed with fusion. Charcot's arthropathy has a high failure rate. Avascular necrosis of the shoulder is managed by arthroplasty.

The optimum position for arthrodesis is 25°–40° of abduction, 20°–30° of flexion and 25°–30° of internal rotation. This is sometimes simplified as 30° flexion, 30° abduction and 30° internal rotation (30–30–30).

A contoured plate along the spine of the scapula, acromion and proximal humerus provides stable support following arthrodesis.

Elbow Arthrodesis

Elbow arthrodesis in indicated in patients with chronic infections or post-traumatic arthritis, and in severely comminuted fractures in young patients. Elbow arthroplasty provides good function, but limited long-term survival of the implant makes arthrodesis a viable option in younger patients.

The optimum position for fusion is individualised to the needs of the patient and varies from 70° to 90° of flexion.

Arthrodesis is performed by debridement of the joint and bone grafting. A tibial graft can be used to supplement. Cancellous screws or plates and external fixators can be used to stabilise the fusion until bone healing.

Wrist Arthrodesis

Wrist arthrodesis is indicated for post-traumatic arthritis in young patients, chronic infection, tumours, paralytic disorders, salvage of Kienbock's disease and failed wrist arthroplasty. It is contraindicated in patients with an open physis (i.e., aged <17 years).

The optimum position for wrist fusion is 10°–20° of extension, with the long axis of the third metacarpal lined up with the long axis of the radius in the sagittal plane. Dorsiflexion improves grip strength. In rheumatoid patients, a neutral position or flexion of 10° can be used.

The preferred method of fusion is iliac crest bone grafting along with internal fixation with a plate. The plate extends from the long finger metacarpal to the distal radial shaft. The wrist is splinted postoperatively for 6–8 weeks.

Amputation

The aim of amputation is to remove diseased or non-functional parts of an extremity to reduce morbidity and mortality; and enable restoration of function.

Indications for amputations are:

- Peripheral vascular disease—irreversible ischaemia in a limb is an absolute indication for amputation.
- Trauma with an insensate limb.
- Uncontrolled infection. Necrotising fasciitis is a situation which may require an urgent amputation as a life saving measure.
- Thermal injury—burns or frostbite.
- Tumour.
- Congenital anomalies.

Peripheral vascular disease is the most common indication for amputation. Revascularisation techniques may avoid the need for amputation and an assessment must be made for this possibility. Infection should be treated and the nutritional status optimised prior to amputation.

An irreparable vascular injury as a result of trauma and an insensate foot due to tibial nerve injury are indications for amputation. The Mangled Extremity Severity Score (MESS) (Table 12.1) helps surgeons to make an objective decision as to whether limb salvage is worthwhile.

A score of greater than 7 indicates a high likelihood of amputation. A score of 6 or less correlates with a salvageable limb. The decision to amputate or salvage is based on multiple factors, including the extent of the injury, the feasibility of reconstruction, the expected function after sal-

Table 12.1 The Mangled Extremity Severity Score (MESS)

Feature	Score
Skeletal soft tissue injury	
Low-energy injury	1
Medium-energy injury	2
High-energy injury	3
Very high-energy injury	4
Limb ischaemia	
Pulse reduced, but normal perfusion	1
Pulseless, reduced capillary refill	2
Cool, paralysed, insensate	3
Shock	
Systolic blood pressure > 90 mmHg	1
Transient hypotension	2
Persistent hypotension	3
Age	
<30 years	1
30–50 years	2
>50 years	3

A score >7 indicates a high likelihood of amputation; ≤6 correlates with a salvageable limb

vage, the cost and time involved in salvage and, importantly, the views of the patient.

Johansen K, Daines M, Howey T, et al. Objective criteria accurately predict amputation following lower extremity trauma. J Trauma 1990;30:568–72. A retrospective study of 25 patients and prospective application of the MESS in 26 patients. A score of more than 7 was 100% predictive of amputation.

Burns are managed with immediate aggressive debridement, grafting, flap cover, release of contracture or amputation as necessary. Frostbite is managed by re-warming and pain management in the initial stage. Amputation is delayed by 2–6 months until demarcation is clear.

Patient Assessment

Locally, signs of impaired circulation are a weak or absent pulse, reduced skin temperature and reduced transcutaneous oxygen tension. The ankle–brachial index indicates the healing potential of lower limbs and an arteriogram will demonstrate the distal circulation.

A thorough evaluation of the general condition of the patient is carried out. Laboratory tests include haematocrit, white cell count and serum albumin levels. The serum albumin level should be higher than 3.5 g/dL and the absolute lymphocyte count higher than 1500 cells/μL.

Glycaemic control is instituted and cardiac and renal functions are assessed. The nutritional condition of the patient should be assessed and deficiencies corrected as needed. Preoperative counselling and the use of support groups are helpful for early rehabilitation.

Surgical Technique

The level of amputation is decided based on a balance between the preservation of useful limb and the removal of non-functional limb. A proximal level allows disease clearance, while a more distal level allows better function. Transtibial amputations allow better walking speed and greater energy efficiency than transfemoral amputations.

The optimum amputation level for the tibia is a minimum of 2.5 cm for each foot of height of the patient. Commonly, it is 12.5–15 cm below the medial joint line of the tibia. Amputations in the lower third of leg have poor soft tissue cover and are avoided. Transfemoral amputations are planned in the middle third of the femur. A minimum of 15 cm space should be allowed above the knee joint for fitting the prosthesis.

Transradial amputations are planned at the junction of the proximal two-thirds and distal third of the forearm. Transhumeral amputations are performed in the mid third of the arm.

The skin flaps should be marked out, and the combined length of the flaps should be slightly more than the diameter of the planned stump. The base of the flaps should be level with the bone resection (Fig. 12.4). The flaps should be full thickness. The scar should not be adherent to the underlying bone.

In ischaemic limbs, the posterior flap in the leg is long and the anterior flap is kept short to maximise the blood supply to the suture line.

Muscles should be attached to bone at their resting length (myodesis) instead of suturing muscle to its antagonist (myoplasty). Myoplasty is preferred in vascular insufficiency.

The Ertl technique involves creating an osteoplasty to seal the medullary canal with an osteo-

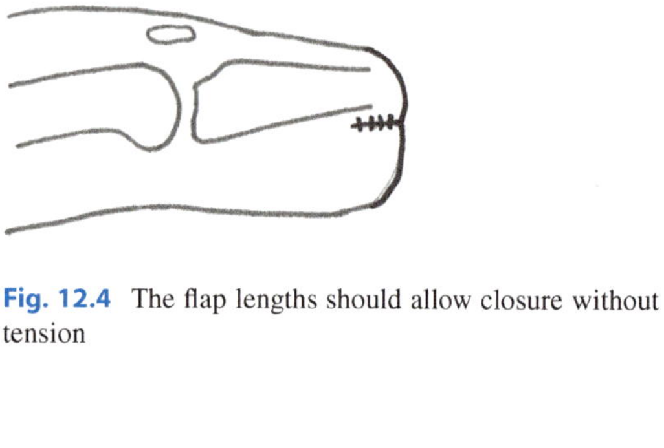

Fig. 12.4 The flap lengths should allow closure without tension

periosteal graft. In transtibial amputations, a bone bridge is created between the tibia and fibula to increase the bony surface area for weight bearing.

Neuromas can be reduced by avoiding injury to the nerves and dividing them as proximal as possible with a sharp knife. The major vessels are ligated and hemostasis achieved. A suction drain is inserted and skin closure is achieved without tension.

Postoperatively, compression dressings are provided and avoidance of contractures is paramount through patient education and physiotherapy. Early prosthetic fitting is the goal, and a definitive cast for prosthesis can be provided once the stump is mature.

Complications

Early complications after amputation include haematoma, infection and necrosis of the skin margin. Infections are more common in those with diabetes and peripheral vascular disease.

Late complications are contractures, neuroma formation and phantom limb pain. Residual limb pain is often due to a poorly fitting cast and can be addressed by altering the cast to avoid pressure. Phantom sensation is very common and gradually resolves (known as 'telescoping'). Phantom pain is less common and is difficult to treat.

Children undergoing amputation may experience terminal bone overgrowth. This is due to appositional growth at the end of the bone. It is common in the humerus and the fibula and in severe cases may penetrate the skin, requiring excision.

Prosthetics

A prosthesis is a replacement of a body part. A limb prosthesis has the following components:

- Socket—the interface between the prosthesis and the stump.
- Suspension system—to hold the socket in place.
- Joint mechanism
- Terminal device—for example a hook, foot or hand.

Further Reading

Aderinto J, Lulu OB, Backstein DJ, Safir O, Gross AE. Functional results and complications following conversion of hip fusion to total hip replacement. J Bone Joint Surg Br. 2012;94(11 Suppl A):36–41.

Charnley J, Lowe HG. A study of the end results of compression arthrodesis of the knee. J Bone Joint Surg Br. 1958;40(4):633–5.

Gougoulias NE, Agathangelidis FG, Parsons SW. Arthroscopic ankle arthrodesis. Foot Ankle Int. 2007;28:695–706.

Johansen K, Daines M, Howey T, et al. Objective criteria accurately predict amputation following lower extremity trauma. J Trauma. 1990;30:568–72.

MacDonald JH, Agarwal S, Lorei MP, Johanson NA, Freiberg AA. Knee arthrodesis. J Am Acad Orthop Surg. 2006;14(3):154–63.

Morris JB. Charnley compression arthrodesis of the hip. J Bone Joint Surg Br. 1966;48(2):260–79.

Razii N, Abbas AM, Kakar R, Agarwal S, Morgan-Jones R. Knee arthrodesis using a long intramedullary nail as limb salvage for complex periprosthetic infections. Eur J Orthop Surg Traumatol. 2016;26(8):907–14.

Smith R, Wood PL. Arthrodesis of the ankle in the presence of a large deformity in the coronal plane. J Bone Joint Surg Br. 2007;89:615–9.

Paediatric Disorders 13

Clare Carpenter

Legg–Calvé–Perthes Disease

Legg–Calvé–Perthes (LCP) disease is idiopathic avascular necrosis (AVN) of the femoral head in childhood.

The condition was initially described by Professor Henning Waldenström in 1909, who thought the condition was a form of tuberculosis of the hip. Soon after, in 1910, Arthur Legg (from the USA), Jacques Calvé (France) and Georg Perthes (Germany) independently described the same disease, proposing that it was *not* tuberculosis.

Epidemiology

The annual prevalence is 5–10 per 100,000 children per year. There is a well-described regional variation in the UK: the prevalence is 5.5 per 100,000 in Wessex and 11.1 per 100,000 in Liverpool.

LCP disease is more common in temperate climates, and Caucasian population, as opposed to Afro-Caribbeans. Other risk factors are passive smokers (odds ratio 5.3), short stature and children with delayed bone age.

Children aged 4–8 years are usually affected, but the age range can vary from 2 to 12 years. Boys are four to five times more commonly affected than girls.

The disease is bilateral in 10% of patients, although both sides usually do not present at the same time.

LCP disease is generally not related to irritable hip. Only 3% children with a single episode of irritable hip go on to develop LCP disease. Recurrent irritable hip may, however, constitute a risk factor, especially if it is associated with delayed bone age.

Keenan WN, Clegg J. Perthes disease after irritable hip: delayed bone age shows the hip is a "marked man". J Bone Joint Surg Br 1996;16(1):20–3. 13 children with recurrent irritable hip. Only those with more than 2 years delay in bone age were found to be in early stage of Perthes disease.

Aetiology

The underlying cause is ischaemia of variable duration. This is followed by a repair process that leads to femoral head deformity. Several causes of the initial ischaemia have been proposed (Table 13.1) although the exact cause may be multifactorial and remains unproven.

A link to maternal smoking, abnormalities in insulin like growth factor-1 pathway and type II

C. Carpenter (✉)
University Hospital of Wales, Cardiff, UK
e-mail: clare.carpenter2@wales.nhs.uk

S. Agarwal (ed.), *Current Orthopaedic Practice*, https://doi.org/10.1007/978-3-030-78529-1_13

Table 13.1 Theories on aetiology of Perthes disease

Thrombophilia theory	Underlying coagulation disorder e.g.—deficiency of protein C or S, resistance to activated protein C, or increased APTT
Vascular theory	Repeated occlusion of the lateral circumflex femoral artery. This may also explain the delayed bone age
Hormonal theory	Abnormal levels of insulin-like growth factor binding-protein 3

APTT activated partial thromboplastin time

collagen mutation have been proposed as possible etiological factors.

Hresko MT et al. Prospective reevaluation of the association between thrombotic diathesis and legg perthes disease J Bone Joint Surg Am 2002;84(9):1613–8. Found no relationship in a prospective study comprising consecutive patients.

Szepesi K. The most severe forms of perthes disease associated with the homozygous Factor V Leiden mutation. J Bone Joint Surg Br 2004;86(3):426–429. Found homozygous factor V Leiden was associated with most severe form of LCP disease.

Pathogenesis

The sequence of events is summarized in Fig. 13.1.

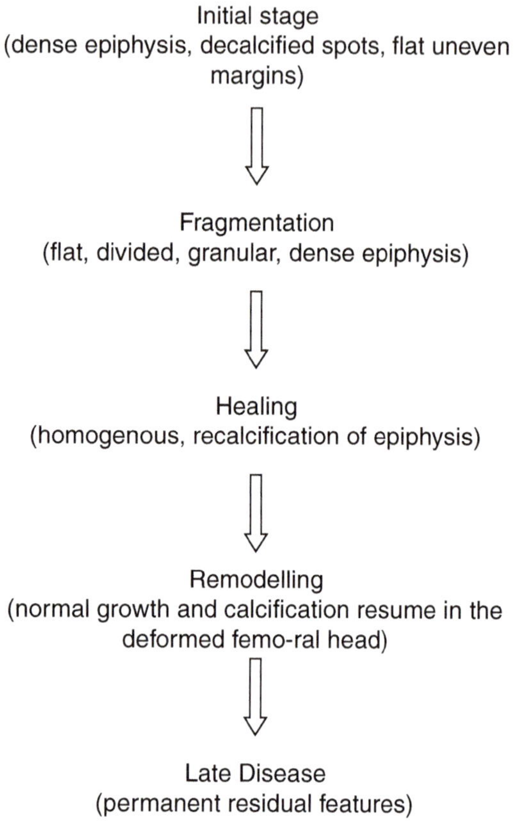

Fig. 13.1 Pathogenesis of Perthes disease

Pathology

The pathologic changes are illustrated in Fig. 13.2.

Natural History

After healing, the pain resolves. An elevated trochanter deformity leads to a limp. The leg-length shortening is usually less than 2 cm. Most patients are symptomatic after the age of 40 years and 50% are expected to have significant arthritis by the age of 45 years.

Clinical Features

Children can present with a painless limp, or intermittent episodes of pain in the hip, or referred pain in the ipsilateral knee.

Gait typically demonstrates an antalgic limp initially. Later, a Trendelenburg gait develops due to trochanteric overgrowth and a flattened femoral head.

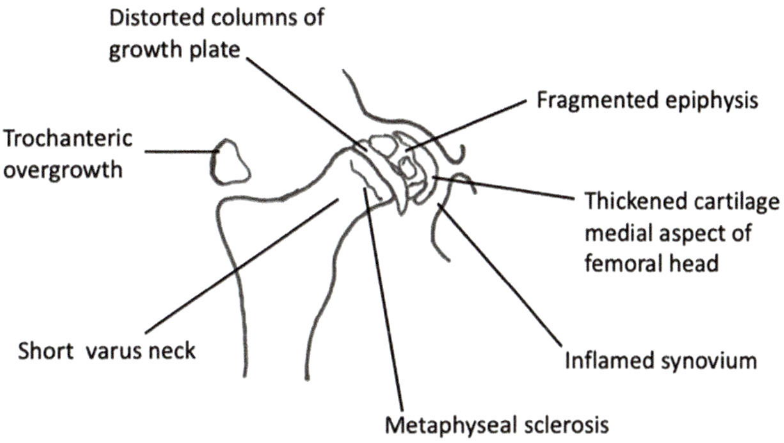

Fig. 13.2 Pathologic changes in Perthes disease

On flexion, the hip goes into abduction and external rotation. The presence of adduction contracture is a sign of severe disease.

Differential Diagnosis

If symptoms and signs are bilateral, differential diagnoses to consider are:

- Hypothyroidism.
- Spondyloepiphyseal dysplasia, multiple epiphyseal dysplasia.

If presentation is unilateral:

- Down's syndrome.
- Renal dysfunction.
- Infection—tuberculosis hip, subacute septic arthritis, osteomyelitis of the femoral neck.
- Blood disorders—sickle cell disease, haemophilia, leukaemia.
- Eosinophilic granuloma.
- Gaucher's disease.
- Lymphoma.
- Steroid therapy, immunosuppressed patient.

Imaging

Initial imaging is anteroposterior (AP) view and frog-leg lateral—in abduction, flexion and, external rotation of the hip. For follow-up, an AP view of the pelvis is adequate. AP of the wrist can be done for bone age, if in doubt.

Ultrasound scan shows persistent distension of the capsule for more than 6 weeks and thickened cartilage.

Arthrography can be done to see the shape of the femoral head and containment.

A pinhole collimated Tc-99 bone scan can be done to detect revascularisation.

Magnetic resonance imaging (MRI) demonstrates the changes in the bone and flattening of the femoral head.

Classification

Different classification systems have been proposed, of which the Catterall and Herring systems are commonly used (Table 13.2 and Fig. 13.3).

The Herring system (Fig. 13.4) is based on the height of the lateral pillar of the femoral physis at the beginning of the fragmentation phase. The lateral pillar is defined as the lateral 15–30% of the femoral head in the anteroposterior view. The central pillar is the middle 50% while the medial pillar is the medial 20–35%.

The height of the lateral pillar serves as a guide to severity.

A borderline B/C group has also been defined for the Herring system:

- A very narrow lateral pillar (2–3 mm) >50% height.
- A lateral pillar with very little ossification but >50% height.
- A lateral pillar exactly 50% height, depressed relative to the central pillar.

Legg-Calve-Perthes disease Part I: classification of radiographs with use of modified lateral pillar and Stulberg classification. Herring JA, Kim HT, Browne R. J Bone Joint Surg Am 2004;86(10):2103–20. The lateral pillar is demarcated from the femoral head by a radiolucent line of fragmentation and can be 5–30% of the head on the AP view. If there is no demarcation then the head is the lateral quarter.

Table 13.2 The Catterall classifications

I Anterocentral	Visible in lateral view Only the anterior part of the femoral head is involved No collapse, loss of height, metaphyseal changes
II Centrosuperior	Collapse with dense sequestrum AP view—density between medial and lateral pillar Lateral view—V sign
III Centrosuperior lateral	Anteroposterior—head within head appearance on radiographs Broad femoral neck, metaphyseal changes
IV Whole femoral head	Epiphysis mushrooms anteriorly and posteriorly

Another classification system has been proposed by Salter and Thompson, based on the crescent sign. Group A is where less than 50% of the femoral head is involved (equivalent to Catterall groups I and II). In group B, more than 50% of the femoral head is involved (Catterall groups III and IV).

Stulberg has devised a classification to describe late changes in the hip joint. This system is applicable at skeletal maturity and has high correlation with clinical symptoms. The classification can also be used to predict arthritis (Table 13.3).

Salter RB, Thompson GH. Legg-Calve-Perthes disease. The prognostic significance of the subchondral fracture and a two group classification of the femoral head involvement. J Bone Joint Surg Am 1984;66(4):479–89.

Stulberg SD et al. The natural history of Legg-Calve-Perthes disease. J Bone Joint Surg Am 1981;63(7):1095–108.

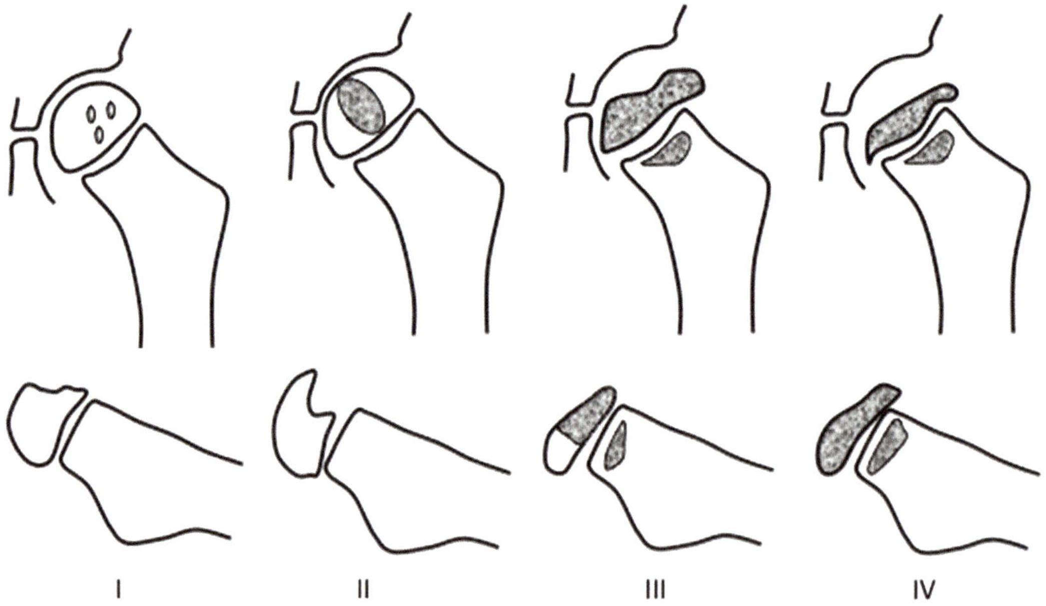

Fig. 13.3 Diagrammatic representation of the Catterall classification

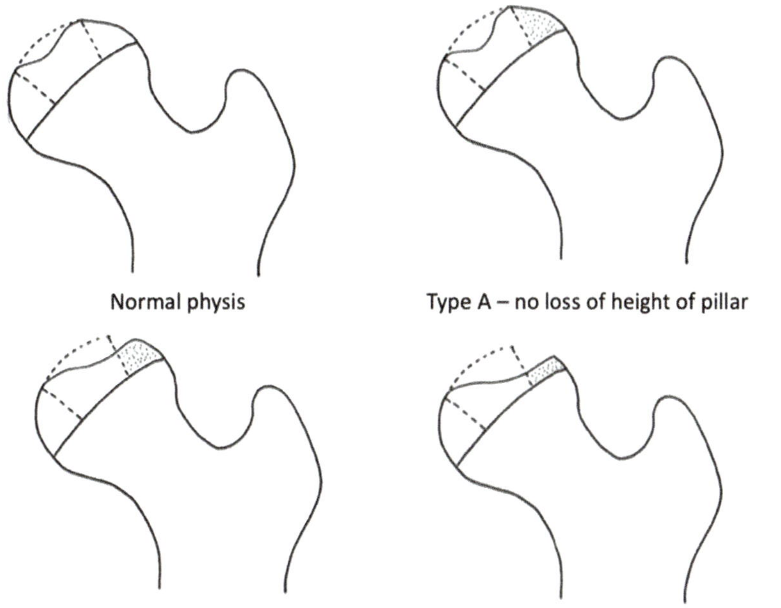

Fig. 13.4 Herring classification for Perthes disease

Table 13.3 The Stulberg classification of late changes in the hip joint and the predictability of arthritis

Group	Description	Arthritis prediction
I	Normal articulation	Spherical head, congruous—no early arthritis
II	Spherical head but larger (coxa magna) or short neck (Coxa Brevis)	
III	Aspherical head—ovoid/mushroom shape + type II, not flattened	Aspherical head, congruous—moderate early arthritis
IV	Flat femoral head and abnormal neck and acetabulum	
V	Flat femoral head and normal neck and acetabulum, loss of congruence	Aspherical head, incongruous—severe early arthritis

Mose proposed a sphericity measurement, whereby more than 2 mm deviation from a perfect circle on the AP and lateral views is considered abnormal.

Herring JBJS Am Oct 2004—circle fit—2 mm. Less than 2 mm on Mose sphericity. The widest diameter of femoral head is drawn. The perpendicular to widest point is drawn and circle drawn. The same diameter is used on lateral view to see for sphericity.

Femoral Head 'At-Risk' Signs

Clinical indicators of an at-risk femoral head include obesity, a decreasing range of movement and adduction contracture due to lateral subluxation of the head.

Radiological signs may also be seen (Fig. 13.5).

The V-shaped lytic area in the lateral epiphysis and metaphysis (Gage sign) indicates hinged abduction. Calcification lateral to the epiphysis may be caused by ossification of the extruded head, which is mushroomed out. Diffuse metaphyseal reaction indicates non-ossified nests of cartilage. Lateral subluxation of the femoral head is caused by thick cartilage medially on the femoral head and acetabulum. A horizontal growth plate indicates the hip is lying in external rotation.

Prognostic Factors

The poor prognostic factors are summarised in Fig. 13.6. Based on Herring classification, in type A, almost all patients have a good result. In type B, two-thirds have a good result, in Herring B/C,

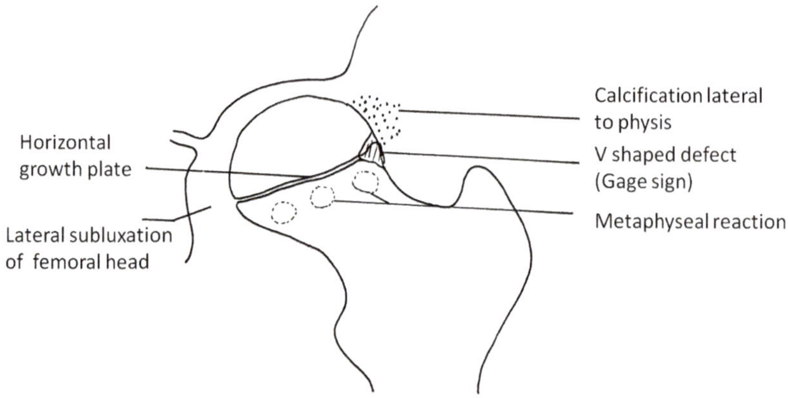

Fig. 13.5 Diagrammatic representation of 'head at risk' signs

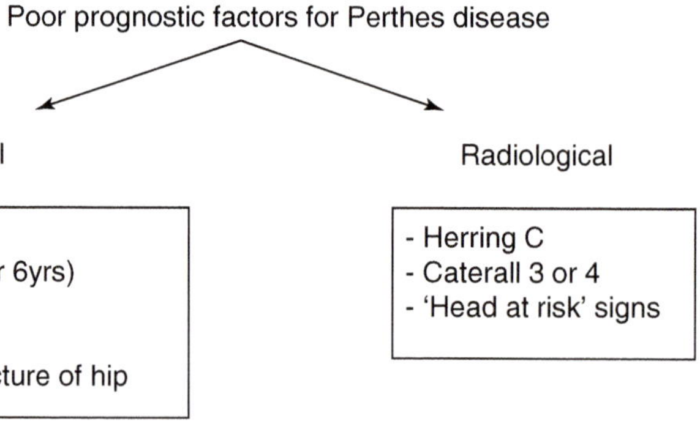

Fig. 13.6 Poor prognostic factors in Perthes disease

a quarter have a good result and in Herring C, one-eighth have a good result.

Under the age of 8 years, 8% have a poor result while over the age of 8 years, 26% have a poor result.

Management

Fifty to 60% of children have a good prognosis regardless of management. The rest will require hip replacement or hip salvage surgery when adults, usually in middle age.

The aim of management is to contain the femoral head within the acetabulum.

Treatment of acute painful episodes is by short-term bed rest, traction, an abduction cast and anti-inflammatory medication (NSAIDs).

Bracing

Bracing (e.g., Atlanta Scottish Rite brace) keeps the hip in over 30° abduction but allows flexion and extension. The brace should be worn at all times, with removal only for 1 h for a bath and for maximum of 3 h for swimming in a day. An arthrogram is performed before bracing to check containment in abduction. The patient should be followed-up with X-rays every 3–4 months. Bracing continues until the lateral column ossifies and sclerotic areas of epiphysis disappear.

Decreased hip movements indicate a worsening prognosis. The period in the brace varies from 3 months to 3 years. In modern practice, bracing is rarely advised.

Herring JA, Kim HT, Browne R. Legg Calve Perthes disease. Part I. Prospective multicentre study on the effect of treatment on outcome. J Bone Joint Surg Am 2004;86(10):2121–34. Treatment has little influence on outcome. Outcome depends on Herring grade and age of onset, regardless of treatment. Brace is not effective.

Adductor Tenotomy and Petrie Cast

Adductor tenotomy addresses the tight adductors and improves abduction range. A Petrie cast keeps the knees flexed and the hips in internal rotation with a bar between the legs. Forty degree abduction is maintained at the hips. However, a cast is rarely used in modern practice.

Surgical Containment

The recommendations for surgery are summarised in Table 13.4.

Herring JA, Kim HT, Browne R. Legg-Calve-Perthes disease. Part II: Prospective multicenter study of the effect of treatment on outcome. J Bone Joint Surg Am 2004;86-A:2121–34. This prospective, multicentre study was started in 1984. A total of 438 patients, aged 6–12 years at disease onset, were enrolled. This amounted to 451 affected hips, and 345 hips were studied at maturity. The conclusions are summarised in Table 13.4.

Redirectional procedures include femoral varus osteotomy and Salter's osteotomy (Figs. 13.7 and 13.8). A comparison of these two approaches is presented in Table 13.5.

Table 13.4 Recommendations for surgery based on the Herring classification

Herring classification	Age <8 years	Age >8 years
A	No need for surgery	
B	No need for surgery	Surgery
B/C	No need for surgery	Surgery
C	Surgery has no effect of treatment	

Böhm P, Brzuske A. Salter innominate osteotomy for the treatment of developmental dysplasia of the hip in children: results of seventy-three consecutive osteotomies after twenty-six to thirty-five years of follow-up. J Bone Joint Surg Am 2002;84-A:178–86. In this study, conducted Salter's osteotomy on 73 hips in patients with a mean age of 4 years at surgery and a 31-year follow-up. Overall, mean age 4 years at surgery. 21% had poor results.

Non-redirectional procedures include the shelf procedure and Chiari osteotomy. The latter is indicated in an enlarged incongruous epiphysis in an older patient.

Late Sequelae

Hinge abduction is a late sequel. It can be managed with valgus osteotomy or cheilectomy. In valgus extension osteotomy, 20° valgus will relieve pain for few years. An anterolateral approach is used in cheilectomy as the protuberance is usually anterolateral.

Yoo WJ, Choi IH, Chung CY, et al. Valgus femoral osteotomy for hinge abduction in Perthes' disease. Decision-making and outcomes. J Bone Joint Surg Br 2004;86:726–30. In this study of 21 hips, with a mean patient age of 9.7 years and a 7.1-year follow-up, the mean hip score improved from 66 to 92 following valgus femoral osteotomy.

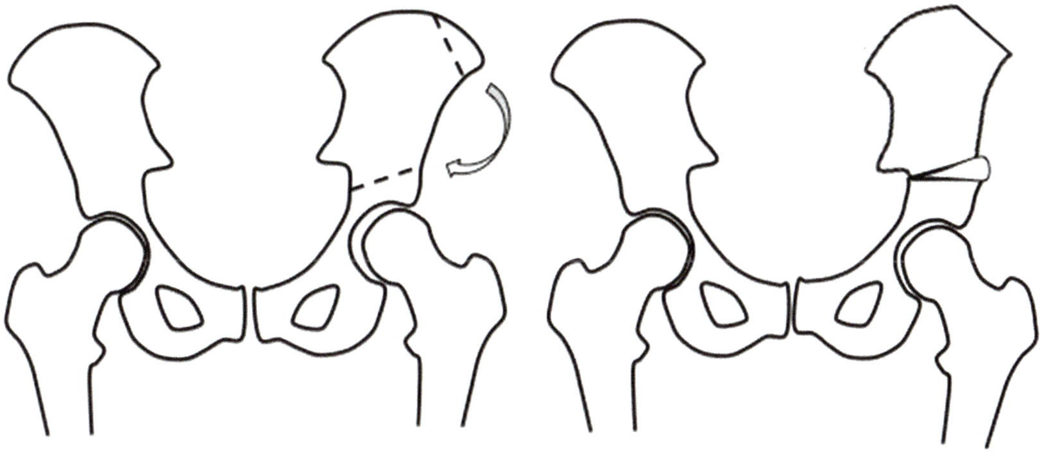

Fig. 13.7 Principle of the Salter osteotomy

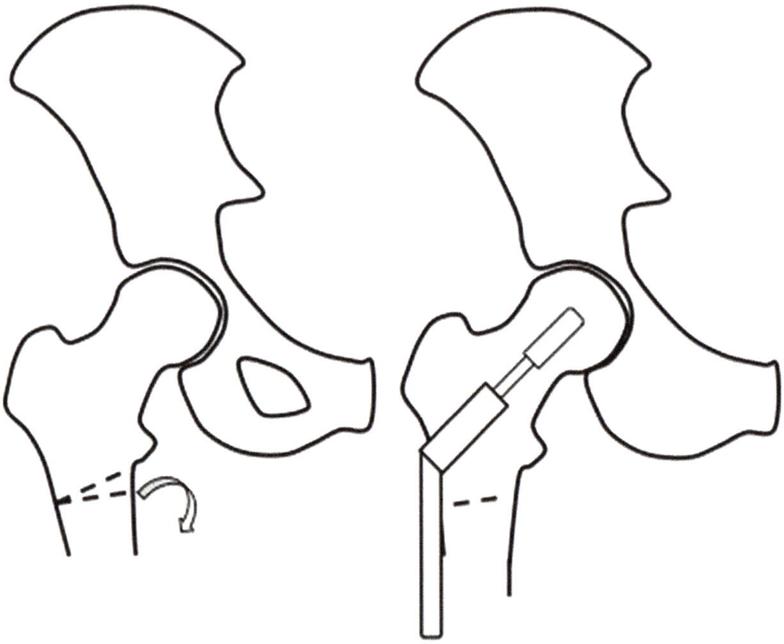

Fig. 13.8 Principle of medial closing wedge femoral varus osteotomy

Table 13.5 Comparison of femoral varus osteotomy and Salter's osteotomy

Procedure	Indications	Notes
Femoral varus osteotomy	Age 8–10 years No leg-length discrepancy Uncovered femoral head on arthrogram Reduced angle of Wiberg	Causes additional shortening The varus remodels in 3 years The neck shaft angle should not be reduced below 115° A 20° abnormal angle is restored with growth
Salter's osteotomy	Age >6 years Full range of motion Round femoral head Reasonable congruence in abduction Subluxation in weight bearing >50% head involvement	No shortening Avoids varus

Herring reported nonoperative treatment of Perthes in a prospective study with 20 years follow up.

Noelle Larson A, Sucato DJ, Herring JA, Adolfsen SE, Kelly DM, Martus JE, Lovejoy JF, Browne R, DeLaRocha A.A Prospective Multicenter Study of Legg Calve Perthes Disease. J Bone Joint Surg Am 2012;94:584–92. 56 patients, mean 20 year follow up. 26% no hip arthritis, 30% mild arthritis, 44% had moderate to severe arthritis. Stulberg classification correlated with clinical score.

Developmental Dysplasia of the Hip

The term 'developmental dysplasia of the hip' (DDH) includes prenatal teratologic dislocation, postnatal instability and adolescent acetabular dysplasia. Teratologic dislocation is a severe form with dislocated hip at birth and is associated with neuromuscular syndromes like arthrogryposis and Larsen syndrome.

Epidemiology

The male to female ratio of DDH is 7:1. The left side is more commonly affected than the right. Incidences of a positive Barlow or Ortolani test is one in 250 live births; frank dislocation is one in 1000 live births. Incidence of late dislocation or dysplasia is 1 in 250 live births.

Aetiology

The family history is positive in 34% of patients. Other factors associated with DDH are breech presentation, oligohydramnios, congenital dislocation of the knee, congenital torticollis and metatarsus adductus.

Pathology

The pathology is illustrated in Fig. 13.9. The acetabular labrum is enlarged and may infold, preventing reduction of the femoral head. The transverse acetabular ligament (TAL) occupies the lower part of the acetabulum and blocks reduction of the femoral head. The acetabulum fills with pulvinar, a fibrofatty tissue. The hamstring, glutei and psoas tendons are contracted. The psoas tendon causes an hourglass constriction in the joint capsule seen on arthrograms.

Natural History

Ninety percent of unstable hips stabilise within 2 months. If unreduced, the joint will develop osteoarthritic changes at ages 20–60 years.

Screening

Routine ultrasound screening for newborns is not practiced in the UK. All newborn are examined clinically at birth, and at 6–10 weeks. An ultrasound examination is performed at age 6 weeks or X-ray at age 4 months is performed for those at risk of DDH. This includes children with a family history, breech presentation, foot deformities or abnormal examination of hip.

The arguments against general screening are that it results in a higher treatment rate and has a negative cost–benefit analysis.

Wirth T, Stratmann L, Hinrichs F. Evolution of late presenting developmental dysplasia of the hip and associated surgical procedures after 14 years of neonatal ultrasound screening. J Bone Joint Surg Br 2004;86:585–9. General neonatal ultrasound screening was found to reduce surgical procedures and late presentations. The authors strongly recommended general screening. With selective screening, the splintage rate is 4–10 per 1000 live births. With general screening, the splintage rate is 49 per 1000 live births.

Lewis K, Jones DA, Powell N. Ultrasound and neonatal hip screening: the five-year results of a prospective study in high-risk babies. J Pediatr Orthop 1999;19:760–2. Selective ultrasound

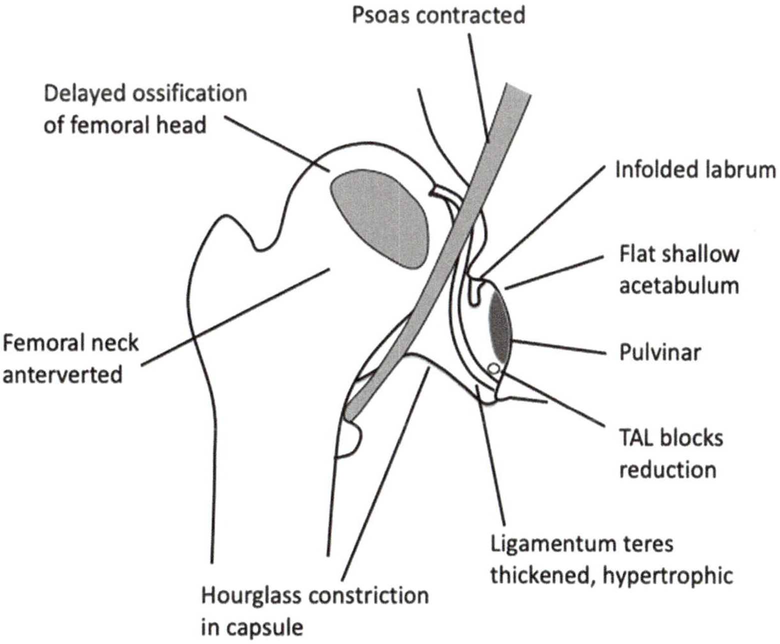

Fig. 13.9 Pathology in DDH

screening reduced late DDH cases from 2.2 to 0.34 per 1000 live births. The authors recommended general screening.

Clinical Features

Examination focuses on the Barlow and Ortolani tests.

In Barlow test, the examiner attempts to dislocate a reduced hip. The hip is flexed and adducted, and the thigh pushed axially in a proximal direction in an attempt to dislocate the hip. An unstable hip will be felt as a click as the femoral head slips out of the acetabulum.

In the Ortolani test, the examiner attempts to reduce a dislocated hip. The hip is flexed and adducted. The examiner's thumb is placed on the medial side of thigh and fingers around the greater trochanter. The hip is then abducted and an attempt made to gently reduce the hip. The presence of a clunk or sensation of reduction is a positive test.

Both of these tests are negative after 3 months because a dislocated hip (Ortolani-positive) cannot be reduced, and a hip that is reduced in a position of rest (Barlow-positive) tends to stabilise by 3 months.

These tests are 60% sensitive and 90% specific, so are poor screening tests.

Other clinical features of a dislocated hip are

- Galeazzi sign—shortened femur.
- Asymmetry of the skin folds—a non-specific sign.
- Telescoping of the thigh.
- If the child is walking, clinical signs of DDH are excess lordosis, pelvic obliquity, Trendelenburg gait and hip flexion contracture.

A 'clicky hip' is not related to DDH. Rather, it has a soft tissue aetiology.

Bond CD et al. Prospective evaluation of newborn soft-tissue "clicks" with ultrasound. J Pediatr Orthop 1997;17(2):199–201. 50 infants over the age of 3 months with clicky hips had a stable hip on dynamic ultrasound examination.

Imaging

X-ray

In a fixed irreducible hip dislocation, an X-ray of the pelvis in the AP view should be performed to assess the presence of teratologic dislocation.

Several parameters should be assessed on X-rays (Fig. 13.10).

Perkin's line is a vertical line at the superolateral margin of the acetabulum. Hilgenreiner's line is a horizontal line at the level of the triradiate cartilage.

Based on these two lines, the femoral head should be in the inferomedial quadrant. The presence of the femoral head in the superolateral quadrant indicates hip dysplasia.

Other parameters are illustrated in Fig. 13.11.

Acetabular index is normally less than 30° at age 1 year. Shenton's line is a continuous curve from the inferior border of the femoral neck to the inferior border of the superior pubic ramus. The centre-edge angle should be more than 25° in children older than 8 years.

Ultrasound

Ultrasound is used to document and monitor reduction. It is useful before the age of 6–8 months because it can identify the non-osseous part of the femoral head, the acetabulum and soft

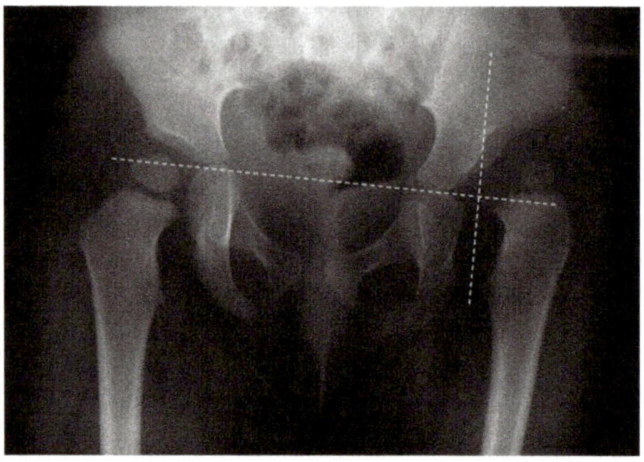

Fig. 13.10 A radiograph showing developmental dysplasia of the left hip. The femoral physis is lateral to Perkin's line (vertical line through the superior margin of the acetabulum) and superior to Hilgenreiner's line (horizontal line through the triradiate cartilage). The acetabular index is high and the Shenton's line is discontinuous

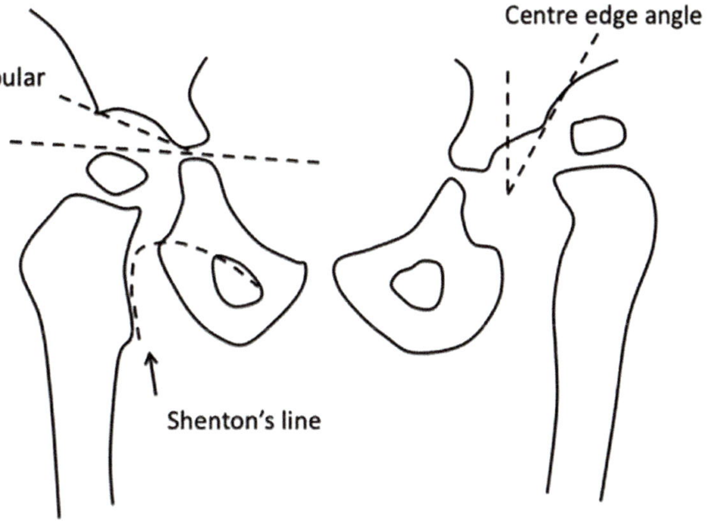

Fig. 13.11 Indicators of hip dysplasia

Table 13.6 Grading based on the static (Graf's) method

Type	Alpha angle	Description
I	>60°	Normal
II	43°–59°	Normal if age <3 months Indicates delayed ossification if age >3 months
III	<43°	Dislocation
IV	<43°	Dislocated with the labrum interposed between femoral head and acetabulum

tissue structures such as the labrum and capsule. It may, however, overdiagnose dysplasia.

In the static (Graf's) method, the hip is assessed in the coronal plane. A straight line of the ilium indicates the scan is through the centre of the acetabulum. The alpha angle is the angle between the outer cortex of the ilium and the bony acetabulum, and measures the depth of the acetabulum (Table 13.6 and Fig. 13.12). It should be more than 60° in children older than 3 months.

The beta angle reflects the cartilaginous roof and the position of the femoral head and should be less than 55°.

In the dynamic (Harcke's) method, measurement is performed in the transverse plane and the joint is stressed while imaging.

Arthrography

Arthrography is the gold standard. The 'rose-thorn sign' indicates the labrum is not interposed between the femoral head and the acetabulum. The medial pooling should be less than 5 mm and the image should demonstrate a deep concentric reduction.

Computed Tomography Scan

A computed tomography (CT) scan is useful to document a reduction in spica after open or closed reduction. A limited scan of the hip is sufficient to demonstrate reduction.

Magnetic Resonance Imaging

The role for MRI is uncertain at present.

Management

Closed Reduction with a Pavlik Harness

Closed reduction in a Pavlik harness is an option generally up to the age of 6 months, although it may be used satisfactorily up to 12 months. The harness works as a dynamic splint to maintain flexion and abduction. It can be used for a hip that is initially not reducible (negative Ortolani test), but this treatment must be abandoned if the hip does not reduce within 3 weeks.

Hip flexion is kept between 100° and 110°, and abduction between 50° and 70° (Safe zone of Ramsey). Excess abduction causes AVN, excess adduction can lead to dislocation and excess flexion can damage the femoral nerve. Reduction is confirmed by ultrasound and the patient should

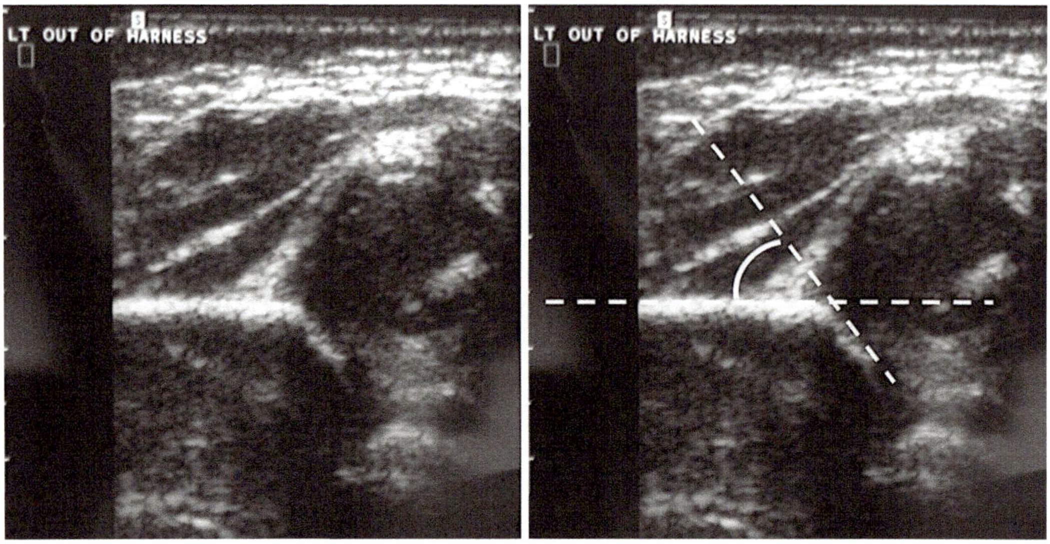

Fig. 13.12 Ultrasound image demonstrating the alpha angle. The image on the left shows the view obtained when the lateral cortex of the ilium appears as a straight line. The angle measurement is shown in the image on the right

be followed-up again after 1 week to ensure the parents can manage the harness effectively. Follow-up is with ultrasound every 4–6 weeks. The harness is worn continuously until the hip is stable, and this is checked on ultrasound. Bracing is continued part time until acetabular remodelling is complete.

Bracing is effective in 90% of patients and the risk of AVN is less than 5% if bracing is started within 6 weeks of birth. Teratologic hip is a contraindication for bracing. The following factors are associated with a poor prognosis:

- Bracing started after age 7 weeks.
- A negative Ortolani test.
- Bilateral hip involvement.

Nakamura J, Kamegaya M, Saisu T, et al. Treatment for developmental dysplasia of the hip using the Pavlik harness: long-term results. J Bone Joint Surg Br 2007;89:230–5. This study looked at 115 patients, with 130 complete dislocations of the hip, over 14 years of follow-up. A Pavlik harness was applied at age 1–12 months and the average duration was 6.1 months. Overall, 83% patients were treated with the harness alone and the rest required supplementary surgery. The outcome was satisfactory in 91.5% and AVN was seen in 12.3% of patients.

Closed Reduction in Traction

There is no evidence that traction is useful.

Closed Reduction with Hip Arthrography

Closed reduction with hip arthrography is performed under general anaesthetic and image intensifier control. A medial approach is used. Using the medial groin crease as a landmark, the needle entry site is posterior to the adductor longus. A spinal 22G needle is aimed towards the ipsilateral shoulder or iliac spine, keeping the needle parallel to the table (horizontal). Once in the joint, 2–4 mL of saline is injected. The saline should flow back. Needle placement is checked with an image intensifier, and then 1 mL of Omnipaque iohexol 240 mg/mL is injected.

The following are assessed on the arthrogram:

- The amount of medial pooling—should be less than 5 mm.
- Deep concentric reduction indicates the hip is congruent.

- Rose-thorn sign—indicates the labrum has folded outwards and is associated with a good prognosis.
- The safe zone (of abduction)—percutaneous tenotomy of the adductor longus can be performed to increase the safe zone.

Obstruction to closed reduction can be caused by several structures as illustrated in Fig. 13.13.

Reduction is acceptable when the limbus is not interposed and there is less than 5 mm contrast between the femoral head and the acetabulum.

Spica cast is applied in the human position: 90° flexion and 30°–60° abduction. Congruence is checked with a CT scan. Spica is continued for 4 months, changed every 6 weeks and followed by night-time abduction bracing.

Kiely N, Younis U, Day JB, Meadows TM. The Ferguson medial approach for open reduction of developmental dysplasia of the hip. A clinical and radiological review of 49 hips. J Bone Joint Surg Br 2004;86:430–3. This study looked at 49 hips in patients aged 6–23 months, with a 4-year follow-up. Three redislocations occurred. AVN in Kalamchi and MacEwen group I was seen in four hips, group II in two hips and group III in one hip.

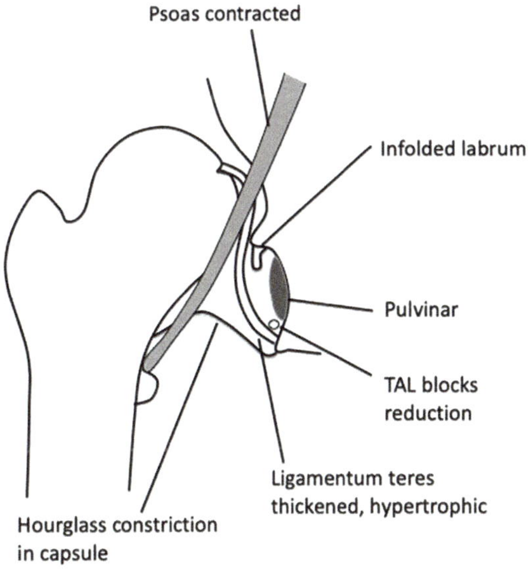

Fig. 13.13 Structure obstructing reduction of femoral head

Open Reduction

Open reduction is indicated where reduction is non-concentric.

Open reduction in the anterior approach can be performed at any age. It gives versatile, excellent exposure. Capsulorrhaphy and pelvic osteotomies can be performed through same approach. A bikini incision is made from middle of the iliac crest, centred on the anterior superior iliac spine. The interval between the sartorius and the TFL (tensor fascia lata) is developed. The lateral femoral cutaneous nerve is protected and retracted medially.

The iliac apophysis is split. The sartorius is divided and retracted distally. The psoas tendon is recessed. Tenotomy of the rectus femoris is performed 1 cm distal to the anterior inferior iliac spine and the muscle is retracted distally. A T-capsulotomy is performed excising the ligamentum teres. Multiple T incisions are made in the hypertrophied labrum. Excision of the labrum may damage the lateral acetabular physis, resulting in dysplasia. The deep transverse acetabular ligament is divided and fat cleared from the acetabulum.

If the femoral head is stable, a double breast of the capsule is performed, suturing the lateral flap as far medially as possible. A postoperative CT scan will confirm reduction in spica.

The medial (Ludloff) approach is applicable for infants aged less than 1 year. If capital epiphysis is not seen on X-rays, a higher risk of AVN is present. There is no access to the labrum and capsulorrhaphy cannot be performed.

The anteromedial approach goes anterior to the adductor brevis, while the posteromedial approach is posterior to the adductor brevis.

The transverse incision is centred over the adductor longus. The adductor longus is divided. The plane of dissection is anterior to the adductor brevis, protecting the anterior division of the obturator nerve. The iliopsoas is divided, taking care to avoid damage to medial circumflex femoral artery.

Femoral Shortening

Femoral shortening is required in children older than 2 years. A lateral approach is used and the amount of overlap of the femur indicates the degree of resection. Excess anteversion and varus can be corrected and the osteotomy is fixed with a plate and screws.

In children older than 3 years, open reduction, femoral osteotomy and redirectional pelvic osteotomy can be performed simultaneously with good results. There is no increase in the risk of AVN.

Pelvic Osteotomy

Pelvic osteotomies are considered in children older than 3 years. Acetabular remodelling is highest in those younger than 4 years, unpredictable between 4 and 8 years and non-existent in those older than 8 years. Maximal remodelling occurs within 1 year of hip reduction.

Pelvic osteotomy improves contact and reduces point loading. Osteotomies can be redirectional, reshaping or salvage.

Redirectional procedures involve complete cuts through the innominate and fixation in a corrected position (Table 13.7). These are Salter's, Steel and Ganz osteotomies.

Reshaping can be with the Pemberton or Dega procedures (Table 13.8). These aim to improve the shape of the acetabulum by hinging the superior half of the acetabulum on the triradiate cartilage.

Salvage Procedures

An extra-articular buttress of bone is fashioned over the subluxed femoral head. These rely on fibrocartilaginous metaplasia of the joint capsule. Examples of salvage procedures are Chiari osteotomy and Staheli shelf osteotomy (Table 13.9)

Macnicol MF, Lo HK, Yong KF. Pelvic remodelling after the Chiari osteotomy. A long-term review. J Bone Joint Surg Br 2004;86:648–54. This study involved a long-term follow-up of 215 Chiari osteotomies at a mean of 18 years after surgery (range 5–30 years). Only 20% of procedures were converted to a total hip arthroplasty. The centre-edge angle improved from 2.5° to 41.8° postoperatively, and was maintained at 38.5° on follow-up. Remodelling did not reverse the medialisation produced by the osteotomy.

Complications

Failed reduction is generally due to inadequate capsular release or inadequate capsulorrhaphy, and a repeat open reduction. Poorer results and higher rates of AVN are seen with repeat attempts at reduction.

AVN can occur with any treatment method and the incidence is same for open or closed treatment. It is caused by compression of the vascular supply due to excessive abduction or repeat surgery.

Radiological evidence of avascular necrosis:

- Failure of appearance of the ossific nucleus within 1 year.
- Increased radiographic density and fragmentation.
- Deformity of the femoral head and neck.
- Broadening of the femoral neck.

The changes may involve part or all of the femoral head. Kalamchi and MacEwen proposed a classification system for avascular changes (Table 13.10).

Kalamchi A, MacEwen GD. Avascular necrosis following treatment of congenital dislocation of the hip. J Bone Joint Surg Am 1980;62:876–88. Classification of avascular changes.

Treatment options of avascular necrosis include proximal femoral varus osteotomy, trochanteric epiphysiodesis and distal transfer of the trochanter.

Table 13.7 Redirectional pelvic osteotomies

Salter osteotomy-Ideal for providing anterolateral coverage Provides 20°–25° lateral and 10°–15° anterior coverage Hinges on the pubic symphysis	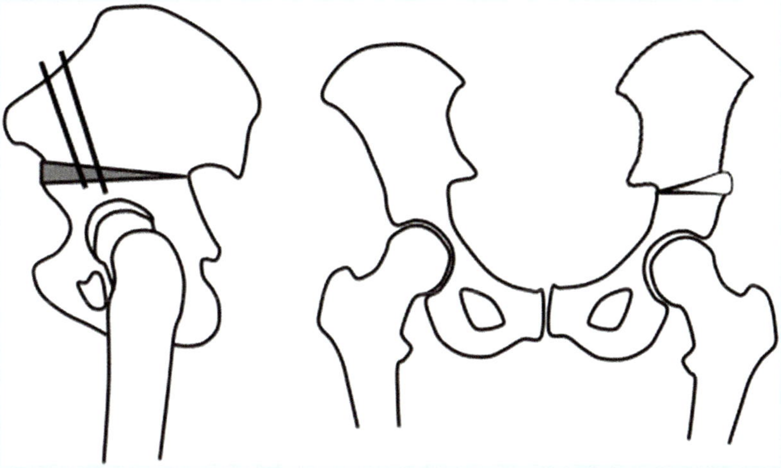
Steel osteotomy—Used in older (beyond 8 years of age) patients with limited mobility of the pubic symphysis This is a triple osteotomy.	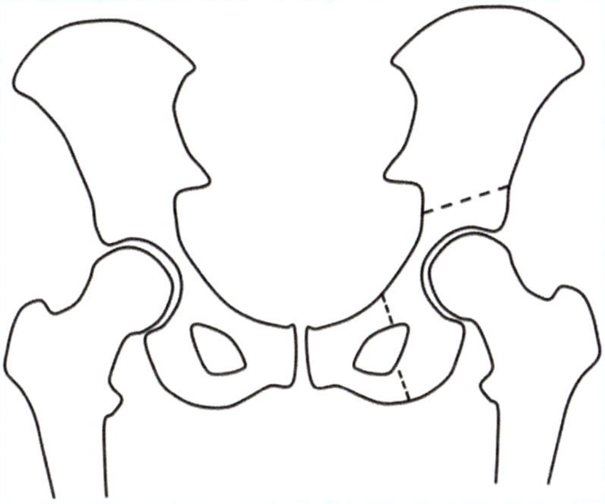
Ganz periacetabular osteotomy This is an osteotomy of all three bones and vertical osteotomy of the posterior column The osteotomy is inherently stable as the posterior column is intact A periacetabular osteotomy is contraindicated if the triradiate cartilage is open Technically, this is a demanding procedure	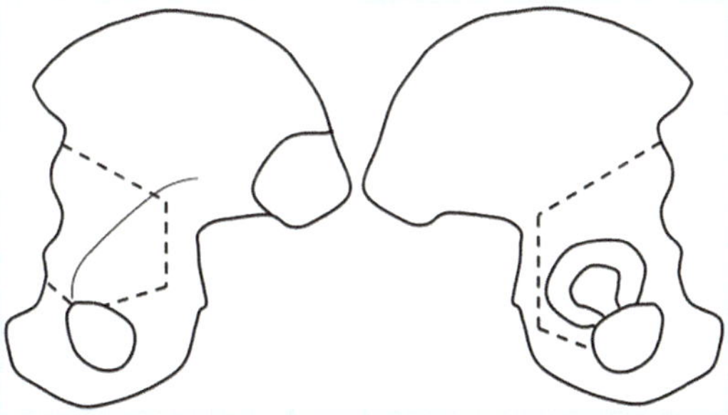

Table 13.8 Reshaping pelvic osteotomies

Pemberton osteotomy Incomplete extracapsular cuts are made 1 cm above the joint capsule This can be performed in the age range of 2–10 years This helps to decrease the volume of the acetabulum Both the outer and inner table of the ilium are cut, beginning 5 mm above the joint capsule	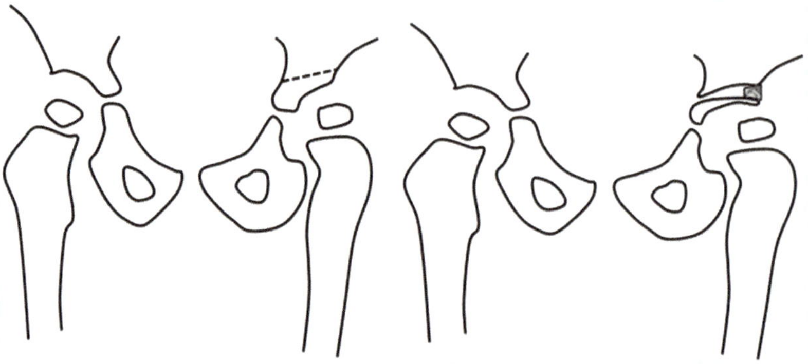
Dega The osteotomy is through the outer table of ilium only	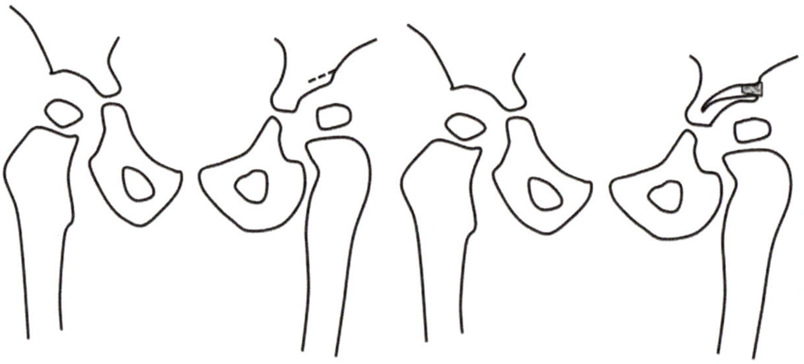

Table 13.9 Salvage procedures for DDH

Chiari osteotomy The ilium is divided inclined cephalad 20° through both outer and inner surfaces The osteotomy is between the joint capsule and the reflected head of the rectus The acetabulum is displaced medially	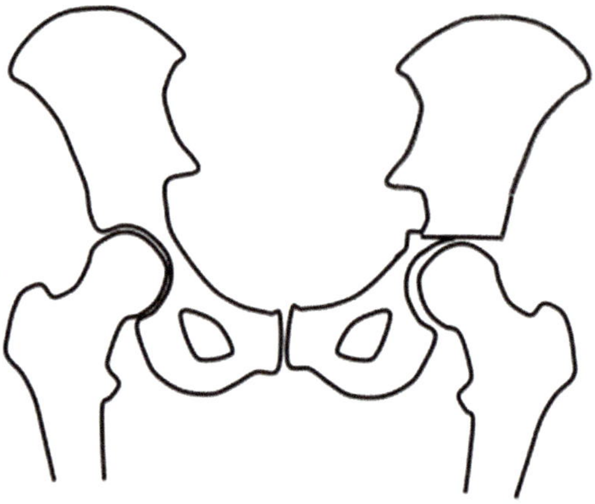

Table 13.9 (continued)

Staheli's shelf augmentation
A corticocancellous bone shelf is made over the femoral head
It relies on fibrocartilaginous change between the femoral head and the bone graft

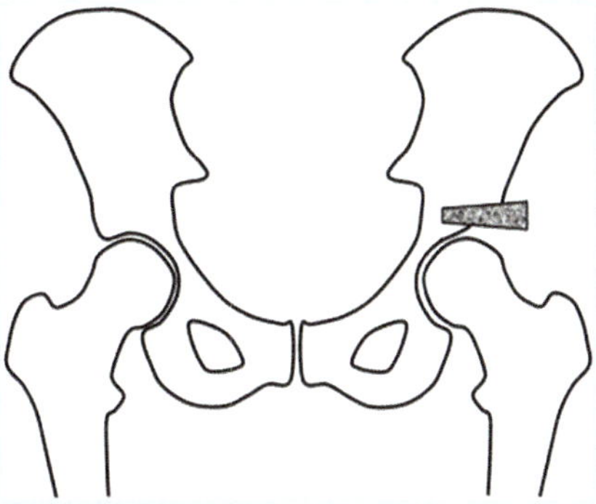

Table 13.10 Kalamchi and MacEwen classification for AVN hip in DDH

Group I	Change affects the ossific nucleus
Group II	Lateral physeal damage
Group III	Central physeal damage
Group IV	Total damage to the head and physis

Clinical Decision Scenarios

Scenario 1

Newborn with hip positive for Ortolani test (hip is dislocated but reducible)
↓
Pavlik harness
↓
Re examine at 2 weeks to ensure hip is reduced
↓
Discontinue brace when hip is stable

Scenario 2

Newborn with hip positive for Barlow test (hip is unstable)
↓
Review with ultrasound scan at 6 weeks
↓
Hip stable — no treatment
Hip unstable — Pavlik harness, as in Scenario 1

Scenario 3

3 month old with a stable hip but reduced alpha angle on scan
↓
No treatment needed
X ray at 6 months

Scenario 4

6 month old with a dislocated hip

↓

Examination Under Anaesthesia, arthrogram ± adductor tenotomy

↓

Spica for 4 months

Change every 6 – 8 weeks

Scenario 5

6 month old with a subluxed hip

↓

As for Scenario 4

Consider a Denis Browne splint

Scenario 6

6 month old with dysplasia

↓

X ray in 6 months

↓

Consider Salter's osteotomy at age 4 or 5 years

Scenario 7

1 year old with a dislocated hip

↓

EUA, arthrogram, adductor tenotomy / open reduction and spica

Scenario 8

2 years or older with a dislocated hip

↓

EUA, arthrogram, adductor tenotomy / open reduction and spica

Femoral osteotomy

Scenario 9

8 year old with a dislocated hip

↓

EUA, arthrogram, adductor tenotomy, femoral osteotomy, Salter's osteotomy and spica for 2 months

Scenario 10

12 year old with dysplasia

↓

Consider a periacetabular or triple osteotomy or observe

If painful, perform an osteotomy

If painless, an operation is controversial

Slipped Upper Femoral Epiphysis

Epidemiology

A slipped upper femoral epiphysis (SUFE or SCFE—slipped capital femoral epiphysis) is more common in boys and Polynesian and Afro-Caribbean children. There is a link with obesity, and more than 60% of affected children are over the 90th percentile for weight. SCFE is also linked to short stature and delayed growth-plate closure.

SUFE is disruption of the proximal femoral growth plate. Pedantically, the epiphysis stays in place, it is the metaphysis which displaces.

Presentation is usually between the ages of 9 and 16 years.

Aetiology

The development of SUFE is multifactorial. Possible contributory factors include mechanical factors and hormonal influences (Table 13.11).

Pathophysiology

The slip occurs due to failure at the junction of the zone of hypertrophy and the zone of provisional calcification. A wide physis, deep acetabulum and increased retroversion increase stress across the physis. Interconnections of chondrocytes provide resistance to shear. Thinning of the perichondrial ring of la Croix is considered as a contributing factor to the occurrence of slip.

Clinical Features

Fifteen percent of patients have pain in the distal thigh and knee only, while 22% have bilateral slip. In bilateral slip, 60% patients have a simultaneous slip while the remaining present with symptoms on the other side in the following 18–24 months.

Acute slip is defined as one with less than 3 weeks of symptoms. 85% of slips are chronic, implying more than 3 weeks' duration. Chronic slip presents as an out-turning of the affected leg. Acute-on-chronic slip is diagnosed when there is a sudden change in pain with a chronic slip.

The Loder classification divides SUFE into stable or unstable. An unstable slip is present if the child is unable to bear weight. In a stable slip, the child can walk with or without crutches.

Table 13.11 Etiological factors for SUFE

Mechanical factors	Hormonal influences
The orientation of the physis changes from horizontal to more oblique in early adolescence.	Increased levels of growth hormone stimulate widening of the physis
Increased femoral retroversion causes more stress across the physis	Testosterone stimulates widening and then closure of the physis
Normal femoral anteversion is about 10°. In obese children, it has been reported to be as low as 0.4°.	Estrogen stimulates closure of the physis Thyroid hormone, vitamin D and calcium are also needed for closure
A deeper acetabulum may play a role. The centre-edge angle of Wiberg is 37° in children with SUFE compared with 33° in unaffected children	Hypothyroidism Hypogonadism Renal osteodystrophy Klinefelter syndrome

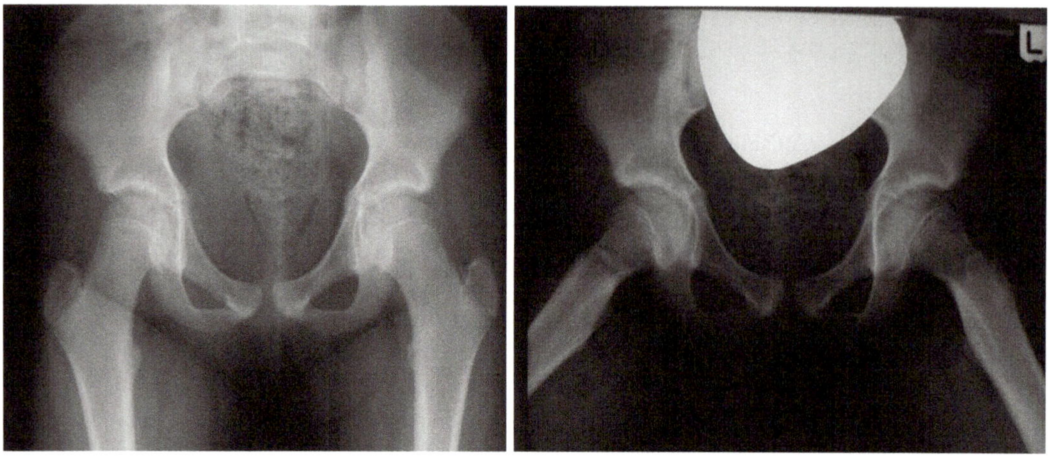

Fig. 13.14 Radiographs showing left sided SUFE. The anteroposterior view of the pelvis (left) does not show an obvious slip, while the frog-leg lateral view in the same patient (right) shows the mild slip

There is a 50% risk of osteonecrosis in unstable SUFE, compared to 4% in stable SUFE.

'Preslip' is mild hip pain with no radiologic slip.

On physical examination, children will experience pain on internal rotation. There is decreased hip flexion and internal rotation. On flexing the hip, there is an increase in external rotation. All children presenting with knee pain should also have a hip examination to rule out SUFE.

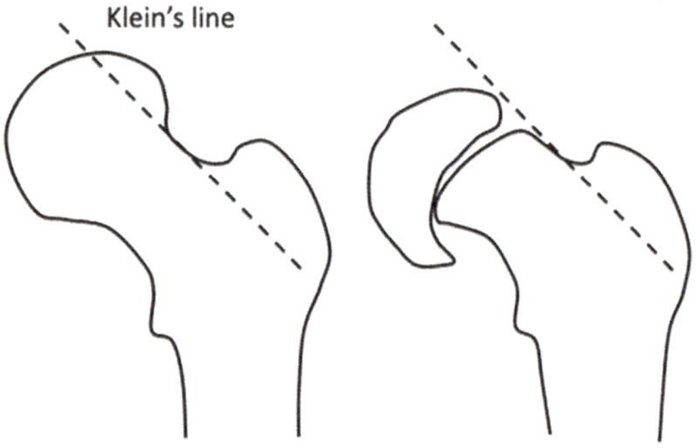

Fig. 13.15 Trethowan's sign on radiograph of the hip

Imaging

In an early slip, widening of the physis on AP radiograph and periphyseal irregularity may be the only abnormalities (Fig. 13.14). A frog leg view should always be obtained.

Klein's line is drawn along the superior border of the femoral neck (Fig. 13.15). In a normal hip, it should intersect with the lateral edge of the epiphysis. If the line passes lateral to the epiphysis (Trethowan's sign), it indicates slipped physis. Steel's sign is density in the femoral neck due to overlap on the slipped physis. The ischium normally overlaps the femoral neck metaphysis. Loss of this overlap is known as Scham's sign.

Southwick method is to measure the head shaft angle on AP and lateral views (Figs. 13.16 and 13.17). The normal angle is 145°. A difference between 2 sides of 30° is mild slip, 30°–60° is moderate slip and over 60° difference is a severe slip. On the lateral view, the normal angle is 10°.

In later stages, new bone formation at the medial edge of the physis and rounding off of the exposed superior edge may be evident.

The accuracy of imaging for diagnosis on AP view radiograph is 66%, and increases to 80% with addition of a frog-leg lateral view.

Ultrasound scan is 95% sensitive while an MR is diagnostic.

Grading of Slip Severity

The severity is graded as shown in Table 13.12.

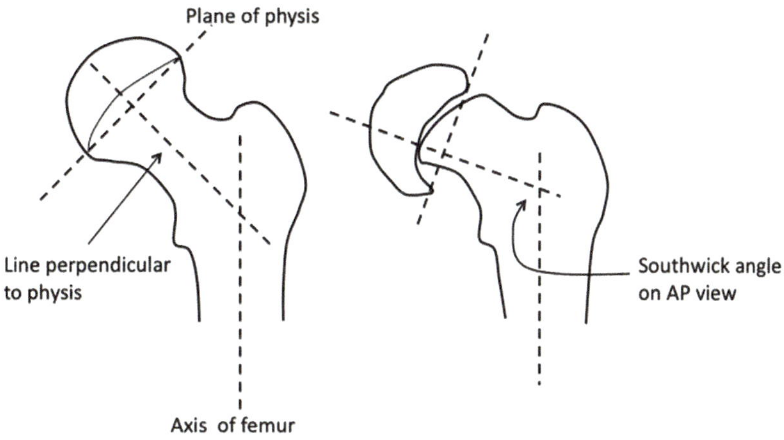

Fig. 13.16 Southwick angle on AP view

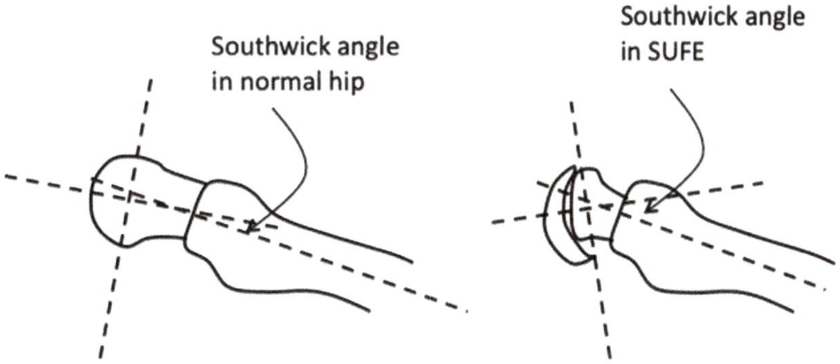

Fig. 13.17 Southwick angle on lateral view

Table 13.12 Grading of slipped capital femoral epiphysis

Factor	Grade of slip	Description
Absolute displacement	–	Complete displacement of the physis
Percentage epiphyseal displacement	Mild	Displacement is less than third of the neck width
	Moderate	Displacement is a third to a half of the neck width
	Severe	Displacement is more than half of the neck width
Slip angle on frog-leg lateral view	Mild	Slip angle <30°
	Moderate	Slip angle 30°–50°
	Severe	Slip angle >50°

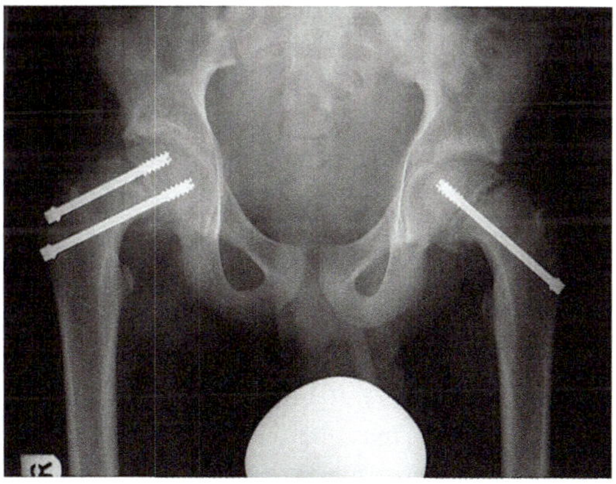

Fig. 13.18 A mild slip on the left side treated with a single partially threaded screw. Moderate slip on the right has been managed with two screws

Management

The immediate management of mild and moderate SUFE slipped upper femoral epiphysis is *in situ* pinning. A single partially threaded cancellous screw is used to stabilise the slip and prevent progression (Fig. 13.18). The location of the screw is marked preoperatively by triangulation and is inserted percutaneously. The screw should

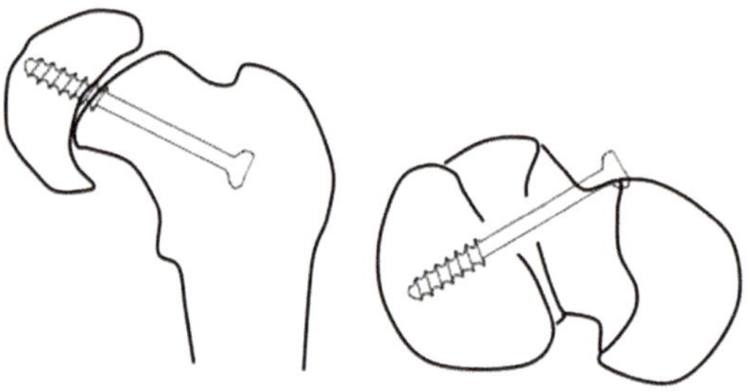

Fig. 13.19 Screw placement in SUFE

be at least 5 mm from subchondral bone and perpendicular to the epiphysis. The posterosuperior quadrant of the femoral head should be avoided as this may damage the lateral epiphyseal artery, causing AVN. Brodetti demonstrated that a central placement of the screw is ideal to avoid injuring this vessel.

The screw often has to be inserted from the front of the neck so as to be perpendicular to the plane of the physis (Fig. 13.19). Entry from the lateral cortex of femoral shaft will not provide adequate fixation in the physis and there will be risk of head penetration.

Transient pin penetration does not cause damage, but the screw should not penetrate into the hip joint. The screw position is checked thoroughly by rotating the image intensifier. An arthrogram can be conducted through the cannulated screw to confirm articular cartilage has not been penetrated. Alternatively, a postoperative CT scan will show the exact screw position.

Transient penetration of the hip during in situ cannulated—screw fixation of slipped capital femoral epiphysis. Zionts LE et al. J Bone Joint Surg am 1991;73(7):1054–60.

Two screws may be used for severe slip (Fig. 13.18). This gives a 33% increase in shear resistance but a tenfold increase in the complication rate.

The traditional view is that the slip should not be reduced prior to fixation. Serendipitous reduction while positioning on the operating table does not adversely affect the outcome. In severe slip, however, reduction may be attempted in specialist units. This aims to minimise the abnormal morphology of the femoral head and avoid problems due to impingement in adulthood.

Peterson MD, Weiner DS, Green NE, Terry CL. Acute slipped capital femoral epiphysis: the value and safety of urgent manipulative reduction. J Pediatr Orthop 1997;17:648–54. AVN was 7% with reductions performed within 24 h of symptoms and 20% with reductions performed after 24 h.

Carney BT, Birnbaum P, Minter C. Slip progression after in situ single screw fixation for stable slipped capital femoral epiphysis. J Pediatr Orthop 2003;23:584–9. Slip progresses if fewer than five screw threads are in the epiphysis

O'Brien ET, Fahey JJ. Remodeling of the femoral neck after in situ pinning for slipped capital femoral epiphysis. J Bone Joint Surg Am 1977;59:62–8. This study reported on the remodelling potential of the proximal femur in SCFE. The proximal femur remodels and range of motion improves after pinning, but the hip develops arthritis earlier and arthroplasty is needed.

Moderate and severe slips lead to degenerative disease. If the patient presents within 24 h then gentle manipulation can be attempted. If not, skin traction is applied for 3 weeks and may reduce the slip to a mild slip, which allows pinning in situ. If the patient remains a high grade slip, then osteotomy should be considered.

Screw removal is advisable, although practices vary in different units. This is sometimes difficult and a reverse cutting thread on the screw, or a fully threaded screw makes removal easier. Removal is done after skeletal maturity.

Reconstructive Osteotomies

Severe slips lead to a metaphyseal bony prominence. This can be removed through open or arthroscopic methods—known as osteoplasty. This reduces the incidence of impingement.

Osteotomy to correct the deformity is an option in severe slip.

Huber H et al. Adolescent slipped capital femoral epiphysis treated by a modified Dunn osteotomy with surgical hip dislocation. J Bone Joint Surg Br 2010;93(6):833–8. 30 hips, 3.8 years follow up. Anatomical or near anatomical reduction achieved in all cases. One avascular necrosis.

Carney BT, Weinstein SL, Noble J. Long-term follow-up of slipped capital femoral epiphysis. J Bone Joint Surg Am 1991;73:667–74.

Uglow MG, Clarke NM. The management of slipped capital femoral epiphysis. J Bone Joint Surg Br 2004;86:631–5.

In severe slips, the area of contact decreases and the chances of vascular injury increase with pinning. There may therefore be a role for subcapital osteotomy (Dunn or Fish osteotomy), basal neck (Kramer) or intertrochanteric osteotomy (Southwick or Imhauser) (Fig. 13.20). The subcapital osteotomy removes a wedge of bone just distal to the physeal plate. The femoral head is reduced onto the neck and stabilised with screws. Subcapital cuneiform osteotomy has a 20–35% risk of AVN.

Fish JB. Cuneiform osteotomy of the femoral neck in the treatment of slipped capital femoral epiphysis. J Bone Joint Surg Am 1984;66:1153–68. Fish reported a 4.5% rate of AVN with cuneiform osteotomy.

Base of neck osteotomy is best for moderate deformities. The degree of correction is limited, but the risk of AVN and chondrolysis is less than with subcapital cuneiform osteotomy.

Intertrochanteric (Southwick) osteotomy carries a 10% risk of AVN. The osteotomy can be fixed internally. The aim is a triplane correction, with valgus, flexion and internal rotation of the distal fragment. Imhauser is a two plane correction with flexion and internal rotation of the distal fragment.

The ability to correct the deformity is highest with subcapital osteotomy, but the risk of AVN is highest as well. With intertrochanteric osteotomy, the risk of AVN is low, and ability to correct is lower as well.

The Berne unit (reference below) has described a capital reorientation procedure through a surgical dislocation approach for patients with moderate and severe slip.

Ziebarth K, Zilkens C, Spencer S, et al. Capital realignment for moderate and severe SCFE using a modified Dunn procedure. Clin Orthop Relat Res 2009;467:704–16. Forty patients underwent capital realignment and were followed for 1–3 years. No patient had osteonecrosis or chondrolysis. The slip angle was corrected to 4°–8°. Articular cartilage damage, full-thickness loss and delamination were observed at the time of surgery.

Management of the Contralateral Hip

If the hip is clinically and radiologically normal, simple observation is advised. Fixation is advised if the slip is associated with renal osteodystrophy, endocrine abnormality, or if there are x ray changes. If symptomatic, fixation is advised.

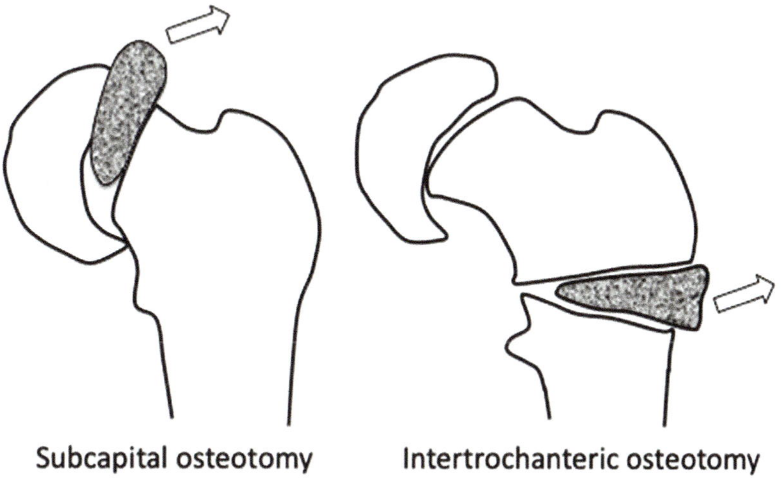

Fig. 13.20 Reconstructive osteotomies for severe SUFE

Long Term Outcomes

Internal fixation helps alleviate the pain. The deformity of the proximal femur persists and results in an externally rotated leg. Patients with mild slips have good long-term results. The presence of an angular deformity at the neck leads to impingement and there is an increasing trend towards hip arthroscopy to alleviate this.

Fraitzl CR, Käfer W, Nelitz M, Reichel H. Radiological evidence of femoroacetabular impingement in mild slipped capital femoral epiphysis: a mean follow-up of 14.4 years after pinning in situ. J Bone Joint Surg Br 2007;89:1592–6. Mild slip was fixed in situ in 16 patients. All hips were abnormal radiologically. None of the hips had a normal head—neck ration and average alpha angle was 86 degrees in AP view and 55° in lateral cross table view.

Complications

Chondrolysis is acute arthritis of unknown aetiology characterised by the rapid loss of articular cartilage. It can also occur after fracture, infection or inflammatory conditions, or after spica for SUFE, severe slip, or fracture. Penetration of the head while pinning is associated with increased risk. Patients present with hip pain and adduction contracture, and radiographs show reduced joint space and juxta-articular osteoporosis. Histologically, there is non-specific cartilage necrosis and joint synovitis. Treatment is with range of motion exercises and non-steroidal anti-inflammatory drugs (NSAIDs). Chondrolysis may improve over time but usually causes stiffness and pain. Half of all patients have a poor prognosis.

The risk of AVN is 50% in unstable SCFE and 3% in chronic SCFE. Incidental reduction of SCFE does not increase the risk. AVN presents with recurrence of hip pain several months after SCFE. The treatment plan relies on rest, NSAIDs and crutches. AVN may require an osteotomy or arthrodesis.

Pathologic fracture through the metalwork site is rarely seen.

Approximately 10% patients develop osteoarthritis of the hip and a pistol-grip-shaped femoral head is found in 40% patients. Remodelling of up to 60° can occur in SCFE.

Congenital Pseudarthrosis of the Tibia

Epidemiology

The prevalence of congenital pseudarthrosis of the tibia is about one in 200,000 live births. Most cases (50–70%) are associated with neurofibromatosis type 1, while 10% of patients with neurofibromatosis type 1 have pseudarthrosis of the tibia.

Clinical Features

Pseudarthrosis of the tibia manifests as a short leg with an anterior bow in the distal third evident at birth. Rarely, it is bilateral. Café-au-lait spots or neurofibromas may be present. The foot is in a calcaneus position.

Differential Diagnosis

The differential diagnosis includes fibrous dysplasia, osteogenesis imperfecta, rickets and campomelic dysplasia.

Classification

Boyd's classification is used (Fig. 13.21).

Management

Prior to Fracture

An ankle–foot orthosis or an onlay graft can be considered. Realignment osteotomy should not be performed due to an extremely high risk of non-union.

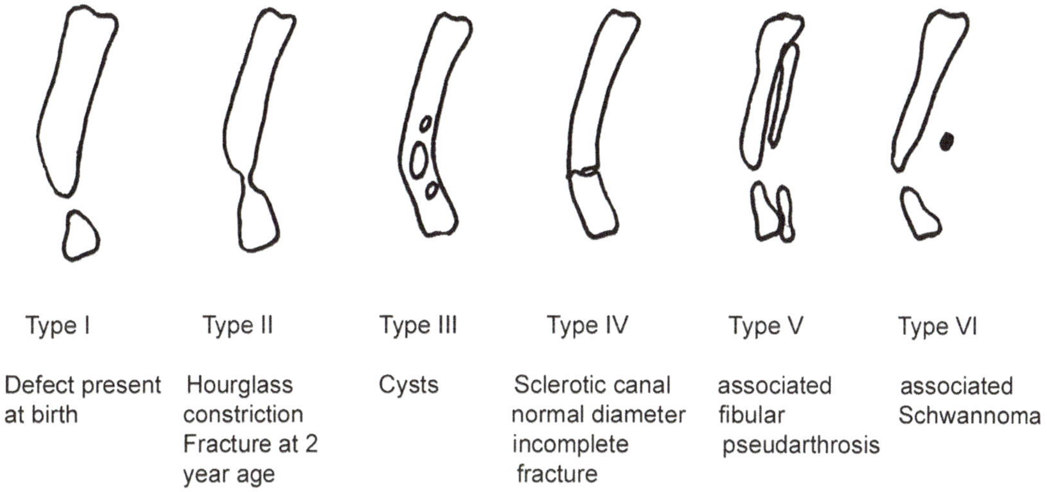

Fig. 13.21 Boyd classification for congenital pseudarthrosis of the tibia

Post Fracture

Resection, bone grafting and Williams intramedullary telescoping nail has 90% success. A rod can be inserted retrograde through the foot if the distal fragment is small.

Free fibular grafting using contralateral normal fibula is an option. There is a risk of refracture with this.

Ring fixators (Ilizarov or Taylor Spatial frame) can achieve union in up to 80% of patients. They correct angulation and restore length. However, risk of refracture remains.

Below-knee or Syme's amputation can be considered for failed reconstructions. The Syme's amputation makes use of the heel pad for weight bearing as the calf musculature and tissues are often poor quality in these patients.

Bone grafting and plating has almost a 100% failure rate.

Boero S, Catagni M, Donzelli O, et al. Congenital pseudarthrosis of the tibia associated with neurofibromatosis-1: treatment with Ilizarov device. J Pediatr Orthop 1997;17:675–84. In 21 patients treated with Ilizarov external fixator, 66% had good results at 2 years or more after the treatment. The prognosis was better for children aged 5 years or older.

Spire AS et al. Combined treatment of congenital pseudarthrosis of the tibia including recombinant human bone morphogenetic protein 2: a case series. J Bone Joint Surg Br 2011;93(5):695–9. Five patient, mean age 7.4 years treated by intramedullary rod, rhBMP-2 and four had additional Ilizarov fixator. All healed within 3.5 months.

Congenital Posteromedial Bow of the Tibia

Congenital posteromedial bow is a benign condition compared to anterolateral bowing of the tibia.

Aetiology

It is thought to be a 'uterine packing disorder' caused by the position of the foetus in the uterus.

Clinical Features

The foot is in a calcaneovalgus position with excessive dorsiflexion. The posteromedial bow is at the junction of the middle and distal one third of the tibia. The condition is almost always unilateral.

Differential Diagnosis

Calcaneovalgus foot has no tibial bow and resolves spontaneously.

Fibular hemimelia has a valgus limb but less ankle dorsiflexion. There may be hypoplasia of the lateral rays of the foot.

Distal motor paresis (L5 myelomeningocele)—a dorsiflexed foot, but the tibia is straight.

In congenital vertical talus, the deformity is at the midfoot.

Imaging

The bones have a normal appearance with no sclerosis of the canal. There may be some cortical thickening on the concave cortex.

Management

The natural course is spontaneous correction before the age of 2 years in 50% of patients. If correction does not occur by the age of 4 years then it is unlikely to correct spontaneously thereafter. Patients may have limb shortening of up to 4 cm at skeletal maturity.

Patients without spontaneous correction should be followed-up and undergo epiphysiodesis for limb-length discrepancy. Limb lengthening should be performed with deformity correction.

Blount's Disease

Blount's disease is characterised by reduced growth at the medial and posterior aspects of the proximal tibial physis resulting in abrupt angulation of the medial proximal tibial metaphysis.

It is associated with obesity, female gender and Afro-Caribbean ethnicity. The family history is positive in up to 40% patients. Histologically, there is disordered endochondral ossification.

Clinical Features

Children present with internal tibial torsion, shortening of tibia and pronation of the feet. There is a progressive varus deformity of the knee.

In normal physiological development, the knees have varus alignment at birth and become neutral at age 18 months. A physiological valgus develops at 30–36 months. Varus that persists at the age of 24 months indicates genu varum deformity.

The varus angulation in Blount's disease is sharp and there may be a varus thrust while walking. This thrust is absent in physiological bowing.

Differential Diagnosis

- Physiologic bowing—bowing occurs both in the femur and tibia.
- Rickets.
- Osteomyelitis.
- Trauma.
- Ollier's disease.
- Focal fibrocartilaginous dysplasia—shows indentation on the medial side of the tibia at the junction of the metaphysis and diaphysis. It improves spontaneously.

Imaging

Imaging is of the lower limb with the hip and ankle on the same plate (long-leg view). The radiographic features are:

- Beaking of the medial wall with a straight lateral cortex.
- Drennan angle is between a line joining the metaphyseal beaks and the long axis of the tibia (Fig. 13.22). It represents the metaphyseal–diaphyseal angle, and an angle of more than 16° is diagnostic for Blount's. Six-

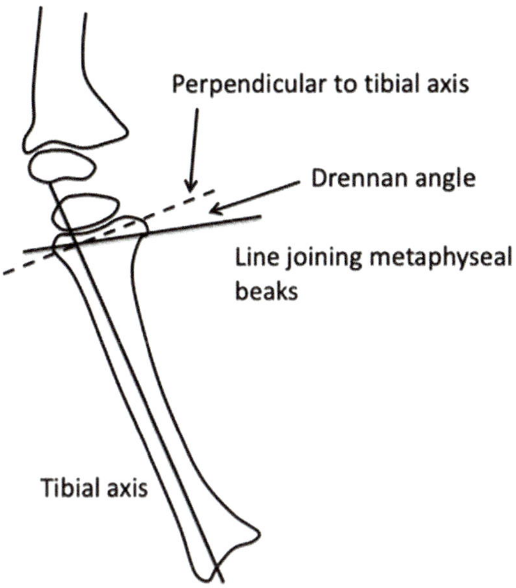

Fig. 13.22 Drennan angle

monthly monitoring is advised with an angle of 11°–16°.

- The upper tibial epiphysis slopes medially, while the physeal plate is narrow medially and wide laterally.

Classification

Three types are recognised:

- Infantile, age under 3 years.
- Juvenile, ages 3–8 years.
- Adolescent, age over 8 years.

The infantile form has a similar appearance to physiologic bowing. However, in physiologic bowing the varus occurs equally in the distal femur and proximal tibia.

Infantile Blount's disease is bilateral in 60% of patients and will sometimes resolve spontaneously. The adolescent type is usually unilateral and may be associated with femoral varus.

Langenskiold proposed six radiological stages. The first stage is seen around age 2–3 years and stage 6 corresponds to changes at puberty. Stage 6 has a bony bar and a vertical tibial physis.

Langenskiold A. Tibia vara. A critical review. Clin Orthop 1989;246:195–207.

Management

Bracing is effective for infantile disease in Langenskiold stage I to II. It is advised if the metaphyseal-diaphyseal angle (Drennan angle) is more than 16°. Bracing is also advised if the Drennan angle is more than 11° in the presence of female sex, obesity, progression or laxity. The brace is a knee–ankle foot orthosis worn during weight bearing. The efficacy of bracing is 65–90%.

Richards BS, Katz DE, Sims JB. Effectiveness of brace treatment in early infantile Blount's disease. J Pediatr Orthop 1998;18:374–80. Bracing was effective in 65% of 37 stage II limbs.

Tibial osteotomy is indicated for progressive deformity. An oblique or dome osteotomy can be performed. Overcorrection is performed to 5°–10° of valgus. Osteotomy should be performed before the age of 4 years; there is a high risk of recurrence after this point.

Chotigavanichaya C, Salinas G, Green T, et al. Recurrence of varus deformity after proximal tibial osteotomy in Blount disease: long-term follow-up. J Pediatr Orthop 2002;22:638–41. Children under the age of 4 years had lower recurrence of varus after corrective osteotomy.

For stage IV disease or higher, a MRI scan is performed to view the medial bar. If the bar is present, it should be excised or an epiphysiodesis performed on the lateral side to avoid recurrent deformity. The effectiveness of epiphysiodesis is questionable and this should be used only for mild deformities.

An external fixator and hemicallotasis is useful for those with moderate to severe deformity.

Lateral hemiepiphysiodesis can be performed in adolescents, if sufficient growth remains. The growth of the medial side is unpredictable.

The use of external fixation—like an Ilizarov ring fixator or a Taylor spatial frame allows correction of the deformity without compromising bone length.

Internal Torsion of the Tibia or Femur

Torsional deformities of the lower limb are generally due to uterine molding and resolve with time.

After formation of limb buds, the upper limb undergoes external rotation and the lower limb undergoes internal rotation *in utero* at 8 weeks. Abnormal rotation in this phase causes torsional abnormalities.

Internal torsion results in in-toeing. With the child standing erect with patella facing forward, the feet will turn inward. The reverse is seen with external tibial torsion.

Clinical Features

The following features should be assessed:

- Hip rotation in a prone position. Internal rotation of more than 70° indicates medial *femoral* torsion.
- Foot progression angle. This is the angle between the long axis of foot and line of walking. Internal torsion of femur or tibia will lead to internal rotation of the foot.
- Thigh–foot angle. This is the angle between the axis of the foot and the longitudinal axis of the thigh. It is best assessed in the prone position with the knee bent to 90°. The foot points medially in newborns and gradually achieves a 10° lateral thigh–foot angle. The thigh foot angle indicates *tibial* torsion; and deviation from the normal is a measure of the severity of deformity.

In persistent femoral anteversion, the patella point inwards when the child is standing with the feet parallel to each other. There is increased internal rotation of the hip with a consequent reduction in external rotation. Secondary tibial torsion may be present in these children.

Ryder test measures the rotational angle (anteversion) of the femur. In the prone position with the knee flexed, the leg is rotated until the greater trochanter is felt prominently. The angle between the leg and the horizontal indicates the angle of femoral anteversion.

Imaging

CT scans provide the most accurate measurement of rotational alignment.

Management

The femoral deformity usually corrects with age. Derotation femoral osteotomy is indicated for deformities that persist after the age of 10 years. The osteotomy can be performed at the subtrochanteric, diaphyseal or supracondylar level. An excessive (>35°) external rotation deformity of the tibia will be accentuated while correcting internal rotation of the femur, and this should be taken into consideration.

Tibial torsion also tends to resolve with age. Supramalleolar osteotomy is required in patients with a medial thigh–foot angle of more than 10° or a lateral thigh–foot angle of more than 35°.

Fibular Hemimelia

Fibular hemimelia is longitudinal deficiency of the fibula. It can be partial or complete.

Associated Conditions

- Proximal femoral focal deficiency.
- Absence of cruciate ligaments.
- Equinovarus foot.
- Ball-and-socket ankle.
- Tarsal coalition.
- Absence of lateral rays of the foot.

Imaging

Standard radiographs are diagnostic.

Management

Management is based on correcting the deformity and equalising the leg-length discrepancy. Prosthetics allow optimum mobility.

Genu Varum and Valgum

Angular deformities at the knee are common in children. Genu varum and valgum present as transient physiologic changes in knee alignment.

The alignment of the knee is varus at birth and becomes neutral by the age of 18 months. There is an increase in valgus up to the age of 3 years, after which the alignment returns to physiologic valgus (Fig. 13.23). This pattern of development was first proposed by Salenius.

Salenius P, Vankka E. The development of the tibiofemoral angle in children. J Bone Joint Surg Am 1975;57:259–61.

The causes of persistent genu varum and valgum are shown in Table 13.13.

Management of genu valgum is based on the age of the child and degree of deformity. Mild deformity can simply be monitored periodically, while a deformity of more than 12°–15° indicates surgical correction (proximal tibial osteotomy, distal femoral osteotomy or lateral epiphysiodesis). Distal femoral osteotomy is the preferred option after skeletal maturity. Most patients do not require surgery.

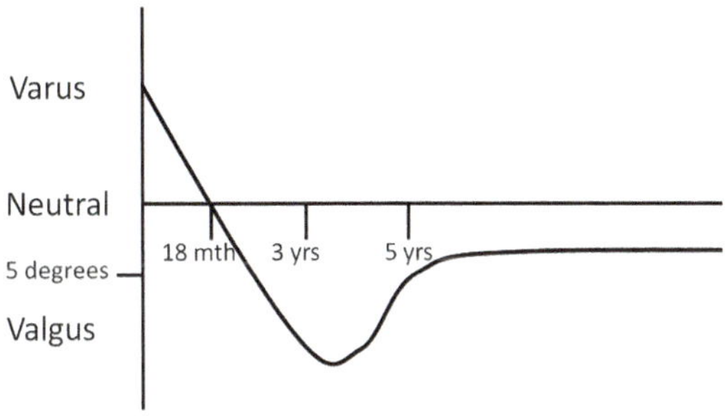

Fig. 13.23 Change in alignment of the knee with age—Salenius curve

Table 13.13 Causes of genu varum and valgum

Genu varum	Genu valgum
Physiologic Asymmetric growth • Tibia vara—Blount's disease • Partial physeal arrest due to trauma, infection or tumour Metabolic • Renal disease • Rickets Bone dysplasia • Achondroplasia • Multiple epiphyseal dysplasia • Enchondromatosis Osteopenia • Juvenile rheumatoid arthritis • Osteogenesis imperfecta	Primary genu valgum Trauma Tumour Infection Metabolic • Renal osteodystrophy • Developmental Dysplasia Absent fibula Contracture of the iliotibial band

Ballal MS, Bruce CE, Nayagam S. Correcting genu varum and genu valgum in children by guided growth: temporary hemiepiphyseodesis using tension band plates. J Bone Joint Surg Br 2010;92(2):273–6. 25 children, 37 legs were corrected using extraperiosteal two hole titanium plate. Mean age 11.6 years, mean deformity 8.3 degrees, and mean time for correction 16 months. Mean correction was 0.7° per month in femur, 0.5° per month in tibia and 1.2° if both were done concurrently. One child had rebound deformity, but there were no physeal tethers.

Congenital Knee Dislocation

Congenital dislocation of the knee can be an isolated entity or associated with breech presentation, Larsen syndrome, arthrogryposis, myelodysplasia, clubfoot or congenital hip dislocation.

Patients have fibrosis of the quadriceps and anterior subluxation of the tibia. The suprapatellar pouch is absent and the patella is underdeveloped. The cruciate ligaments may be absent. The knee is hyperextended and flexion of the knee is restricted.

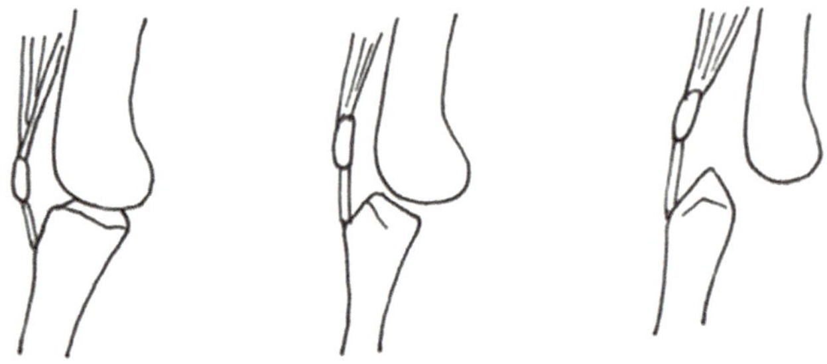

Fig. 13.24 Types of congenital knee dislocation

Congenital knee dislocation can present with varying severity. Three types are described (Fig. 13.24).

Type I resolves spontaneously, but type II requires serial casting. A Pavlik harness is quite helpful once adequate knee flexion is achieved to maintain and improve flexion. Type III carries the worst prognosis and quadricepsplasty and open reduction are needed to realign the knee. This should be performed before the age of 6 months. Isolated knee dislocation carries a better prognosis.

Congenital Patellar Dislocation

Congenital patellar dislocation is anterolateral displacement of the extensor mechanism. The patella is fixed to the lateral aspect of the distal femur with contracture of the iliotibial band and the lateral capsule. The vastus medialis is atrophic and the trochlea is shallow. An external rotation and valgus deformity of the tibia may be evident.

Congenital patellar dislocation is not reducible and requires surgical correction before the age of 1 year. The lateral structures are released and the medial structures are reefed. Associated syndromes are myelodysplasia and arthrogryposis.

Bipartite Patella

Bipartite patella is usually an incidental finding. It is more common in boys.

Saupe's classification is used (Fig. 13.25).

Symptoms may arise from repetitive overuse or trauma. The differential diagnosis includes acute fractures. Sinding–Larsen disease may mimic inferior pole bipartite patellae.

Thrombocytopenia with Absent Radius (TAR) Syndrome

As the name suggests, thrombocytopenia and absent radii are the features of this syndrome. Knee abnormalities are in the form of meniscal hypoplasia, instability and ball-and-socket medial tibiofemoral articulation.

Nail Patella Syndrome

Nail patella syndrome comprises nail dysplasia, patellar absence or hypoplasia, radial head instability and iliac horns. It is often associated with nephritic syndrome.

Larsen Syndrome

Patients with Larsen syndrome have bilateral congenital knee dislocation along with hip dislocation, clubfoot, cervical kyphosis and laryngeal flaccidity. Deformities usually require operative correction.

Osgood–Schlatter Disease

Osgood–Schlatter disease is the result of submaximal repeated avulsion fractures of the patellar tendon from the tibial tubercle. The resulting inflammation causes pain, swelling and local ten-

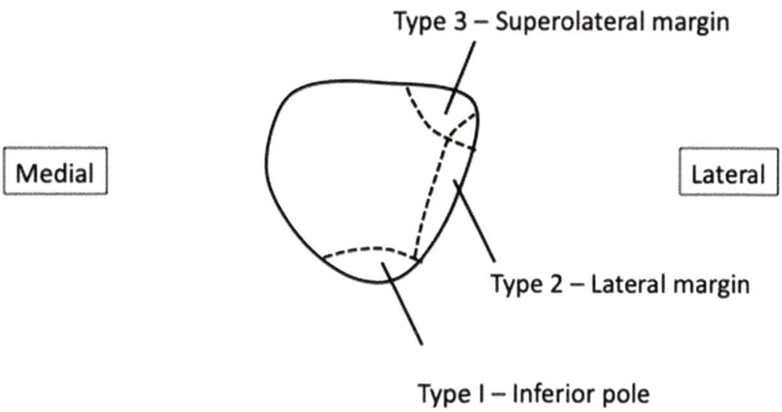

Fig. 13.25 Saupe classification of bipartite patella

derness. It is more common in boys and is bilateral in a quarter of patients.

Patients experience intermittent pain related to activity and the tibial tubercle is enlarged in size and tender. Ossification within the tendon may be seen on radiographs, but more than half of patients have normal radiographs. Fragmentation of the ossicle may be a normal variant and is not diagnostic of Osgood–Schlatter disease.

Management is symptomatic. The symptoms resolve with bone maturity and surgery is rarely needed. If required, surgical intervention aims to enucleate the ossicle and debulk the tubercle. However, this should not be performed before skeletal maturity.

Sinding–Larsen–Johansson Disease

Sinding–Larsen–Johansson disease is similar to Osgood–Schlatter disease and affects the inferior pole of the patella. Radiographs may show ossification in the patellar tendon and the condition should be differentiated from bipartite patella. Management is symptomatic.

Baker's Cyst

Baker's cyst develops in the popliteal fossa, commonly between the semi-membranous and the gastrocnemius. It is painless but is noticed because of the visible swelling. The cyst is transilluminant. Aspiration can be diagnostic but is not therapeutic. Most cysts resolve spontaneously and excision is not indicated. There is a high recurrence rate following excision.

Table 13.14 Grading of metatarsus adductus

Mild deformity (85%)	Forefoot can be passively abducted beyond the midline of the foot
Moderate deformity	Forefoot can be abducted up to the midline but not beyond
Severe deformity	No abduction is possible

Congenital Radial Head Dislocation

Congenital dislocation is characterised by a dysplastic trochlea and lack of concavity in the proximal articular surface of the radial head. Function is generally good and relocation is not indicated. Development of arthritis of the humeroulnar joint is a possibility.

Metatarsus Adductus

In metatarsus adductus, the forefoot is adducted and lateral border of the foot is convex. The heel is unaffected, which differentiates this condition from clubfoot. A few children (1–5%) have associated DDH. Metatarsus adductus can also present as a residual deformity following the correction of clubfoot. The grading of metatarsus adductus is shown in Table 13.14.

Differential Diagnosis

A skew foot is associated with lateral translation of the midfoot and hindfoot valgus in addition to forefoot adduction. It is difficult to correct by casting and surgery is more difficult.

Management

If the deformity is passively correctable then passive stretching exercises are advised. Serial manipulation and casting are conducted in patients with rigid deformity. The treatment should preferably start before the age of 2 years.

Kite has proposed three criteria for determining the adequacy of correction:

- The convexity of the lateral border of the foot is corrected.
- Prominence at the base of the fifth metatarsal is corrected.
- The active abduction is as strong as the active adduction.

In the older child (over 4 years), multiple tarsometatarsal osteotomies and medial release of the abductor hallucis and medial capsule is an option. Metatarsal osteotomy is associated with a risk of damage to the physis of the first metatarsal. Dome-shaped osteotomies are performed after the age of 4 years.

A closing-wedge osteotomy of the cuboid and opening wedge of the first cuneiform, as described by McHale and Lenhart, gives good results.

McHale, Lenhart. Treatment of residual clubfoot deformity—the 'bean shaped' foot—by opening wedge medial cuneiform osteotomy and closing wedge cuboid osteotomy. J Pediatr Orthop 1991;11(3):374–81.

Clubfoot

Clubfoot is congenital malalignment of the talocalcaneal-navicular and calcaneocuboid axis of the foot. It is associated with calf atrophy.

Aetiology

Genetics

There is significant evidence for a role of genetics in the aetiology of clubfoot:

- A second child has a one in 30 chance of having clubfoot if the first child is affected.
- A second child has a one in four chance of having clubfoot if the first child and a parent are affected.
- A monozygotic twin has a one in three chance of having clubfoot if the other twin is affected.
- A dizygotic twin has a 3% chance of having clubfoot if the other twin is affected.
- Males are 2.5 times more likely to be affected.
- An affected female child increases the risk for both male and female subsequent children.
- Patients have a family history in 25% of cases.
- The incidence of clubfoot is 0.39% in those of Chinese descent, 1.2% in Caucasians and, 6.8% in those of Polynesians descent.

Histologic

Possible underlying factors are as follows:

- An increase in the type I to type II muscle fibre ratio—(possible primary nerve abnormality).
- A germplasm defect of bone.
- Increased collagen synthesis.
- Deformity of the talus.
- Reduced cell number and cytoplasm in the posterior tibial tendon sheath—(regional growth disturbance).

Vascular

Hypoplasia of the anterior tibial artery.

Anomalous Muscles

An anomalous flexor muscle in the calf, possibly an accessory soleus muscle, has been proposed as a cause.

Intrauterine Factors

- Intrauterine pressure is not considered to be an etiologic factor.

- Arrested foetal development has been proposed, but there is little evidence for this.
- Amniocentesis and fluid leakage can cause clubfoot.
- Intrauterine retroviral infection may be a cause.

Pathoanatomy

The underlying abnormality is a deformed talus with the anterior part flexed and medially deviated. The navicular often articulates with the medial malleolus. Posteromedial structures are shortened. The talus forces the calcaneus into plantar flexion. The calcaneus rotates into varus and the cuboid and navicular move medially.

Examination

Examination findings are summarised in Fig. 13.26.

Assessment of equinus is performed in flexion and extension, while assessment of varus is performed at the subtalar joint. The lateral border of the foot is measured and compared with the medial border.

Prenatal Diagnosis

The false positive rate on ultrasound is 40%.

Differential Diagnosis

Postural clubfoot due to intrauterine malposition must be differentiated from congenital clubfoot. Postural clubfoot is a benign, self-correcting condition.

Associated Conditions

- Proximal femoral focal deficiency.
- Arthrogryposis.
- Amniotic-band syndrome.
- Myelodysplasia.
- Diastrophic dwarfism.
- Pierre Robin syndrome.
- Larsen syndrome.
- Möbius syndrome.
- Freeman–Sheldon syndrome.

Imaging

Radiographs are obtained in the position of best correction and weight bearing or simulated weight bearing. The beam is focused on the hindfoot.

AP Radiograph

The AP talocalcaneal angle is less than 20° in clubfoot (Fig. 13.27). The talo–first metatarsal angle is normally 30° valgus, but is varus in clubfoot. Medial displacement of the cuboid ossific nucleus on the calcaneus is seen.

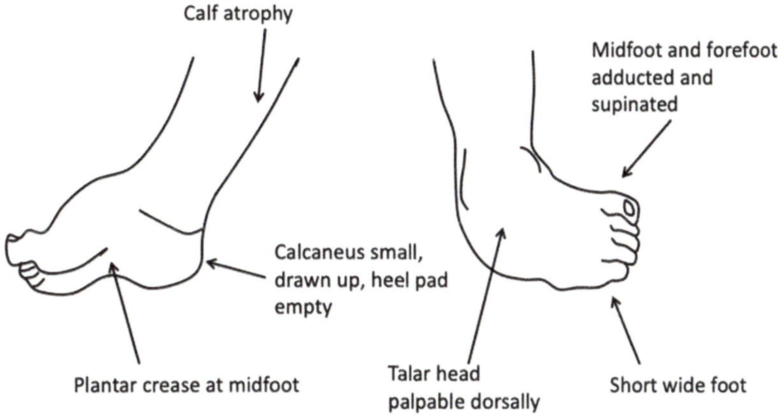

Fig. 13.26 Examination findings in clubfoot

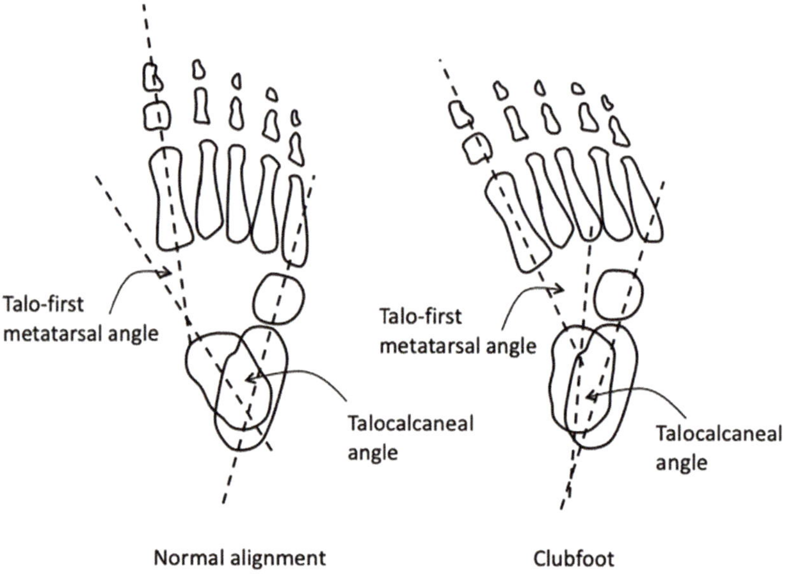

Fig. 13.27 AP radiograph alignment parameters

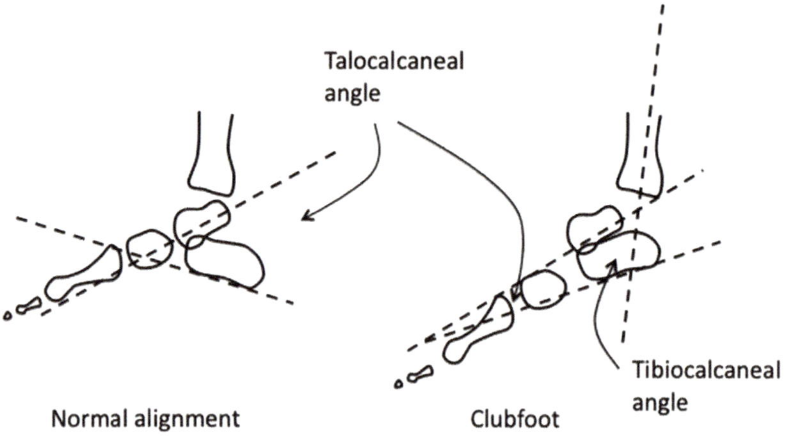

Fig. 13.28 Lateral radiograph alignment parameters

Lateral Radiograph

This is performed in maximum dorsiflexion but with no pronation. The plate is placed laterally. Lateral talocalcaneal angle is less than 25° in clubfoot (Fig. 13.28). Plantar flexion of the forefoot on the hindfoot indicates clubfoot. A tibiocalcaneal angle of more than 90° indicates equinus contracture.

Classification

There is poor interobserver reliability among the different scoring systems. The Dimeglio classification (Table 13.15) has an inter-observer *k* of 0.83.

Management

Non-operative management of clubfoot, if successful, leads to a more supple foot. Historically, plaster-cast treatment was proposed by Guerin in 1836, while Kite emphasised the importance of gentle manipulation in 1932. More recently, the widespread use of the Ponseti method has dramatically reduced the rate of operative interventions for clubfoot deformity.

Table 13.15 The Dimeglio 20-point scale for the classification of clubfoot

Feature	Points
Equinus	4 points
Heel varus	4 points
Internal torsion	4 points
Adduction	4 points
Posterior crease	1 point
Medial crease	1 point
Cavus	1 point
Poor muscle condition	1 point
Grade	
I (score 1–5)	Mild or postural, not requiring surgery
II (score 5–10)	Considerable reducibility
III (score 10–15)	Resistant but partially reducible
IV (score 15–20)	Teratologic

In the Ponseti method, the talonavicular joint is reduced by placing the thumb in the sinus tarsi over the head of the talus and pushing the navicular onto the talus with the index finger of the same hand. Lateral pulling of the forefoot corrects adduction. The foot is externally rotated and an above-knee cast applied. Serial casting produces stress relaxation and helps elongation by viscoelasticity.

Equinus is corrected after forefoot adduction and varus, otherwise a rocker-bottom foot will result. Sequence of correction is adduction—varus—equinus. Percutaneous tendo-Achilles lengthening is often needed to correct equinus.

Ponseti reported good or excellent result at 30 years in 89% of cases. Seventy percent of children had Achilles tenotomies and the duration of cast treatment was 2–4 months, with weekly cast changes. A Dennis Brown splint is applied until the child is walking and night splintage continues until the age of 2–4 years. Recurrence is increased with non-compliance with foot orthosis.

Herzenberg JE, Radler C, Bor N. Ponseti versus traditional methods of casting for idiopathic clubfoot. J Pediatr Orthop 2002;22:517–21. Posteromedial soft tissue release was required in 3% of patients following with treatment with the Ponseti method versus 94% of patient not having serial casts. Tendo-Achilles lengthening was required in 91% of Ponseti patients.

Dobbs MB, Rudzki JR, Purcell DB, et al. Factors predictive of outcome after use of the Ponseti method for the treatment of idiopathic clubfeet. J Bone Joint Surg Am 2004;86-A:22–7. The cases of 51 patients with 86 idiopathic clubfeet were examined retrospectively. Recurrence was related to parent compliance and education level. The severity of the deformity and age at treatment initiation were not related to recurrence.

Janicki JA et al. A comparison of ankle foot orthoses with foot abduction orthoses to prevent recurrence following correction of idiopathic clubfoot by the Ponseti method. J Bone Joint Surg Br 2011;93(5):700–4. Less recurrence is seen in children managed by boot and bar, as compared to ankle foot orthosis only. Hence Denis Browne boot and bar is more effective.

Other Non-operative Measures

A Dennis Brown splint helps in dynamic correction. This is advised after serial casts to maintain correction until child is walking.

Historical measures included daily manipulation by physical therapist and taping for 30 min for 8 months proposed by Bansahel. Dimeglio recommended daily manipulation and continuous passive motion for 8 h a day and then splintage in the remaining time.

The French method was a regimen of stretching exercises. Delgado used the French technique along with botulinum toxin-A injection into the gastrocnemius-soleus and tibialis posterior muscles. These methods are rarely used in modern practice.

Operative Management

The extent of surgery depends on the residual deformity.

Timing

Early surgery at the age of 4–6 months is associated with greater remodelling potential. However, surgery at the age of 9–12 months age is easier and the anatomy is more obvious. In addition, walking helps with spontaneous correction. Simons suggested the foot should be 8 cm long at the time of surgery, which makes identification of anatomy easier.

Simons GW. The diagnosis and treatment of deformity combinations in clubfeet. Clin Orthop 1980;150:229–44.

Incisions

Various incisions have been described:

- Hockey Stick posteromedial incision (Turco)—this crosses the medial skin crease. It may be difficult to reach the lateral structures (calcaneofibular ligament and plantar fascia).
- Cincinnati—a circumferential posterior incision. Exposure of the Achilles tendon is difficult and there may be problems with skin closure but not wound healing. The eventual scar is good, even if skin edges are not approximated primarily.
- Carroll—a two-incision technique: one posterior and one medial.

Medial Release

The abductor hallucis is released from the calcaneus and reflected distally. Attachment of the abductor hallucis to the sustentaculum tali is also released. The motor branch from the medial plantar nerve can be cut. The laciniate ligament is divided, exposing the medial plantar neurovascular bundle. The lateral plantar bundle is identified. Neurovascular structures are protected by a Penrose drain. The origin of the plantar fascia and short toe flexors is divided.

The flexor hallucis longus (FHL) and flexor digitorum longus are identified from the ankle joint to the master knot of Henry. The retinaculum under which the FHL passes under the sustentaculum tali is divided. The peroneus longus is protected as it passes around the lateral border of the foot at the level of the calcaneocuboid joint.

The calcaneocuboid joint is released plantarly and medially. The spring ligament is divided, helping to identify the medial portion of the talonavicular joint. The talocalcaneal capsule is released.

The deep deltoid ligament is not divided and damage to the sustentaculum tali is avoided.

Z-plasty of the tibialis posterior is performed above the ankle joint. Slips of the tibialis posterior extending to the cuneiforms and metatarsals are divided, if needed.

The talonavicular joint capsule is completely divided dorsally, plantarly and medially.

Posterior Release

Z-plasty of the Achilles tendon is performed, dividing the medial part distally. The sural nerve is protected. The talocalcaneal joint is released posteriorly and laterally. The calcaneofibular ligament is divided to allow the calcaneus to rotate back. The cuboid is reduced onto the calcaneus and stabilised with a pin.

Intraoperative Assessment

If the toe cannot be brought back to the neutral position, the FHL and flexor digitorum longus can be lengthened.

The foot should be plantigrade and the thigh foot axis should be deviated 20° externally.

Closure

The skin can be closed and the foot kept in equinus for 1–3 weeks to relieve tension on the closure. The cast is then changed to neutral. Alternatively, a gap of up to 2–3 cm may be left between the skin margins. This still leads to good healing and minimal scarring. A bivalved above-knee cast is applied.

Postoperative Management

Pain relief is with caudal block or an epidural. A wound check and change of cast is performed after 1 week. The cast is changed after 4–6 weeks, and then pins are removed.

Recurrence

Recurrence (commonly forefoot adduction and supination) occurs in 25% of patients.

Residual Forefoot Adduction

Forefoot adduction is the most common residual deformity. It is caused by failure to release the calcaneocuboid joint. Options for management of forefoot adduction are summarised in Table 13.16.

Lampasi M et al. Transfer of the tendon of tibialis anterior in relapsed congenital clubfoot: long term results in 38 feet. J Bone Joint Surg Br 2010;92(2):277–83. Mean age at surgery 4.8 years. Tendon was transferred to third cuneiform, base of third metatarsal or base of fourth metatarsal. Mean follow up 24.8 years. 11 were regarded as failures. 23 had moderate or severe stiffness. The transfer should be considered in patients where muscle imbalance is an underlying factor in the pathogenesis of clubfoot.

Management of Other Residual Deformities

The options are summarised in Table 13.17

Table 13.16 Management of residual forefoot adduction

Age less than 2 years	Repeat soft tissue release can be performed
Age 2–4 years	Calcaneocuboid joint cartilage is excised and joint fused along with medial release Enucleation of the cuboid
Age older than 4 years	The distal part of the calcaneus is excised and the calcaneocuboid joint fused Evans (1961)—calcaneocuboid wedge resection. This may overcorrect and lead to decreased growth of the lateral border of the foot Fowler (1959)—open-wedge osteotomy of the medial cuneiform, plantar release and transfer of the tibialis posterior to the dorsum of the first metatarsal for children aged over 8 years McHale and Lenhart (1991)—open-wedge osteotomy of the medial cuneiform and closing-wedge osteotomy of the cuboid ('flip-flop' procedure) Metatarsal osteotomies—when the deformity is distal to the navicular Lateral transfer of the tibialis anterior to the third cuneiform or split transfer to the fourth metatarsal

An overcorrected foot can result from the release of deep deltoid or interosseous subtalar ligaments. Treatment is as follows:

- Over 4 years, correctable—ankle–foot orthosis.
- Over 4 years, rigid—soft tissue release.
- Over 10 years—triple arthrodesis.

Tarsal Coalition

Tarsal coalition results from congenital failure of differentiation and segmentation of the primitive mesenchyme. It is the most common cause of a rigid flat foot.

Epidemiology

Tarsal coalition is inherited as an autosomal dominant condition with almost full penetrance. It affects 1% of the population.

It may be associated with fibular hemimelia, Apert syndrome or Nievergelt–Pearlman syndrome.

Talocalcaneal and calcaneonavicular coalition are the most common types, comprising 90% of all coalitions. The condition is bilateral in 50–80% of patients.

Pathology

Initially there is fibrous coalition, transforming to synchondrosis or synostosis. This leads to progressive valgus of the hindfoot and flattening of the medial arch. About 25% of feet with coalition are symptomatic.

Calcaneonavicular coalitions become symptomatic by 8–12 years and talocalcaneal coalition presents around 12–16 years. The onset of symptoms coincides with metaplasia from cartilage to bone.

Table 13.17 Management of residual deformities

Residual cavus	Release of the plantar fascia from the calcaneus can be performed In children aged over 6 years, options include Japas midfoot osteotomy or Jahss osteotomy at the level of tarsometatarsal joint
Heel varus	In children aged over 4 year, a Dwyer lateral closing-wedge osteotomy is an option
Heel valgus	In children aged 4–10 years, an extra-articular Grice procedure can be done
Supple recurrent clubfoot	Transfer of the tibialis anterior is an option for children over the age of 6 years. Prerequisites for this procedure are passively correctable deformity, weak peroneals on electromyography and absence of active abduction or eversion
Residual toe-in	Supramalleolar osteotomy or talocalcaneal osteotomy
Dorsal bunion	This results from plantar contracture of the first metatarsophalangeal joint and dorsiflexion contracture of the tarsometatarsal joint The underlying cause is a strong FHL and tibialis anterior and weak peronei and Achilles. Treatment is with the reverse Jones procedure—transfer of the FHL to the head of the first metatarsal
Age over 10 years	Triple arthrodesis Distraction histogenesis using Ilizarov principles or the Taylor Spatial frame can be performed

Clinical Features

A rigid flat foot is evident. Pain may be aggravated by activity and relieved by rest. Pain may be due to ligament sprain, muscle spasm, subtalar joint irritation or impingement in the sinus tarsi.

Examination

Talocalcaneal coalition is associated with a flat foot and lack of subtalar motion. In calcaneonavicular coalition, the flat foot is less rigid. There is adaptive shortening of the peroneal tendons due to hindfoot valgus, but actual spasm of the muscle is debatable.

Due to rigidity, the arch does not appear on toe-standing or toe-raising tests.

Imaging

AP, lateral, oblique and axial views are obtained on X-ray (Table 13.18).

On a CT scan, coronal slices demonstrate the coalition. MRI can help detect fibrous coalitions.

Management

Asymptomatic coalitions require no treatment.

Non-operative measures include activity modification, NSAIDs and shoe inserts. A walking below-knee cast for 4–6 weeks can be worn if the pain does not settle.

The aim of surgery is pain relief. A summary is presented in Fig. 13.29.

Cavus Foot

The anatomical abnormalities are illustrated in Fig. 13.30.

Causes

- Charcot–Marie–Tooth disease.
- Dejerine–Sottas disease.

Table 13.18 Radiological signs of tarsal coalition

C sign	Talocalcaneal coalition	Continuous curve formed by the talar dome and the inferior border of the sustentaculum tali on a lateral heel radiograph
Anteater nose sign	Calcaneonavicular coalition	Elongated process of the anterior calcaneus
Dorsal beaking of the talar head	Talocalcaneal coalition	Traction spur due to the pull of the dorsal talonavicular ligament
	Talocalcaneal coalition	Broad and round lateral process of talus and narrow posterior talocalcaneal facet

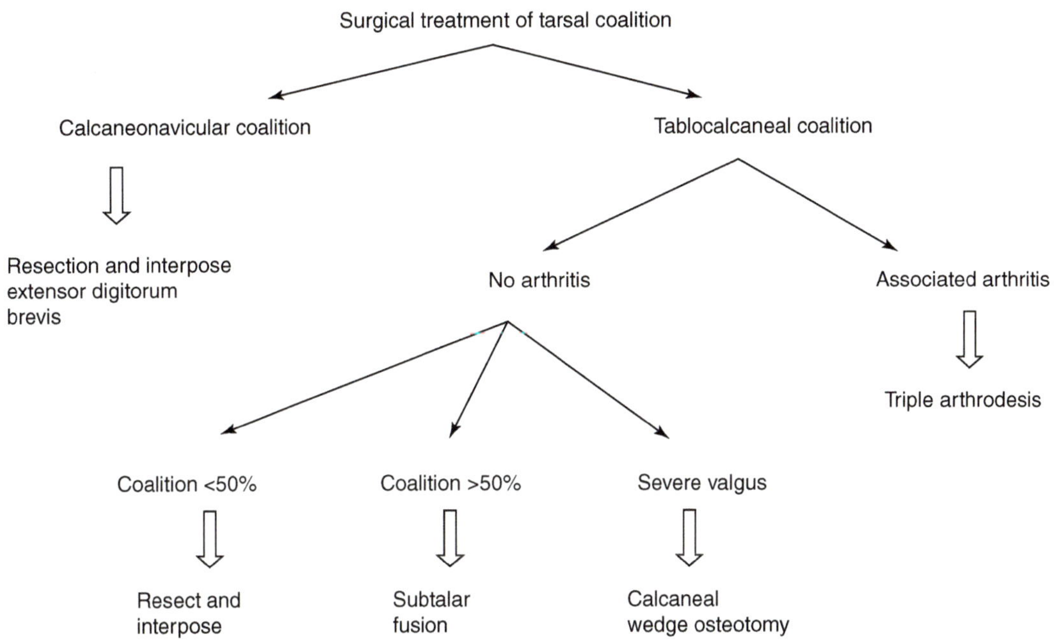

Fig. 13.29 Surgical management of tarsal coalition

Fig. 13.30 Anatomical abnormalities in pes cavus

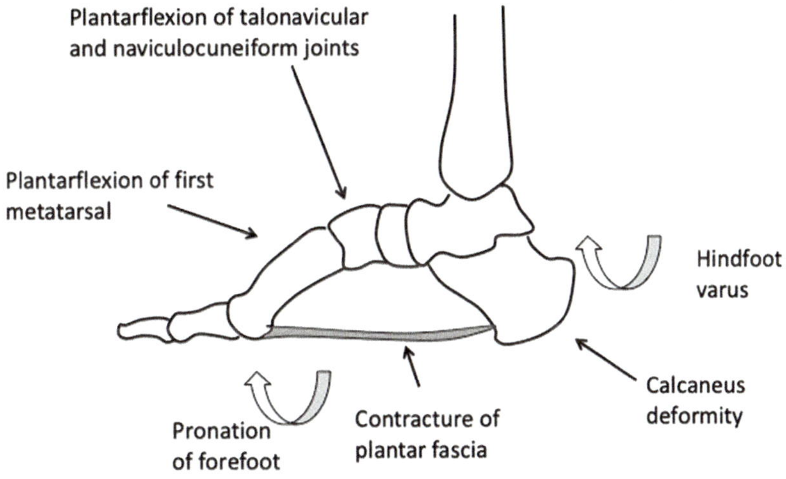

- Refsum disease.
- Spina bifida.
- Tethered cord.
- Polio.

Symptoms

The main symptoms are pain and difficulty in wearing shoes due to altered shape of foot.

Examination

- Arch in standing and walking.
- Colman block test.
- Range of motion of ankle and subtalar joint.
- Hindfoot varus.
- Clawing of toes.

Indications for surgery are pain and difficulty with wearing shoes.

Management

Non-operative management includes shoe modifications, molded orthoses and stretching exercises.

Surgical options include

- Plantar fascia release.
- Tibialis posterior transfer to the dorsum of the foot.
- Dorsal closing-wedge osteotomies of all metatarsals.
- Tarsometatarsal wedge osteotomies.
- Triple arthrodesis.

Accessory Navicular

An accessory navicular can present as a small ossicle in the tendon of the tibialis posterior, or as a prolongation of the medial end of the navicular with a thin zone of fibrocartilage interposed between the two.

These are usually asymptomatic and the findings are incidental. A Tc99 bone scan will show increased uptake in symptomatic patients and an MRI can demonstrate an accessory navicular before it ossifies and becomes visible on plain radiographs.

Management is largely symptomatic and most patients are symptom-free on skeletal maturity. For those with persistent pain, excision of the ossicle and repair of the tibialis posterior tendon to the navicular is performed.

Congenital Vertical Talus

Congenital vertical talus is a congenital dislocation of the talonavicular joint whereby the talus is plantarflexed and the navicular articulates with the dorsum of the talus. Clinically, it gives the appearance of a flat, valgus foot, which is known as a 'rocker-bottom foot'. The talonavicular joint is not reducible by manipulation

Congenital vertical talus can present as an isolated entity. It can also be associated with arthrogryposis multiplex congenita, neurologic anomalies such as myelomeningocele, tethered cord and sacral agenesis, Larsen syndrome, nail patella syndrome, neurofibromatosis and chromosomal anomalies.

Clinical Features

The clinical features are illustrated in Fig. 13.31. Patients walk with a 'peg-leg gait' due to limited toe push off.

Differential Diagnosis

- Oblique talus—the talonavicular joint is reducible on plantar flexion.
- Flexible flat foot—the arch of the foot is reduced but deformity is correctible.
- Rigid flat foot.
- Peroneal spastic flat foot.

Imaging

A lateral radiograph of the foot in dorsiflexion and plantarflexion is obtained. This demonstrates the dislocated talonavicular joint, fixed hindfoot equinus and lack of correctability on plantarflexion. The AP view shows an increased talocalcaneal angle.

Management

The initial treatment is aimed at stretching the contracted tissues with serial casts, which will aid open reduction. Surgery is needed to lengthen the contracted tendons and reduce the talonavicular joint.

Untreated dislocation in the older child requires talectomy or fusion.

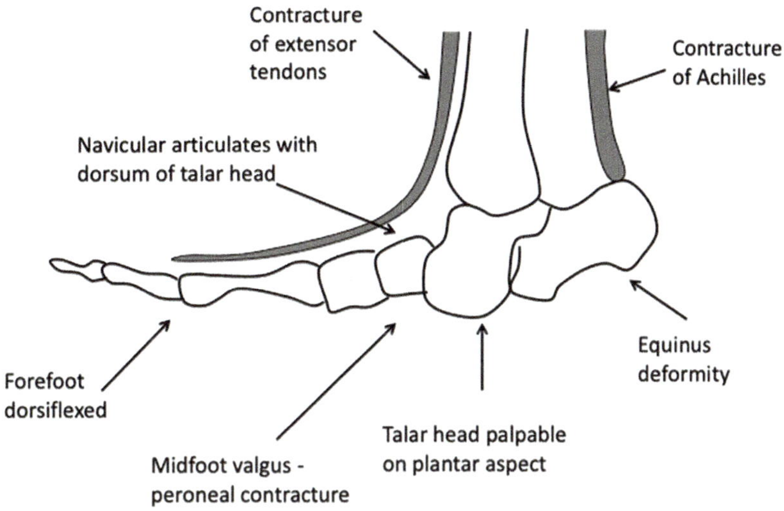

Fig. 13.31 Pathoanatomy of congenital vertical talus

Sever's Disease

Sever's disease is inflammation of the calcaneal apophysis. It affects skeletally immature children and causes tenderness around the calcaneal tuberosity.

Differential diagnosis includes Achilles tendonitis, plantar fasciitis, stress fracture, tarsal tunnel syndrome, cysts and tumours. Radiographs are helpful to rule out other causes of pain. Sclerosis of the apophysis is not consistently related to symptoms.

Acute symptoms are managed by rest or a short period in a cast. Once symptoms settle, Achilles tendon stretching exercises are commenced.

Polydactyly

Polydactyly is usually an isolated, autosomal dominant condition, but may occur as part of genetic abnormality syndromes. It is occasionally associated with syndactyly. The accessory digit can be preaxial or postaxial. Management involves excision of the accessory digit.

Macrodactyly

Macrodactyly is hypertrophy of one or more toes. It may be associated with neurofibromatosis or haemangiomatosis. Treatment aims to achieve cosmetic correction and enable shoe fitting.

Treatment options include soft tissue debulking with osteotomy or epiphysiodesis, or ray amputation.

Curly Toes

'Curly toe' describes a flexion deformity of the metatarsophalangeal and interphalangeal joints of the small toes due to contracture of the flexor digitorum longus (FDL) muscle. The affected toe is deviated under the adjoining medial toe. It commonly involves the third toe.

Most of these resolve and do not interfere with walking. Percutaneous tenotomy of the FDL corrects the deformity.

Torticollis

Congenital muscular torticollis or 'wry neck' is associated with unilateral shortening of the sternomastoid due to fibrosis.

Trauma to the sternomastoid at the time of birth leads to fibrosis and contracture. Other possible etiologies are vascular injury, infection or intrauterine positioning. A nodule or muscle enlargement may be palpable. The mass is palpable within 2 weeks of birth and can disappear by the age of 1 year. Persistent thickening predisposes to congenital muscular torticollis.

The condition may be associated with metatarsus adductus, clubfoot and dysplastic hips.

Treatment in infancy is with passive stretching. Deformities persisting beyond the age of 1 year are managed by release of the sternomastoid muscle. In mild deformities, a unipolar release (distal only) is sufficient. Z-plasty of the lower pole offers better cosmetic result and can be combined with upper pole release (known as bipolar release) for severe deformities. Endoscopic release has also been described.

Rigid torticollis results from atlanto-occipital injuries or congenital disorders.

Klippel–Feil Syndrome

Klippel–Feil syndrome is characterised by a triad of fusion of two or more cervical vertebrae, short neck and low hair line. Restricted cervical movement is evident on examination.

Associated findings include facial asymmetry, torticollis, Sprengel's shoulder and neck webbing. Neurologic compromise may be present.

Radiographs and MRI scans aid the diagnosis. Non-operative management is with avoidance of contact sports and analgesia as required. Decompression or fusion is performed for neurologic compromise or cervical instability.

Sprengel's Shoulder

Sprengel's shoulder is an abnormal superior position of the scapula, which is hypoplastic and misshapen. It is associated with Klippel–Feil syndrome, cervical ribs, scoliosis and diastematomyelia.

The omovertebral bone is a quadrangular accessory bone extending from the superior angle of the scapula to the cervical vertebrae. It is present in about one third of patients and must be excised at the time of correction.

In mild disease, the limitation is minimal. In severe disease, however, there is a cosmetic as well as functional disability.

Treatment is based on release of the vertebral scapular muscles, excision of the supraspinous part of the scapula, moving the scapula down and repairing the inferior muscles to retain the scapula in the corrected position. This was first described by Green. Associated scarring of the soft tissues may compromise the results of surgery.

Woodward procedure involves the transfer of the trapezius inferiorly on the spinous process.

The operation to correct the deformity should be performed around the age of 3 years. Injury to the brachial plexus is a risk in older children.

Congenital Pseudarthrosis of the Clavicle

Congenital pseudarthrosis of the clavicle is present at birth and affects the middle third of the clavicle. Failure of the two ossification centres to fuse may be related to pressure from the underlying subclavian artery.

Functional limitation, pain and cosmetic deformity indicate operative intervention, which is internal fixation by plate and bone grafting. The operation is performed between the ages of 3 and 5 years and the plate can be removed after 1–2 years. The potential for healing is better than for pseudarthrosis of the tibia.

Congenital Dislocation of the Radial Head

Congenital dislocation of the radial head is suspected when there is no associated ulnar injury. The radial head lacks the proximal concavity and appears misshapen. The radial shaft is longer.

Attempts at reduction are futile because there is an insufficient soft tissue envelop to retain the head in place and the bony anatomy is abnormal.

Excision of the head is an option to relieve pain, once skeletal growth is complete.

Congenital Pseudarthrosis of the Radius and Ulna

Congenital pseudarthrosis of forearm bones is extremely rare. It may be related to neurofibromatosis. The radial non-union is in the distal third and is managed by dual-onlay bone grafting or a free vascularised fibular transfer. Pseudarthrosis of the ulna is more resistant to treatment and options include bone grafting with internal fixation, creation of one-bone forearm, a free vascularised fibula graft or the use of ring fixators and bone transport.

Congenital Radioulnar Synostosis

Synostosis of the radius and ulna usually affects the proximal third of diaphysis. Wilkie has described two types. In type I, the fusion is extensive and the medullary canals of the radius and ulna are connected. In type II, the fusion is limited and the proximal end of the radius is dislocated.

Resection of fusion to restore pronation and supination is not successful. Operative intervention is indicated to correct the hyperpronation deformity if it is greater than 90°.

Madelung Deformity

Madelung deformity results from premature fusion of the ulnar half of the distal radial growth plate. The deformity can be congenital or the result of trauma. Congenital deformities present in the early teenage years with pain and cosmetic impairment. Ulnar deviation of the wrist is seen.

Radiologically, there is widening of the radio-ulnar distance, the ulna is long compared with the radius and the distal radial epiphysis appears triangular.

Treatment is by shortening the ulna and performing a dorsolateral closing-wedge osteotomy of the radius.

Osteogenesis Imperfecta

Epidemiology

Osteogenesis imperfecta affects one in 25,000 people.

Pathogenesis

A mutation in the *COL1A1* gene on chromosome 17 or in the *COL1A2* gene on chromosome 7 leads to osteogenesis imperfecta. These genes code for pro-alpha chains, which form type 1 procollagen. The mutations are generally point mutations resulting in the substitution by glycine, which compromises the stability of the helix.

Patients with type I disease have an 80% quantitative reduction in collagen due to presence of a null allele. This is the mildest form of the disease. Patients with type II, III and IV disease have abnormal collagen.

Clinical Features

- Multiple fractures. Fractures tend to reduce with age. Bone healing is not compromised but remodelling is impaired.
- Osteopenia.
- Skeletal deformities.
- Blue sclera.
- Dentinogenesis imperfecta.
- Joint laxity.
- Middle-ear deafness.
- Microcephaly, triangular facies.
- Short stature.
- Chest-wall deformities, kyphoscoliosis.
- Spinal curves of greater than 60° may result in a forced vital capacity (FVC) below 50%, which can lead to respiratory compromise.

Cod fish vertebra are a feature of OI, due to compression.
- Post-traumatic intracranial bleeding is common.

Antenatal Diagnosis

Osteogenesis imperfecta types II and III can be diagnosed by the age of 16–20 weeks. Type I and IV cannot be diagnosed in the antenatal period. Chorionic villus sampling is useful if there is a positive family history.

Classification

Osteogenesis imperfecta is classified according to Sillence (Table 13.19).

Osteogenesis imperfecta: an expanding panorama of variants. Sillence D. Clin Orthop 1981;159:11–25.

Management

The aim of treatment is to maximise function and prevent fractures. Acute fractures are usually managed non-surgically. Surgery, if required, is with an intramedullary nail and realignment osteotomy. Multiple osteotomies of the bone may be needed in order to pass an intramedullary device.

Table 13.19 Sillence classification of osteogenesis imperfecta

Type	Inheritance	Colour of sclera	Features
I	AD	Blue	Type IA—normal teeth Type IB—dentinogenesis imperfecta Type IC—a severe form of Type IA
II	AR	Blue	Lethal *in utero* or perinatal, beaded ribs
III	AR	White	Multiple fractures at birth, dentinogenesis imperfecta
IV	AD	White	Type IVA—normal teeth Type IVB—dentinogenesis imperfecta

AD autosomal dominant, *AR* autosomal recessive

Telescoping rods have been designed to allow lengthening with bone growth and may increases the time span between repeat surgeries. However, some studies have reported a higher complication rate with these rods.

Spinal deformity causes respiratory compromise. The presence of six biconcave vertebrae predicts the development of severe scoliosis. Fusion is considered for curves of more than 50°.

Basilar invagination is the cause of death in patients with type III and IV osteogenesis imperfecta. Symptoms are headache, cranial nerve dysfunction, hyperreflexia, ataxia and nystagmus. Occipitocervical fusion may not be able to halt progression and a long-term Minerva brace may be needed.

Medical treatment is with bisphosphonates, which may help to reduce bone fragility.

Gene therapy and bone marrow transplantation are not yet in clinical use.

Saldanha KA, Saleh M, Bell MJ, Fernandes JA. Limb lengthening and correction of deformity in the lower limbs of children with osteogenesis imperfecta. J Bone Joint Surg Br 2004;86:259–65. This study compared distraction histogenesis with monolateral and Ilizarov frames in osteogenesis imperfecta. Six children were included, with a mean age of 14.3 years. The average lengthening achieved was 6.26 cm. Fixators were well tolerated and regenerate bone formed normally.

Leg-Length Discrepancy

Causes

Causes can be congenital or acquired and are summarised in Table 13.20.

Assessment

Standing

Look for scoliosis, pelvic obliquity and contracture of the hip and knee joints. Flexion contrac-

Table 13.20 Causes of leg length discrepancy

Congenital causes	Acquired causes
Femur	Inflammatory
– Proximal femoral focal deficiency	– Juvenile rheumatoid arthritis
– Congenital short femur	– Haemophilia
– Hypoplastic femur	Infection
Leg	– Physeal arrest
– Fibular hypoplasia	– Meningococcal septicaemia
– Tibial hypoplasia	Trauma
General	– Physeal injury
– Hemihypertrophy, hemiatrophy	– Compensatory overgrowth of diaphyseal fractures
– Klippel–Trénaunay–Weber syndrome	– Radiation
– Proteus syndrome	– Burns
– Neurofibromatosis	Neurologic
Bone diseases	– Cerebral palsy
– Diaphyseal aclasis	– Congenital hemiplegia
– Dysplasia	– Polio
– Enchondromatosis	
– Congenital coxa vara	
– Chondrodysplasia punctata	

tures of the hip and knee can cause apparent leg-length inequality.

Look for hairy patches, vascular markings, muscle wasting and neurofibromas.

Stand the patient on premeasured blocks and reassess for scoliosis or pelvic obliquity.

Symmetry of lateral flexion is checked.

Assessment of gait is done.

Sitting

Scoliosis that corrects in the sitting position indicates a functional cause.

Supine

In Galeazzi's test, the patient places the heels together with the knees flexed. Assessment can be done whether shortening is in the thigh or the leg.

Measurement of true leg lengths is performed with the pelvis square (a line joining the anterior superior iliac spine is perpendicular to the trunk) and both legs in an identical position. Measurement is performed from the anterior superior iliac spine to the medial malleolus. The true length indicates the actual difference in leg length. Segmental leg lengths should be measured to compare the lengths of the supratrochanteric region (the anterior superior iliac spine to the tip of the greater trochanter), femur (the tip of the greater trochanter to the lateral joint line) and tibia (the medial joint line to the tip of the medial malleolus).

Apparent leg length is measured with the patient asked to lie straight with the legs parallel to each other. Measurement is performed from a fixed point in the midline (umbilicus). On comparing this with the true length, pelvic tilt and flexion contractures of the hip and knee may be assessed.

Movements of the hip and knee joints should be assessed.

In patients with hemihypertrophy, screening with abdominal ultrasound and alpha-fetoprotein is performed till the age of 6 years to screen for Wilms' tumour.

The block method is the most accurate clinical test. This takes into account the foot height as well. The pelvis is made level by placing blocks of appropriate height under the short leg.

Imaging

A scanogram shows the entire extremity on a single film. An X-ray tube moves linearly to show all of the bone structure. An orthoroentgenogram is a multiple-exposure radiograph. It shows an AP view of the hips, knees and ankle. The CT scanogram is the most accurate imaging modality to assess leg-length differences.

Prediction of Leg-Length Discrepancy

Menelaus 'rule of thumb' is applicable in girls and boys older than 8 and 10 years, respectively. Menelaus 'rule of thumb' states that the distal femoral physis grows at the rate of 10 mm/year and contributes 70% of femoral growth. The proximal tibial physis grows at the rate of 6 mm/year and contributes 60% of tibial growth. The total adult height is twice the height at the age of

Total discrepancy = Current discrepancy + (years remaining x discrepancy per year)

Fig. 13.32 Meneleus estimation of limb length discrepancy

2 years. Skeletal growth ceases at 14 years in girls and 16 years in boys.

In Menelaus 'rule of thumb' the current discrepancy is measured and the time remaining for growth (girls: 14 years minus current age; boys: 16 years minus current age) is calculated (Fig. 13.32).

Green Anderson growth-remaining charts can also be used to predict leg-length discrepancy.

Moseley straight-line graph relies on at least three measurements over 4-month intervals. It is useful in predicting the effect of epiphysiodesis.

The Greulich and Pyle atlas for bone age was compiled in 1940s and is still occasionally used for determining bone age.

Moseley CF. A straight line graph for leg length discrepancies. J Bone Joint Surg Am 1977;59(2):174–9.

Management

Management depends on the extent of discrepancy and is summarised in Table 13.21.

The current discrepancy and the final expected discrepancy should be predicted accurately. The procedure should not result in different knee heights. Weight bearing is allowed as tolerated postoperatively. Surgery can be performed as an open or closed procedure.

Epiphyseodesis

Contraindications to epiphyseodesis include inadequate growth remaining and short stature (relative contraindication).

Acute Shortening of the Femur

This is performed as the child nears skeletal maturity so that the correction is not lost. The correction achieved is 2–5 cm. Problems include oedema, muscle weakness, compartment syndrome and neurovascular compromise.

Shortening can be conducted as an open procedure (subtrochanteric osteotomy) or by closed intramedullary nailing. In the latter, a segment of the femur is divided into halves and separated, and the nail fixes the remaining proximal and distal fragment after acute docking. An intramedullary saw is used to divide the femur.

Table 13.21 Management options for limb length discrepancy

0–2 cm	Generally no treatment is needed. A shoe lift is adequate, if symptomatic
2–5 cm	Epiphyseodesis/physeal bar resection/ distraction lengthening or acute shortening
5–18 cm	Distraction lengthening
Over 18 cm	Multiple distraction lengthening/ contralateral epiphysiodesis/amputation

Lengthening

Lengthening is indicated in patients with shortening of more than 5 cm or shortening of less than 5 cm with severe deformity.

Tissue distraction techniques are used. The correction is 1 mm per day, achieved in three or four turns of the distraction screw. Monolateral or ring fixators can be used. Monolateral frames are easier to apply, have fewer pin sites, are less bulky and cause less muscle transfixion. Ilizarov and other circular frames are more versatile, allow full weight bearing, and can correct severe deformities, but are bulky.

Physeal Bar Resection

Physeal bar resection is indicated if the child has significant growth remaining. CT and MRI help to define the bar. Resection is advisable only for bars involving less than 50% of the physis.

Peripheral bars can be resected but the recurrence rate is higher than central bars. Central bars are resected through a metaphyseal window and fat is interposed. The physis may not achieve normal growth and osteotomy may be needed.

Real-time three dimensional computer assisted surgery may help improve accuracy of resection.

Amputation or Rotationplasty

Amputation or rotationplasty may be performed for Aitken C or D proximal femoral focal deficiency (see below).

Lengthening for Short Stature

Indications:

- Achondroplasia
- Hypochondroplasia
- Familial short stature

Arthritic/unstable joints (e.g., diastrophic dysplasia, pseudoachondroplasia, epiphyseal dysplasias) are a contraindication.

Bilateral tibial lengthening is performed to increase height.

Proximal Femoral Focal Deficiency

Proximal femoral focal deficiency is malformation of the proximal femur.

Classification

The Aitken classification is used (Fig. 13.33). Proximal femoral focal deficiency may be associated with fibular hemimelia, absent lateral rays of the foot and tarsal coalition.

Management

In patients with type A and B, varus corrective osteotomy will help restore alignment. The gross shortening of the extremity due to loss of growth at the proximal end of the femur can be compensated for with knee fusion and a prosthetic limb. Rotationplasty is an option.

Types C and D respond poorly to surgery; a prosthesis is a viable option.

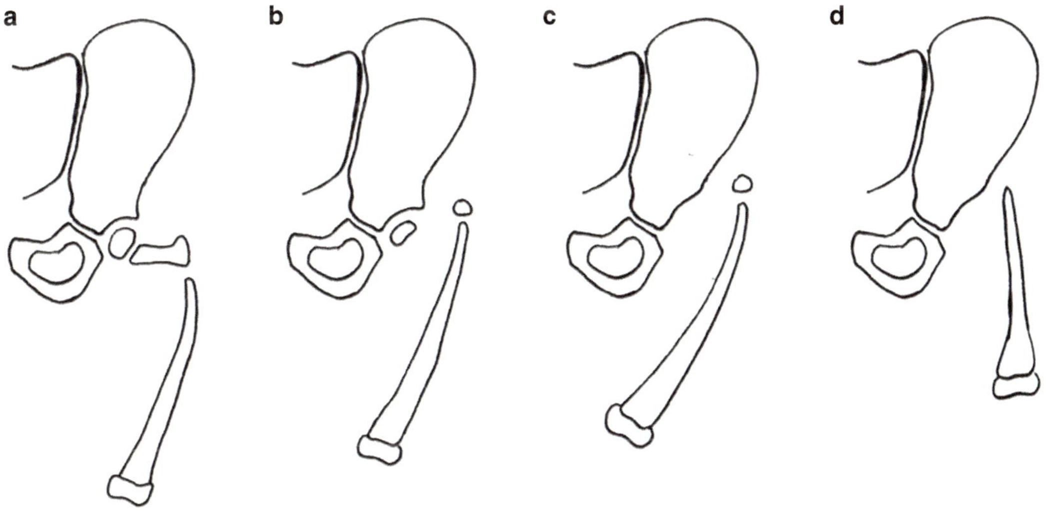

Fig. 13.33 Diagrammatic representation of Aitken classification. (**a**) Type A: gap at the proximal half of femur, which ossifies by skeletal maturity. (**b**) Type B: as for Type A, with a hypoplastic femoral head and shallow acetabulum. (**c**) Type C: an absent femoral head and proximally migrated femoral shaft remnant; (**d**) Type D: complete absence of the femoral head and acetabulum

The Limping Child

The assessment of the limping child can be divided based on age group (Table 13.22).

Children with septic arthritis present with fever (over 38.5 °C), inability to bear weight, white cell count >12,000/mm^3, an increased erythrocyte sedimentation rate (ESR) over 40 mm/hr and C-reactive protein (CRP) level >20mg/L. Movements of the hip joint are painful. Ultrasound scan shows effusion and X-rays may show increased joint space. A bone scan shows increased local uptake and an MRI will demonstrate bone marrow changes. Aspiration is diagnostic, and over 80,000 white blood cells/mm^3, and more than 75% polymorphs indicates infection. Culture of aspirate helps to identify the causative organism, which is usually *Staphylococcus* and rarely *Streptococcus*.

Transient synovitis is more common in children older than 3 years and presents with pain, a limp and reduced range of motion. Fever is not a feature and ESR and CRP are near normal. Aspirate has 5000–15,000 white blood cells/mm^3 with less than 25% polymorphs. Transient synovitis generally resolves spontaneously over 7–10 days.

Table 13.22 Common causes of limping child based on age

Age 1–3 years	
Painful limp	*Painless limp*
Septic arthritis	Developmental dysplasia of the hip
Transient synovitis	Congenital coxa vara
Discitis	Cerebral palsy
Fracture	Muscular dystrophy
Inflammatory disorders	
Neoplasm	
Age 4–10 years	
Transient synovitis	
Perthes disease	
Discoid lateral meniscus	
Limb-length discrepancy	
Age 11–15 years	
Hip (SUFE, dysplasia of the hip, idiopathic chondrolysis)	
Knee (overuse syndromes such as Osgood–Schlatter disease or jumper's knee, or Osteochondritis dissecans)	
Foot (tarsal coalition)	

Singhal R et al. The use of CRP within a clinical prediction algorithm for the differentiation of septic arthritis and transient synovitis in children. J Bone Joint Surg Br 2011;93(11):1556–61. CRP >20mg/L and inability to weight bear were the strongest independent variables in differentiating septic arthritis from transient synovitis.

Discitis can present between the ages of 6 months and 4 years. The child will have pain on bending forwards. ESR and CRP are raised and a bone scan will be positive after 1 week. X-rays are positive after 2–6 weeks. The usual causative organism is *Staphylococcus aureus*.

Fractures of the tibia, fibula, calcaneum or metatarsals can present with a painful limp.

Juvenile arthritis can present at 2 years of age with swelling, raised local temperature and multiple joint involvement. The most common joints involved are the knee, ankle and subtalar joint.

Acute leukaemias may present with a limp. The usual age group is 2–6 years. Clinical features are local pain, raised temperature and enlarged lymph nodes, liver and spleen. Myeloblasts are seen in blood film. X-rays may show metaphyseal bands.

Developmental dysplasia of the hip causes a painless limp with increased lumbar lordosis, shortening and positive Galeazzi sign. X-rays are diagnostic.

Congenital coxa vara presents with poor abduction and a painless limp. X-rays are diagnostic.

Cerebral palsy is sometimes noticed when a child starts walking. The tone is increased and hyperreflexia is seen. The limp is accentuated when the child runs. There may be a history of problems at the time of birth.

Cerebral Palsy

Cerebral palsy describes a group of permanent disorders of the development of movement and posture causing activity limitation(s) that are attributed to non-progressive disturbances that occurred in the developing foetal or infant brain.

Although the neurological insult is non-progressive, the increasing functional demands of the growing child may make the neurological manifestations of the condition appear to progress.

Rosenbaum P, Paneth N, Leviton A, et al. A report: the definition and classification of cerebral palsy April 2006. Dev Med Child Neurol Suppl 2007;109:8–14.

Incidence

Cerebral palsy has an incidence of 1–7 per 1000 live births. This incidence has not changed in the last 10 years. Improvements in neonatal care have resulted in the increased survivorship of preterm infants, with associated long-term sequelae.

Aetiology

A large number of causes have been identified, although no risk factors can be identified in 30% of patients. The causes are shown in Table 13.23.

Neuropathology

Children with cerebral palsy exhibit upper motor neuron signs. The management of the child should address both the negative and positive features of the condition.

Kerr Graham H, Selber P. Musculoskeletal aspects of cerebral palsy. J Bone Joint Surg Br 2003;85(2):157–66. A description of the constellation of positive and negative features that interact to produce the musculoskeletal manifestations of cerebral palsy.

Table 13.23 Causes of cerebral palsy

Prenatal	Congenital malformation, intrauterine infection (cytomegalovirus, toxoplasmosis)
Perinatal	Birth trauma/asphyxia, kernicterus
Postnatal	Infection, non-accidental injury, cerebral haemorrhage

Cerebral palsy results in several problems for the child:

- Muscle weakness.
- Spasticity.
- Muscle contractures.
- Lengthened muscles.
- Bony deformities—torsional problems, subluxation and dislocations.
- Premature degenerative changes.

Spasticity is a velocity-dependent increase in tone that is caused by the loss of central inhibitory control on anterior horn cells within the spinal cord.

Neurological Classification

Cerebral palsy may be spastic, ataxic, athetoid, hypotonic or mixed.

Spastic

Spastic cerebral palsy is the most common type, accounting for 80% of all cases. Thirty percent of patients with other forms of cerebral palsy will have a spasticity element to their condition. Children have a generalised increased tone as a result of damage to the pyramidal system, corticospinal tract or motor cortex.

Spastic cerebral palsy is further classified by the distribution of the body involvement:

- Monoplegia—paralysis of a single limb, usually an arm. This is the mildest form of cerebral palsy and can affect just one muscle group or muscle. Children generally have a good prognosis.
- Diplegia—paralysis of the lower extremities with little or no upper-body spasticity. This is the most common of the spastic forms. Children are usually fully ambulatory, but may require assistive devices and have a scissor-type gait. Flexion contractures of the knees and hips to varying degrees are common. Hip dislocations and strabismus (three-quarters of those with spastic diplegia) can

also be present. The children are usually of normal intelligence.
- Hemiplegia—one side of the body is affected. Children with spastic hemiplegia are typically the ambulatory, although there may be dynamic equinus on the affected side.
- Quadriplegic/whole-body involvement—all four limbs are affected equally. Children with spastic quadriplegia are the least likely to be able to walk, if they are ambulatory. Often their muscles are too tight and require large energy expenditure to ambulate.

Ataxia

Ataxic-type symptoms are attributed to cerebellar damage. Ataxic cerebral palsy accounts for 10% of cases. Fine motor skills and balance are affected, especially while walking. Children may also be hypotonic, but hip dysplasia is rare.

Athetoid/Dyskinetic

Athetosis or dyskinesia accounts for 10–20% of cerebral palsy cases and is notably difficult to treat. The damage occurs to the extrapyramidal motor system and basal ganglia. In the past, kernicterus was a cause of athetoid cerebral palsy, with untreated high bilirubin levels in the blood of newborn infants resulting in damage to the basal ganglia.

Patients have abnormal movement. Children have trouble holding themselves in an upright, steady position for sitting or walking, and often show involuntary movements. Because of the mixed tone and trouble maintaining a steady position, they may not be able to hold objects (e.g., a toothbrush or pencil).

Hypotonia

Children appear limp and have generally poor mobility.

Mixed

Some children exhibit a mixed pattern of neurological compromise. The individual functional deficits will determine treatment.

Gross Motor Function Classification System

The Gross Motor Function Classification System for cerebral palsy is a useful system for describing the usual functional levels of an affected child. It gives generalised descriptions of five functional levels (Table 13.24).

Each of these levels further contains a separate description for the age groups less than 2 years, 2–4 years, 4–6 years, 6–12 years and 12–18 years.

Palisano R, Rosenbaum P, Walter S, et al. Development and reliability of a system to classify gross motor function in children with cerebral palsy. Dev Med Child Neurol 1997;39:214–23.

Specific Gait Abnormalities in Cerebral Palsy

Several specific gait abnormalities are commonly seen in children with cerebral palsy (Table 13.25).

Examination

General Inspection

A general inspection will contribute the major part of the complete assessment. The examination should be tailored to the age and functional abilities of the child. Consider the following points:

- Is the child ambulant or chair-bound?
- Does the child use any walking aids?

Table 13.24 Gross motor function classification system

Level I	Walks without limitations
Level II	Walks with limitations
Level III	Walks using a hand-held mobility device (e.g., walker, crutches, cane)
Level IV	Self-mobility with limitations; may use powered mobility
Level V	Transported in a manual wheelchair

Table 13.25 Types of gait patterns in cerebral palsy

Toe walking	Commonly seen in hemiplegic cerebral palsy as a consequence of dynamic equinus and spasticity in the gastrosoleus complex
Crouch gait	Increased knee flexion in stance due to hamstring spasticity
Scissoring gait	Caused by adductor spasticity
Jump gait	Involves a decrease in flexion at the hip and knee from initial contact to late stance, with equinus in late stance, giving the appearance that the child is jumping up and down
Stiff knee gait	Decreased knee flexion during swing associated with rectus femoris tightness
Foot drop	Excessive equinus in swing caused by weakness of the tibialis anterior or gastrosoleus contracture

- Is the child able to communicate either verbally or using aids?
- Does the child have good head control?
- Does the child make any involuntary movements?
- Is the child positioned adequately in his/her chair?
- Does the child use any splints, orthotics, special footwear or Lycra suits?

Gait
Watch the child walk and attempt to follow a straight line. Does the child have a recognisable gait pattern? If the child can run, do the upper limbs elevate? If so, this is a characteristic of diplegic cerebral palsy.

Spine
Assess for a scoliosis. If present, determine if this is postural (due to leg-length discrepancy). Consider whether the curve be corrected to be held in a brace or seating modification.

Upper Limbs
Check the general tone and passive movements of the joints. Are deformities fixed or correctable?

Lower Limbs
Again, check the general tone and passive movements of the joints. Is the hip painful or in abduction? Measure any leg-length discrepancy. Conduct a Thomas test for hip flexion contracture, a Gage or Staheli's test for the rotational profile and Ely's test for a tight rectus femoris. Assess hamstring tightness and the popliteal angle.

Foot and Ankle
The Silfverskiold test differentiates an isolated gastrocnemius from a gastrosoleus contracture when there is increased dorsiflexion of the foot between an extended and flexed knee.

Management Principles

Each treatment regimen should be individualised to the child, including his/her functional requirements and neurological deficits. A multidisciplinary approach is necessary to rationalise the number of hospital attendances.

- Define the end product in terms of the long-term treatment objectives.
- Identify the patient's problems, both immediate and future.
- Analyse the potential effects of growth.
- Consider all treatment alternatives, including non-treatment.
- Treat the whole child, not just the motor skeletal parts.

Management of Spasticity

Management aims to limit the joint contractures associated with chronic spasticity. Control of generalised spasticity is non-surgical, with popular agents including baclofen and diazepam. These can be administered orally, although there is a role for intrathecal baclofen in children with severe generalised spasticity. Botulinum toxin-A (BTX-A) and phenol are indicated for the control of localised spasticity in muscle groups.

BTX is a potent neurotoxin produced from the bacterium *Clostridium botulinum*. It is commercially available as two preparations: Dysport and Botox. The mechanism of action is binding of the neurotoxin to the cholinergic nerve endings, inhibiting the release of presynaptic vesicles containing acetylcholine. Its effects are dose dependent and last for approximately 3 months, due to the growth of new nerve terminals. The beneficial effects of BTX-A for both upper and lower limb spasticity are well established within the literature.

Hoare BJ, Wallen MA, Imms C, et al. Botulinum toxin A as an adjunct to treatment in the management of the upper limb in children with spastic cerebral palsy (UPDATE). Cochrane Database Syst Rev 2010;(1):CD003469. This Cochrane review found high-level evidence supporting the use of BTX-A as an adjunct to managing the upper limb in children with spastic cerebral palsy. The review recommended that BTX-A should be accompanied by occupational therapy.

Surgical treatment with selective dorsal rhizotomy aims to reduce spasticity by interrupting the stretch reflex. Sectioning the dorsal rootlets between L1 and S1 reduces the stimulatory input from muscle spindles, helping to balance muscle tone.

Management of Orthopaedic Problems

Spine

Posterior and/or anterior spinal fusion is performed for severe rigid deformities.

Shoulder

Adduction and internal rotation is caused by subscapularis and pectoralis major transfer. This is addressed by muscle lengthening or release and humeral derotation osteotomy.

Elbow

Flexion contracture is caused by contracture of the biceps, brachialis and brachioradialis. It is treated by serial casting, BTX-A injections or surgical release.

Pronation of the forearm is caused by contracture of the pronator teres and quadratus. These can be released surgically.

Wrist

Wrist flexion contracture is caused by a tight flexor carpi ulnaris or radialis, which can be released. In severe flexor spasticity, the flexor carpi ulnaris can be transferred to the extensor compartment (Green's transfer). Wrist fusion is an option.

Hand

Adductor pollicis contracture causes thumb-in-palm. Contractures can be released and unstable joints stabilised. For finger clawing, the flexor carpi ulnaris or radialis can be transferred to the extensor compartment. Spasticity of the finger flexors can be corrected by fractional lengthening of flexor digitorum superficialis and profundus in the forearm. Proximal row carpectomy is an option.

Swan-neck deformities can be managed by splinting or surgical correction.

Hip

Hip dislocation occurs in 1% of patients with spastic hemiplegia, 5% of those with spastic diplegia and 35–55% of those with quadriplegia. Contributory factors include muscular imbalance, acetabular dysplasia, pelvic obliquity, excess femoral anteversion, coxa valga and the absence of weight bearing. Problems are a continuum starting from the hip at-risk, progressing through to subluxation and dislocation. Reimer's migration index (also known as femoral extrusion index) is a useful guide to the progression of the uncovered hip (Fig. 13.34). It is the percentage of femoral head that lies outside the acetabular roof. A progression of more than 15% in 30 months is an indicator that 50% of hips will dislocate.

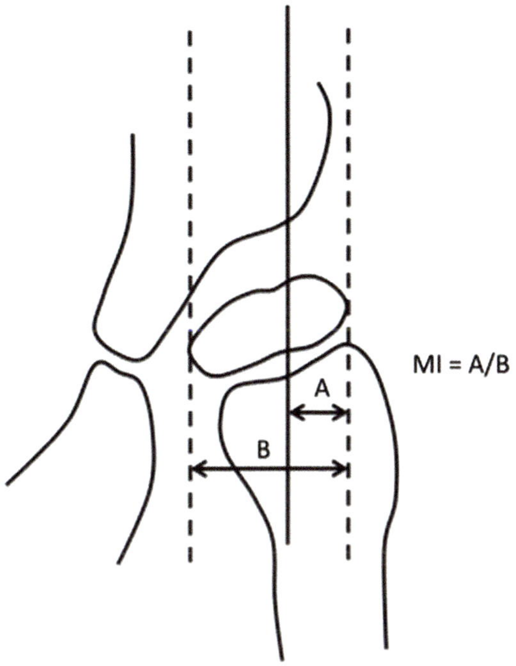

Fig. 13.34 Reimer migration index (MI). A vertical line is drawn from the superolateral margin of the acetabular roof (Perkin's line). The index is the ratio of the femoral head lateral to Perkin's line (**a**) and the total width of the femoral head (**b**)

Indications for surgical treatment include pain, perineal hygiene associated scoliosis, difficulty in sitting and to enable transfers. The principles of surgery include soft tissue release or lengthening in combination with a proximal femoral varus osteotomy and/or a pelvic osteotomy to redirect or augment the posterior–superior deficiency of the acetabulum. Other options involve excision or arthrodesis of the proximal femur.

Flexion contractures of the hip are managed by release of the psoas. In-toeing is the result of increased femoral anteversion and this can be addressed by derotation femoral osteotomy. Adduction contractures cause scissoring, and can be managed by BTX-A injection or release.

Hip subluxations are managed by a femoral varus derotation osteotomy with or without a pelvic osteotomy. Hip dislocations can be managed similarly. In severe cases, hip arthrodesis or replacement using constrained implants is considered. Proximal femoral resection helps in achieving abduction in wheelchair-bound patients with chronic hip dislocation.

Knee

Flexion contractures of the knee are managed by release of the posterior capsule and hamstrings or distal femoral extension osteotomy.

Ankle

Equinus at the ankle results from an overactive gastrosoleus and weak tibialis anterior. This is managed by BTX-X injections or lengthening of the Achilles tendon. Spastic tibialis anterior is managed by transfer of the muscle or SPLATT (Split anterior tibial tendon transfer).

Foot

A planovalgus foot is managed by calcaneal osteotomy or subtalar fusion. An overactive adductor hallucis can lead to hallux valgus, which can be managed with soft tissue release or osteotomy.

Dwarfism

Dwarfism is defined as an adult height of less than 4 feet 10 inches. Dwarfism can be either proportional or disproportionate (Fig. 13.35).

Proportionate dwarfism is commonly due to glycogen storage diseases.

Achondroplasia is the commonest type of dwarfism. 80% of cases are the result of a mutation. Transmission is autosomal dominant. Risk of homozygous achondroplasia is 25% if both parents have heterozygous achondroplasia. Homozygous achondroplasia is almost always fatal in utero. As with Mendelian inheritance, parents with heterozygous achondroplasia have a 25% chance of having an offspring with average stature.

The mutation affects the Fibroblast Growth Factor Receptor 3.

Features are short stature with rhizomelic disproportion. Head size is large and midface is flattened. There is thoracolumbar kyphosis and lower lumbar hyperlordosis.

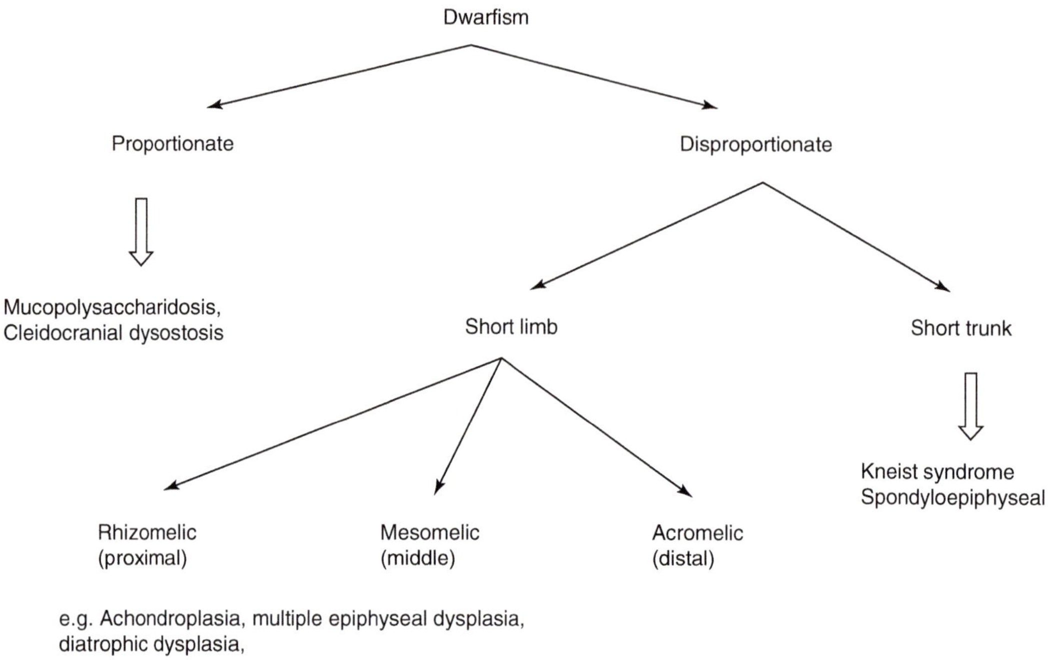

Fig. 13.35 Types of Dwarfism

Suboccipital compression of cord can be life threatening and requires decompression. Spinal deformities may require surgical correction.

Further Reading

Ballal MS, Bruce CE, Nayagam S. Correcting genu varum and genu valgum in children by guided growth: temporary hemiepiphyseodesis using tension band plates. J Bone Joint Surg Br. 2010;92(2):273–6.

Boero S, Catagni M, Donzelli O, et al. Congenital pseudarthrosis of the tibia associated with neurofibromatosis-1: treatment with Ilizarov device. J Pediatr Orthop. 1997;17:675–84.

Böhm P, Brzuske A. Salter innominate osteotomy for the treatment of developmental dysplasia of the hip in children: results of seventy-three consecutive osteotomies after twenty-six to thirty-five years of follow-up. J Bone Joint Surg Am. 2002;84-A:178–86.

Bond CD, et al. Prospective evaluation of newborn soft-tissue "clicks" with ultrasound. J Pediatr Orthop. 1997;17(2):199–201.

Carney BT, Weinstein SL, Noble J. Long-term follow-up of slipped capital femoral epiphysis. J Bone Joint Surg Am. 1991;73:667–74.

Carney BT, Birnbaum P, Minter C. Slip progression after in situ single screw fixation for stable slipped capital femoral epiphysis. J Pediatr Orthop. 2003;23:584–9.

Chotigavanichaya C, Salinas G, Green T, et al. Recurrence of varus deformity after proximal tibial osteotomy in Blount disease: long-term follow-up. J Pediatr Orthop. 2002;22:638–41.

Dobbs MB, Rudzki JR, Purcell DB, et al. Factors predictive of outcome after use of the Ponseti method for the treatment of idiopathic clubfeet. J Bone Joint Surg Am. 2004;86-A:22–7.

Fish JB. Cuneiform osteotomy of the femoral neck in the treatment of slipped capital femoral epiphysis. J Bone Joint Surg Am. 1984;66:1153–68.

Fraitzl CR, Käfer W, Nelitz M, Reichel H. Radiological evidence of femoroacetabular impingement in mild slipped capital femoral epiphysis: a mean follow-up of 14.4 years after pinning in situ. J Bone Joint Surg Br. 2007;89:1592–6.

Herring JA, Kim HT, Browne R. Legg-Calve-Perthes disease Part I: classification of radiographs with use of modified lateral pillar and Stulberg classification. J Bone Joint Surg Am. 2004a;86(10):2103–20.

Herring JA, Kim HT, Browne R. Legg Calve Perthes disease. Part I. Prospective multicentre study on the effect of treatment on outcome. J Bone Joint Surg Am. 2004b;86(10):2121–34.

Herzenberg JE, Radler C, Bor N. Ponseti versus traditional methods of casting for idiopathic clubfoot. J Pediatr Orthop. 2002;22:517–21.

Hoare BJ, Wallen MA, Imms C, et al. Botulinum toxin A as an adjunct to treatment in the management of the upper limb in children with spastic cerebral palsy (UPDATE). Cochrane Database Syst Rev. 2010;1:CD003469.

Hresko MT, et al. Prospective reevaluation of the association between thrombotic diathesis and legg perthes disease. J Bone Joint Surg Am. 2002;84(9):1613–8.

Huber H, et al. Adolescent slipped capital femoral epiphysis treated by a modified Dunn osteotomy with surgical hip dislocation. J Bone Joint Surg Br. 2010;93(6):833–8.

Janicki JA, et al. A comparison of ankle foot orthoses with foot abduction orthoses to prevent recurrence following correction of idiopathic clubfoot by the Ponseti method. J Bone Joint Surg Br. 2011;93(5):700–4.

Kalamchi A, MacEwen GD. Avascular necrosis following treatment of congenital dislocation of the hip. J Bone Joint Surg Am. 1980;62:876–88.

Keenan WN, Clegg J. Perthes disease after irritable hip: delayed bone age shows the hip is a "marked man". J Bone Joint Surg Br. 1996;16(1):20–3.

Kerr Graham H, Selber P. Musculoskeletal aspects of cerebral palsy. J Bone Joint Surg Br. 2003;85(2):157–66.

Kiely N, Younis U, Day JB, Meadows TM. The Ferguson medial approach for open reduction of developmental dysplasia of the hip. A clinical and radiological review of 49 hips. J Bone Joint Surg Br. 2004;86:430–3.

Lampasi M, et al. Transfer of the tendon of tibialis anterior in relapsed congenital clubfoot: long term results in 38 feet. J Bone Joint Surg Br. 2010;92(2):277–83.

Langenskiold A. Tibia vara. A critical review. Clin Orthop. 1989;246:195–207.

Lewis K, Jones DA, Powell N. Ultrasound and neonatal hip screening: the five-year results of a prospective study in high-risk babies. J Pediatr Orthop. 1999;19:760–2.

Macnicol MF, Lo HK, Yong KF. Pelvic remodelling after the Chiari osteotomy. A long-term review. J Bone Joint Surg Br. 2004;86:648–54.

McHale L. Treatment of residual clubfoot deformity—the 'bean shaped' foot—by opening wedge medial cuneiform osteotomy and closing wedge cuboid osteotomy. J Pediatr Orthop. 1991;11(3):374–81.

Moseley CF. A straight line graph for leg length discrepancies. J Bone Joint Surg Am. 1977;59(2):174–9.

Nakamura J, Kamegaya M, Saisu T, et al. Treatment for developmental dysplasia of the hip using the Pavlik harness: long-term results. J Bone Joint Surg Br. 2007;89:230–5.

Noelle Larson A, Sucato DJ, Herring JA, Adolfsen SE, Kelly DM, Martus JE, Lovejoy JF, Browne R, Delarocha A. Prospective multicenter study of Legg Calve Perthes disease. J Bone Joint Surg Am. 2012;94:584–92.

O'Brien ET, Fahey JJ. Remodeling of the femoral neck after in situ pinning for slipped capital femoral epiphysis. J Bone Joint Surg Am. 1977;59:62–8.

Palisano R, Rosenbaum P, Walter S, et al. Development and reliability of a system to classify gross motor function in children with cerebral palsy. Dev Med Child Neurol. 1997;39:214–23.

Peterson MD, Weiner DS, Green NE, Terry CL. Acute slipped capital femoral epiphysis: the value and safety of urgent manipulative reduction. J Pediatr Orthop. 1997;17:648–54.

Richards BS, Katz DE, Sims JB. Effectiveness of brace treatment in early infantile Blount's disease. J Pediatr Orthop. 1998;18:374–80.

Rosenbaum P, Paneth N, Leviton A, et al. A report: the definition and classification of cerebral palsy April 2006. Dev Med Child Neurol Suppl. 2007;109:8–14.

Saldanha KA, Saleh M, Bell MJ, Fernandes JA. Limb lengthening and correction of deformity in the lower limbs of children with osteogenesis imperfecta. J Bone Joint Surg Br. 2004;86:259–65.

Salenius P, Vankka E. The development of the tibiofemoral angle in children. J Bone Joint Surg Am. 1975;57:259–61.

Salter RB, Thompson GH. Legg-Calve-Perthes disease. The prognostic significance of the subchondral fracture and a two group classification of the femoral head involvement. J Bone Joint Surg Am. 1984;66(4):479–89.

Sillence D. Osteogenesis imperfecta: an expanding panorama of variants. Clin Orthop. 1981;159:11–25.

Simons GW. The diagnosis and treatment of deformity combinations in clubfeet. Clin Orthop. 1980;150:229–44.

Singhal R, et al. The use of CRP within a clinical prediction algorithm for the differentiation of septic arthritis and transient synovitis in children. J Bone Joint Surg Br. 2011;93(11):1556–61.

Spire AS, et al. Combined treatment of congenital pseudarthrosis of the tibia including recombinant human bone morphogenetic protein 2: a case series. J Bone Joint Surg Br. 2011;93(5):695–9.

Stulberg SD, et al. The natural history of Legg-Calve-Perthes disease. J Bone Joint Surg Am. 1981;63(7):1095–108.

Szepesi K. The most severe forms of perthes disease associated with the homozygous Factor V Leiden mutation. J Bone Joint Surg Br. 2004;86(3):426–9.

Uglow MG, Clarke NM. The management of slipped capital femoral epiphysis. J Bone Joint Surg Br. 2004;86:631–5.

Wirth T, Stratmann L, Hinrichs F. Evolution of late presenting developmental dysplasia of the hip and associated surgical procedures after 14 years of neonatal ultrasound screening. J Bone Joint Surg Br. 2004;86:585–9.

Yoo WJ, Choi IH, Chung CY, et al. Valgus femoral osteotomy for hinge abduction in Perthes' disease. Decision-making and outcomes. J Bone Joint Surg Br. 2004;86:726–30.

Ziebarth K, Zilkens C, Spencer S, et al. Capital realignment for moderate and severe SCFE using a modified Dunn procedure. Clin Orthop Relat Res. 2009;467:704–16.

Zionts LE, et al. Transient penetration of the hip during in situ cannulated—screw fixation of slipped capital femoral epiphysis. J Bone Joint Surg am. 1991;73(7):1054–60.

14 Hip and Knee Replacement

Sanjeev Agarwal

Total Hip Replacement

Total hip replacement, or total hip arthroplasty is one of the most successful operative procedures in orthopaedic surgery. Over 75,000 hip replacements are carried out annually in the UK.

Indications for Hip Replacement

The primary indication for Total Hip Replacement (THR) is to relieve pain from an arthritic joint and consequently, to improve function.

The vast majority of hip replacements are performed for hip osteoarthritis. Other indications include rheumatoid arthritis, posttraumatic arthritis, avascular necrosis, dysplastic hip in skeletally mature patients, failed fracture fixations and tumours.

Total hip replacement is the preferred treatment in active patients over the age of 65 years with displaced intracapsular femoral neck fractures.

Blomfeldt R, Törnkvist H, Ponzer S, Söderqvist A, Tidermark J. Comparison of internal fixation with total hip replacement for displaced femoral neck fractures. Randomised, controlled trial performed at 4 years. J Bone Joint Surg Am. 2005;87(8):1680–8. 102 patients with femoral neck fracture were studied. All were over 70 years and with intact cognitive function. At 4 years, mortality was 25% in both groups. THR group had 4% complication and 4% reoperation rate. Fixation group had 42% complication rate and 47% reoperation rate. Hip function was better in arthroplasty group.

Lee BP, Berry DJ, Harmsen WS, Sim FH. Total hip arthroplasty for the treatment of an acute fracture of the femoral neck. J Bone Joint Surg Am 1998; 80(1):70–5. 126 hip replacements for femoral neck fractures, 10 year follow up. 5% revised for aseptic loosening. 95% 5 year survival.

Contraindications to Total Hip Replacement

Active infection in the hip is a contraindication to hip replacement. Active infection at remote sites is a contraindication as well for elective total hip replacement. Relative contraindications include poor abductor function, severe impairment due to medical conditions or immobility, an immature skeleton and progressive neurologic disease.

Despite infection being a contraindication, in some situations of septic arthritis of the native hip in adults, a hip replacement may be undertaken as part of debridement and to provide a high dose of local antibiotics and a functioning joint. This is

S. Agarwal (✉)
University Hospital of Wales, Consultant Orthopaedic Surgeon, Cardiff, UK

S. Agarwal (ed.), *Current Orthopaedic Practice*, https://doi.org/10.1007/978-3-030-78529-1_14

similar to the first stage of a two-stage revision for infection.

Surgical approach for Hip Replacement

The commonest approach for hip replacement surgery in the UK is the posterior approach, used in 68% of hip replacements in 2018 (NJR annual report 2019). Other approaches include the Hardinge's approach in 31%. The direct anterior approach (DAA) and trochanteric osteotomy were used in less than 1% patients.

The DAA is often publicized in non-peer reviewed media, but scientific evidence to support its superiority over posterior approach is sparse.

Meermans G, Konan S, Das R, Volpin A, Haddad FS. The direct anterior approach in total hip arthroplasty. A systematic review of the literature. Bone Joint J 2017; 99: 732–40. There is little evidence for improved outcome with DAA in terms of complications, length of stay and outcomes. Systematic review of 42 studies.

Preoperative Assessment and Investigations

Preoperative assessment should include a detailed history and examination to confirm that the hip joint is the source of pain. Abductor function, shortening of the limb and any neurovascular deficit should be documented.

Full blood count, renal function and electrolytes are checked. Crossmatching for blood transfusion is done, although need for blood transfusion after hip replacement is rare in most centres, especially with routine use of tranexamic acid preoperatively. Urine analysis for infection used to be routine, but has limited value in asymptomatic patients. Asymptomatic bacteriuria is not necessarily a contraindication for surgery. Symptomatic urine infections should be treated before surgery.

Nasal and perineal swabs for MRSA (Methicillin Resistant Staphylococcus Aureus) and MSSA (Methicillin Sensitive Staphylococcus Aureus) are routinely done. Skin lesion in psoriasis should be treated or avoided in the surgical approach. Electrocardiogram and chest X-ray is done, if medically indicated.

X-ray of the anteroposterior (AP) view of the pelvis includes an AP view of the hip performed in 20° of internal rotation for templating; and a horizontal beam lateral view of the hip. At some centres, a shoot through lateral view of the hip is also obtained. Visualisation of the ischial spine on the AP view and a crossover sign indicate retroversion of the acetabulum.

Lateral cervical spine flexion and extension views are done for patients with rheumatoid arthritis to check cervical spine stability. A difference of over 10 mm in the atlanto-dens interval (ADI) on flexion—extension indicates instability. The space available for cord (SAC) should be over 14 mm.

Preoperative templating is extremely helpful and gives the surgeon an idea about implant sizes and positioning, level of neck resection, leg length discrepancy and offset.

Informed Consent

The procedure should be explained to the patient, along with all the risks of surgery. These are described later in the section on complications. The consent should be obtained in advance of the procedure and information provided has to be clearly documented.

Cemented Femoral Component Design

In the early days of hip arthroplasty, the femoral prostheses were made out of cast stainless steel. This was not strong enough to sustain prolonged physiological loading and instances of stem fracture led to development of cold-forged implants.

Cemented femoral components are now made of stiffer materials—cobalt chrome or stainless steel. Titanium stems in cement transfer more load to the cement because titanium is relatively more elastic (less stiff). This leads to early cement fatigue and failure.

A broad medial border on the prosthesis reduces the load on the cement. In cross section, the prosthesis should have a flat medial surface as opposed to a medial border. The diamond-shaped Muller prosthesis, which had a narrow medial border, is not considered an ideal shape. The Thompson prosthesis, which was commonly used in hemiarthroplasty, was also diamond-shaped in cross-section with a narrow medial border.

Modern cemented femoral components should have a broad medial surface to reduce strain on the proximal medial cement mantle (zone 7). The C stem (DePuy, Warsaw, USA) was designed on the principle of loading cement in compression; and is thicker laterally and thinner medially (Fig. 14.1). This is known as the third taper and this loads the medial cement mantle, which is desirable.

Tapered stems (e.g., the Exeter system) help to transfer the load to cement evenly. Cement is stronger in compression. The flanged Charnley stem is also broader laterally and helps to load the cement in compression.

Anteversion of the cemented femoral stem can affect the survival. Reproducing normal anteversion (10–25°) gives the best outcome, while less than 10° anteversion can lead to progressive retroversion and loosening of the stem.

Kiernan S, KL, Wagner P, L, Flivik G. The importance of adequate stem anteversion for rotational stability in cemented total hip replacement. Bone Joint J 2013;95(1):23–30. Reduced version leads to greater failure rate. 60 patients, 10 year RSA analysis with post op CT scan for rotational profile.

Offset

The offset of the stem is the perpendicular distance between the centre of the prosthetic femoral head and the longitudinal axis of the femoral stem (Fig. 14.2). A high offset produces higher stress in the femoral stem and can lead to failure of the cement or metal. A high offset gives mechanical advantage to the hip abductors because of an elongated lever arm. Increasing offset also improves stability without changing leg length. The offset of the prosthesis selected should normally reproduce the original offset of the patient.

Most femoral prostheses have a high-offset option. For instance, the Charnley stem provides an offset of 40 or 45 mm and the Exeter stem allows 35.5 mm, 37.5 mm or 44 mm offset options. In some implant systems where a range of stem sizes is available, the offset increases with increasing stem size. Increasing the neck length also results in a higher offset, as well as increasing leg length.

Implanting a femoral stem in varus alignment effectively increases the offset. However, this is disadvantageous in cemented stems as it leads to an inadequate cement mantle in zones 3 and 7 and may lead to early failure. A cementless stem implanted in varus will be undersized and have less contact with the endosteum.

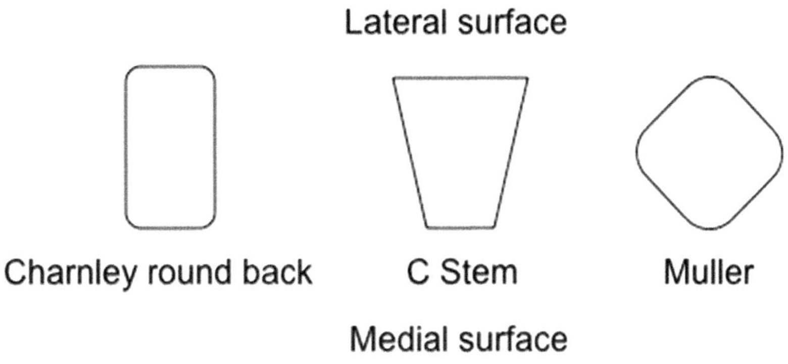

Fig. 14.1 Different cross sectional shapes of cemented stem designs

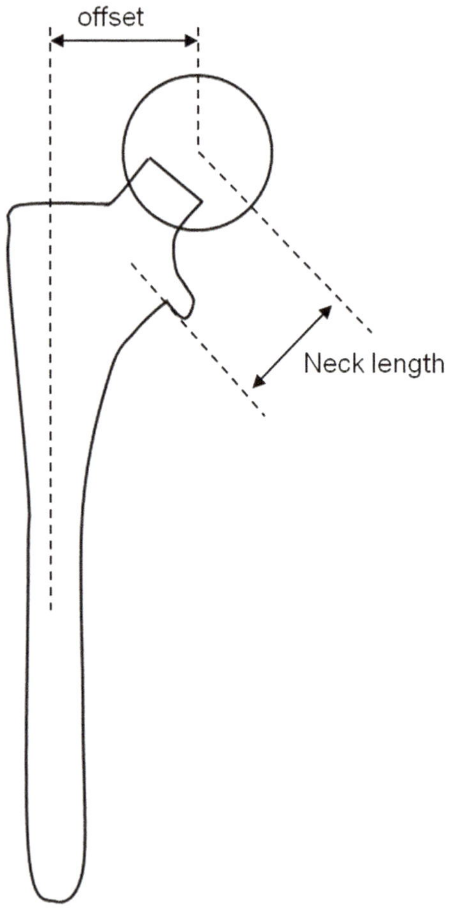

Fig. 14.2 Offset and neck length of femoral components

Offset can be altered during surgery by:

- Using a high-offset stem—this will increase offset without increasing leg length.
- Using a longer neck length—this will add to offset as well as leg length.
- Using an offset liner with a cementless socket. The centre of rotation is placed more laterally in offset liners compared to standard liners.
- Lateral placement of the acetabular component. Reducing the medial reaming will lateralize the acetabular component.

Table 14.1 Development of cementing techniques.

First generation	Second generation (1975 onwards)	Third generation
Finger packing	Cement gun	Vacuum mixing
Cast stem	Pulse lavage	Pressurisation
Open bowl mixing	Canal brush and dry	Precoated stems
	Cement restrictor	Rough surface finish
	Forged stem	Centraliser
	Broad round medial border	
	Collared stem	

Cementing Techniques

A summary of cementing techniques is presented in Table 14.1.

Fourth-generation techniques involve using a proximal centraliser in addition to a distal centraliser. The centraliser cuts through the cement as the stem is inserted and this may have a detrimental effect on the cementation. This has to be balanced against the benefit of having a centraliser to achieve a circumferential cement mantle. Distal centralisers are routinely used in cemented stems.

Vacuum mixing and porosity reduction are intended to improve the strength of cement. Vacuum mixing reduces pores and voids. However, pore-free cement may shrink and this can compromise the strength of the cement bond in vivo. The benefits are debatable.

A varus or valgus positioning of the femoral stem by more than 5° is related to increased stress in the cement mantle and a higher failure rate (Fig. 14.3).

'Creep' is the deformation of viscoelastic materials under constant load and is time dependent. The viscoelastic nature of cement is responsible for creep. Creep leads to stress relaxation, which is the change in stress due to constant strain. As a result of stress relaxation, tensile stress in the cement reduces and this improves longevity.

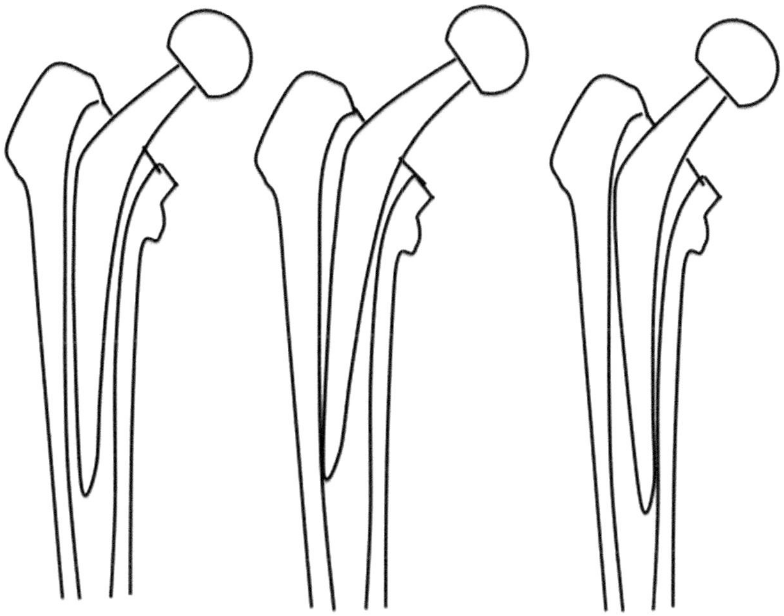

Fig. 14.3 Stem malpositioning

Surface Finish

The roughness of surface finish is described as R_a (average roughness). This is the average of all variations from the central line of the roughness profile. Rough surfaces adhere well to cement and prevent subsidence, while the bonding of a smooth polished stem to cement is weaker. If loose within a cement mantle, a rough stem generates greater wear debris.

Fixation

Fixation of cemented femoral components can be described under two mechanisms—'composite beam' or 'sliding taper'. In the composite beam mechanism, the stem is not intended to subside and a collar is useful to prevent subsidence. The stem is matt-finished or grit-blasted to allow a good interface between the metal and cement. The Charnley stem is based on composite beam principle. Subsidence in a Charnley stem is a sign of loosening (Fig. 14.4).

In the sliding taper mechanism (e.g., Exeter stem or the CPT stem), the stem is polished and tapered and is intended to subside to a stable position. The stem generates 'hoop stress' within the cement mantle and loads the cement uniformly in compression. Such a stem is described as a 'collarless polished tapered' stem. These are stable despite subsiding 1–2 mm, and the mode of failure is often related to rotational stresses.

The Exeter V40 stem has a polished finish. In 1980 the surface was changed to a matt finish, resulting in a high failure rate. A non-polished stem that subsides within the cement mantle will produce a large amount of cement debris and lead to early failure. The surface finish was changed back to smooth in 1988 and the results since have been excellent.

'Composite beam' stems fail because of micromotion between the stem and cement, leading to generation of wear debris. The 3M femoral component in the 1990s was a Charnley design stem but made of titanium. The higher elasticity of the stem within the cement mantle led to excess micromotion, excessive wear debris formation and failure. Failure of sliding taper stems is due to rotational movement or axial loading.

A precoated stem has a layer of Poly Methyl Meth Acrylate (PMMA) that substantially improves the cement–metal interfaces strength when the stem is implanted. These stems have a

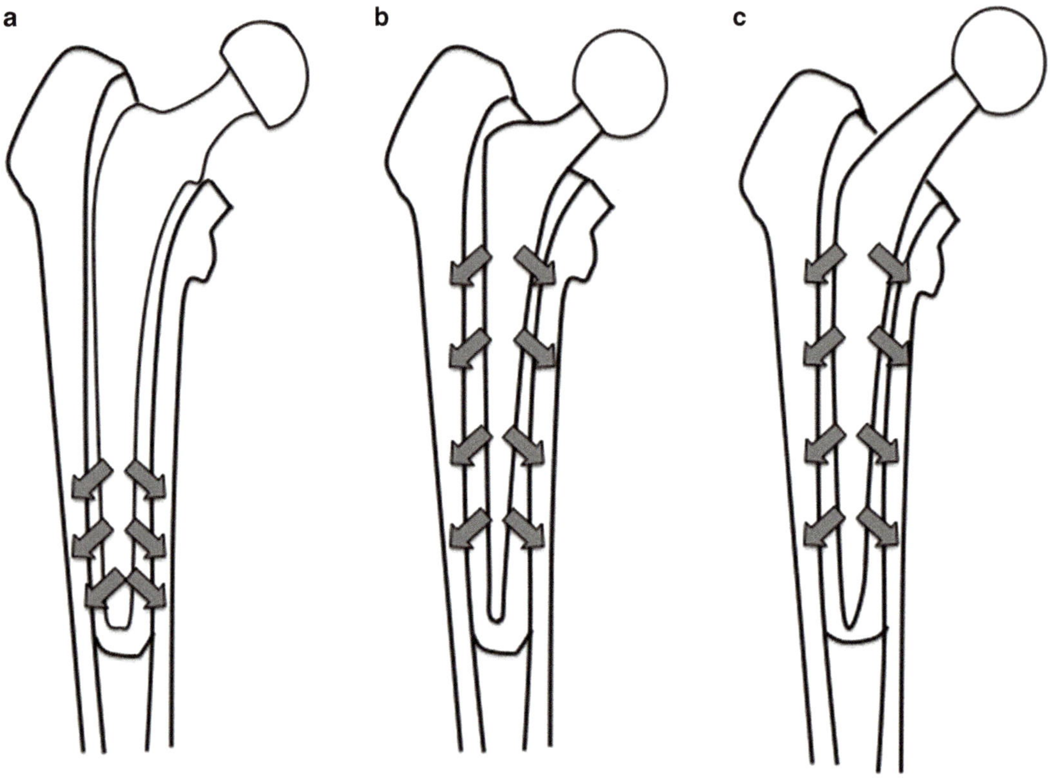

Fig. 14.4 Differences in fixation principles between distally fixed stem (**a**), the polished tapered stem (**b**) and the C stem (**c**)

rough surface finish (Ra 30–60 micro inches) and are not designed to subside. Hence, the composite beam principle is the method of fixation. Micromotion between the stem and the cement leads to generation of cement debris and eventual failure.

Collar

A collar is desirable if subsidence is not intended. A collar pressurises the proximal cement and prevents subsidence of the stem in the event of loosening. In polished, tapered stem, a collar is not desirable—hence the name Collarless Polished Tapered (CPT stem).

Centralisers

A circumferential cement mantle of 1–2 mm should be present. Centralisers were introduced in third-generation cementing techniques to keep the stem central within the cement mantle. Distal centralisers are used more often than proximal centralisers. Problems with centralisers include voids around the centraliser, failure of the interface and impingement of the centraliser against the cortex.

Chambers IR, Fender D, McCaskie AW, Reeves BC, Gregg PJ. Radiological features predictive of aseptic loosening in cemented Charnley femoral stems. J Bone Joint Surg Br 2001: 83(6): 838–42. Inadequate cementing (grade C and D) had an odds ratio of 9.5 for risk of loosening and failure.

Table 14.2 Grades of femoral cementing

Type A	Complete filling of the femoral canal with no distinguishable border between cement and bone ('white out')
Type B	Near complete filling with some demarcation between cement and bone Radiolucency at the cement–bone interface is <50%
Type C1	More than 50% lucency at the cement–bone interface
Type C2	The cement mantle is <1 mm or the prosthesis is in contact with the bone
Type D	Gross deficiency or large voids

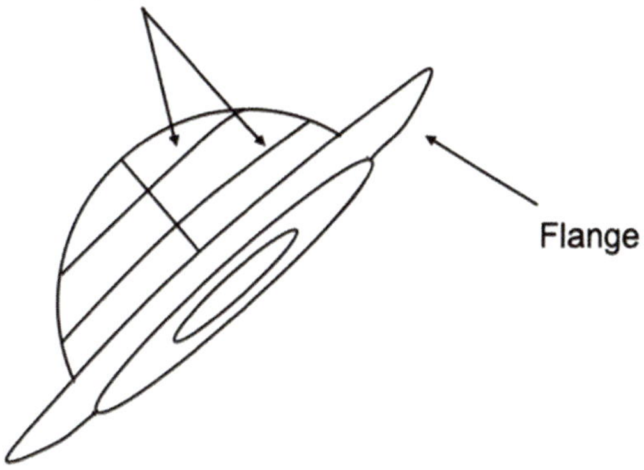

Fig. 14.5 Cemented acetabular component design

Grades of Femoral Cementing

The grade of femoral cementing was proposed by Barrack and Harris (Table 14.2).

A thin cement mantle leads to fatigue failure of the cement and loosening of the component. Poor cementing—type C or D and a mantle less than 2 mm—is correlated with early failure.

Barrack RL, Mulroy RD, Harris WH. Improved cementing techniques and femoral component loosening in young patients with hip arthroplasty. A 12 year radiographic review. J Bone Joint Surg Br 1992;74(3);385–9.

Cemented Acetabular Component Design

All-polyethylene acetabular cups are used in preference to metal-backed cemented cups as a thicker polyethylene can be used. Cemented acetabular components are useful in elderly patients with osteopenic bone.

The outer surface of the cup has grooves for interlocking with the cement (Fig. 14.5). A metal wire marker is placed in one of the grooves on the outer aspect of the component that allows positioning assessment on postoperative radiographs.

Flanged cups allow better pressurisation of cement mantle around the acetabular component compared to nonflanged cups. The Ogee Charnley cup has a flange that can be cut to the required size so as to pressurise the cement. 'Ogee' is an architectural term used to describe the shape of the flange. The aim is to pressurise the cement around the component so as to achieve a good cement–bone interface.

The minimum thickness of polyethylene recommended for an all-polyethylene cup is 8 mm. With thinner cups, the stress transfer to acetabular bone is not uniform and may lead to failure. The subchondral bone should be preserved in cemented acetabular components.

A thicker polyethylene reduces the stress transmitted to the cement mantle.

Cementless Femoral Component Design

The cementless femoral component design should provide adequate primary stability to resist physiologic loads until biologic ingrowth or ongrowth occurs and provides long-term stability. It should prevent axial subsidence, mediolateral and anteroposterior displacement, and rotation in all three axes.

Good contact with bone will facilitate biologic integration. A wide range of sizes is available to achieve a good fit with the femur. Some implants have a collar for additional axial stability. Some revision implants allow the matching of different metaphyseal components to different diaphyseal stems to gain maximum contact.

Micromotion should be less than 50 μm. Over this limit, fibrous tissue forms in the implant–bone interface.

Osseo-integration of cementless components can take place through bone ongrowth or bone ingrowth. For ongrowth, the surface is coated with Hydroxyapatite (HA), or is grit blasted.

Hydroxy apatite (HA) is a ceramic—$Ca_{10}(PO_4)_6(OH)_2$. HA is osteoconductive and allows bone ongrowth to takes place right up to the surface of the implant, providing stable fixation. The thickness of the coating is between 50 and 100 μm. The ideal pore size is 100–400 μm.

Grit blasting involves exposing the surface of the implant to a spray of particles that makes pits and roughens the surface.

Examples of coatings for bone ingrowth include a porous coating of titanium wire mesh, cobalt chrome or titanium beads, or plasma spray. Bone ingrowth surfaces may have an additional coating of HA to further enhance integration. HA reduces the time to reach final shear strength by 50%. Cortical bone provides predictable bone ingrowth.

Some earlier designs (e.g., Harris–Galante, Omniflex) had patch-porous coating instead of circumferential porous coating. This resulted in some areas that were not bonded to bone. These smooth areas acted as conduits through which wear particles could reach the distal part of the stem (Fig. 14.6), leading to stem loosening and failure. All modern stem designs have circumferential porous coating.

The extent of coating may be either proximal only, or extensive (Fig. 14.7). Proximal porous-coated stems depend on good metaphyseal contact and demonstrate good fixation, as do extensively coated stems. Extensively coated stems such as the Furlong (JRI, London, UK) and the Corail (DePuy, Warsaw, Indiana) may result in distal load transfer through the tip of the stem and proximal stress shielding due to reduced forces on the femur proximal to the load-bearing tip of the stem.

Proximally coated stems usually have coating in the proximal part of the femoral component,

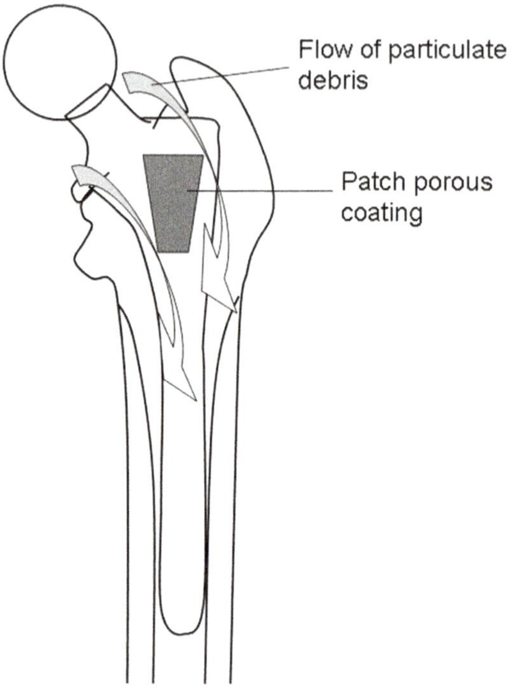

Fig. 14.6 Particle access path along smooth areas of non-circumferential coating of femoral stems

with grit blasting of the stem distal to the coating. The removal of proximally coated stems at revision surgery is generally easier compared to extensively coated stems.

Cobalt chrome cementless stems (e.g., Porous coated anatomic—Howmedica, Rutherford, New Jersey) are commonly coated with sintered beads, while titanium stems (e.g., Zimmer; VerSys, Warsaw, Indiana) have wire mesh. The Furlong and Corail stems have HA coating.

Femoral implants may be of four different shapes:

- Metaphyseal filling wedge-shaped—these gain stability within the metaphysis.
- Wedge-shaped and relatively flattened AP—to gain stability in the metaphysis.
- Tapered stems fixing at the diaphyseal-metaphyseal junction.
- Distally fixing cylindrical stems with flutes or porous coating.

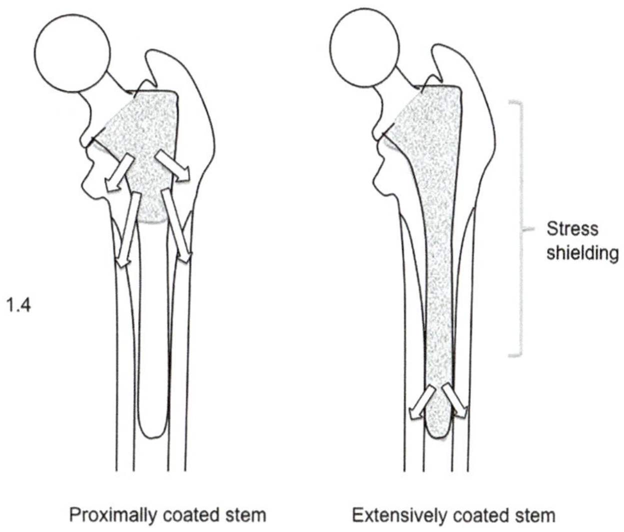

Fig. 14.7 Partial (proximally) versus fully coated stems

Proximal porous coating is adequate when a metaphyseal fit is aimed for. For femoral components intended for diaphyseal fixation, the stem must be coated to allow bone integration. Modular implants allow matching different stems and proximal components but introduce a risk of failure at the modular junction and corrosion.

Titanium is not used to make femoral heads because of poor wear characteristics. Femoral heads are made of cobalt chrome or ceramics. A common combination is a cobalt chrome head over a titanium stem. This can lead to galvanic corrosion, fretting at the Morse junction and third-body wear. Clinically significant problems as a direct result of modularity are not common.

Stress shielding happens when a femoral component is well fixed distally such that load is transferred from distal part of the stem. The proximal femur is inadequately loaded and undergoes bone resorption. This makes revision difficult due to loss of bone stock. A stiff, thick, fully porous coated stem fixed distally will led to stress shielding. It is less common in cemented stems. Avoiding tight fitting diaphyseal cylindrical stems can reduce stress shielding. Titanium stems, tapered distally, or fluted stems help reduce stress shielding.

Presence of a collar in cementless stems may impede full seating of the stem, resulting in an inadequately fixed stem. On the other hand, a well seated collar will help load the proximal femur and reduce stress shielding.

Thigh pain in cementless femoral stems may be due to a loose stem or stress concentration. A stiff, proximally coated femoral component with micromotion between the implant and bone when the femur is loaded can be a cause of thigh pain. In order to reduce the stress concentration at the tip of a well-fixed stem, the tip of the stem is tapered. Alternatives are a stem design with flutes, or hollow stems to reduce the stiffness.

Cementless Acetabular Component Design

The principles of biological integration with cementless acetabular component design are similar to those with femoral components.

The most commonly used acetabular components are hemispherical cups. The implants are HA coated (e.g., Furlong) or porous coated—which can be titanium mesh (e.g., Harris–Galante, Trilogy; Zimmer) or beads (PCA). These are usually made of titanium, as the Young's modulus of titanium is comparable to that of cancellous bone. Trabecular metal components made of tantalum have porosity similar to cancellous bone, and these are useful in revision situations, but not generally needed for primary surgery.

A press fit of 1–2 mm generally gives adequate primary stability. Press fit by 2 mm implies the cup is 2 mm bigger than the last reamer used. A cup significantly larger than the last reamer will have only equatorial fit and this should be avoided (Fig. 14.8). Equatorial contact cups are prone to loosening as the hoop stress reduces. There is also a risk of fracture if the cup is tight fitting and forceful impaction is attempted. Polar contact happens when the selected acetabular component is smaller than the last reamer, and this will not provide adequate stability. A well seated component is desirable when using uncemented acetabular components.

An alternative to press fit is 'line to line' reaming, whereby the size of the acetabular component is same as the size of the last reamer. This relies on porous coating to provide adequate stability and is known as frictional fit or scratch fit or interference fit. Screws can be used to augment the initial fixation.

The choice between press fit and line to line reaming depends on bone quality and type of component selected. For instance, the Trilogy trabecular metal acetabular (Zimmer, Warsaw, USA) components are used with line-to-line reaming while the Trilogy HA coated porous acetabular components are designed for a press fit.

A minimum thickness of 6 mm for the polyethylene insert should be allowed in metal-backed acetabular components. The liners can be polyethylene, ceramic or rarely, metal. The locking mechanism between the liner and the metal shell should minimise micromotion, to reduce backside wear.

Screws are optional and may be used to augment primary stability. Screw holes may act as passage routes for the wear debris to the pelvic bone and screws may themselves contribute to wear debris through corrosion and fretting.

Wasielewski has described the safe quadrant for screw insertion. A line is drawn from the anterior superior iliac spine to the centre of the acetabulum. Another line is drawn perpendicular to this line through the centre of the acetabulum, thus dividing the cup into four quadrants. Screws in the postero-superior quadrant are relatively safe (Fig. 14.9).

Wasielewski RC, Cooperstein LA, Kruger MP, Rubash HE. Acetabular anatomy and the trans-acetabular fixation of screws in total hip arthroplasty. J Bone Joint Surg Am 1990:72(4);501–8. An anatomical and radiographic study to determine the safe quadrant for placement of screws in cementless acetabular component insertion.

Concerns with metal-backed cementless cups are backside wear, dissociation of the liner from the metal backing and osteolysis.

Lipped liners are available which can improve stability in one direction (Fig. 14.10). These increase risk of impingement on the lipped side, and can lead to loosening of the acetabular component.

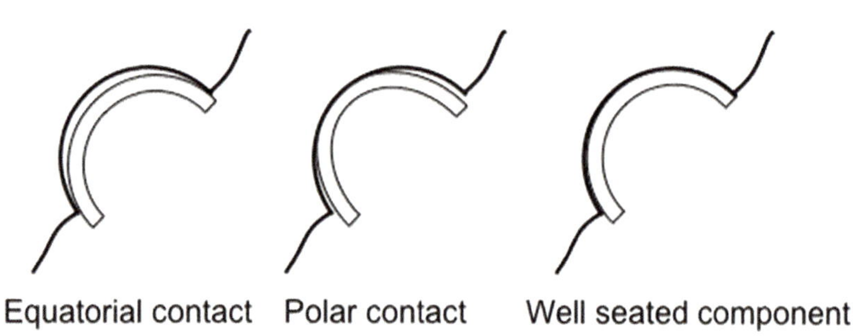

Fig. 14.8 Polar and equatorial contact of the acetabular component

Threaded cups have been abandoned due to a higher failure rate, possibly resulting from increased stresses at the point of contact of the threads.

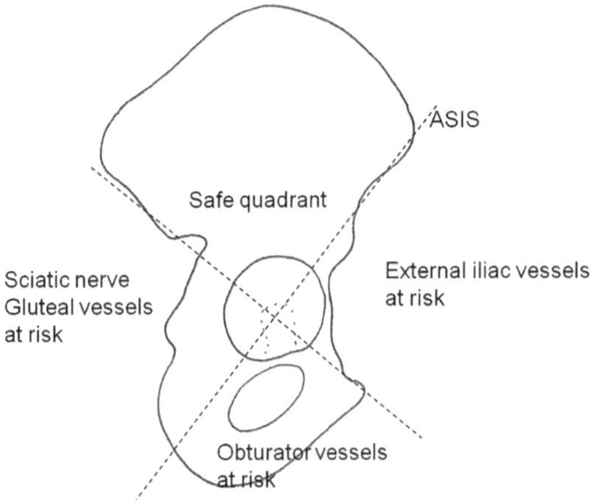

Fig. 14.9 Safe quadrant for screw placement in the acetabulum

Effect of Head Size

Sir John Charnley, in his concept of low friction arthroplasty in the early 1960s used a 22-mm head (22.225 mm), which reduced the moment arm on the head. As a result, the distance the head has to move for a certain degree of movement of the hip was reduced. This head size gave a reduced frictional torque and generated less wear particles. The low-friction torque led to the nomenclature 'low-friction arthroplasty'.

Over the years, various head sizes have been used. The introduction of the highly cross-linked polyethylene, which had a significantly lower wear rate in joint simulators, and the use of ceramic articulations and metal-on-metal implants have enabled the use of bigger head sizes while keeping a low wear rate.

A larger head size allows a greater arc of movements and is more stable (Fig. 14.11). The stability is the result of a higher 'jump distance'. The jump distance is the amount of translation of

Fig. 14.10 Elevated lip liners

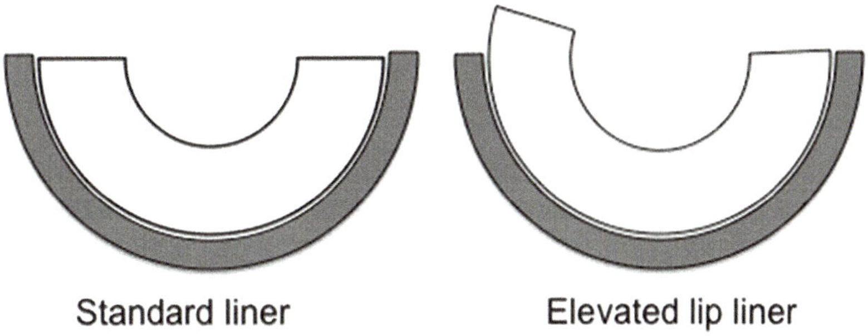

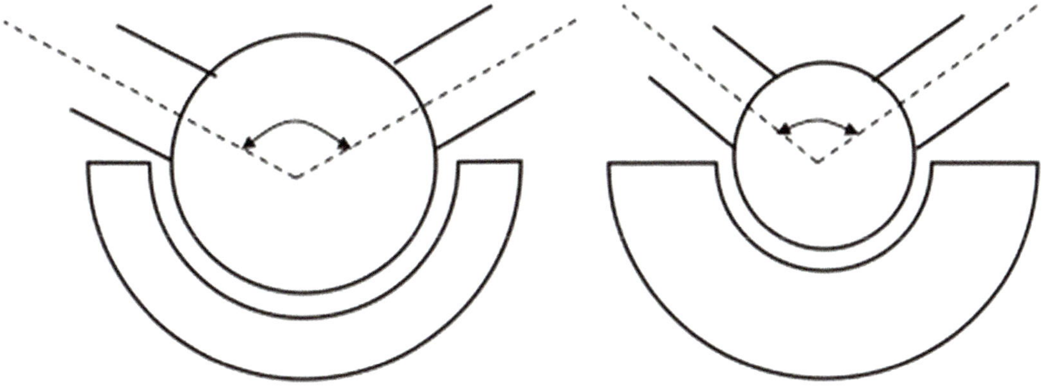

Fig. 14.11 Arc of movement related to head size. Larger head has greater arc of movement

the femoral head required for dislocation of the hip, and equals the radius of the head. A larger head will have a greater jump distance.

A larger head generates more wear particles due to greater volumetric wear. For the same arc of movement, a point on the surface of a larger head covers a longer distance against the polyethylene compared to small heads (Fig. 14.12).

Hence, the volume of wear particles and volumetric wear are greater. A larger head puts more stress on the Morse taper between head and stem. This is a factor leading to fretting corrosion at the Morse taper junction.

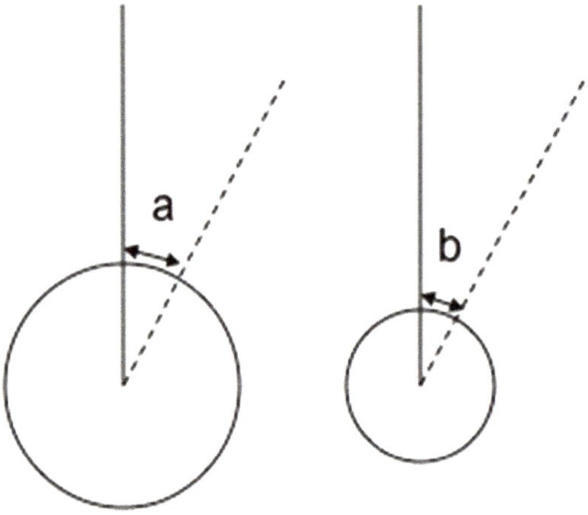

Fig. 14.12 The excursion of a point on the head is greater in a larger head for the same arc of movement

Trunnion Problems

The Morse taper between the femoral stem and the femoral head may be a source of corrosion and particle generation. Larger diameter heads produce larger torque and have a high rate of 'trunnionosis'. This was a particular problem with large diameter metal on metal bearings. Titanium stems coupled with metal heads are predisposed while ceramic heads have lower of trunnionosis.

Trunnionosis is the price for modularity of the femoral head.

Serum cobalt level greater than 1 ppb (part per billion) suggests trunnionosis in patients without other cause.

Stability in Hip Arthroplasty

Stability in hip replacements depends on implant factors, surgeon factors and patient factors (Table 14.3).

A larger head has a lower dislocation rate.

Berry DJ, von Knoch M, Schleck CD, Harmsen WS. Effect of femoral head diameter and operative approach on risk of dislocation after primary total hip arthroplasty. J Bone Joint Surg Am 2005;87(11):2456–63. 21,047 hips over 30 years. Risk of dislocation 2.2% in 1st year, 3% at 5 years, 6% at 20 years. Larger femoral head diameter was associated with lower dislocation rate.

Table 14.3 Determinants of stability in hip replacement

Implant design-related factors	Surgical factors	Patient-related factors
Larger femoral head is more stable Larger acetabular component has lower risk of impingement Skirt on the femoral head (present in long-neck versions) predisposes to impingement Elevated lip liners can lead to impingement on the opposite side A narrow offset may cause impingement	Posterior approach without capsular repair may have higher risk Component malposition Abductor muscle dysfunction/poor repair Inadequate offset restoration Trochanteric non-union Surgeon's experience Secondary impingement from osteophytes and retained excess cement may lever the head out Impingement of the greater trochanter against the ilium can lead to dislocation	Noncompliance or cognitive impairment Previous surgery: revision hip surgery has twice the dislocation rate of primary surgery Hip replacement for femoral neck fractures Poor muscular balance or neuromuscular diseases Infection leads to effusion, capsular distension and dislocation

A skirt on the femoral head (seen in long-neck versions) predisposes to impingement and dislocation (Fig. 14.13).

Elevated lip liners can lead to impingement and lever the head out from the opposite side (Fig. 14.14). The elevated lip is placed posterosuperiorly when hip replacement is performed through a posterior approach to reduce risk of posterior dislocation. However, the combination of an elevated lip and an excessively anteverted cup can lever the femoral head anteriorly, leading to anterior dislocation.

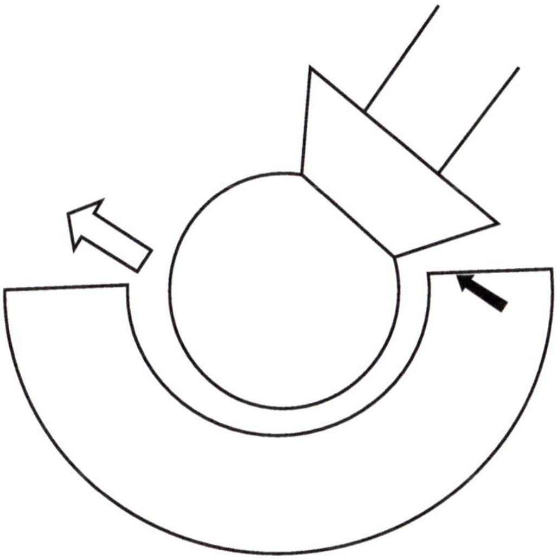

Fig. 14.13 The effect of skirted heads on impingement

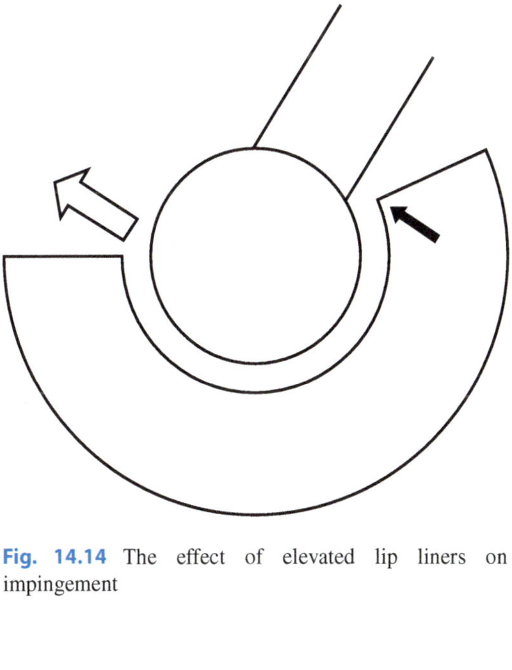

Fig. 14.14 The effect of elevated lip liners on impingement

The posterior approach has been blamed for a higher dislocation rate, but an enhanced repair reduces the dislocation rate comparable to direct lateral approach.

Pellici PM Bostrom M, Poss R. Posterior approach to total hip replacement using enhanced posterior soft tissue repair. Clin Orthop 1998; 355: 224–228. Dislocation rate of 6.2% was reduced to 0.8% in 124 hips with the enhanced repair.

Retroverted acetabular components predispose to posterior dislocation and excess anteversion predisposes to anterior dislocation. A more vertical cup alignment may also predispose to dislocation. Femoral anteversion over 15° can contribute to anterior instability. The combined anteversion of the femoral component and the acetabular component should be 30°. Cup inclination should be 35–45°.

The direction of dislocation is commonly posterior, even in a hip that has been performed from a direct lateral approach. Patient compliance may be an important factor in outcomes, as some studies have shown no difference in the position of the acetabular component between patients experiencing a dislocation and those with a stable prosthesis.

Complications in Total Hip Arthroplasty

Infection

Infections can be inadvertently introduced at the time of surgery and may spread through the bloodstream. Those with rheumatoid arthritis, psoriasis and diabetes are at higher risk for infection.

Philips JE, Crane TP, Noy M. The incidence of deep prosthetic infections in a specialist orthopaedic hospital. A 15 year prospective survey. J Bone Joint Surg Br 2006;88(7):943–8. Study from the Royal Orthopaedic Hospital, Birmingham. 10,735 patients having primary hip or knee replacement. Infection rate 0.57% in hips and 0.86% in knees. The commonest organism was coagulase negative staphylococcus. 72% were sensitive to routine antimicrobial prophylaxis. 29% infections were diagnosed within 3 months, 35% between 3 months and 1 year and 36% after 1 year of surgery. Most were detected acutely and treated aggressively and infection was eradicated in 96%.

Early postoperative infection (EPOI) occurs within 4 weeks of surgery, while infections after 4 weeks are classified as late chronic infections (LCI). Acute haematogenous infection (AHI) occurs as a late event with acute onset. Late haematogenous spread may develop following dental, gynaecological, abdominal or urologic procedures.

The American Musculoskeletal Infection Society laid down the diagnostic criteria for prosthetic joint infection. One of the three criteria should be present for infection. (Table 14.4).

Workgroup convened by the musculoskeletal infection society. New definition for periprosthetic joint infection. J Arthroplasty 2011;26:1136–8.

Prevention

Infection risk can be minimised by:

- Preoperative antibiotics given 30 min before start of surgery (commonly cefuroxime, Augmentin and/or Teicoplanin). The rationale for postoperative antibiotic therapy is debatable, and some studies suggest that a single dose before start of surgery is adequate.

Table 14.4 MSIS criteria for diagnosis of infection

1	Presence of sinus communicating with the prosthesis
2	Isolation by culture of a pathogen from two or more separate samples from the affected joint
3	Four of the following six: (a) Elevated ESR > 30 mm/h and CRP > 10 mg/L (b) Elevated synovial leucocyte count > 3000 cells/μL (c) Elevated synovial PMNs > 80% (d) Purulent joint fluid (e) Isolation of microorganisms in one culture of periprosthetic tissue or fluid (f) More than 5 PMN per High power field observed on histologic examination of periprosthetic tissue at ×400 magnification

- Vertical laminar air flow.
- Antibiotic-loaded cement—the use of gentamicin with bone cement has been shown to reduce the infection rate. Adding 2 g gentamicin to 40 g cement powder does not significantly compromise the mechanical strength of the cement.

Preoperative screening is done for active infection elsewhere. Symptomatic bacteriuria is a contraindication for elective implant surgery, although asymptomatic bacteriuria does not significantly increase the risk of implant infection.

Laminar air flow and preoperative intravenous antibiotics are considered mandatory for hip arthroplasty.

Diagnosis

Clinical suspicion of an infection should be raised by the presentation of pain at rest. Infections should be considered in patients with dislocation of the hip due to distension of the capsule.

Investigations

The ESR and CRP level are commonly used blood parameters in investigating infection. The ESR returns to normal 3 months after hip arthroplasty, while the CRP level normalises in 2–3 weeks. Elevation of both ESR and CRP has a high predictive value (>95%) for diagnosis of infection.

Yi PH, Cross MB, Moric M, Sporer SM, Berger RA, Della Valle CJ. The 2013 Frank Stinchfield Award: Diagnosis of infection in the early postoperative period after total hip arthroplasty. Clin Orthop Relat Res. 2014;472(2):424–9. Synovial fluid white cell count, CRP and synovial fluid differential were the best tests for diagnosis of PJI.

Maniar RN, Navaneedhan G, Ranvir S, Maniar AR, Dhiman A, Agrawal A. What Is the Normal Trajectory of Interleukin-6 and C-reactive Protein in the Hours and Days Immediately After TKA? Clin Orthop Relat Res. 2019;477(1):41–6. IL-6 peaks at 12 h post op and returns to near normal at 4 days. CRP reaches peak at 4 days and returns to normal at 2 weeks.

The white blood cell count has poor sensitivity and specificity for hip infections. Many studies have shown it to be elevated in only 15–26% of infected hip arthroplasties.

IL-6 is a highly sensitive marker for PJI. Combination of CRP and IL-6 carries a high positive predictive value. Procalcitonin has a high specificity for infection.

Glehr M, Friesenbichler J, Hofmann G, Bernhardt GA, Zacherl M, Avian A, Windhager R, Leithner A. Novel biomarkers to detect infection in revision hip and knee arthroplasties. Clin Orthop Relat Res. 2013;471(8):2621–8. A procalcitonin cut-off level of 0.35 ng/mL had a sensitivity of 80% and specificity of 37%. An IL-6 cut-off level of 2.55 pg/mL had a sensitivity of 92% and specificity of 59%.

On X-ray, irregular endosteal scalloping, a lacy periosteal reaction, early loosening and rapidly progressive radiolucent lines indicate infection. Radiological signs are generally a late feature in infection.

On radionuclide imaging, a Tc-99 scan may be positive in aseptic loosening. An indium-111 leukocyte scan is more specific that the Tc-99 scan. An indium-111 leukocyte scan has a nearly 100% sensitivity and 60% specificity for infection. When interpreted in combination with Tc-99 sulphur colloid imaging, however, the sensitivity remained high and the specificity is improved to 97%.

Preoperative joint aspiration has a sensitivity and specificity of 85% for infection in the hip. It also identifies the organism and helps determine sensitivity to antibiotics prior to revision surgery.

Partridge DG, Winnard C, Townsend R, Cooper R, Stockley I. Joint aspiration, including culture of reaspirated saline after a 'dry tap', is sensitive and specific for the diagnosis of hip and knee prosthetic joint infection. Bone Joint J. 2018;100(6):749–54. Retrospective study of 580 hips. Sensitivity and specificity of aspirate 84 and 85%. Saline injection and aspiration had similar accuracy.

Intraoperative frozen section is another method of identifying infection. Samples should be obtained from areas of inflammation surrounding the prosthetic joint. More than 5 polymorphonuclear (PMN) leucocytes per high-power field indicate infection with a sensitivity of 100% and specificity of 96%. The experience of the pathologist is an important factor.

Finally, culture of intraoperative samples is the gold standard for the diagnosis of joint infections. Multiple samples should be obtained, with different studies advising three to seven samples. Two or more samples should grow the same pathogen for diagnosis of infection.

Treatment

Superficial infections may be treated with antibiotics, with or without joint washout and retention of components. Deep infections, however, usually require removal of all metalwork and cement and reimplantation—either as single-stage or two-stage procedure.

Single-stage surgery is indicated when the organism is known and the organism is of low virulence and susceptible to antibiotics. The success of surgery may be compromised if the infecting organism is resistant (e.g., MRSA), the patient is immunocompromised or significant bone defects impair the stability of the implant. The advantages of single-stage are a reduced hospital stay, lower morbidity, faster return to mobility and lower cost.

Kunutsor SK et al. One- And Two-Stage Surgical Revision of Peri-Prosthetic Joint Infection of the Hip: A Pooled Individual Participant Data Analysis of 44 Cohort Studies. Eur J Epidemiol 2018;33(10):933–46. Similar results following one stage and two stage revision.

Kunutsor SK, Whitehouse MR, Blom AW, Beswick AD; INFORM Team. Re-Infection Outcomes following One- and Two-Stage Surgical Revision of Infected Hip Prosthesis: A Systematic Review and Meta-Analysis. PLoS One. 2015 Sep 25;10(9):e0139166. Similar results following one stage and two stage revision.

Callaghan JJ, Katz RP, Johnston RC. One stage revision surgery of the infected hip. A minimum 10 year follow up study. Clin Orthop 1999;369:139–143. 24 one stage revisions. 8.3%

reinfection rate. Criteria were—no draining sinuses, no immunocompromise, good bone stock after debridement and 3–6 months of postoperative oral antibiotic therapy.

In a two-stage revision, the first stage is removal of all metalwork, cement, infected tissue and infected bone. An antibiotic-loaded spacer is left in situ to provide a high local concentration of antibiotics. The second stage is generally performed 3 or more months later. During this stage, components are inserted once the inflammatory markers and signs of infection have settled. Two-stage revision allows the use of specific antibiotics. Patients can be monitored for control of infection and the optimum time for reimplantation can be planned.

Hsieh PH, Shih CH, Chang YH. Treatment of deep infection of the hip associated with massive bone loss: two stage revision with an antibiotic-loaded interim cement prosthesis followed by reconstruction with allograft. J Bone Joint Surg Br 2005;87(6): 770–5. 24 patients, two stage revision for infection, 4.2 year follow up, No recurrence of infection.

PROSTALAC (prosthesis with antibiotic-loaded acrylic cement) is a prosthesis used between the first and second stages to allow mobilisation, prevent shortening of the leg and provide a high dose of local antibiotics. Commercial prostheses are available although are often expensive. An option to these is using a cemented hip implant inserted without cement pressurisation. Lack of pressurization allows easier removal at the time of second stage, and the implant works like a hip replacement in the time between first and second stage. Many patients are able to continue with the temporary implant for a prolonged period without the need for a second stage operation.

Antibiotics can be mixed in the cement based on sensitivity, and a very high local concentration of antibiotics can be achieved, which would not be possible with parenteral dosage. Only heat stable antibiotics are used e.g. Vancomycin, gentamicin and tobramycin. Commercial preparations with antibiotic mixed in cement are available, although expensive. Presence of antibiotics weakens the cement and a general upper limit would be 3.2 g of tobramycin and 4 g of Vancomycin in 40 g of cement. If mixed in operation theatre, vacuum mixing is not done as higher porosity of cement encourages elution of antibiotics.

Local antibiotic delivery options exist through the use of absorbable calcium compounds. The advantage is elution of entire antibiotic as opposed to only surface elution when the antibiotics are mixed in cement. The setting of the calcium compound is not an exothermic reaction. Consequently, heat sensitive antibiotics and antifungal agents can be delivered. Data on their use is limited to case series at present.

Other options for treatment of infections include excision arthroplasty, antibiotic suppression and surgical debridement without removal of components. Excision arthroplasty helps control of infection, but the functional result is often poor. Antibiotic suppression can be considered for patients who are not medically well enough, or for those who refuse surgery. For antibiotic suppression, a well-fixed prosthesis, absence of systemic sepsis and presence of an organism sensitive to a well-tolerated antibiotic are required. Antibiotic therapy may be effective in early infection confined to the soft tissues, but formation of a biofilm on the implants significantly impairs the efficacy of antibiotics.

DAIR—Debridement, Antibiotics and Implant Retention is an option in acute onset infection (under 3 weeks). The parts of the implant fixed to the bone—acetabular component and the femoral stem are not removed. The acetabular liner and femoral head, if modular, are exchanged and a thorough debridement is undertaken. Post operative antibiotics are continued for 3–6 months.

Glycocalyx is a layer of protein and polysaccharide secreted by the bacteria which allows them to adhere to the surface of the implants. Biofilm is due to the bacteria multiplying in the glycocalyx layer. These bacteria are inaccessible to the antibiotics and resistant to phagocytosis. The biofilm forms in about 4 weeks after onset of infection. By this stage, removal of implant is necessary to treat infection.

Dislocation of Hip

Reported dislocation rates vary from less than 1% in reports from specialist centres to up to 5% in data from joint registries. Most dislocations happen in the 1st year and there is a slow and steady increase in this percentage with time. The risk of dislocation is higher in women and in those with inflammatory arthritis, non-union of femoral neck or avascular necrosis. The risk of dislocation rises over long term follow up.

Fender D, Harper WM, Gregg PJ. Outcome of Charnley total hip replacement across a single health region in England: the results at 5 years from a regional hip register. J Bone Joint Surg Br 1999;81(4):577–81. 1198 hips, aseptic loosening 2.3%, deep infection 1.4%, dislocation 5.0% and revision 3.2%. 9% failure rate at 5 years.

Berry DJ, von Knoch M, Schleck CD, Harmsen WS. . The Cumulative long term risk of dislocation after primary Charnley total hip arthroplasty. J Bone Joint Surg Am 2004; 86(1):9–14. Over 6000 patients over 15 years. All 22 mm cemented. 1% risk of dislocation at 1 month; 1.9% risk of dislocation at 1 year; 1% risk for every 5 years and 7% at 25 years. Higher risk in females, inflammatory arthritis, nonunion femoral neck and avascular necrosis.

A third of patients who have a dislocation do not have a second episode; another third may have two or three episodes and then stabilise without surgical intervention; and the remaining third may continue to have recurrent dislocations and require intervention.

The presence of an identifiable cause of dislocation improves the success rate of corrective surgery.

Revision hip where exchange of the liner in modular cementless acetabular components (leaving the metal shell in situ) is done has been shown to have a higher dislocation rate.

Blom AW, Astle L, Loveridge J, Learmonth ID. Revision of an acetabular liner has a high risk of dislocation. J Bone Joint Surg Br 2005;87(12):1636–8. 38 liners revised for wear. 11 (28.9%) of these exchanged liners had a dislocation within 4.5 year follow up.

Management of a First Time Dislocation of Hip Replacement

The history of events leading to dislocation is elicited and the neurological status is checked. Specifically, sciatic nerve function is documented.

X-rays of the pelvis in the AP view and the hip in the lateral view are obtained to assess the direction of the dislocation, the type and position of components, and whether there are signs of impingement or trochanteric problems.

Infection may be an underlying cause for dislocation and it should be ruled out by checking the erythrocyte sedimentation rate (ESR) and C-reactive protein (CRP) levels. Aspiration of the hip is not required unless inflammatory markers are elevated with no other obvious cause.

A manipulation under anaesthetic is undertaken. Posterior stability is assessed by flexion to 90° and internal rotation. Anterior stability is checked in extension and external rotation. Telescoping the leg is used to check laxity of abductors. Screening in the image intensifier is done to check the anteversion of the acetabular component and version of the femoral component.

Management of Recurrent Hip Dislocation

In addition to relocation of the hip as described, patients with an identifiable cause for instability, or those experiencing more than two or three episodes of dislocation should be considered for revision surgery. The underlying cause should be determined preoperatively, if possible. Plain X rays, evaluation of previous imaging of the hip, screening under image intensifier and CT scans are helpful in this respect.

In the presence of infection, management is according to infection guidelines.

The aim of surgery for recurrent dislocation is to remove any cause for impingement (e.g., cement, osteophytes or soft tissues).

Malalignment of components is corrected. Offset and the neck length are restored.

A larger head size or an elevated lip liner may improve stability.

Dual mobility liners provide stability through a larger femoral head but have the disadvantage of an additional bearing surface within the head. It is increasingly popular with evidence for relatively low complication rate.

Darrith B, Courtney PM, Della Valle CJ. Outcomes of dual mobility components in total hip arthroplasty: a systematic review of the literature. Bone Joint J 2018;100(1):11–19.

Over ten thousand dual mobility sockets, 1.3% aseptic loosening, 1.1% intraprosthetic dislocation and 0.46% dislocation. 98% survivorship at 8.5 years.

Constrained liners (Fig. 14.15) are available which can be cemented into the existing shell, or exchanged into the metal shell if the shell is compatible. These liners may predispose to loosening because the restrictions on head movement are transmitted to the implant–bone interface as a shear force.

Revision to a bipolar hemiarthroplasty is an option as a larger head is more stable. Postoperative pain is a problem in these patients.

If all fails, or if patient is medically unfit for major reconstruction, excision arthroplasty can be considered.

Ekelund J. Trochanteric osteotomy for recurrent dislocation of total hip arthroplasty J Arthro 1993;8(6):629–32. 17 out of 21 patients had no further dislocation. Indicated when no cause can be found.

Parvizi J, Morrey BF. Bipolar hip arthroplasty as a salvage treatment for instability of the hip. J Bone Joint Surg Am 2000;82(8):1132–9.

Goetz DD, Bremner BR, Callaghan JJ, Capello WN, Johnston RC. Salvage of a recurrently dislocation total hip prosthesis with use of a constrained acetabular component. J Bone Joint Surg Am 2004;86(11):2419–23. 55 patients, 10.2 year follow up, 7% had subsequent dislocation, 4% revised for aseptic loosening, one hip revised for osteolysis.

Venous Thromboembolism

The incidence of venous thromboembolism (VTE) in those undergoing hip replacement has been reported to range from 8 to 70%. The risk of non-fatal PE is 1% and risk of fatal PE is less than 1%.

A diagnosis of pulmonary embolism (PE) should be suspected in patients with shortness of breath, chest pain or mental status changes. Oxygen saturation may fall and analysis of blood gas will show respiratory failure. Investigations for diagnosis include chest X-ray and a computed tomography (CT) scan with pulmonary angiography.

Prophylaxis is with warfarin, low molecular weight heparin or fondaparinux. The newer oral anticoagulants rivaroxaban and dabigatran have

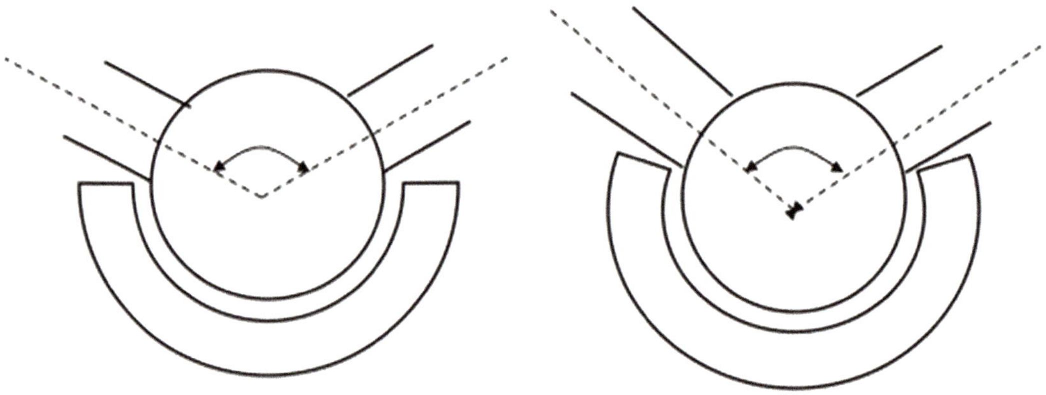

Fig. 14.15 A standard liner is hemispheric or less than a hemisphere. Constrained liners extend beyond the equator of the femoral head

been approved by NICE for postoperative anticoagulation and can be continued following discharge from hospital. Mechanical prophylaxis is provided in addition to chemical prophylaxis by foot or calf pumps. The chemoprophylaxis should continue for a period of 5 weeks following hip replacement surgery.

Treatment is with warfarin for 3 months (in patients with VTE) or 6 months (in patients with proven PE.

Heterotopic Ossification

Patients with ankylosing spondylitis, posttraumatic arthritis, extensive soft tissue dissection, hypertrophic arthritis (extensive osteophytes) and hip arthrodesis for conversion to total hip replacement are at higher risk for heterotopic ossification (HO). Clinically, HO rarely restricts motion.

HO may be classified by the Brooker classification (Table 14.5).

Table 14.5 Classification of heterotopic ossification: Brooker staging

Grade	Description	
I	Islands of bone within soft tissues	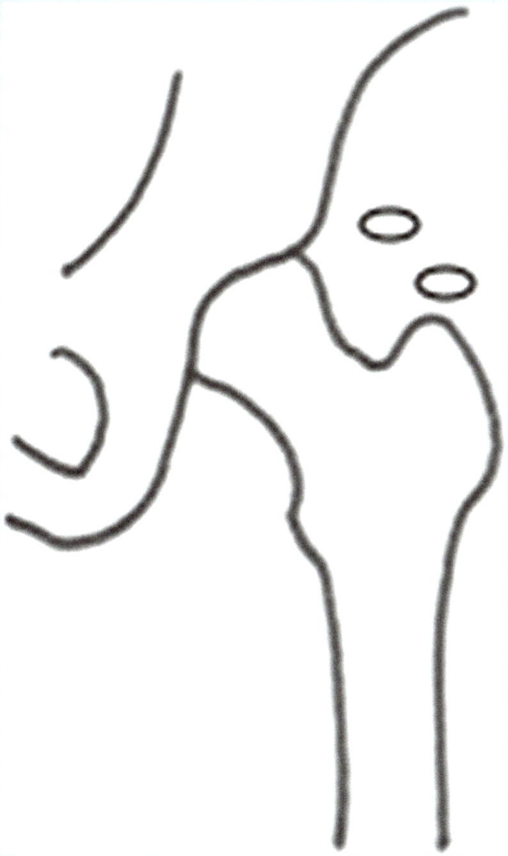

(continued)

Table 14.5 (continued)

Grade	Description	
II	Bone spurs on femur or pelvis with >1 cm gap between opposing surfaces	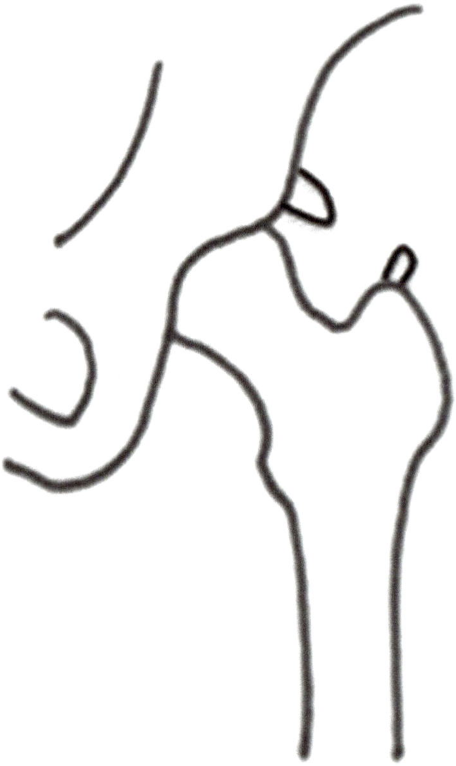
III	Bone spurs on femur or pelvis with <1 cm gap between opposing surfaces	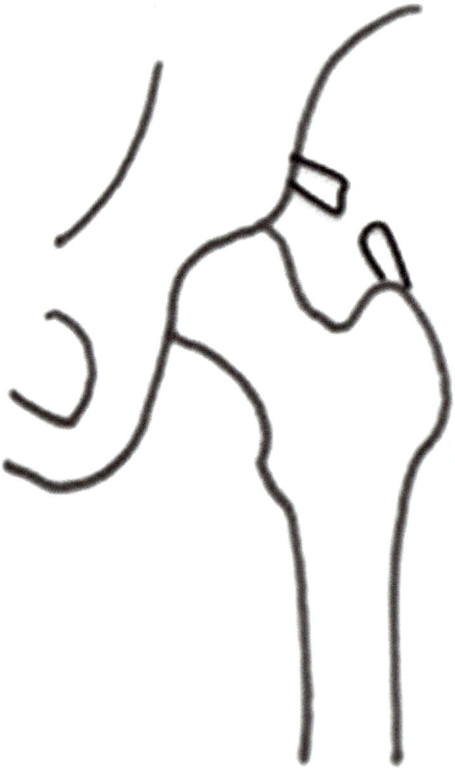

Table 14.5 (continued)

Grade	Description
IV	Apparent bony ankylosis

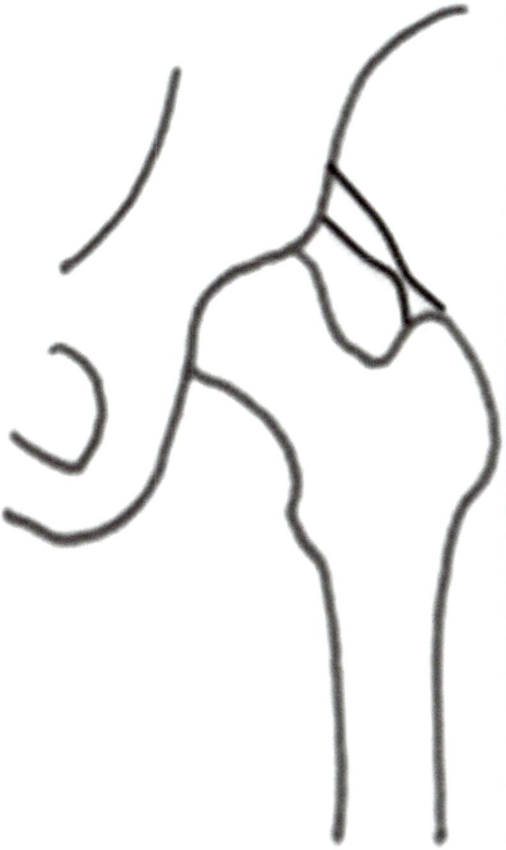

A limitation of the Brooker classification is that it is a two-dimensional description of a three-dimensional event. The AP view of the pelvis may show spurs close to each other, but those spurs may be in different coronal planes. However, the system is easy to use and gives some idea of the amount of heterotopic bone.

HO can be prevented with radiation or indomethacin. Radiation therapy is with single dose of 750 rads postoperatively before discharge. Cementless prostheses must be shielded to avoid interference with bone ingrowth. Indomethacin 75 mg once daily for 6 weeks is another option. Indomethacin is not advisable for uncemented prostheses, however, as it may interfere with bone ingrowth.

Leg Length Discrepancy

Leg length discrepancy is minimised by careful preoperative planning. This should take into account the preoperative leg length difference, the planned position of the acetabular component, the planned level of the neck cut, the size and position of the femoral component and the neck length and offset.

The operating surgeon should have a fairly accurate estimate of the implant type and size required before starting surgery. Intraoperative checks include assessment of tension in the soft tissues, comparing the position of knees or other methods to compare preoperative and postoperative length.

Lengthening of up to 5 mm may be tolerated well. Beyond this, a shoe raise can be used on the other side to balance the difference. A very small percentage of patients may require revision for leg length inequality, generally for difference greater than 10 mm.

Fracture of Femur

Fractures are more common with cementless stems, which fit snugly into the femur, and virtually unknown with cemented stems.

Fractures at the proximal end of femur that are detected while impacting the prosthesis can be managed with cerclage wiring and restricted postoperative weight bearing.

Unstable fractures near the tip of the femoral component should be managed with a long stem implant that bypasses the fracture site by more than two cortical diameters. Additional cerclage or cable plate may be needed for stability.

Acetabular fractures may occur in cementless components that are press fit.

Trochanteric Non-union

Trochanteric non-union is a complication of trochanteric osteotomy. The traditional trochanteric osteotomy is rarely done for primary hip replacements.

Revision surgery sometimes necessitates a transtrochanteric approach, but the extended trochanteric osteotomy has a better healing potential and provides excellent access, with a very low risk of non-union. Diaphyseal fixation of femoral component is needed when using the transtrochanteric approach.

Failure of Components

Historically, femoral stems failed due to poor metallurgy, high offset and a thin cross-section, or a combination of these. Breakage of the femoral component is now uncommon. Failure usually initiates on the anterolateral aspect, which is the tension side in the stem.

Factors contributing to stem fracture are:

- A higher body weight exerts more stress on the stem and can lead to failure of thin stems.
- Thin stems have lower ultimate strength.
- A long neck or higher offset increases the lever arm on the stem.
- Varus positioning of the stem in effect increases the lever arm due to an increased distance between the centre of the femoral head and the axis of the femur.
- Type IV failure, where the stem is firmly fixed distally but is loose proximally, leads to toggle of the stem and early failure.
- Poor metallurgy means weaker stems.

Currently, most manufacturers advise a maximum patient weight that should not be exceeded for a particular stem size. This is a consideration when using very small stem sizes.

Stem failure can be diagnosed before actual fracture by comparing the most recent radiographic films with the postoperative films. Any evidence of bending of the stem is a sign of impending failure and an indication for revision. Fracture of the stem can be a subtle finding on postoperative radiographs.

Limp

A Trendelenburg gait can be due to abductor damage, damage to the superior gluteal nerve resulting in abductor palsy or trochanteric non-union. In addition, a short or a long leg following surgery can result in a limp. An antalgic gait can be due to a painful arthroplasty because of infection or loosening.

Nerve or Vessel Injury

The nerve most commonly at risk is the sciatic nerve in the posterior approach. The risk is higher in patients with developmental dysplasia of the hip or those undergoing revision surgery.

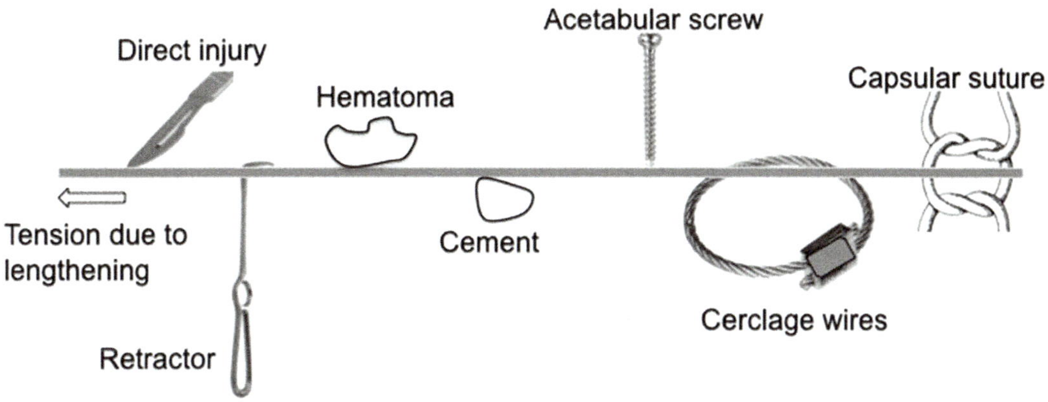

Fig. 14.16 Illustration of causes of sciatic nerve injury

Schmalzreid TP, Amstutz HC. Update on nerve palsy associated with total hip replacement. Clin Orthop Relat Res 1997;344:188–206. Femoral nerve has more predictable recovery than sciatic. 15% have a poor outcome and 44% have a complete or near complete recovery.

Nerve injury may be due to various causes as illustrated in Fig. 14.16.

The maximum lengthening permitted intraoperatively in developmental dysplasia of the hip is approximately 2.5 cm. Beyond this limit, the nerve is at risk for stretch injury. In dysplastic hips, the nerve is short and has never been as long as the contralateral normal hip.

In acquired shortening, for instance after excision arthroplasty in adulthood, maximum lengthening is 4 cm.

Patients with post operative nerve palsy should have an urgent CT scan, which can help delineate a hematoma around the sciatic nerve or a screw in close contact with the nerve. Postoperative nerve palsy should be managed by early exploration to rule out hematoma and to check for any direct injury

Kyriacou S, Pastides PS, Singh VK, Jeyaseelan L, Sinisi M, Fox M. Exploration and neurolysis for the treatment of neuropathic pain in patients with a sciatic nerve palsy after total hip replacement. Bone Joint J 2013;95:20–22. 56 patients with postoperative sciatic nerve palsy after primary, revision or resurfacing hip arthroplasty. Improvement in neuropathic pain VAS was seen after neurolysis. Recommend neurolysis as opposed to conservative treatment.

Femoral nerve injury is rare and may be due to improper retractor placement, or correction of severe fixed flexion deformity.

Aseptic Loosening of the Prosthesis

A number of factors determine the loosening of an implant over time. In cementless implants, stability is determined by the initial stability achieved at insertion, degree of porous coating, extent of bone ingrowth/ongrowth, response to wear debris and effective joint space. Cemented femoral implants have two potential interfaces for loosening: the metal–cement interface and the cement–bone interface.

Loosening is diagnosed on radiographs by criteria described by Harris. The features that indicate definite loosening are:

- Progressive or complete radiolucency at the cement–bone or implant–bone interface.
- Migration of the component.
- Fracture of the component.
- Fracture of the cement mantle.
- Debonding.

Debonding, which is lucency at the metal–cement interface commonly seen in Gruen zone 1, is predictive of loosening in cemented stems.

Debonding is not a sign of loosening in polished taper stems such as the Exeter as these stems are designed to subside in the cement mantle. A flanged Charnley is not intended to subside and debonding indicates loosening.

Probable loosening is defined as complete radiolucency at the cement–bone interface, while possible loosening is the presence of radiolucency of more than 50% but not complete at the cement–bone interface.

A pedestal may be present just distal to the tip of an unstable subsiding stem. This is a bridge of bone that forms to provide some stability to the stem.

Indicators of a stable implant are as follows:

- Absence of radiolucency at the implant bone interface.
- Proximal stress shielding, indicating that the stem that is well-fixed distally.
- Presence of 'spot weld'—areas of dense bone extending from the ingrowth surface of the implant to the endosteal surface of cortex of bone.

The acetabular zones have been described by DeLee and Charnley (Fig. 14.17). Gruen's zones of demarcation are used to define the extent of loosening of femoral components (Fig. 14.18).

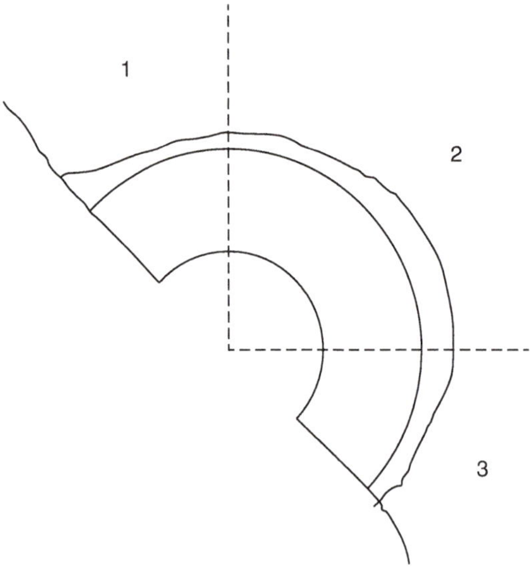

Fig. 14.17 Delee Charnley zones for acetabular loosening. The vertical and horizontal lines are drawn through the centre of the acetabulum

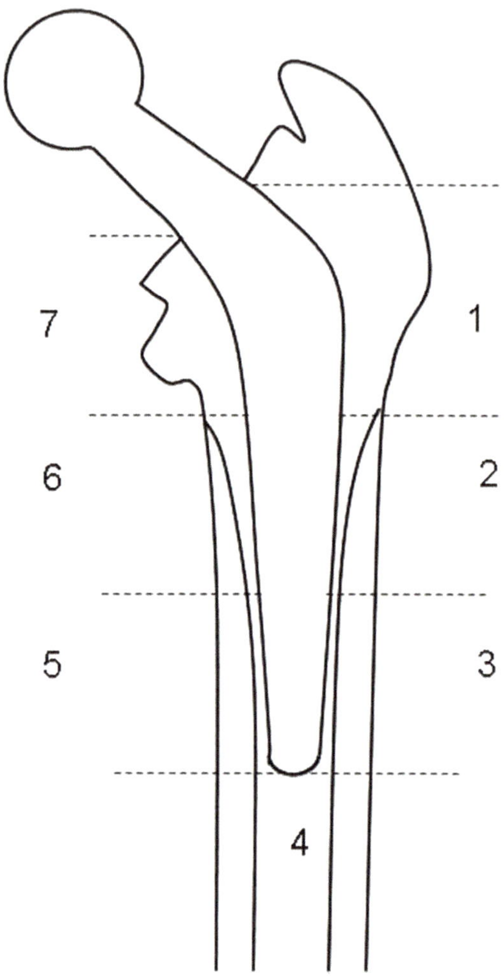

Fig. 14.18 Gruen zones for femoral component loosening

Gruen TA, McNeice GM, Amstutz HC. "Modes of failure" of cemented stem-type femoral components: a radiographic analysis of loosening. Clin Orthop Relat Res 1979;141:17–27.

DeLee J, Charnley J. Radiological demarcation of cemented sockets in total hip replacement. Clin Orthop 1976;121:20–32.

Modes of Failure of Femoral Component

Gruen described four modes of failure of cemented femoral components that are summarised in Table 14.6.

Table 14.6 Gruen modes of failure of femoral components

Mode of failure	Mechanism	Illustration
1a—Pistoning of stem within cement mantle	Inadequate bonding at metal-cement interface Fracture of zone 4 cement Lucency in zone 1 and 7	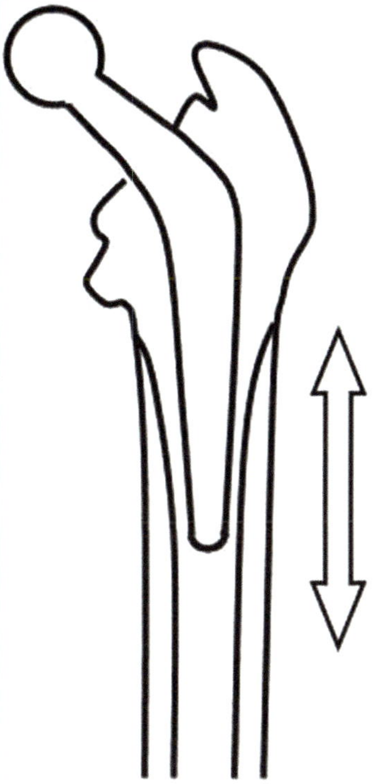
1b—Pistoning of cement mantle within bone	Due to inadequate cementation Lucency in all zones	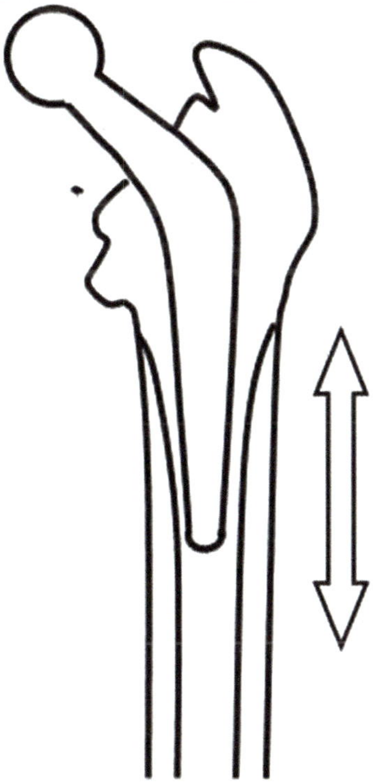

(continued)

Table 14.6 (continued)

Mode of failure	Mechanism	Illustration
2—Mid stem pivot	Inadequate cementation in zone 7 and zone 3 Stem tilts into varus	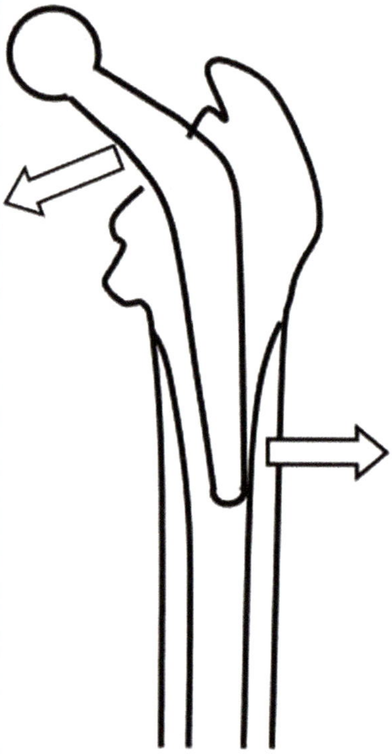
3—Calcar pivot	Due to poor distal cementation Well fixed calcar cement, but windshield wiper effect seen at tip of stem	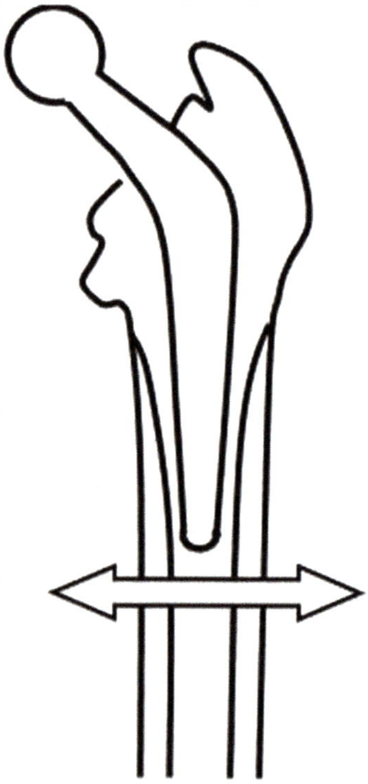

Table 14.6 (continued)

Mode of failure	Mechanism	Illustration
4—Cantilever bending	Stable distal fixation but poor proximal fixation Stem may bend and eventually fractures	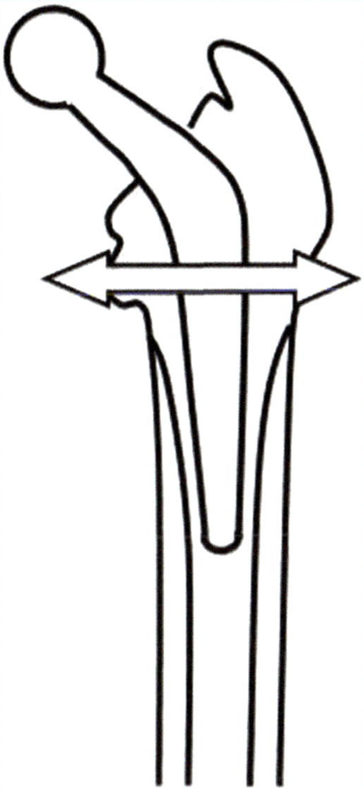

Wear of Bearing Surface

The hip prosthesis is subject to wear over time. The mechanism of wear can be of three types:

1. Adhesive wear—the articulating surfaces bind to each other under load and movement results in material being pulled off the weaker surface.
2. Abrasive wear—asperities from the harder surface physically cut through the weaker surface removing material from the weaker surface.
3. Fatigue wear—the repeat stresses exceed the failure strength of the material.

Modes of Wear

The modes of wear can be divided into four types (Table 14.7).

Mode I wear is integral to a functioning joint. The other types may be present to varying extents and may progress with time. Mode III is called third body wear. Mode II and IV are not intended.

Table 14.7 Modes of wear

Mode	Mechanism	Example
Mode I	Wear due to motion between two bearing surfaces that are intended to articulate against each other	The femoral head against the polyethylene
Mode II	Wear due to motion between a bearing surface and a non-bearing surface	The femoral head against the acetabular metal shell; or femoral condyle against the tibial base plate
Mode III	Wear between primary bearing surfaces with interposed particles. This is known as 'third body wear'	The particles may be cement, polyethylene, metal or HA
Mode IV	Wear due to motion between two non-bearing surfaces	The femoral neck against the acetabular metal shell or motion between the polyethylene insert and the metal shell in acetabular components (backside wear)

Quantification of Wear

Wear can be measured as linear penetration of the femoral head measured on radiographs; or as volumetric wear.

The AP radiograph only measure wear in the coronal plane (Fig. 14.19) and completely ignores wear in planes different from that of the radiograph. Combining the AP and the lateral view of wear analysis improves this assessment as it considers wear in two planes. However, lateral radiographs are not always performed and may not be adequate for wear analysis.

While making wear measurements, it is important to consider that other factors may contribute to migration of the femoral head within the acetabulum. Creep in the polyethylene and 'bedding in' of the insert in the metal shell occur in the same direction as wear and can influence measurement of wear on postoperative radiographs.

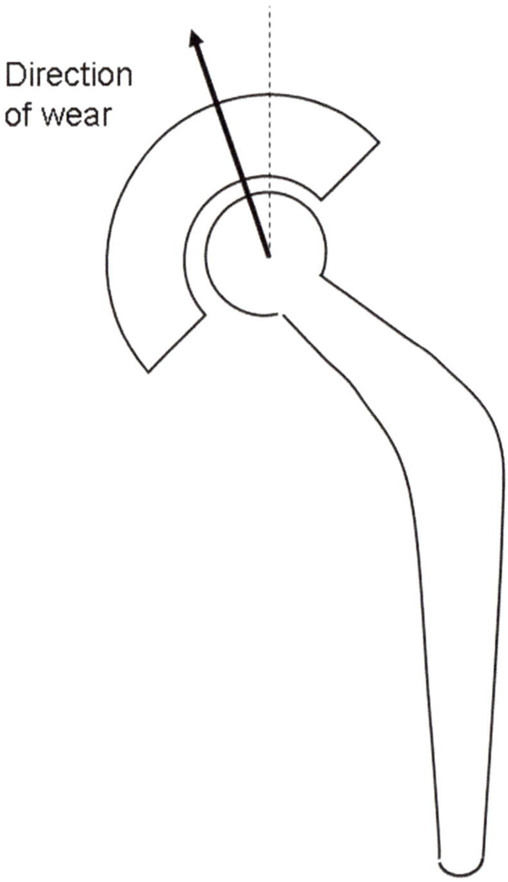

Fig. 14.19 Direction of wear in hip arthroplasty in the coronal plane

Volumetric wear is the product of linear penetration and the diameter of the head. For the same distance worn, volumetric wear will be greater for larger femoral head.

Radiostereometric analysis (RSA) or Ein Bild Roentgen Analysis (EBRA) are used to measure wear postoperatively.

Choice of Bearing Surface

The options available to the surgeon for bearing surface in total hip replacement are

(a) Metal/ceramic femoral head with standard/highly cross-linked polyethylene liner for the acetabulum
(b) Ceramic femoral head and ceramic acetabular liner
(c) Metal femoral head and metal acetabular liner.

Titanium is not a good material for femoral heads. It scratches easily and a scratched titanium head will damage the polyethylene insert leading to rapid wear. Zirconia ceramic heads increase in roughness over time through a process called phase transformation. These were used in the past but are no longer considered suitable material for femoral head.

Delta ceramic femoral head with a polyethylene liner is a good articulation.

Highly cross linked polyethylene continues to be a popular choice. Polyethylene used to be sterilized in air. The radiation led to breakage of polyethylene chains with formation of free radicals. In the presence of oxygen (air), free radicals combined with oxygen to form oxidized polyethylene, which had poor wear characteristics. Polyethylene is now sterilised in inert environment. The polyethylene is exposed to electron beam (5–15 Megarads) that causes the chains to cross link. This is cross linked polyethylene (XLPE), and has improved wear characteristics. Addition of vitamin E to the polyethylene is also considered to reduce the impact of free radicals.

The rate of wear of conventional UHMWPE is 0.1–0.2 mm/year. Cross linking with electron beam reduces the rate of wear although makes the polyethylene brittle.

Kuzyk PRT, Saccone M, Sprague S, Simunovic N, Bhandari M, Schemitsch EH. Cross linked versus conventional polyethylene for total hip replacement: a meta-analysis of randomized controlled trials. J Bone Joint Surg Br 2011;93(5):593–600. Significantly low wear rate with highly cross-linked polyethylene.

Squeaking from the articulation is sometimes seen in patients with ceramic on ceramic bearings. It may be related to component positioning. The implant positioning factors associated with squeaking are:

(a) High acetabular component inclination
(b) High femoral offset
(c) Lateralization of the hip centre
(d) High or low acetabular anteversion.

Patient characteristics associated with squeaking are tall, heavy and young. Increased mechanical force across the hip joint and edge loading are associated with squeaking.

Sexton SA, Yeung E, Jackson MP, Rajaratnam S, Martell JM, Walter WL, Zicat BA, Walter WK. The role of patient factors and implant position in squeaking of ceramic on ceramic total hip replacements. J Bone Joint Surg Br 2011;93(4):439–42. 2406 ceramic hips, 10 year follow up, 3.1% incidence of squeaking. Associated factors—as detailed in text.

Metal on metal bearings demonstrate wear rates of 2–5 μm/year. Adverse reaction to metal debris has dramatically reduced the usage of metal on metal articulations.

Low-Friction Arthroplasty

When developing the hip arthroplasty procedure, Sir John Charnley used a 22.225 mm head to reduce friction torque at the metal–polyethylene interface. A smaller head size was supposed to reduce torque and an added advantage was the use of a thicker polyethylene, which distributed the torque over a large surface area.

Over the years, the wear particles have assumed a greater significance than the torque generated. Charnley's concept still holds good because a smaller head generates a lower volume of wear particles. However, the use of surfaces with low wear characteristics—such as highly cross-linked polyethylene or ceramic—may allow the use of larger-diameter heads.

Wroblewski BM, Siney PD, Fleming PA. Wear of the cup in Charnley LFA in the young patient. J Bone Joint Surg Br 2004;86(4):498–503. High wear seen in men, osteoarthritis, valgus stem position. Varus stem position correlated with low wear.

Osteolysis

Osteolysis is resorption of bone. With regards to joint replacement, it is initiated as a chemico-immunological reaction to particulate material resulting in absorption of bone around the implant.

In 1977, Willert and Semlitsch demonstrated the presence of macrophages in response to wear debris. Goldring described the synovial-like character of the interfacial membrane and demonstrated the presence of prostaglandin E_2 (PGE_2) and collagenase secretion from the cells. Observations of osteolysis in cemented implants led to a general belief that osteolysis was related to the acrylic cement and the term 'cement disease' was introduced.

A functioning hip joint generates wear particles. The most biologically active particle are sized between 0.5 and 1.0 μm. Polyethylene particles are the predominant type among the various types of particles found in the wear debris and account for 70–90% of the debris volume. Other particles may be of cobalt chrome, polymethylmethacrylate, bone, titanium alloys, ceramics or stainless steel.

Larger particles (>50 μm) induce fibrous encapsulation, while smaller particles (<7 μm) are phagocytosed and lead to macrophage activation and release of a variety of cytokines such as interleukins, TNF-α, PGE_2 and metalloproteases. Small irregular particles of polymethylmethacrylate have greater reactivity than spherical particles of the same size.

The effective joint space is the entire region within a prosthetic joint that is exposed to the joint fluid and consequently the wear particles. A patch-porous coated stem allows particles to pass distally in the intramedullary canal leading to osteolytic bone resorption. A prosthesis with a good fit proximally, and which is cemented or circumferentially porous-coated, will resist this particle flow.

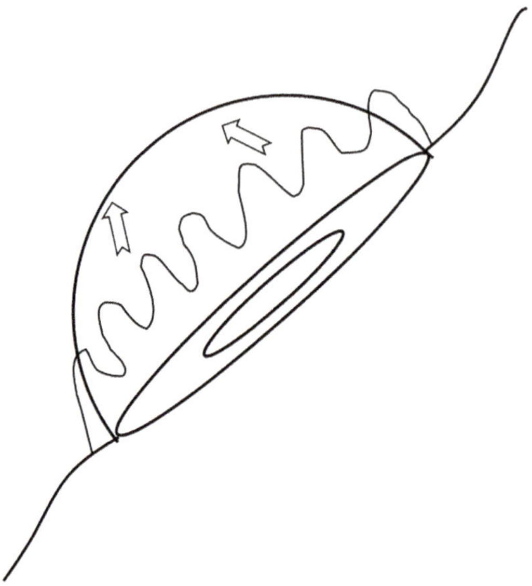

Fig. 14.20 Formation of histiocytic membrane at cement bone interface from the equator to the pole of the cup. This is characteristic of cemented acetabular components

Clinical Presentation

Osteolysis is a silent process and, in itself, does not cause any symptoms. The symptoms may arise from the sequelae of osteolysis—which can be loosening or pathologic fracture through an area of resorbed bone. Osteolysis is diagnosed by serial radiographic follow-up or CT scans.

Radiological Assessment

The extent of osteolysis is frequently underestimated on plain radiographs and a CT scan gives a more accurate assessment. The site of osteolysis around the hip joint depends on the access of particles to the area and is determined, in turn, by the fixation of the implant.

In cemented cups, failure is through formation of a histiocytic membrane from the rim to the dome of the cup (Fig. 14.20). The membrane forms at the cement–bone interface. The subchondral bone acts as a barrier to ingress of wear particles, resulting in a linear pattern of bone resorption. This pattern is known as linear osteolysis.

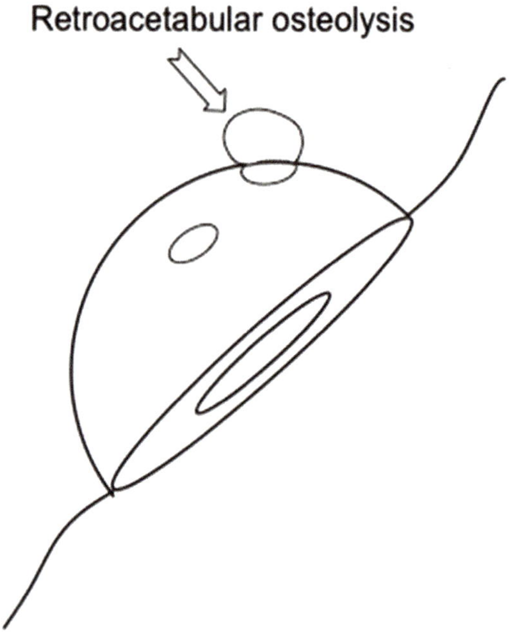

Fig. 14.21 Pattern of osteolysis in well fixed cementless acetabular components. The access of particles is through the screw holes in the metal shell

In cementless components, the particles gain access to the retroacetabular area through the screw holes (Fig. 14.21). Cementless acetabular components show localised areas of osteolysis that represent areas of particle collection. These are described as balloon osteolysis. 'Spot welds' (areas of strong fixation of the cementless component to the bone by dense trabeculae) act as barriers to particle access—hence the localised nature of the osteolysis.

In cementless stems, the patch-porous coating used in historical implants allowed particle access to the distal end of the stem (Fig. 14.6). All modern implants now have circumferential coating in the proximal part of the stem to achieve firm fixation. Circumferential osseointegration in the proximal femur will restrict particle access to the distal aspect of the femoral component, thus reducing the 'effective joint space'.

Other Causes of Bone Loss/ Radiolucency Around Femoral Implants

Osteolysis is only one cause of bone loss or radiolucency around femoral implants. Other causes may be:

- Non-filling of cement. This describes gaps between the cement and the bone that did not fill with cement at the time of implantation. These areas will be apparent on the initial postoperative radiographs.
- Adaptive remodeling with formation of a neocortex. Over a period of many years in elderly patients, the femur expands due to osteoporosis. A new layer of bone forms adjacent to the cement surface, providing stability. Lucency will be visible on the radiographs between the cement and the bone. This will remain the same on follow-up because the stem is stable.
- Stress shielding. This is commonly seen in distally coated femoral stems. Stress shielding occurs when there is distal stability and the proximal femur is bypassed with regards to weight-bearing forces. This results in diffuse loss of bone in the proximal femur with dense cortical bone distally, which is where the load is being transferred between the prosthesis and bone. A stiff distally fixed stem will lead to greater stress shielding.

Table 14.8 Guidelines for management of acetabular osteolysis in metal backed acetabular components

Type	Clinical situation	Recommended solution
I	Metal shell is stable, in a good position and has a good track record. The locking mechanism is intact A replacement liner is available	Replace liner, graft lytic lesion
II	The shell is stable, but a liner is not available or the above criteria are not met	1. Revise shell Or: 2. A polyethylene liner can be cemented into the stable metal shell. The outer surface of liner is scored to improve the cement bond
III	Metal shell is loose	Revise metal shell

Management of Osteolysis

Osteolysis resulting in loosening of components is an indication for revision surgery.

Guidelines for management of acetabular osteolysis are shown in Table 14.8.

Maloney W, Paprosky W, Engh CA, Rubash HE. Surgical treatment of pelvic osteolysis. Clin Orthop Rel Res 2001;393:78–84.

Metal on Metal Hip Arthroplasty

Metal on metal (MoM) hip replacements gained popularity on the premise of low wear and high postoperative activity level.

These are hard bearings and particles generated are of the size of 50–100 nm, which are substantially smaller than polyethylene debris particles, but much more in number. The bearing surface is 'self polishing' and resistant to abrasive wear. Particle generation is maximal in the first 2 years.

Metal on metal articulation are subject to adhesive wear and have fluid film lubrication. Historical MoM had equatorial bearing and had a high torque and poor lubrication.

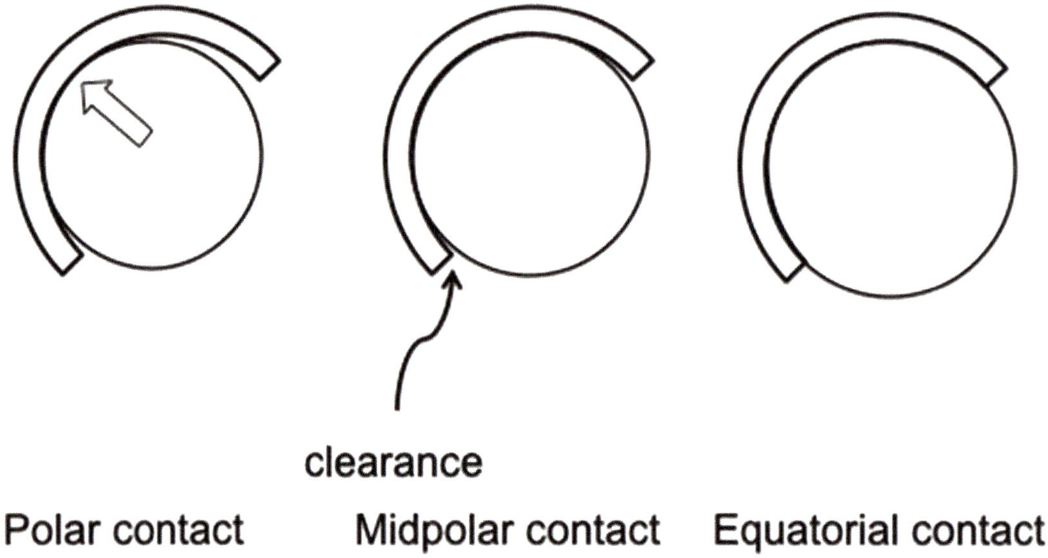

Fig. 14.22 Contact between acetabular liner and femoral head in metal on metal bearings

Clearance is the difference between cup internal radius and the head radius (Fig. 14.22). Polar contact allows a much lower torque but excess stress concentration and wear. Mid polar contact is preferable with a 90–200 μm clearance. Equatorial contact leads to lockout of the fluid film and is not desirable.

The problems with MoM hips are metal ion release in the periarticular tissues and systemic effects.

Adverse Reaction to Metal Debris (ARMD) is a term which includes metallosis, ALVAL (aseptic lymphocytic vasculitis associated lesions) and pseudotumours. The mechanism of ARMD can either be direct cytotoxicity from metal ions, or a type 4 hypersensitivity reaction. Hypersensitivity is ascribed to sensitivity to Nickel ions in the metal articulation and is seen in the early period after implantation.

The metal particles generated are nanometer size compared to macron size in polyethyelene articulation, but are in much greater number. Accumulation of particles in the joint space causes increased levels in blood and urine.

Ingestion of these particles by macrophages leads to cell death. Metallosis is black staining of the tissues from the metal particles. Pseudotumours can be solid or cystic and have a biologically active membrane which secretes collagenase, IL-1 and TNF.

Systemic metal ions are excreted through the kidneys. Concerns over carcinogenesis and teratogenicity remain but robust scientific evidence of this is lacking.

Resurfacing Hip Arthroplasty

The use of large-diameter metal-on-metal articulation has been attempted at various stages of the development of total hip arthroplasty. Initial attempts in the 1950s were, however, overshadowed by the development of the successful Charnley hip arthroplasty.

In 1988 there was a resurgence of interest in hip resurfacing with the development of cobalt chrome alloy bearings. McMinn introduced resurfacing in 1991. The initial design was a smooth press fit, but this had a high incidence of aseptic loosening. Cemented components were introduced and the acetabular component again had a high loosening rate. In 1994, a HA-coated acetabulum and cemented femoral component was developed. From 1994 to 1996, McMinn hip resurfacing used a smooth HA cup and cemented femur. In 1996, the Birmingham hip resurfacing

(BHR) system was introduced, using a porous HA-coated cup and cemented femoral component.

Most of the current resurfacings have a high carbon-content cobalt chrome alloy, with a cemented femoral component and cementless acetabular component. The components of a wrought cobalt chrome alloy are harder and show better wear resistance. Cast cobalt chrome alloy requires postcasting heat treatment.

Double heat treatment of the components leads to a high rate of wear and failure. The heat treatment depletes the carbon, and the reduced percentage of carbide leads to poor wear resistance.

Daniel J, Ziaee H, Kamali A, Pradhan C, Band T, McMinn DJ. Ten year results of a double heat treated metal on metal hip resurfacing. J Bone Joint Surg Br 2010;92(1):20–27. 184 hips done in 1996 in Birmingham. 16% revisions at 7 years, 24% had signs of failure on X rays. High rate of wear due to double heat treatment.

Advantages

The advantages and disadvantages are summarised in Table 14.9.

Hip resurfacing involves limited removal of bone on the femoral side but removal of acetabular bone is similar to conventional hip replacements.

Table 14.9 Pros and cons of hip resurfacing

Advantages of hip resurfacing	Disadvantages of hip resurfacing
Better reproduction of hip biomechanics Avoids stress shielding of the proximal femur Allows a higher level of activity due to hard bearing and low wear Allows a greater range of motion (ROM) and a lower risk of dislocation compared to conventional hip replacement Conservative procedure with limited removal of bone on the femoral side.	High failure rate with certain designs Risk of ARMD Femoral neck fractures in 1–2% Avascular necrosis of the femoral head Femoral neck thinning Learning curve for surgeons

Vendittoli J, Lavigne M, Girard J, Roy AG. A randomised study comparing resection of acetabular bone at resurfacing and total hip replacement. J Bone Joint Surg Br 2006;88(8):997–1002. 210 hips randomly assigned. Uncemented press fit cups compared to resurfacing. No difference in amount of acetabular bone removed between the two groups.

Avascular necrosis of the femoral head may lead to loosening of the prosthesis or periprosthetic fracture. Femoral neck thinning may be due to altered stress distribution in the femoral neck, possibly related to the presence of the femoral stem.

Fixation of an acetabular component may not be as secure as usual titanium cementless total hip replacement components, as the cobalt chrome component in hip resurfacing is stiffer and has different mechanical properties. In addition, screws cannot be placed in hip resurfacing acetabular components to augment fixation.

Indications for Hip Resurfacing

Ideally, hip resurfacing is indicated in young patients with osteoarthritis, and most surgeons would prefer relatively normal bone geometry. Patients with avascular necrosis, secondary arthritis from developmental dysplasia of the hip, Perthes' disease and slipped upper femoral epiphysis may also be indications for hip resurfacing.

Contraindications for Hip Resurfacing

Metal hypersensitivity, impaired renal function and proximal femoral osteoporosis in elderly patients are contraindications for hip resurfacing. Large cysts in the proximal femur, severe acetabular bone loss, grossly abnormal proximal femoral geometry and inflammatory arthritis are also relative contraindications for the procedure.

Hip resurfacing is contraindicated in women of childbearing age, and the use of a head size less than 46 mm is also not advised.

De Smet K, Campbell PA, Gill HS. Metal on Metal resurfacing. A consensus from the advanced hip resurfacing course, Ghent, June 2009. J Bone Joint Surg Br 2010;92:335–6.

Causes of Failure of Hip Resurfacing

1. Component size

   The size of the components of resurfacing may have an influence on the survival of the prosthesis, as suggested by data from the Australian National Joint Register. The report suggested that femoral components of less than 44 mm correlated with fivefold risk of revision.

   Shimmin AJ, Walter WL, Esposito C. The influence of the size of the component on the outcome of resurfacing arthroplasty of the hip: a review of literature. J Bone Joint Surg Br 2010;92(4):469–76. Suggested the cause of failure may be multifactorial. Femoral component size less than 44 mm have a five-fold higher risk of revision compared to hips with femoral components more than 55 mm size.
2. Component design

   The arc of the acetabular component is less than a hemisphere in resurfacing arthroplasty and may range from 145 to 170°. A smaller arc increases the risk of edge loading, especially if the component is placed in a more open position.
3. Component orientation

   Steeply placed acetabular components are at risk of edge loading and this correlates with a higher rate of wear and early failure (Fig. 14.23).

   De Haan R, Pattyn C, Gil HS. Correlation between inclination of the acetabular component and metal ion levels in metal on metal hip resurfacing replacement. J Bone Joint Surg Br 2008; 90: 1291–1297. An arc of cover of over 10 mm has less wear rate compared to components which cover the femoral head by less than 10 mm.

   The acetabular component should provide adequate cover superiorly over the femoral

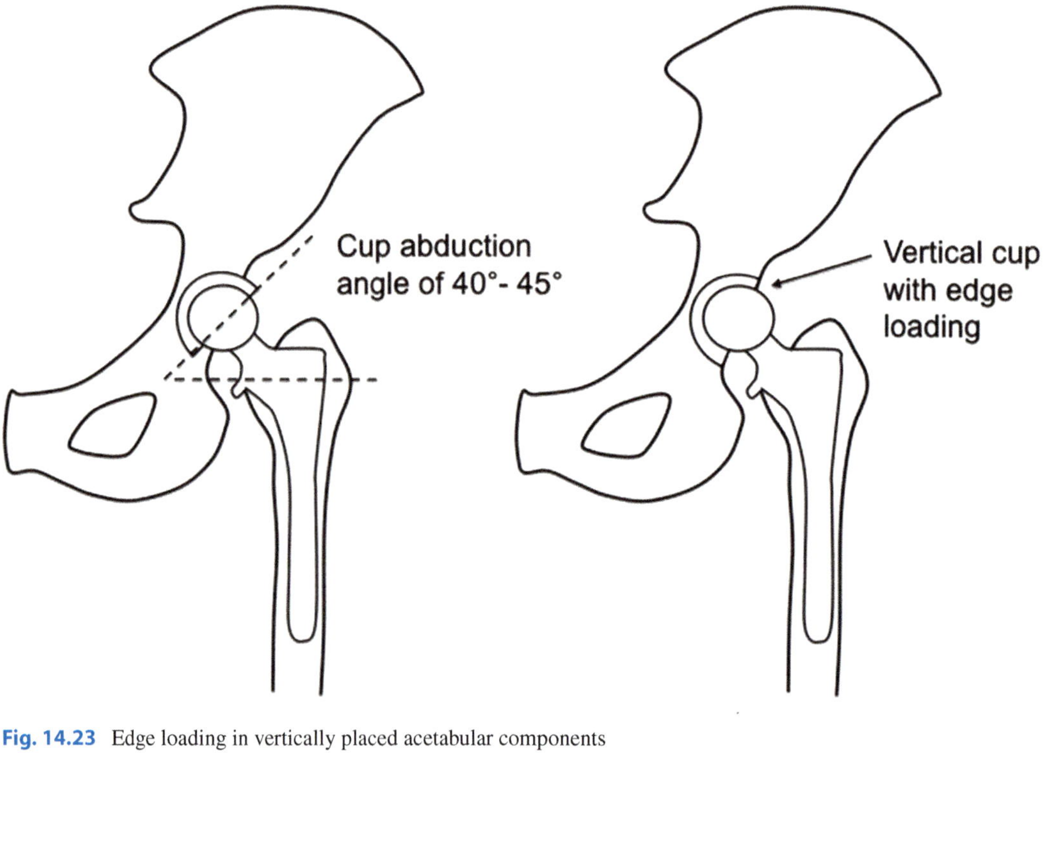

Fig. 14.23 Edge loading in vertically placed acetabular components

head: components that cover the femoral head by more than 10 mm have a lower wear rate than those that cover the femoral head by less than 10 mm. Coverage is measured from a vertical line drawn through the centre of the femoral head.

Similarly, varus positioning of the femoral component can cause high load and fracture of the femoral neck.

4. Stress shielding in the proximal part of femoral neck.

   The presence of a stiff cobalt chrome femoral stem causes stress shielding of the proximal neck, which may predispose to late neck fracture. In a smaller sized femoral component, the degree of stress shielding may be greater.

5. ARMD

   Metal ions released as a result of movement can lead to a local tissue reaction known as ARMD. This causes local tissue destruction.

   Formation of inflammatory pseudotumours has been reported.

   Glyn Jones S, Pandit H, Kwon YM. Risk factors for inflammatory pseudotumour formation following hip resurfacing. J Bone Joint Surg Br 2009;91:1566–74. Out of 1419 hip resurfacings, 1.8% had a revision for pseudotumours, with pseudotumours being more common in women. The study authors recommended that resurfacing be carried out with caution in women.

6. Ion levels in blood

   Resurfacing hip components are made of cobalt chrome alloy and there is an increase in the ion levels in the body following resurfacing. The levels rise rapidly following operation and after 12–18 months, a steady state is reached. There have been reports of further increase in levels after 5–10 years.

   DeSouza RM, Parsons NR, Oni T, Dalton P, Costa M, Krikler S. *Metal ion levels following resurfacing arthroplasty of the hip. Serial results over a 10 year period. J Bone Joint Surg Br 2010;92(12):1642–7. Rise in levels noted initially and then at 5–10 year follow up after surgery.*

7. Femoral neck fractures

   Femoral neck fractures in hip resurfacing may be due to patient- or surgeon-dependent factors. Patient factors include osteoporosis, small component size, and female gender. Women are twice as likely to have a femoral neck fracture than men. Surgeon factors are notching of the superior neck and varus placement of the femoral component.

   Shimmin AJ, Back D. Femoral neck fractures following Birmingham hip resurfacing: a national review of 50 cases. J Bone Joint Surg Br 2005;87(4):463–4. 3497 Birmingham hips. 50 patients had femoral neck fracture (1.46%). Higher risk in women. Rick factors were varus placement of femoral component and intraoperative notching.

8. Painful resurfacing

   Patients who experience pain during resurfacing should be evaluated with blood test to assess cobalt and chrome levels, MARS (Metal Artifact Reduction Sequence) MRI to view periprosthetic fluid collections or soft tissue masses, and CT scan to assess acetabular component position and angulation.

   Abnormalities in any of these parameters should be taken into consideration while planning revision operations.

   Hart AJ, Sabah S, Henckel J, Lewis A, Cobb J, Sampson B, Mitchell A, Skinner JA. The painful metal on metal hip resurfacing. J Bone Joint Surg Br 2009;91:738–744.

Surveillance of Metal on Metal Bearings

The MHRA (Medicines and Healthcare products Regulatory Agency) in UK has provided guidance on follow up of metal on metal hips. All women, men with femoral head size ≤48 mm, all Depuy ASR resurfacings and all stemmed resurfacing with head size ≥36 mm are followed up annually with serum metal ion levels and hip questionnaire. Any rise in serum ion levels or decline in clinical hip score requires a MARS MRI scan. Revision surgery is considered if there is a decline in hip score, rising ion levels or changes on MR scan. Patients with hip resurfacing head size >48 mm or stemmed hip replacements with head size <36 mm are also followed up regularly and revision considered based on the same indications.

Whole blood metal levels ≥7 ppb (119 nmol/L cobalt or 134.5 nmol/L chromium) indicates need for MR scan.

The Smith and Nephew Birmingham hip resurfacing (48–62 mm head size) has a 10A* ODEP (Orthopaedic Data Evaluation Panel) rating.

Failure of the ASR

The ASR hip resurfacing (Depuy) was designed as a non-hemispheric cup to improve ROM but this led to edge loading, excess metal ion release and very high early failure. 93,000 were implanted worldwide and the implant was withdrawn in August 2010.

The NJR UK reported 13% failure rate at 5 years. Some reports suggested a failure rate of 26% for resurfacing and 55% for stemmed hip replacements at 6 years.

Hip replacement with large metal head and metal liners exhibited very high metal ion levels. The trunnion (junction between the femoral stem and the femoral head) wear contributed to the high metal ion release.

Results of Hip Arthroplasty

The results of hip arthroplasty are related to a variety of factors. Experience of the surgeon is one such key factor.

Charnley Hip

The Charnley hip design has an excellent track record in the long term as exemplified by these reports.

Wroblewski BM, Siney PD, Fleming PA. Charnley low-frictional torque arthroplasty in patients under the age of 51 years. Follow-up to 33 years. J Bone Joint Surg Br. 2002; 84(4):540–3. 1092 patients, 1434 hips. Under 51 years at time of primary. With revision for any indication as the endpoint the survivorship was 93.7% at ten years, 84.7% at 15 years, 74.3% at 20 years and 55.3% at 27 years

Callaghan JJ, Templeton JE, Liu SS, Pedersen DR, Goetz DD, Sullivan PM, Johnston RC. Results of Charnley total hip arthroplasty at a minimum of 30 years. A concise follow-up of a previous report. J Bone Joint Surg Am 2004;86(4):690–5. 27 patients alive at 30 year postop. 88% prosthesis intact at last follow up or at patient's death.

Fender D, Harper WM, Gregg PJ. Outcome of Charnley THR across a single health region in England. J Bone Joint Surg Br 2006;88(10):1293–8. The results at 10 years from a regional arthroplasty register. 1198 consecutive Charnley hips. 1001 hips analyzed. Crude revision rate 6.2%. Survival with revision as end point 93.1%.

Exeter Hip

The Exeter stem based on the sliding taper principle has excellent long term survival. The predominant cause of revision in this group was acetabular component loosening.

Carrington NC, Sierra RJ, Gie GA, Hubble MJW, Timperley AJ, Howell JR. The Exeter universal cemented femoral component at 15–17 years. An update on the first 325 hips. J Bone Joint Surg Br 2009;91:730–7. Hips done between 1988 and 1990. For aseptic loosening, femoral component survival at 17 years was 100% and the acetabular component survival was 90.4%.

Hydroxyapatite-Coated Hip Arthroplasty

More recently, cementless hydroxy-apatite coated stems have shown good long term results.

Shetty AA, Slack R, Tindall A, James KD, Rand C. Results of Hydroxyapatite coated (Furlong) total hip replacement: a 13–15 year follow up. J Bone Joint Surg Br 2005 87(8):1050–

4. 134 consecutive hips. 14.2 year follow up. 6 lost to follow up. 22 died. No cup revised. One stem revised for fracture. No aseptic loosening. 99% survival at 13 years.

Trikha SP, Singh S, Raynham OW, Lewis JC, Mitchell PA, Edge AJ. Hydroxyapatite ceramic coated femoral stems in revision hip surgery. J Bone Joint Surg Br 2005;87(8):1055–60. 120 revision hips in 107 patients. JRI Furlong femoral component. 8 year follow up. No re-revision of femoral component for loosening. No new radiolucent lines in femoral components. With revision or impending revision for aseptic loosening as end point, there was 100% survival at 10 years.

Minimally Invasive/Two-Incision Hip Arthroplasty

Minimally invasive hip surgery implies hip surgery done through a smaller incision with minimal soft tissue damage. In common term, the length of skin incision is 10 cm or less.

Taking this one step further, the two-incision hip technique was devised to insert the acetabular and femoral component through two separate 4–5 cm incisions. This technique uses image intensifier intraoperatively. Advantage is early mobilisation and potentially same day discharge. Concerns remain about the long learning curve, achieving good fixation, and lack of difference compared to conventional hip replacements by 3–6 months postoperative stage.

Berger RA. Total hip arthroplasty using the minimally invasive two incision approach. Clin Orthop 2003;417:232–41. First 100 patients. 1% complication rate—one proximal femoral fracture. No dislocations, no failure of ingrowth. After 12 patients, of the 88, 85% went home same day and 15% went home day after. No readmissions, no complications after discharge. Two incision is safe, rapid recovery, should be done only after proper training.

Bal BS, Haltom D, Aleto T, Barrett M. Early complications of primary total hip replacement performed with a two incision minimally invasive technique. Surgical technique. J Bone Joint Surg Am 2006;88(Suppl 1):221–33. Two incision is technically demanding and has a higher complication rate in the learning curve of the surgeon.

Ogonda L, Wilson R, Archbold P, Lawlor M, Humphreys P, O'Brien S, Beverland D. A minimal incision technique in total hip arthroplasty does not improve early postoperative outcomes. A prospective, randomised, controlled trial. J Bone Joint Surg Am 2005;87(4):701–10. Single incision posterior approach. 219 hips randomised. Patients and staff blinded. Single incision. No difference in post op haematocrit, pain score, early walking ability, function score at 6 weeks.

Antibiotic Cover for Dental Procedures After Hip Arthroplasty

Prophylaxis is not routinely required for the majority of dental procedures following hip arthroplasty. If there is significant risk of bacteraemia, antibiotics (cephalexin or clindamycin) 1 h before and 2 h after the procedure can be considered. Immunocompromised patients are at higher risk and should be considered for prophylaxis.

The disadvantage of routine prophylaxis is the development of drug resistance.

Activity Level After Hip Arthroplasty

An improvement in activity level is reported following hip arthroplasty. A high level of activity following surgery may be associated with development of femoral osteolysis and loosening.

Lubbeke A, Garavaglia G, Barea C, Stern R, Peter R, Hoffmeyer P. Influence of patient activity on femoral osteolysis at 5 and 10 years following hybrid total hip replacement. J Bone Joint Surg Br 2011;93(4);456–63. 433 patients, mean age 67 years. Osteolysis seen in 5.4% patients with low activity, 7.5% with moderate activity and 24.1% with high activity.

Hip Replacement in Patients Under 50–55 Years of Age

Kim YH, Kim JS, Park JW, Joo JH. Comparison of total hip replacement with and without cement in patients younger than 50 years of age: the results at 18 years. J Bone Joint Surg Br 2011;93(4):449–55. 109 hybrid hips mean age 43 years and 79 cementless hips mean age 46 years. Survival of acetabular component 87% versus 84% and survival of femoral component 97% versus 96%.

Total Hip Replacement in Morbidly Obese

Morbidly obese patients may have a higher risk of complications and lower prosthesis survival, and this should be discussed in the informed consent. A higher risk of infection and aseptic loosening are reported. Most patients are unable to lose weight after surgery.

Chee YH, Teoh KH, Sabnis BM, Ballantyne JA, Brenkel IJ. Total hip replacement in morbidly obese patients with osteoarthritis: results of a prospectively matched study. J Bone Joint Surg Br 2010;92(8):1066–71. 55 hips in morbidly obsess matched to 55 in non-obese. 5 year prospective follow up. Survival 90% in obese compared to 100% in non-obese. Dislocation and infection risk higher in obese patients.

McCalden RW, Charron KD, MacDonald SJ, Bourne RB, Naudie DD. Does morbid obesity affect the outcome of total hip replacement. An analysis of 3290 THRs. J Bone Joint Surg Br 2011;93(3):321–5. Slightly higher rate of revision for infection in morbidly obese.

Bariatric surgery prior to hip replacement surgery does not seem to reduce the complication rate.

Smith TO, Aboelmagd T, Hing CB, MacGregor A. Does bariatric surgery prior to total hip or knee arthroplasty reduce postoperative complications and improve clinical outcomes for obese patients. Bone Joint Surg 2016;98:1160–67. Meta-analysis of five studies. Over 22,000 patients. No difference in infections, complications or mortality.

Hip Replacement in Rheumatoid Arthritis

Malviya A, Walker LC, Avery P, Osborne S, Weir DJ, Foster HE, Deehan DJ. The long term outcome of hip replacement in adults with juvenile idiopathic arthritis: the influence of steroids and methotrexate J Bone Joint Surg Br 2011;93(4):443–8. 47 hips in 25 patients with Juvenile idiopathic Arthritis (JIA). Mean age 27 years, follow up 19 years. Survival of prosthesis 54% at 19 years. Survival better in patients on methotrexate and poorer in patients on long term steroids.

Hip Replacement in Ankylosing Spondylitis

Patient with ankylosing spondylitis have loss of lumbar lordosis. Placement of the acetabulum in the normal position can lead to higher functional anteversion. Reducing anteversion of the acetabular component helps reduce the risk of anterior dislocation.

Putnis SE, Wartemberg GK, Khan WS, Agarwal S. A Literature Review of Total Hip Arthroplasty in Patients with Ankylosing Spondylitis: Perioperative Considerations and Outcome. Open Orthop J. 2015;9:483–8.

Hip Replacement for Femoral Neck Fractures

In acute femoral neck fractures, hip replacement is indicated in patients who are cognitively intact, medically well enough to withstand the procedure and independently mobile, or mobile with one stick. Functional outcome following hip replacement is better compared to hemiarthroplasty. Also, patients with Paget's disease, pre-existing arthritis and inflammatory arthritis are better served with a total hip replacement.

Failed fixation of hip fractures may necessitate hip replacement surgery. Problems in these patients include retained metalwork, scarring around the sciatic nerve, abnormal femoral anatomy, shortening, trochanteric nonunion and loss of proximal femoral bone stock. Femoral stem should bypass the most distal screw hole by two cortical diameters.

Technical problems in hip replacement after acetabular fractures include retained metalwork, scarring, tethering of nerves, and bone loss around the acetabulum.

Periprosthetic Fractures

Fractures of the femoral shaft or the acetabulum in association with a total hip arthroplasty are a common indication for revision hip surgery. Poor bone quality, use of uncemented stems, bowing of femur, and trauma are risk factors for femoral periprosthetic fractures.

The Vancouver system (Table 14.10) is commonly used to classify femoral periprosthetic fractures.

Table 14.10 The Vancouver system of classifying femoral periprosthetic fractures.

Type	Description		Treatment
A	Fracture around the trochanter		
A_G	Fracture of the greater trochanter	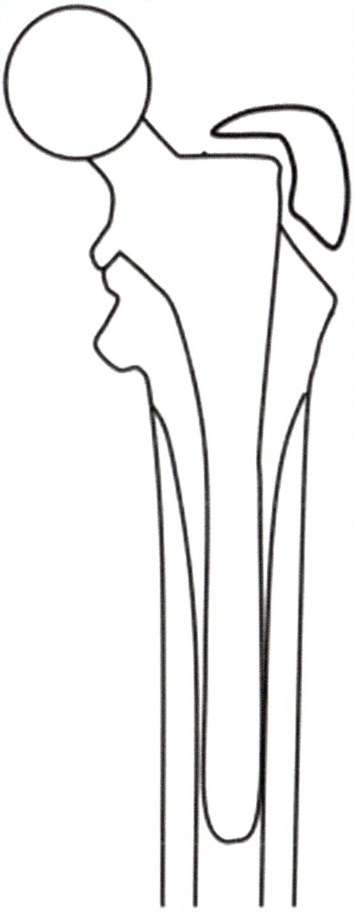	Undisplaced—nonoperative, restricted weight bearing Displaced—fix with claw plate or cerclage wires

(continued)

Table 14.10 (continued)

Type	Description		Treatment
A_L	Fracture of the lesser trochanter	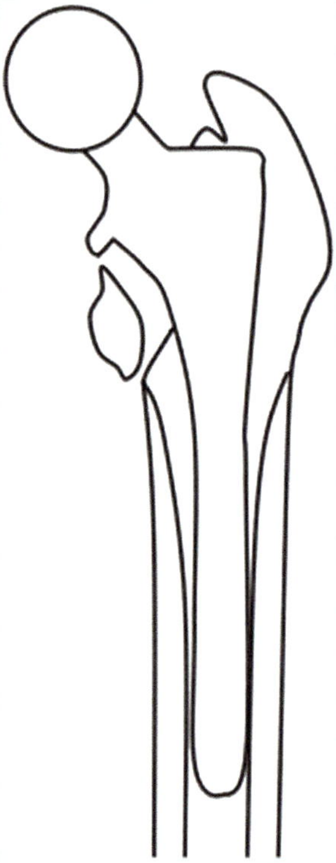	If stem is stable—restricted weight bearing Unstable stem has to be revised
B	Fracture around the stem extending into the region of the tip of the stem		
B1	Fracture with a well-fixed stem	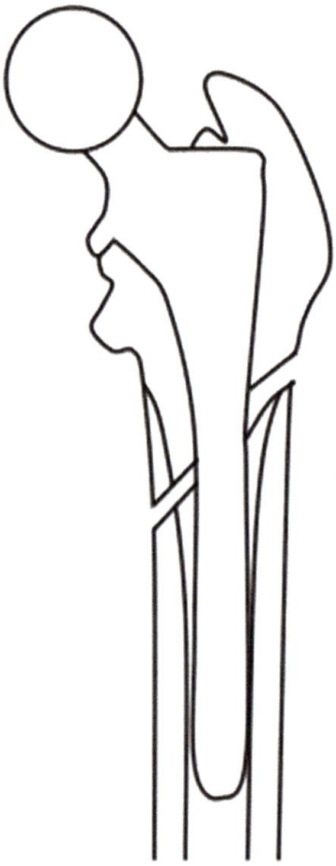	Undisplaced—restricted weight bearing. If unstable/displaced—cerclage wiring

Table 14.10 (continued)

Type	Description		Treatment
B2	Fracture with a loose femoral component	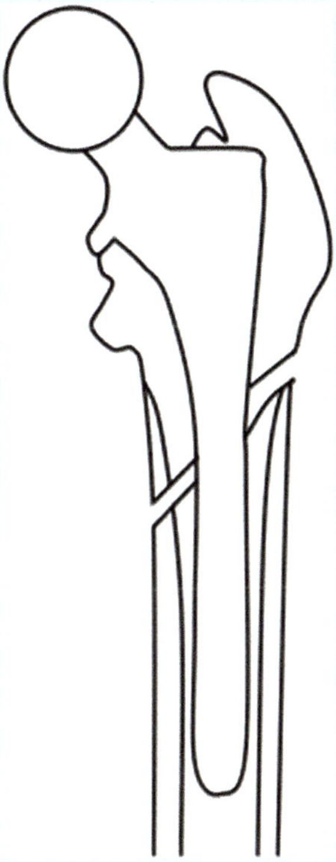	Revision of stem to a porous, fully coated longer stem
B3	Fracture with loose femoral component and loss of femoral bone stock	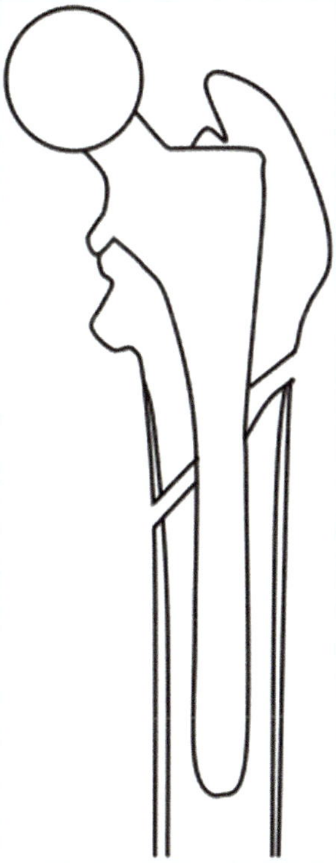	Revision to distally fixed long uncemented stem. Consider allograft, distal locking stems or a megaprosthesis

(continued)

Table 14.10 (continued)

Type	Description		Treatment
C	Fracture of the femoral shaft distal to the tip of the stem	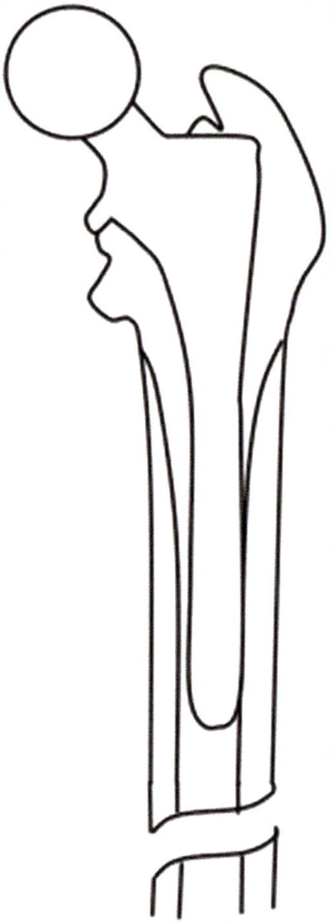	Internal fixation with an overlapping distal plate or revision to distally locked stem

Duncan CP, Masri BA. Fractures of the femur after hip replacement. Inst Course Lect 1995;44:293–304.

Masri BA, Meek RM, Duncan CP. Periprosthetic fractures: evaluation and treatment. Clin Orthop 2004;420:80–95.

Revision femoral stems should have a minimum of 4 cm of cortical contact, also known as scratch fit. These should bypass the distal extent of the fracture by a minimum of two cortical diameters.

Acetabular Periprosthetic Fractures

Acetabular periprosthetic fractures are less common, but may pose significantly more complex management issues. Risk factors for acetabular fracture include uncemented component, press fit of over 2 mm, poor bone quality, postoperative trauma.

Fractures can be intra operative or post operative. Additionally, the acetabular component may be stable or unstable.

Table 14.11 Classification of acetabular periprosthetic fractures

Type I	Undisplaced fracture with stable acetabular component
Type II	Undisplaced fracture with compromise of stability
Type III	Displaced fracture

Peterson and Lewallen proposed a classification system grouping these injuries into two types—Type I with a stable acetabular component, and Type II with a radiologically loose acetabular component. Another classification by Davidson delineates three types (Table 14.11)

The principles of management depend on stability of the component, and the integrity of the pelvic columns. Stable components can be managed with observation and serial radiographs until union of fracture. Displaced fractures with unstable component require restoration of pelvic support using a posterior column plate. An uncemented acetabular component with multiple screws is used.

A liner can be cemented into the shell, which improves the stability provided by the screws. Revision acetabular components with locking screws are an option.

Uncontained defects of the posterior column require augmentation with trabecular metal augments or structural allograft. A cup cage construct is considered in patients with pelvic discontinuity.

Revision Hip Arthroplasty

Indications for revision hip surgery are:

- Pain:
- Pain on beginning to walk (start-up pain) indicates a loose implant. Constant pain or night pain indicates infection. Pain that is unchanged after hip arthroplasty should lead to consideration of other causes of pain such as spine pathology, hernia, trochanteric bursitis or an underlying infection.
- Infection.
- Recurrent dislocation.
- Periprosthetic fracture with a loose implant or loss of bone stock.
- Extensive osteolysis with potential compromise of hip stability.
- Uncommon indications are leg length discrepancy and abductor lurch.

Assessment of Patients for Revision Arthroplasty

Patients who are being considered for revision arthroplasty should undergo a complete history and examination. The following investigations should also be performed:

- X-rays—AP view of the pelvis, AP and lateral views of the femur to include the entire stem and cement mantle, and a shoot -through lateral to assess the acetabular component. Look for alignment, wear, loosening, stress shielding, periosteal reaction and heterotopic ossification. Judet views (45° oblique views) are useful in visualising the anterior and posterior columns and to determine the bone stock.
- CT scan—helpful in assessing bone stock. It may be possible to template and plan implants based on CT scan images. Contrast CT scan is helpful in planning acetabular surgery where close proximity of the cup to the iliac vessels is a concern.
- Tc-99 bone scan—this can provide information about loosening or infection, although it is not used universally.
- Aspiration of the hip—the presence of bacteria in Gram staining or a white cell count greater than 25,000/mm^3 in the aspirate is indicative of infection.
- Blood parameters—an elevated ESR and CRP level are indicative of infection. The white cell count in peripheral blood may be normal despite an infected joint.
- Intraoperative frozen section—the presence of more than 10 white cells per high power field is indicative of acute inflammation.
- Intraoperative culture and histology—multiple culture specimens should be obtained and

a histology specimen sent to check for any rare forms of infection such as fungal infection or tuberculosis.

Preparing for Revision Surgery

The following steps should guide preparations for revision surgery:

- Establish a diagnosis and cause of failure.
- Obtain all previous operation notes and implant details.
- Consider all possibilities and ensure implants are available to deal with such situations. Special instruments for removing cement, power burrs, a range of osteotomes, implant extractors, cerclage cables and wires, bone graft (cancellous and allograft) and cell saver should be available.
- Template. Choose the implant and determine the size of components, level of neck resection, neck length, head size, additional procedures such as trochanteric osteotomy and impaction grafting. Templating is commonly performed with plain radiographs using implant templates and matching the appropriate size implant to the bone geometry. Software is available to template on CT scans using preoperative standardised CT scan images.

Bone Defects

Classification of Femoral Bone Defects

Femoral bone defects can be grouped according to the American Academy of Orthopaedic Surgeons (AAOS) classification (Table 14.12):

Table 14.12 The American Academy of Orthopaedic Surgeons classification of femoral bone defects

Femoral bone defects	
Segmental	Proximal: • Partial or complete • Anterior/medial/posterior Intercalary Greater trochanteric
Cavitary	Cancellous Cortical Ectasia
Combined segmental and cavitary	–
Malalignment	Rotational/angular
Femoral stenosis	–
Femoral discontinuity	–

Management of Femoral Bone Defects

Femoral bone defects may be managed as follows:

- An intact cortical tube can be used for implant fixation.
- Extensive proximal bone loss proximally requires impaction grafting, calcar replacement stems, distally fixed cementless stem or proximal femoral replacement.
- Bone loss extending beyond the isthmus of the femur makes it difficult to achieve fixation distally due to a divergent femoral canal and may require proximal femoral replacement or an allograft.
- Femoral malalignment may require a femoral osteotomy to achieve a straight canal.

Classification of Acetabular Bone Defects

The AAOS classification of acetabular defects is summarised in Table 14.13, and the Paprosky classification of acetabular bone deficiency in Table 14.14.

Management of Acetabular Bone Defects

For minimal or moderate bone defects, a larger cemented or a hemispheric cementless component can be used. Cementless cups rely on adequate host bone contact. An intact posterior column is necessary, as well as anterosuperior or anteroinferior bone. The survivorship of cementless cups is 96% at 15 years in the revision scenario.

Della Valle CJ, Berger RA, Rosenberg AG, Galante JO. Cementless acetabular reconstruction in revision total hip arthroplasty. Clin Orthop 2004;420:96–100.

For larger defects, the options are impaction grafting, structural allograft, placement of a larger hemispheric cementless cup or a smaller cup placed at a higher level (the high hip centre). For stable cementless fixation, 35% of the acetabular component should be ingrown. Over 50% host bone contact is desirable.

In impaction grafting, bone graft, usually allograft, is impacted into the acetabular defect. Ideal graft size is about 1 cm blocks, rather than milled bone. An intact rim is needed and the cup is cemented into the new bed. An uncemented cup can be used but will require adequate host bone contact. Trabecular metal cups are advantageous in this situation due to better osseointegration potential.

Schreurs BW, Bolder SB, Gardeniers JW. Acetabular revision with impacted morsellised cancellous bone grafting and a cemented cup. A 15–20 year follow up. J Bone Joint Surg Br 2004;86(4):492–7. 62 acetabular revisions, 16.5 year follow up. Survival of cup was 79% at 15 years. Includes 2 cups revised or infection and one cup revised along with femoral revision. Excluding these, survival was 84% at 15 years.

Schereurs BW, Keurentjes JC, Gardeniers JW et al. J Bone Joint Surg Br 2009;91:1148–53. 20–25 year result. 62 acetabular revisions, 75% survival at 20 years, 87% survival at 20 years for aseptic loosening.

Table 14.13 The American Academy of Orthopaedic Surgeons classification of acetabular bone defects.

Acetabular bone defects	
Segmental	Peripheral: anterior/superior/posterior Central
Cavitary	Peripheral—anterior/superior/posterior Central
Combined	–
Pelvic discontinuity	–
Arthrodesis	–

Table 14.14 The Paprosky classification of acetabular bone deficiency

Type	Description	
1	Minimal lysis or component migration	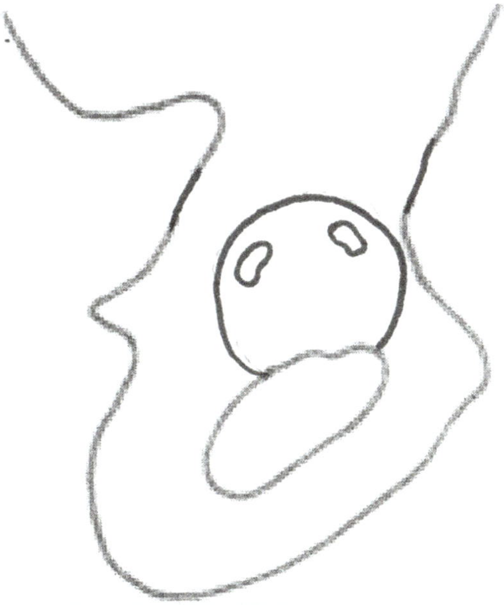

(continued)

Table 14.14 (continued)

Type	Description	
2a	Superomedial migration <2 cm	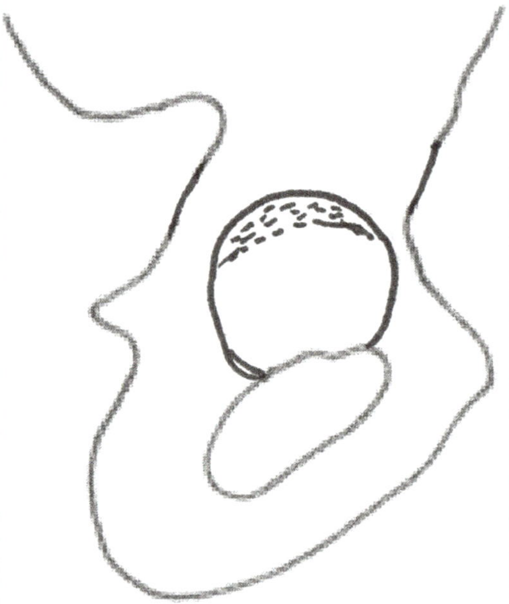
2b	Superolateral migration <2 cm	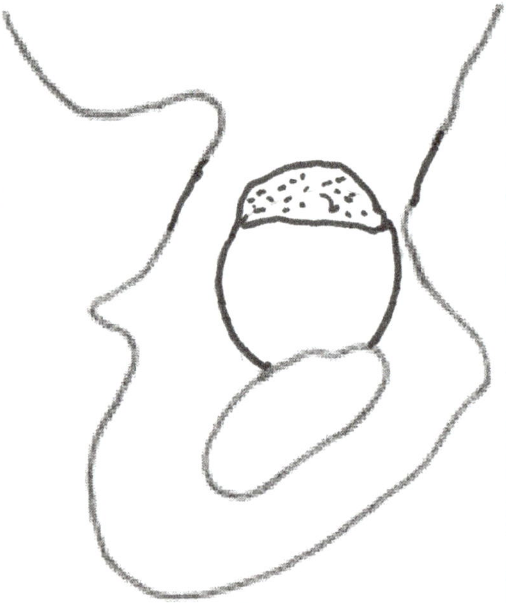

Table 14.14 (continued)

Type	Description	
2c	Teardrop lysis or loss of medial wall	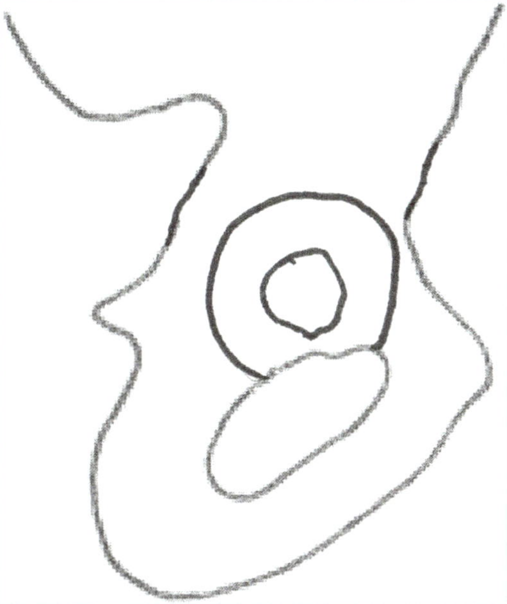
3a	Migration >2 cm, ischial lysis	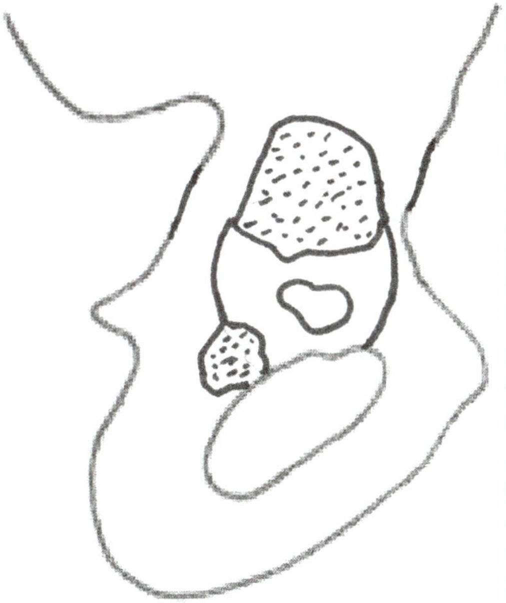

(continued)

Table 14.14 (continued)

Type	Description	
3b	Type 3a plus disruption of Kohler's line, indicating profound medial loss Pelvic discontinuity	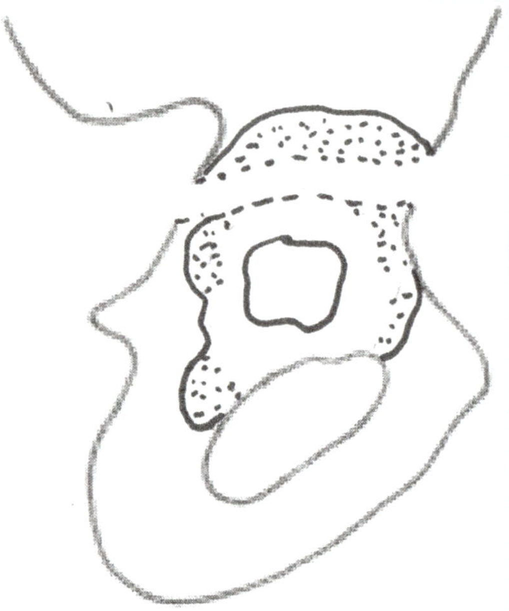

The 'high hip centre' is superior placement of the acetabulum where adequate host bone is available. This has a high risk of impingement and is largely historical.

Defects of the posterior column may require a structural allograft to replace the bone loss along with stabilisation.

Antiprotrusio cages or pelvic reconstruction by plates and grafting may be required if there is pelvic discontinuity (Fig. 14.24). Antiprotrusio cages help protect the bed after impaction grafting. The cage is secured by screws into the pelvis. A polyethylene liner can be cemented into the cage in the desired version and inclination. Acetabular cages are prone to loosening but the advantage is restoration of bone stock, making further revisions easier.

Gill TJ, Sledge JB, Müller ME. The Burch-Schneider anti-protrusio cage in revision total hip arthroplasty: indications, principles and long term results. J Bone Joint Surg Br 1998;80:946.

Trabecular metal augments are made of tantalum with a porosity similar to cancellous bone and can be used for large defects and pelvic discontinuity. Different shapes of augments are available to fill defects and these can be used in patients with pelvic discontinuity to restore the posterior column using a posteroinferior and posterosuperior augment. The metal functions as an internal plate and the acetabular component can be cemented into the reconstructed acetabulum.

Long term results with trabecular metal are not available, but the augments are increasing popular in acetabular reconstruction.

Lingaraj K, Teo YH, Bergman Nl. The management of severe acetabular bone defects in revision hip arthroplasty using modular porous metal components. J Bone Joint Surg Br 2009; 91: 1555–60. 23 reconstruction, 41 month follow up, 21 were well fixed. Short term results were good.

Acetabular rings rely on support from the remaining periphery of the acetabulum. These are not used commonly. Oblong cups can be used to gain maximum host bone contact in patients with superior bone loss. Allografts in the acetabulum are rarely used with the increasing popularity of trabecular metal augments.

Herrera A, Martínez AA, Cuenca J, Canales V. Management of type III and IV acetabular defi-

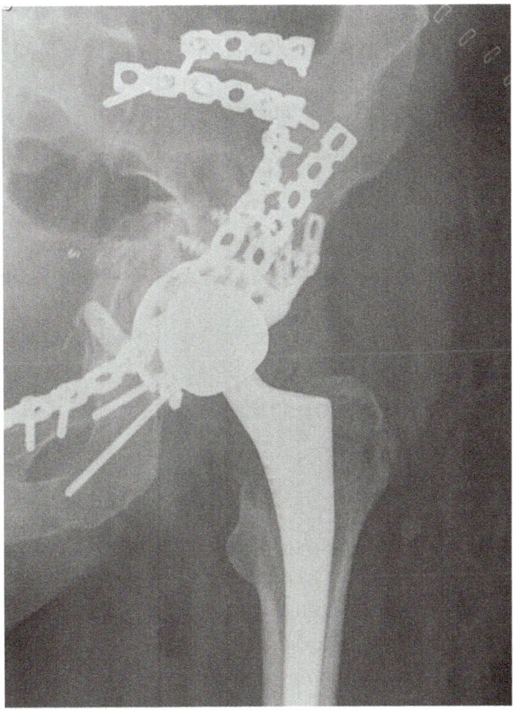

Fig. 14.24 The use of an acetabular cage and impaction grafting to reconstruct a post-acetabulum fracture bone defect

ciencies with the longitudinal oblong revision cup. J Arthro 2006;21:857–64.

Sporer SM. The use of structural distal femoral allografts for acetabular reconstruction. J Bone Joint Surg Am 2005;87:760–5.

Total Knee Replacement

Over 80,000 knee replacements are performed in the UK annually, with primary osteoarthritis being the commonest indication. The prevalence of knee arthritis is about 30% in individuals over the age of 60 years. The prevalence is expected to increase with aging population in the western world.

The etiology of knee osteoarthritis is multi factorial. Generalised causes include age, gender and obesity. Local factors include trauma, recreational abuse, malalignment, and meniscectomy. There is a significant genetic predisposition.

Patient Assessment

Patient assessment for total knee replacement (TKR) should include taking a full history, performing a physical examination and assessing X-rays.

History

Pain is the predominant presenting feature in patients with knee arthritis. The site, severity, onset, course and duration of pain is evaluated. Pain at a night is a feature of arthritis, and can be present in malignant processes and infections as well. It is important to distinguish the hip or spine as a source of pain.

The patient's level of functional ability should be assessed to determine if he or she can undertake activities of daily living (e.g., shopping, cleaning and personal hygiene). The ability to go up and down stairs and kneel on the ground should be noted, and an activity score can be employed to document preoperative mobility. The Oxford Knee Score (OKS) is commonly used for quantifying preoperative and postoperative function.

The patient must also be assessed in terms of prior treatments (e.g., non-steroidal anti-inflammatory drugs [NSAIDs], activity modifications, walking aids, bracing, hyaluronate/steroid injections) and previous surgeries.

Medical co morbidities such as immune compromise (diabetes, renal dysfunction, AIDS) and infective foci (chest infection, urinary tract infection, dental infections, skin infections) should be taken into account.

Examination

Areas for examination are listed in Table 14.15.

Baker's cysts in patients with arthritis knees resolve only in a small number of patients after surgery and may remain symptomatic.

Hommel H, Perka C, Kopf S. The fate of Baker's cyst after total knee arthroplasty.

Table 14.15 Examination for total knee replacement.

Area	Description
Gait	Antalgic Trendelenburg—to rule out hip pathology Valgus/varus thrust, indicating ligamentous laxity
Soft tissues	Previous incisions—location and time since previous surgery Psoriasis patch anteriorly on the knee
Knee joint	Tenderness, effusion, Baker's cyst Range of motion, extensor lag Ligamentous laxity Any deformities—assess if correctable or not
Neurovascular	Rule out radicular pain Check distal pulses
Spine and hip joint areas	Spine, ipsilateral hip as a possible source of pain
Contralateral knee	Assess function

Bone Joint Journal 2016;98:1185–8. 102 patients with MR scan proven cysts followed up with ultrasound after surgery. Cysts resolved in only 15% and were symptomatic in 31%.

X-Rays

The standing AP view and lateral view are routine. The skyline view is taken to assess the patellofemoral joint and patellar tracking, and should also be part of the routine assessment. The AP standing view with knees flexed to 45° (Rosenberg view) may help to identify any loss of joint space that is not otherwise obvious on standing radiographs.

Long leg films may be required to assess alignment if there are significant deformities at the knee or where there is a suggestion of previous fractures, malunions or deformities in the femur or tibia.

The tunnel view can be helpful in detecting osteochondritis and loose bodies in the notch.

Kellgren and Lawrence proposed a scoring system in 1957. Only the AP radiograph of the knee is considered for grading. The five grades described are shown in Table 14.16.

Table 14.16 The Kellgren Lawrence grades

Grade 0	No changes on X rays
Grade 1	Doubtful
Grade 2	Minimal
Grade 3	Moderate
Grade 4	Severe

Kellgren JH, Lawrence JS. Radiological assessment of osteoarthrosis. Ann Rheum Dis 1957;16:494–502.

Contraindications to Knee Arthroplasty

Active local or systemic infection is a definite contraindication to knee replacement.

Relative contraindications are incompetent extensor mechanism, neuropathic joint, knee fusion and peripheral vascular disease. Lack of extensor mechanism leads to instability. It is possible to reconstruct the mechanism with an allograft at the time of arthroplasty, but may result in residual extensor lag, or knee stiffness due to different rehabilitation program for the knee replacement and the allograft.

Neuropathic joints can be due to diabetes, syringomyelia, Charcot–Marie–Tooth disease, spinal dysraphism, amyloidosis or multiple sclerosis. Arthrodesis is an option and hinged arthroplasty can be considered. Problems in neuropathic joints are malalignment, ligamentous laxity, bone loss and infection.

Converting a knee fusion to arthroplasty imposes problems of poor muscle power and ligaments, possible underlying infection if fusion is related to a previous infection and poor postoperative ROM.

Bae DK, Yoon KH, Kim HS, Song SJ. Total knee arthroplasty in stiff knees after previous infection. J Bone Joint Surg Br 2005;87(3):333–6. 32 knee replacements in stiff or partially ankylosed hips. 10 year follow up. Post op range was 75° in knees with complete ankylosis and 98° in partially ankylosed knees. Complications were one superficial and one deep infection, one nerve palsy and one supracondylar fracture.

Peripheral vascular disease can lead to wound complications or ischaemia leading to amputation. Indicators are intermittent claudication, prior vascular surgery, absent distal pulses and the presence of vascular calcification on radiographs. If the ankle–brachial index is less than 0.9 then a vascular surgeon should be consulted. If less than 0.5, preoperative bypass may be necessary. Arterial calcification, by itself, is not a contraindication for the use of tourniquet.

Surgical Approach for Total Knee Arthroplasty

The midline anterior approach is the commonest. The vascularity of the skin is based medially and, consequently, the lateral flap is less well oxygenated. Existing transverse scars should be intersected at a right angle if possible. If there are multiple longitudinal incisions, the most lateral incision is used, if appropriate for access.

The standard approach is the medial parapatellar arthrotomy along the medial third of the quadriceps tendon and curves around the patella leaving a cuff of tissue on the patella for repair. Alternatively, the arthrotomy can be vertically down over the medial aspect of patella with subperiosteal elevation of the extensor mechanism from the medial margin of patella as described by Insall.

The lateral parapatellar approach is indicated for the markedly valgus knee. This preserves the medial blood supply of the patella while achieving a lateral release. A potential problem is lack of familiarity of many surgeons with this approach.

The midvastus approach partly preserves the vastus medialis insertion onto the patella. The proximal extent of the arthrotomy is in line with the fibres of the vastus medialis and the muscle fibres are split rather than cut. This approach can be difficult in obese patients, and where the patella is difficult to evert. The patella can be retracted instead of everted to gain access to the joint.

In the sub vastus approach, the plane of dissection is distal to the vastus medialis. This is used for minimally invasive surgery. Special jigs that make the bone cut from the medial side are used.

The various approaches are illustrated in Fig. 14.25.

Extensile approaches are generally indicated in revision situation to avoid excess tension on the extensor mechanism and to improve access to the joint. This can be achieved by the quadriceps snip or tibial tubercle osteotomy.

The quadriceps snip reduces the risk of injury to the extensor mechanism from over-stretching. The quadriceps tendon is divided at the proximal extent of the medial parapatellar arthrotomy. The tendon can be divided in different ways to gain access (Fig. 14.26).

Meek RM, Greidanus NV, McGraw RW, Masri BA. The extensile rectus snip exposure in revision of total knee arthroplasty. J Bone Joint Surg Br 2003;85(8);1120–2. The rectus snip does not affect the function, pain or satisfaction score compared to the standard medial parapatellar arthrotomy.

For the tibial tubercle osteotomy (TTO), the tibial tubercle along with anterior crest of tibia is divided keeping a length of 8–10 cm (Fig. 14.27).

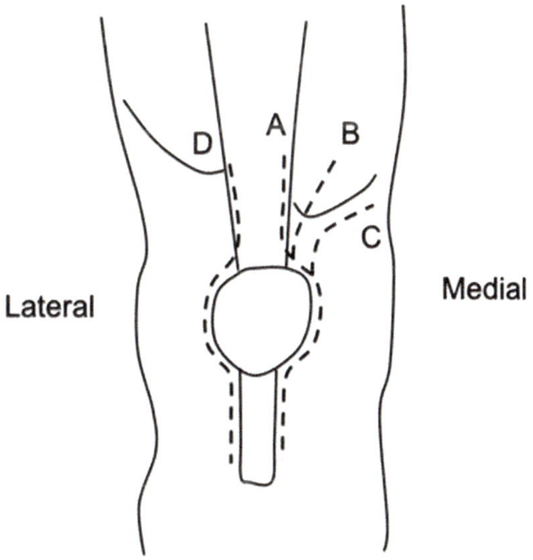

Fig. 14.25 Standard knee joint exposure approaches. (A) Medial parapatellar; (B) midvastus; (C) subvastus; (D) lateral parapatellar. VMO, vastus medialis obliquus

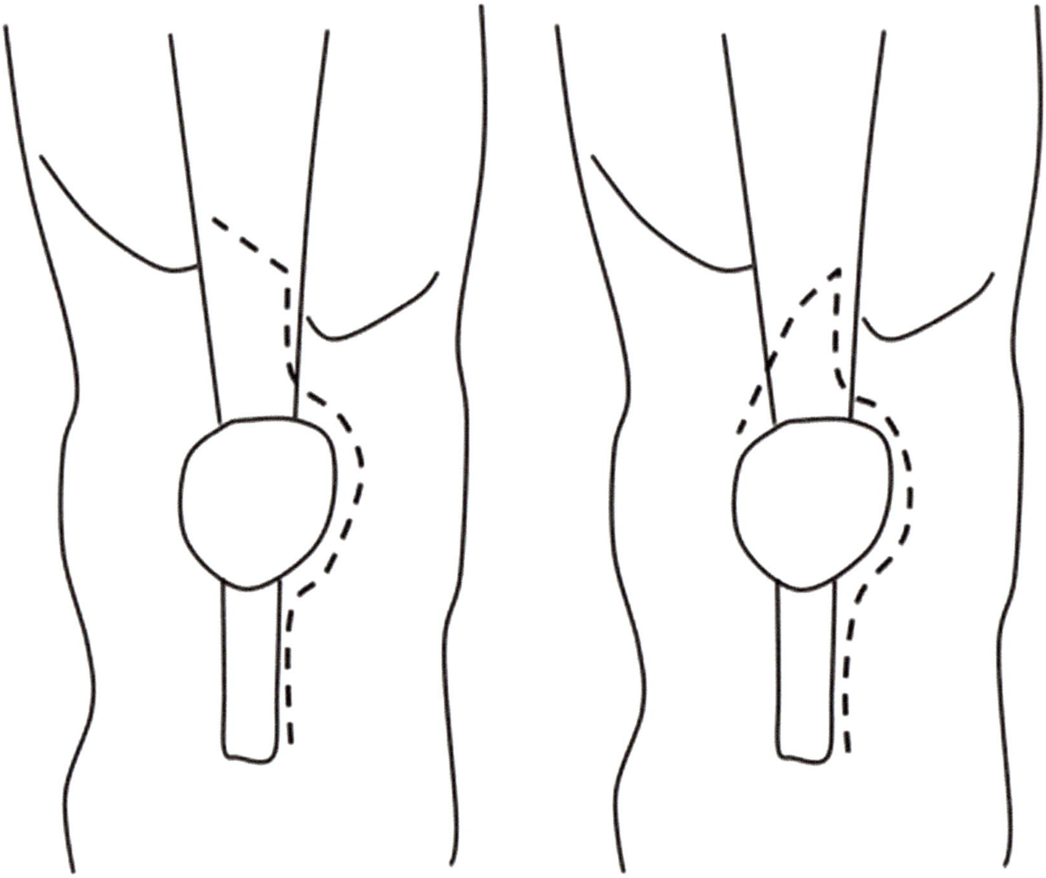

Fig. 14.26 Variations on the quadriceps snip for extensile exposure

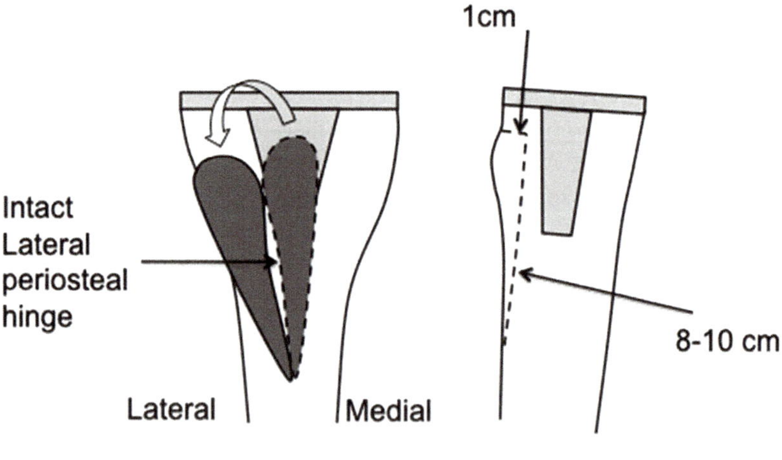

Fig. 14.27 Tibial tubercle osteotomy for extensile exposure

A step cut at the proximal extent reduces the risk of proximal migration of the fragment. The fragment is 1 cm thick proximally and narrows down to the anterior cortex of tibia distally. The lateral periosteal hinge is preserved. Reattachment is done with multiple wires or heavy non-absorbable suture. Originally described by Dolin in 1983, this technique was modified by Whiteside by increasing the length of the osteotomy to 8–10 cm (instead of 4–5 cm) and using wires instead of screws for reattachment.

Either approach does not compromise the function of the extensor mechanism postoperatively and no change in rehabilitation is required. Osteolysis in the region of the tibial tubercle is a contraindication for tibial tubercle osteotomy.

Femoral Components: Design and Materials

In the sagittal plane, the femoral component has differing radii: a larger radius (more flat) distally that articulates with the tibia in extension and a more curved posterior part that comes into contact with the tibial component in flexion. The large radius distributes the load over a larger area, while the smaller radius helps to improve rollback and gives greater flexion (Fig. 14.28).

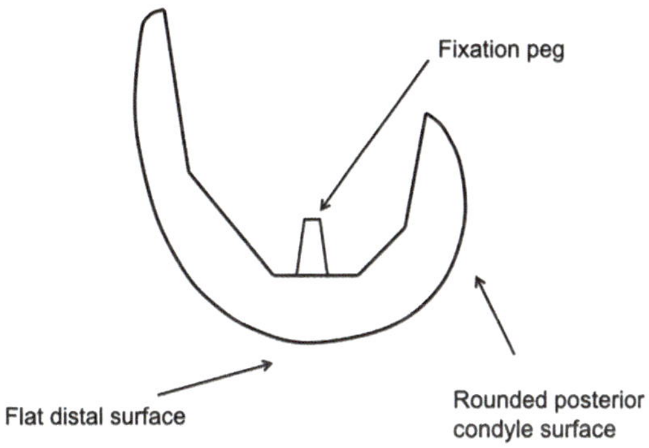

Fig. 14.28 Lateral view of femoral component

Femoral components are made of Cobalt–chromium alloy. Oxidised Zirconium (oxinium) covering of femoral components has been developed to reduce wear. Ceramic femoral components are being trialed.

Femoral components can be cruciate preserving or cruciate substituting. Two pegs are provided in cruciate retaining implants for medial–lateral stability. Cruciate substituting designs have a box in the intercondylar area to accommodate a post from the polyethylene insert (Fig. 14.29). The articulation of the post and the box produces rollback of the femoral component. This is sometimes referred to as the third condyle.

The post and box mechanism can be used to provide stability in varus–valgus place through the use a more conforming post in the box. These are known as varus–valgus constrained (VVC) knees. Greater stability can be achieved in hinged knees, where a hinge mechanism is built into the femoral component.

Cementless fixation in femur is acceptable and has predictable bone ingrowth.

Bassett RW. Results of 1000 Performance knees: cementless versus cemented fixation. J Arthro 1998;13(4):409–13. 1000 Knees, 5.2 year follow up. No difference in clinical results between cemented and cementless. No loosening or osteolysis in either group.

Stems can be used to reduce bending moment at the implant–bone interface in primary knee replacement in the presence large areas of osteonecrosis of the femoral condyle. Notching of the

Fig. 14.29 Design of a cruciate substituting femoral component

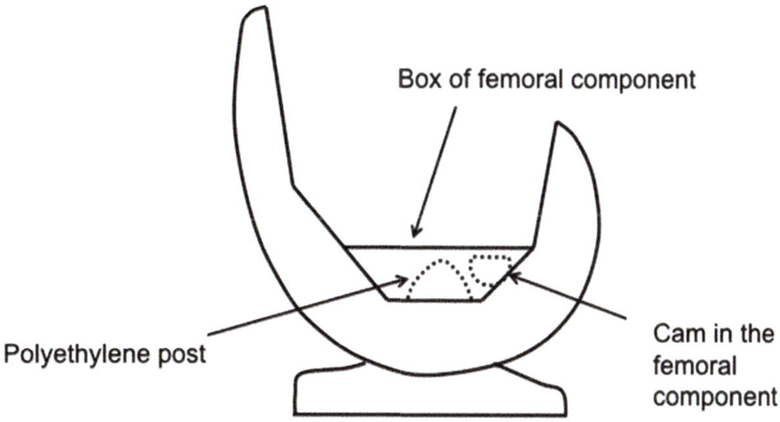

anterior femoral cortex, osteopenia and femoral osteotomies performed along with replacement are indications for stemmed components.

Cemented stems provide secure fixation, but are harder to revise.

Tibial Components

Cemented fixation is much more commonly used for tibial components. Keel is used to augment fixation and this can be cemented. Alternatively, only the superior tibial surface can be cemented leaving the keel uncemented as long as there is adequate cementation on the superior surface of tibia.

Bert, JM, McShane M. Is It Necessary to Cement the Tibial Stem in Cemented Total Knee Arthroplasty? Clin Orthop 1998;356:73–8. Either the keel should be cemented or the tibial cement mantle on the superior cut surface should be 3 mm for adequate stability.

Cementless tibial components have screws or spikes to augment fixation, but these have limited ingrowth on autopsy retrievals.

Tibial components can be made of titanium or cobalt chrome. The Young's modulus of titanium is similar to cancellous bone. Cobalt chrome tibial components have the advantage of a polished surface to reduce backside wear at the articulation with the polyethylene.

Metal-backed trays are associated with backside wear, but allow modularity compared to all-polyethylene trays.

Primary knee replacement implants can be cruciate retaining or posterior stabilised depending on preservation or sacrifice of the posterior cruciate ligament (Fig. 14.30). The polyethylene insert can be locked into the metal tibial component through a locking mechanism (fixed bearing knee replacement) or it can be free to rotate on a highly polished metal tibial surface (mobile bearing tibial component).

Semiconstrained implants have a polyethylene post which fits into the box of the femoral component, providing some degree of varus-valgus stability (Fig. 14.31). These are also known as varus-valgus constrained (VVC). Examples of VVC are the total condylar III (TC-3 by DePuy, Warsaw, Indiana) and the Constrained Condylar Knee (CCK by Zimmer Biomet, Warsaw, Indiana). These substitute the PCL by cam and post mechanism as well as compensate for laxity of the lateral collateral ligament. In the primary arthroplasty setting, it is indicated for large coronal plane deformities and lack of functioning lateral collateral ligament.

Lack of functioning medial collateral ligament generally requires hinged knee prosthesis.

Medial offset stems are useful in patients with a previous high tibial osteotomy, and metal wedges and blocks can be used for congenital or traumatic defects. Blocks produce less shear force at the fixation interface, but require more bone resection compared to wedges (Fig. 14.32).

The advantages and disadvantages of metal-backed tibial components are listed in Table 14.17.

Patellar Component

The vast majority of patellar components are cemented and made of polyethylene.

Cementless patellar components are associated with problems of fracture of metal pegs, dissociation of polyethylene from the metal backing and excess wear due to a relatively thin polyethylene. Using an inset porous coated metal backing that is countersunk below the resected surface of the patella allows a thicker polyethylene to be used.

Both multiple and single peg fixation designs are available. The shape of the implant may be oval, circular, symmetric or anatomic.

The advantages and disadvantages of patella resurfacing are listed in Table 14.18.

Burnett RS, Haydon CM, Rorabeck CH, Bourne RB. Patella resurfacing versus non resurfacing in total knee arthroplasty. Clin Orthop 2004;428:12–25. Prospective RCT 10 year follow-up, 90 patients, 100 knees. Randomised to resurfacing or non resurfacing. No difference in revision rate, knee score, ROM, patient satisfaction, anterior knee pain. However, no group with selective resurfacing.

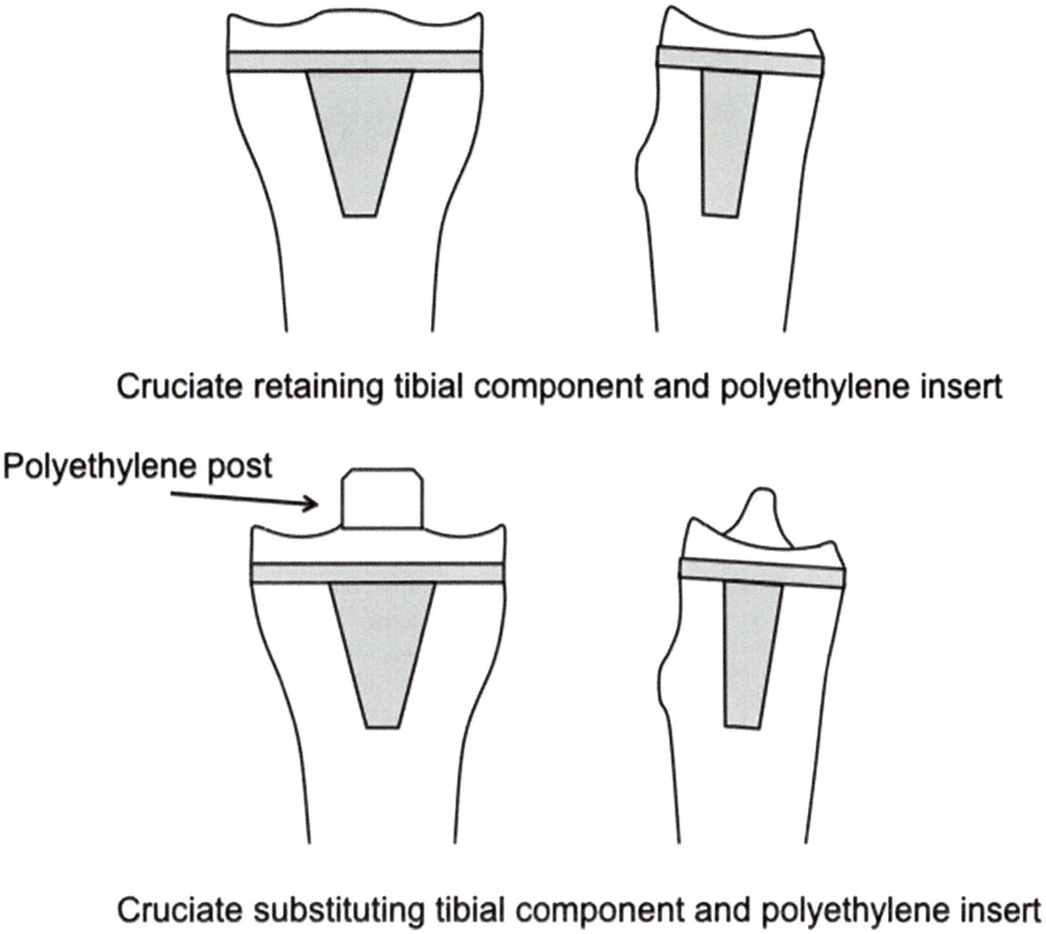

Fig. 14.30 Cruciate retaining and cruciate substituting polyethylene insert designs

Fig. 14.31 Varus valgus constrained knee design

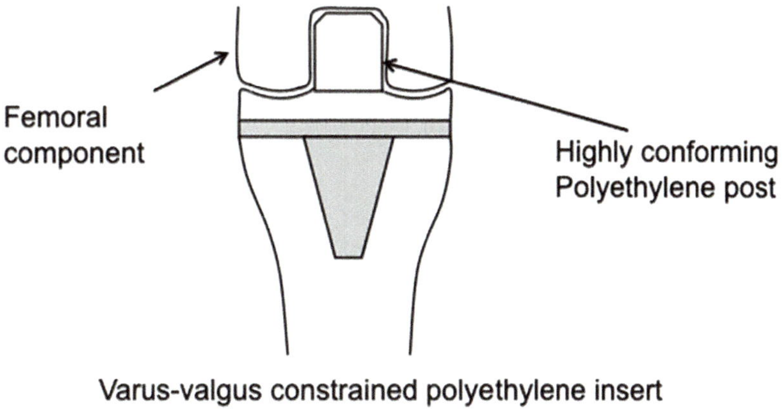

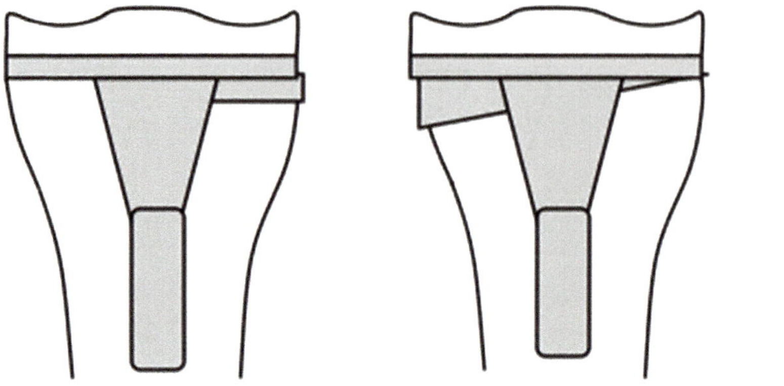

Fig. 14.32 Tibial block and wedge augments

Table 14.17 Advantages and disadvantages of metal-backed tibial components.

Advantages	Disadvantages
Stress transfer to underlying bone is lower and more evenly distributed Permits modularity	The thin polyethylene can lead to increased stress on the insert and catastrophic failure The stiff metal tray can cause stress shielding of the proximal tibia The tray can tilt if eccentrically loaded Generally more expensive than all-polyethylene tibial components

Table 14.18 Advantages and disadvantages of patella resurfacing

Advantages	Disadvantages
Reduces risk of patellofemoral pain Lower reoperation rate for patellofemoral problems after knee replacement Improves tracking	Problems of failure of patella fixation Unsuitable in young patients with high demand due to high joint forces

Pilling RWD, Moulder E, Allgar V, Messner J, Sun Z, Mohsen A. Patellar resurfacing in primary total knee arthroplasty. A meta-analysis. J Bone Joint Surg Am 2012.94(24):227–8. Meta-analysis of 16 RCTs. 3500 knees. 1700 with patella and 1700 without patella. No difference in anterior knee pain or satisfaction. However, higher number of secondary procedures in patients where patella was not resurfaced.

Electrocautery of the patellar rim without resurfacing in an attempt to denervate the patella has no impact on outcome of postoperative patellar symptoms.

S Gupta, Augustine A, Horey L, Meek RM, Hullin MG, Mohammed A. Electrocautery of the patellar rim in primary total knee replacement: beneficial or unnecessary. J Bone Joint Surg Br 2010; 92(9): 1259–61. Retrospective study. No difference in anterior knee pain.

Mobile Bearing Knees

Mobile bearing knees were introduced to reduce backside wear in modular fixed bearing tibial trays. Backside wear occurs at the interface between the polyethylene and the tibial articulation. Even in fixed bearing knees, micromotion at this interface will produce wear debris.

Mobile bearing knees can be meniscal-bearing or rotating platform (Fig. 14.33). The movement on the undersurface of the tibial tray should allow only rotation and not multidirectional movement, as multidirectional movement increases wear and leads to early failure. Advantages and disadvantages of mobile bearing inserts are summarised in Table 14.19.

Chang CW, Lai KA, Yang CY, Lan SM. Early mechanical complications of a multidirectional mobile bearing total knee replacement. J Bone

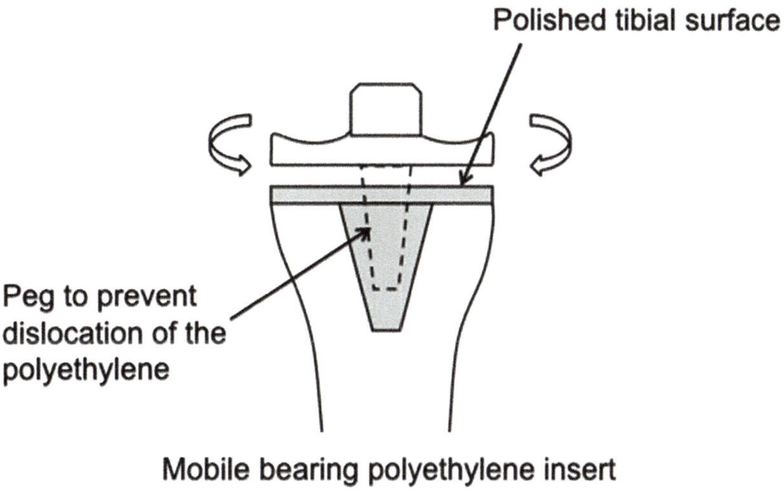

Fig. 14.33 Mobile bearing knee replacement design

Table 14.19 Advantages and disadvantages of mobile bearing inserts

Advantages of mobile bearing inserts	Disadvantages of mobile bearing inserts
Allows more conforming inserts at the femoral interface, thereby reducing wear There is less backside wear due to flat-on-flat articulation between the insert and the tibial tray with unidirectional motion, which therefore increases longevity of the polyethylene The prosthesis accommodates minor degrees of malrotation between the femur and tibia The design allows a better contact area in high flexion	Impingement or dislocation of the bearing may occur. In high flexion, if the PCL is tight, the lateral femoral condyle moves posteriorly and the lateral side of the insert is pushed anteriorly and subluxes—known as bearing spinout Little clinical evidence to prove superiority of mobile bearings over fixed bearings

Joint Surg Br 2011; 93(4): 479–83. 241 knees, 49 month follow up. 7.5% had mechanical complications.

Dislocation (spinout) is more likely in cruciate retaining inserts as compared to posterior stabilised inserts. The peg in posterior stabilized inserts may act as a physical restraint to spinout. Spinout can be due to a tight posterior cruciate ligament (PCL).

Tightness is addressed by releasing anterior and lateral fibres from the femoral side of the PCL. The PCL is checked with the patella relocated in the trochlear groove instead of everted patella. If there is still a tendency to spinout then a larger sized bearing of the same thickness can be used. This gives a larger AP dimension, reducing the chances of dislocation. The rotational excursion will be reduced if a larger insert is used and the contact area will also be slightly reduced, but this generally is not clinically significant. The amount of contact will still be more than with a comparable fixed bearing insert.

Currently, some surgeons prefer mobile bearings for young, active patients. Evidence to support the use of mobile bearings is equivocal.

Namba RS, Inacio MC, Paxton EW, Ake CF, Wang C, Gross TP, Marinac-Dabic D, Sedrakyan A. Risk of revision for fixed versus mobile bearing primary total knee replacement. J Bone Joint Surg Am 2012;94(21):1929–35. Prospective cohort joint registry study, 47,000 knees; 42,000 fixed, 5000 mobile. 1% revision rate (apart from infection). 97.8% survival at 6.7 years. No association with surgeon/case volume/mobile or fixed.

Posterior Cruciate Ligament in Knee Replacements

The PCL extends from the lateral surface of the medial femoral condyle to the posterior part of the intercondylar area of the tibia. It comprises an anterolateral band that is tight in flexion and posteromedial band that is tight in extension. The distal insertion extends below the level of the articular surface and the ligament is extrasynovial.

As the knee flexes from the fully extended position, the first 30° of flexion involves rolling of femoral condyles over the tibial plateau. Beyond 30° the PCL produces a rollback of the femur on the tibia, preventing impingement of the posterior surface of the distal femur against the posterior part of the tibial plateau. As a result of rollback, higher flexion can be achieved.

With femoral rollback the extensor mechanism moves anteriorly, improving the power. The lateral femoral condyle rolls back further than the medial. Normal femoral rollback is not reproduced in the prosthetic knee with or without the PCL.

The forerunner to the cruciate substituting (posterior stabilised) knee was the cruciate sacrificing prosthesis. The stability of the cruciate sacrificing prosthesis depended on equal flexion and extension gaps and intact collaterals with a well-conforming tibial component. An example of this was the total condylar knee. This evolved into the first successful posterior stabilised knee: the Insall–Burstein posterior stabilised knee. The advantages of retaining or substituting the PCL are summarised in Table 14.20.

Checking for PCL Tension

With the trial components in place, it should not be possible to pull out the tibial component from under the femoral component with the knee flexed to 90°. If the tibial component can be pulled out or pushed in with the femoral component in situ, the knee is too loose and a thicker insert must be used.

If flexion of the knee with the trial components causes the front of the tibia trial component to lift off, or the femoral trial to be pushed off distally, the PCL is too tight. A tight PCL pulls the femur backwards and the impingement of the femoral condyle on the back of the tibial tray causes lift off in the front. In this situation, the PCL should be released. This test should be performed with the patella restored to the trochlear

Table 14.20 Advantages of retaining or substituting the PCL

Advantages of retaining the PCL	Advantages of substituting the PCL
Allows the use of a less constrained prosthesis, resulting in less stress transfer to the interface	PCL function is compromised in the arthritic knee and in the absence of the ACL, reproducible femoral rollback does not occur
The PCL acts as an additional tether to prevent an excessively wide flexion gap	Some PCL-retaining knees actually allow the femur to move forwards in flexion instead of backwards (paradoxical roll forward)
Less femur has to be resected to insert cruciate retaining components because the flexion space does not open up as much	Balancing a knee with significant coronal plane deformity of excessive flexion deformity may be easier if the PCL is removed
There is less elevation of the joint line, preserving collateral ligament kinematics	There is less effect of the level of the joint line on the function of the prosthesis
Mid-flexion instability is avoided	It allows more conforming articular surfaces, reducing contact stress
There is no patellar clunk or dislocation of the post	PCL substitution should be considered for severe flexion deformity, ankylosed knee, post-patellectomy knee, inflammatory arthritis, PCL injury, and for patients with chronic patellar dislocation
There is no peg fracture or wear	
There are more options to treat supracondylar fractures above the femoral component	
PCL-substituting designs do not tolerate hyperextension as it leads to impingement of the post	
PCL-substituting implants can have dislocation of the femoral cam anterior to the tibial polyethylene post on hyperflexion (known as 'cam jump'). Reduction of this requires manipulation under general anaesthetic or open reduction	
Retaining PCL allows better proprioception	
PCL retention should be considered in patients with hyperextension, and those who are likely to achieve very high flexion (to reduce risk of cam jump)	

groove and not everted, otherwise the tight quadriceps can cause a false lift off. Posterior femoral osteophytes are also a rare cause of lift off and should be removed.

Hinged Knee Replacement

Hinged knee replacements have a hinge mechanism built into the femoral component. Hinges can be rotating hinge or a fixed hinge. The rotating hinge knees allow rotation of the polyethylene insert on the tibial component. This compensates for lack of rotation in the hinge and for any rotational mismatch between the femoral and tibial component.

Indications for hinged knee replacement include MCL deficiency, hyperextension deformity, tumour resection or massive bone loss.

Cemented/Cementless Technique

Cemented knee replacements are more commonly used than cementless knee replacements.

For cementless knees, the optimum pore size is 400–600 μm. The distance between bone and implant should be less than 50 μm for ingrowth. Micromotion of more than 150 μm results in fibrous tissue formation instead of bone ingrowth. Pegs and screws help to provide initial stability. The undersurface of tibial components should be fully coated to prevent migration of wear particles.

Osteopenic bone may not be able to support cementless fixation and cemented implants should be considered.

Cementless fixation technique requires accurate bone preparation and accurate ligament balancing to avoid early failure.

Park J W, Kim YH. Simultaneous cemented and cementless total knee replacement in the same patient. J Bone Joint Surg Br 2011;93(11):1479–86. 50 patients had simultaneous bilateral knee replacement with one side cemented and other uncemented. No difference in knee society scores, range of movements, patient satisfaction and radiological outcome at 14 years.

Coronal Alignment in Knee Replacement

The mechanical axis is the line joining the centre of the femoral head and the centre of the ankle joint, passing through the centre of the knee. The anatomical axis is the line along the tibial shaft and femoral shaft, making an angle of 5–7° valgus with the mechanical axis (Fig. 14.34).

The mean mechanical axial alignment of the knee is 1–1.5° of varus, hence loading the medial tibial plateau greater than the lateral tibial plateau. Commonly, 60–70% weight transmission takes place through the medial compartment.

Varus knees have high adduction moment, predisposing to medial compartment osteoarthritis. Medial compartment osteoarthritis in turn leads to increased adduction moment, leading to greater varus deformity—a cycle of progression.

Anatomically, the femoral condyle is in 7° of valgus and the tibial plateau is in 3° of varus. In flexion, the medial femoral condyle extends 3° more posteriorly in relation to the lateral condyle.

The aim of distal femoral alignment is to make the resection plane perpendicular to the mechanical axis. A component that is not perpendicular to the mechanical axis will be subject to shear stress on loading. The femoral prosthesis is aligned by intramedullary jigs along the anatomical axis of femur. The distal resection is made at 5–7° valgus angle to the anatomical axis of femur, resulting in a plane perpendicular to the mechanical axis of the limb. Femur alignment should be restored to 5° ± 1–2° of valgus.

For the femur, intramedullary jigs are more accurate than extramedullary jigs. The entry point should be in line with the medullary canal of the femur and slightly medial to the centre of intercondylar notch.

The proximal tibial resection is perpendicular to the mechanical axis of tibia, which is collinear with the anatomical axis of tibia. Extramedullary

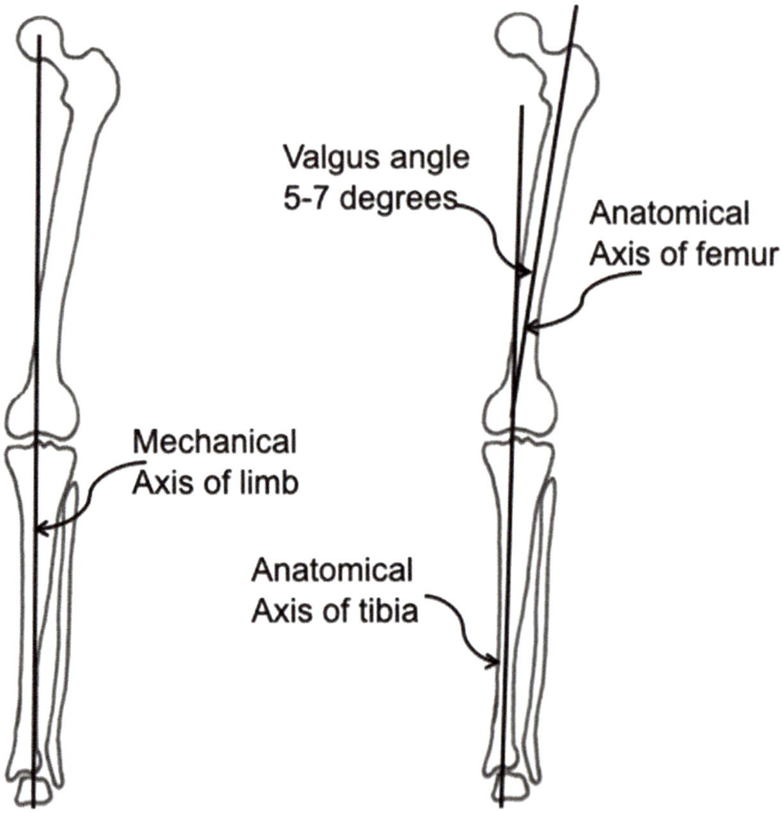

Fig. 14.34 The mechanical axis of the femur makes an angle of 4–7° with the anatomical axis of the femoral shaft

alignment is used for the tibia as the mechanical axis can be clinically assessed. Bowing of the tibial diaphysis can mislead the surgeon if intramedullary rods are used for tibial alignment.

A perpendicular resection of the tibia places the component parallel to the ground, minimising shear stress at the implant interface on weight bearing.

Kinematic alignment is a concept that has gained popularity in the last few years. This moves away from restoring the same mechanical alignment for every individual, and instead aims to reproduce the pre-arthritic alignment. The pre-arthritic alignment is determined on CT or MR scans. Long term results of kinematically aligned knee replacement are under evaluation.

Howell SM, Shelton TJ, Hull ML. Implant Survival and Function Ten Years After Kinematically Aligned Total Knee Arthroplasty. J Arthro 2018;33:3678–84. 222 kinematically aligned knees using patient specific jigs. 78% of tibial components were outlying in terms of varus malalignment. One tibial loosening at 10 years. 98.4% survival at 10 years for aseptic loosening.

Flexion and Extension Gaps

The flexion gap is the distance between the cut surface of the distal femur and the cut surface of the proximal tibia, measured with the knee in flexion; the extension gap is the distance between the cut surface of the distal femur and the cut surface of the proximal tibia, measured with the knee in extension (Fig. 14.35). Both of these gaps should be rectangular—implying equal tension on the medial and lateral side—and should be equal to each other.

Changing the distal femoral resection will influence only the extension gap, while the amount of posterior femoral resection will influence only the flexion gap (Fig. 14.36). Tibial resection will have an effect on both flexion and extension gaps. This is helpful in understanding gap balancing as summarised in Table 14.21.

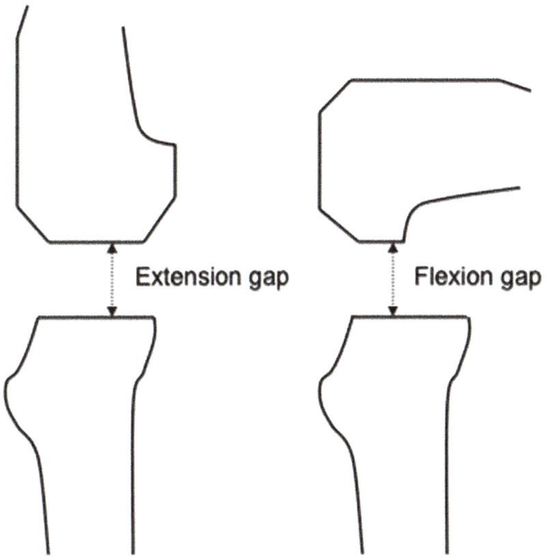

Fig. 14.35 The concept of flexion and extension gaps

Balancing and Sizing of Components

The size of the femoral component can be determined by anterior or posterior referencing. Anterior referencing implies the component selected will be aligned to anterior femoral cortex and posterior referencing means the femoral component is lined with the posterior part of femoral condyles.

Anterior referencing gives an accurate anterior resection—hence avoids notching the anterior femoral cortex and overstuffing the patellofemoral joint. The disadvantage is that measurements that fall in between femur sizes must be downsized (i.e., smaller component is used), which involves removing more posterior condyle, resulting in a potentially bigger flexion gap. Posterior referencing allows accurate flexion gap at the cost of potentially overstuffing the patellofemoral joint or notching the femur.

There are two schools of thought for balancing knee replacement—'measured resection' and 'gap balanced'. The measured resection technique involves removing enough bone from the femur and tibia to allow similar thickness compo-

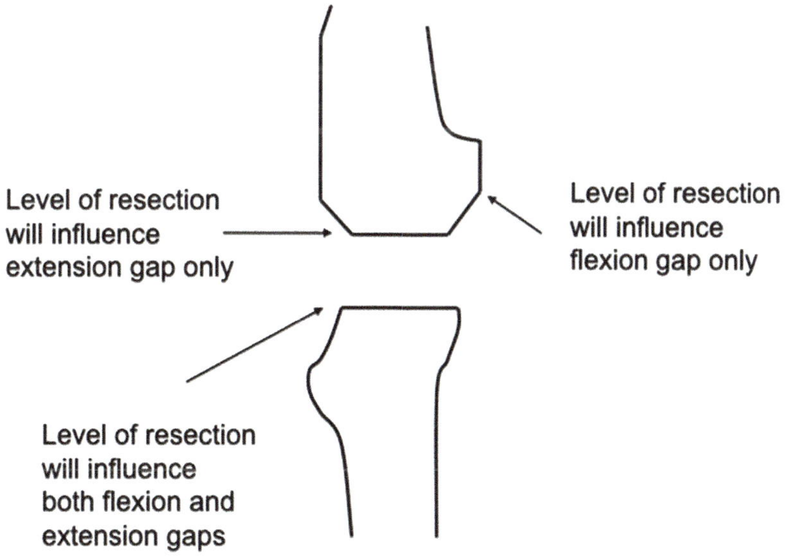

Fig. 14.36 Effect of bone resection on the flexion and extension gaps

Table 14.21 Problems and solutions in soft tissue balancing

Problem	Solutions
Flexion and extension gaps tight	Increase tibial resection
Flexion and extension gaps loose	Use thicker polyethylene insert Augment under tibial tray
Extension gap tight, flexion gap satisfactory	Release posterior capsule from femur Clear the osteophytes at back of femoral condyle Increase distal femoral resection
Flexion gap tight, extension gap satisfactory	Downsize femur (will increase posterior condyle resection) Release posterior cruciate ligament from femoral side Increase posterior tibial slope Increase tibial resection, use thicker insert and treat loose extension gap

nents. The gap balanced technique involves making the proximal tibial cut first and then equalising the flexion and extension gaps by adjusting the rotation of the femoral component.

Joint line restoration is desirable, which means after bone resection and implantation, the level of distal femoral surface matches the normal level for the patient. This allows the collateral ligaments to function at their optimum length.

Femoral component rotation (internal/external rotation) can be assessed by different methods (Table 14.22).

Whiteside L, Arima J. The anteroposterior axis for femoral rotational alignment in valgus knee arthroplasty. Clin Orthop 1995;321:168–72.

If posterior referencing is used, the presence of a hypoplastic lateral femoral condyle in a val-

Table 14.22 Assessment of femoral component rotation

Bony landmarks	Diagrammatic representation
Interepicondylar axis—the anterior and posterior flanges of the component should be parallel to the interepicondylar axis. The epicondylar axis (CD) is the line connecting the lateral epicondylar prominence and the median sulcus of the medial epicondyle Whiteside's line is a line from the deepest part of the trochlear groove to the centre of the intercondylar notch posteriorly (IJ). The femoral component is oriented perpendicular to Whiteside's line Posterior condylar axis extends between the posterior surfaces of femoral condyles (EF). This is unreliable in the presence of bone loss or dysplasia of the condyles Rectangular flexion gap—in the flexed knee, the cut surface of the femur posteriorly (AB) should be parallel to the superior cut surface of the tibia (GH)	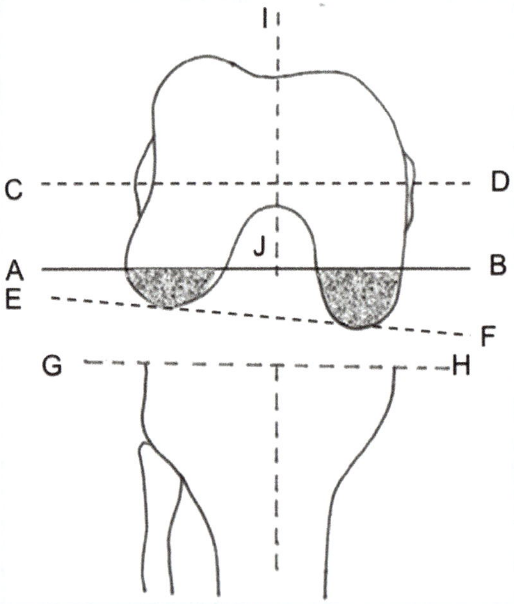 AB—posterior femoral resection plane CD—Inter-epicondylar axis EF—Posterior condylar axis GH—Tibial resection plane IJ—Whiteside's line

Table 14.22 (continued)

Bony landmarks	Diagrammatic representation
More bone is removed from the back of the medial femoral condyle than from the lateral, as the medial femoral condyle extends further posteriorly	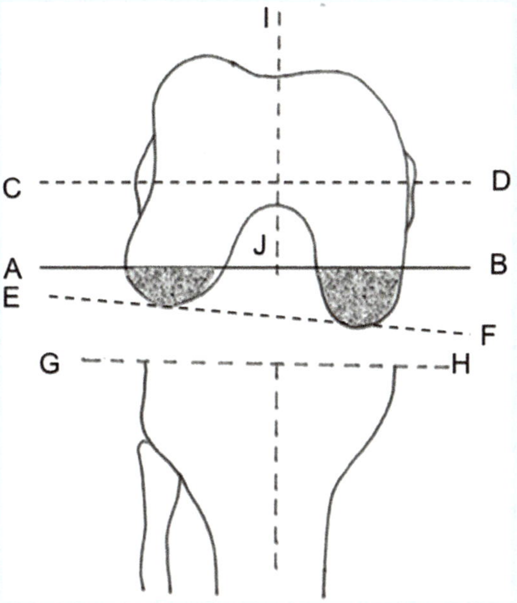
The anterior femoral cut surface should resemble a double curve, with the medial peak lower than lateral peak. This is the 'grand piano sign' or the 'Matterhorn sign'	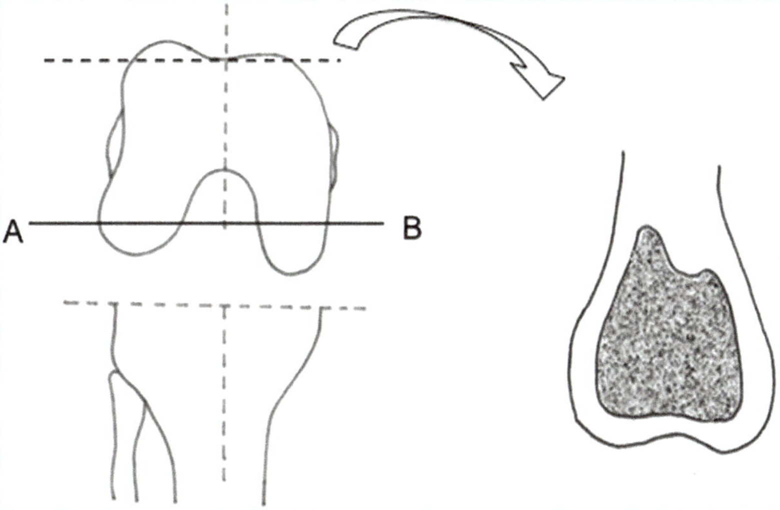

gus knee can lead to excess internal rotation of the femoral component. Excess internal rotation or medialisation of the femoral or tibial component leads to a relative lateral displacement of the extensor mechanism and problems with patellar tracking (Table 14.23).

Excess internal or external rotation of the femoral component can lead to reduced contact with

Table 14.23 Effects of inappropriate rotation of the femoral component

Excess external rotation	Excess internal rotation
Loose medial flexion gap	Tight medial flexion gap
Tight lateral flexion gap	Loose lateral flexion gap
Lateral displacement of patellofemoral groove of the implant	Medial displacement of patellofemoral groove of the implant

the patella, increasing the contact pressure and may lead to early failure of the patellar component.

Verlinden C, Uvin P, Labey L, Luyckx JP, Bellemans J, Vandenneucker H. The influence of malrotation of the femoral component in total knee replacement on the mechanics of patellofemoral contact during gait: an in vitro biomechanical study. J Bone Joint Surg Br 2010;92(5):737–42. Experimental study to prove reduction in patellofemoral contact when the femoral component is malrotated.

The tibial resection is perpendicular to the mechanical axis, which usually coincides with the long axis in the AP view. The tibial cut can be made with the help of extramedullary or intramedullary alignment jigs.

Extramedullary alignment is not affected by tibial deformities or obstruction in the tibial canal. Intramedullary alignment is useful in obese patients, where it may be difficult to palpate bony prominences (required for extramedullary alignment). For intramedullary alignment the starting point is at the junction of attachments of the anterior cruciate ligament (ACL) and the anterior horn of the lateral meniscus. Fluted rods reduce the incidence of fat embolism.

The tibial cut is perpendicular to mechanical axis of the tibia in the AP view, such that the tibial tray is parallel to the ground on weight bearing. A varus cut increases load on the medial side and leads to early failure.

Berend ME, Ritter MA, Meding JB et al. Tibial component failure mechanism in total knee arthroplasty. Clin Orthop 2004;428:26–34. Tibial cut in more than 3° of varus increases failure rate. Varus limb alignment postoperatively increases failure rate.

The extramedullary jig is positioned slightly medial to the midpoint of the ankle along the intermalleolar line so as to avoid a varus cut of the proximal tibia. The upper platform is lined up with the medial third of the tibial tubercle. The normal posterior slope should be reproduced. The thickness of bone removed should match the thickness of components to be inserted and is generally 10 mm from the surface of less arthritic plateau.

Medialisation or internal rotation of the tibial component results in relative lateral positioning of the tibial tubercle. This malaligns the pull of the quadriceps to a more lateral force, and that leads to patellar maltracking. Internal rotation of the tibial component is a possible cause of persistent pain following knee replacements.

Nicoll D, Rowley DI. Internal rotation error of the tibial component is a major cause of pain after total knee replacements. J Bone Joint Surg Br 2010;92(9):1238–44. 22 out of 39 painful knees had internal rotation of the femoral, tibial or both components. 4.6% of all knees in the cohort may have significant internal rotation errors.

If there is a bowing deformity of the tibia, the resection should be perpendicular to the mechanical axis. This may involve removing an asymmetric amount of bone from the medial and lateral tibial plateaus. In severe cases, deformity correction may be required as a separate procedure prior to arthroplasty.

The Varus Knee

In the varus knee the deformity is generally in the tibia. This contrasts to the valgus knee, in which the deformity is often in the femur. Neutral alignment is considered to be between 4 and 9°. Less than 4° is considered varus and more than 9° is valgus.

Varus is a more common deformity than valgus. Rheumatoid patients have a relatively higher incidence of valgus, but the majority still have varus deformity.

A varus deformity can be correctable if medial structures are not contracted. In longstanding deformity, however, contractures may develop. The tibial resection is referenced from the preserved lateral plateau, removing 10 mm from the lateral side. The usual 3° of external rotation of the femur may have to be increased because a hyperplastic medial femoral condyle may distort the posterior referencing.

Using the medial parapatellar approach, osteophytes are removed to the level of the semimembranosus bursa in the plane between the medial tibial plateau and the deep MCL. The deep MCL and tight medial capsule is released. A subperiosteal release of the pes can be done and this can be extended along the proximal medial tibia deep to the superficial MCL. The superficial MCL is preserved in all but the most extreme instances. Release of the superficial MCL will likely require the use of a hinged implant.

A tibial component one size smaller may have to be selected along with excision of bone from the medial tibial margin to slacken the MCL (Fig. 14.37). If the perpendicular distance (difference in height) between the medial and the lateral joint line is more than 15 mm then medial augmentation may be needed. This can be in the form of cement, a bone graft or metal augments. Alternatively, metal metaphyseal sleeves can be used.

The Valgus Knee

In the valgus knee, the lateral femoral condyle may be hypoplastic both distally and posteriorly, affecting femoral component alignment. The lateral structures may be tight and the MCL attenuated or nonfunctional.

The distal femoral cut is aligned to 5° valgus, although the angle can be 3° if there is significant diaphyseal valgus remodeling because the axis of the femoral canal exits more medially to the normal entry point.

Using a 5° valgus cut is a good compromise; a cut of 2 or 3° requires a greater lateral release to balance the knee. A smaller cut (less than 5°) helps to take the strain off the attenuated MCL during weight bearing. A resection of more than 5° valgus will lead to more strain on the already stretched medial structures.

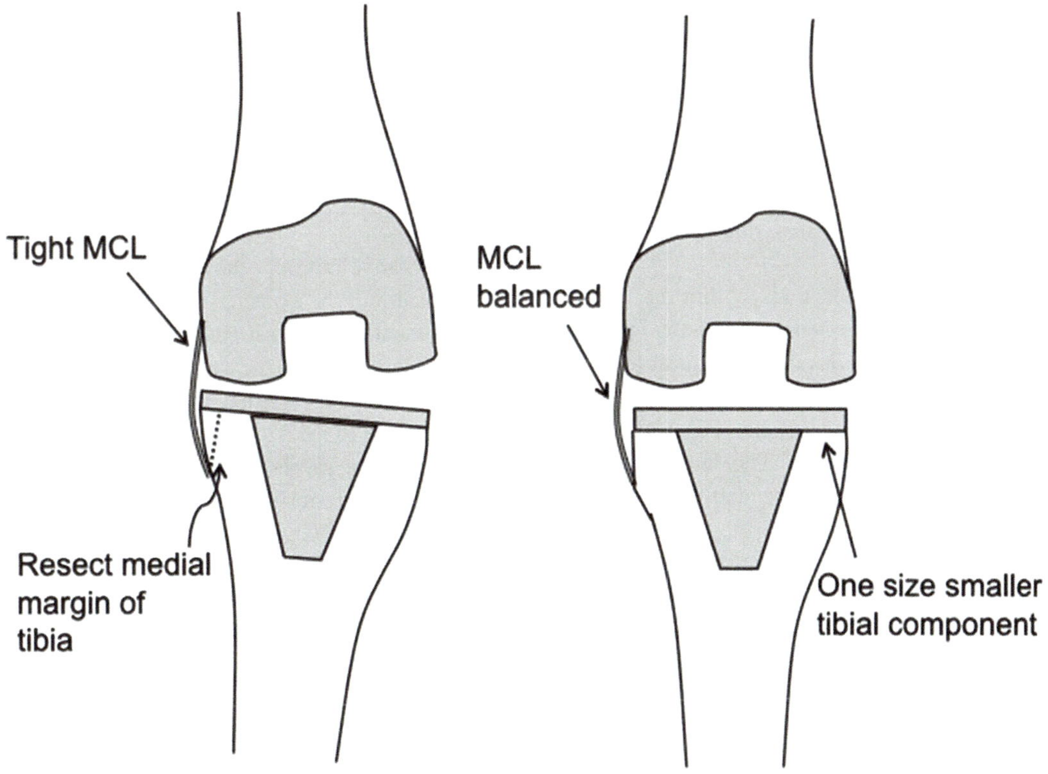

Fig. 14.37 Balancing the MCL by resection of medial margin of tibia

The hypoplastic lateral femoral condyle should be augmented instead of resecting down to the level of the condyle. A distal femoral resection performed at the level of the hypoplastic lateral femoral condyle elevates the joint line, which in turn interferes with the kinematics of the collateral ligaments. Additionally, it creates an excessive extension gap.

Once the femoral and tibial cuts have been made, a rectangular shape of the flexion and extension gaps is achieved by soft tissue balancing. The rotation of the femoral component is adjusted on the basis of flexion gap symmetry.

The lateral release starts with the osteophytes and then the posterolateral capsule. The capsular release is at the level of the tibial resection, extending from the posterior margin of the iliotibial band to the posterior capsule. Any tight bands can be felt and divided.

If still tight, in extension, the iliotibial band can be released by a 'pie-crusting' technique. This involves multiple transverse stab incisions from the deep surface. If the knee is tight in flexion, the popliteus can be released. This is rarely needed.

Release of the lateral collateral ligament from the femoral attachment is possible. If the lateral release results in loss of lateral support, a semi-constrained implant (varus-valgus constrained) is required.

The patella should track within the trochlear groove on knee flexion and remain in contact with both the condyles of the femoral trial component. If it is still tight laterally, a lateral retinacular release should be considered after releasing the tourniquet. The lateral release is through multiple transverse stab incisions on the lateral retinaculum.

The lateral popliteal nerve is at risk of stretch injury when valgus deformity is corrected. If nerve palsy is detected postoperatively, flexing the knee will relieve the stretch on the nerve.

An excessively stretched medial collateral ligament in a valgus knee is an indication for a hinged prosthesis. As a rule of thumb, a gap of 10 mm or more on the medial margin of the knee on weight bearing films should instigate consideration of a hinged implant.

Dealing with Extraarticular Deformity

The impact of an extraarticular deformity on knee replacement surgery depends on the extent of deformity and its distance from the knee joint. Deformities within the distal fourth of femur or proximal fourth of tibia, if more than 20°, should be corrected prior to, or at the time of knee replacement. This is McPherson's one-fourth rule.

Range of Motion After Total Knee Replacement

Different activities require different degrees of knee flexion (Table 14.24). Most patients should regain at least 110° of knee flexion following replacement to enable near normal function.

Stiffness After Total Knee Replacement

Causes of stiffness after TKR are summarised in Fig. 14.38.

.

Preoperative range of movement is an important indicator of the expected postoperative range of movement. Previous surgery, obesity, multiple joint involvement, age, sex and bilateral surgery have not shown a consistent relationship with post-operative ROM.

Tight flexion gap is due to oversized femoral component, posteriorly translated femoral component or a tight PCL.

Table 14.24 Knee flexion requirement for different activities

Action	Degree of flexion required
Walking on level ground	70
Ascending stairs	90
Descending stairs	100
Rising from a chair without using arm support	105

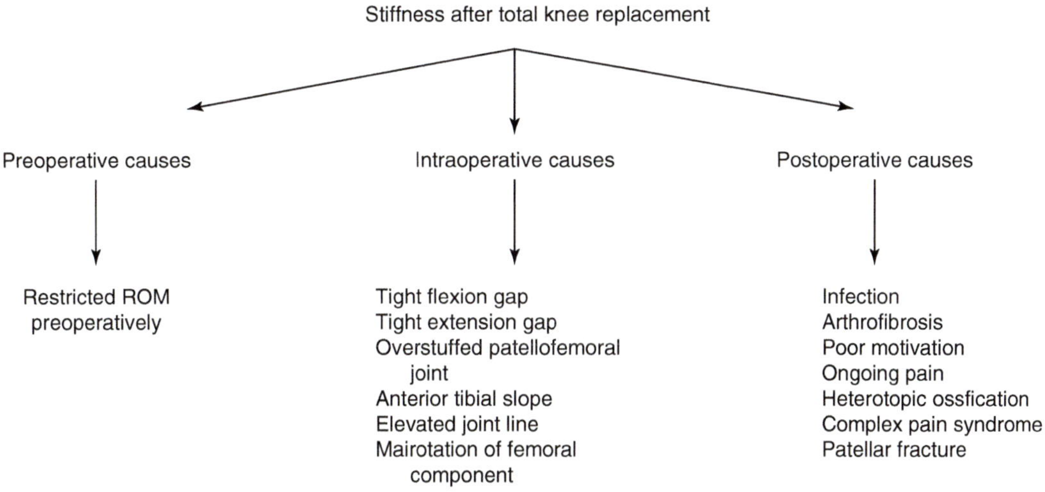

Fig. 14.38 Causes of stiffness after total knee replacement

Tight extension is gap is due to inadequate distal femoral resection, inadequate tibial resection, tight posterior capsule or osteophytes.

Inadequate patellar resection or anterior translation of femoral component will lead to an overstuffed patellofemoral joint.

Anterior tibial slope restricts femoral rollback in flexion. An accurate evaluation of posterior tibial slope should be made for patients with restricted knee flexion.

Elevation of joint line—causes relative patella baja and increased joint forces and stiffness.

Malrotation (internal rotation) of the femoral component can cause an asymmetric flexion gap.

In the absence of an identifiable cause for stiffness, manipulation under anesthetic can be attempted up to 4 months following knee replacement. Improvement in flexion is expected, but it does not improve fixed flexion deformities. In delayed presentations, open adhesiolysis is an option although there is a high risk of recurrent stiffness.

Total Knee Replacement in Presence of Fixed Flexion Deformity

For preoperative flexion contracture, the osteophytes from the intercondylar area and from the posterior part of the femoral condyle are removed. An extensive posterior release is the key to correcting flexion deformity. The PCL is resected for unrestricted access to the posterior capsule.

Increasing the distal femoral resection by 2 mm if the preoperative flexion contracture is more than 15° helps to achieve extension. A further 2 mm extra resection can be done for every further 10° of fixed flexion deformity. This carries the disadvantage of elevating the joint line.

Severe preoperative flexion contractures may require serial casting prior to surgery.

Total Knee Replacement After Failed High Tibial Osteotomy

High tibial osteotomy (HTO) provides good short-term results in 80–90% of patients. The results deteriorate with time, however, and on long-term follow-up only 60% of patients retain good function. Risk factors for early failure include male sex, increased weight, young age at the time of TKR, coronal laxity and preoperative limb malalignment.

Parvizi J, Hanssen AD, Spangehl MJ. Total knee arthroplasty following proximal tibial osteotomy: risk factors for failure. J Bone Joint Surg Am 2004;86(3):474–9. 118 patients, average clinical follow up 15.1 years, high rate of radiographic loosening. Male gender, increased

Table 14.25 Potential problems and solutions with TKR after failed high tibial osteotomy

Problems	Solutions
Existing scars	Conduct preoperative planning to avoid compromising the blood supply Use the most lateral scar if there are multiple longitudinal scars
Existing metalwork	Remove at time of replacement or as a separate procedure prior to replacement
Patella baja	Consider increased tibial resection and shifting the femoral component distally
Nonunion of osteotomy	Stemmed tibial component and bone grafting of non-union
Tibial deformity	Alter bone cuts to correct deformity or correct deformity in a separate procedure
Offset tibial shaft from tibial plateau	Use a smaller component shifted medially or use offset stems
Excess valgus after overcorrected osteotomy	Ensure accurate rotation of the femoral component and avoid excess release of the medial collateral ligament

weight, young age at the time of total knee arthroplasty, coronal laxity, and preoperative limb malalignment were identified as risk factors for early failure.

TKR after failed HTO may present several problems (Table 14.25).

Knee Replacement in Special Situations

Obesity may impose problems of wound healing, poor functional outcome, superficial infection and medial collateral ligament (MCL) avulsion.

Dowsey M, Liew D, Stoney JD, Choong PF. The impact of preoperative obesity on weight change and outcome in total knee replacement. J Bone Joint Surg Br 2010;92:513–20. 529 consecutive patients. Weighed preop and at 1 year post op. 60% were obese or morbidly obese. 12% of the obese patients lost weight at 1 year but 21% gained weight after 1 year. Adverse events in 14% of obese and 35% of non obese.

Diabetes may lead to a higher risk of infection due to immune dysfunction. The use of antibiotic-loaded cement reduces the risk of infection.

Chiu FY, Lin CF, Chen CM, Lo WH, Chaung TY. Cefuroxime-impregnated cement at primary total knee arthroplasty in diabetes mellitus: A prospective, randomised study. J Bone Joint Surg Br 2001;83(5):691–5. Single blind prospective RCT. 78 patients. No infection if cefuroxime was added to cement. 5/37 (13.5%) infection in group without antibiotic cement.

Osteonecrosis can be steroid induced or idiopathic. The poor-quality bone does not adequately support the components and there is a high rate of loosening and revision. The use of cemented implants and stemmed implants, where necessary, improves outcomes.

Mont MA, Rifai A, Baumgarten KM, Sheldon M, Hungerford DS. Total knee arthroplasty for osteonecrosis. J Bone Joint Surg Am 2002;84(4):599–603. 32 knees, mean age 54, mean follow up 108 months, 97% clinically successful outcome with no progressive radiolucency

Haemophilia may be associated with poor bone quality and soft tissue fibrosis. Patients with coexisting AIDS have immunodeficiency. Factor VIII levels should be maintained near 100% peri-operatively. The presence of antibodies against factor VIII is a contraindication to arthroplasty.

Silva M, Luck JV Jr. Long-term results of primary total knee replacement in patients with hemophilia J Bone Joint Surg Am 2005;87:85–91. 38 knees, 16% infection rate. Mechanical failure of prosthesis was not significantly higher.

Goddard NJ, Mann HA, Lee CA. Total knee replacement in patients with end stage hemophilic arthropathy—25 years results. J Bone Joint Surg Br 2010;92(8):1085–9. 70 knees in 57 patients. One deep infection. 94% survival at 20 years.

In patients with Paget's disease, medical management before surgery helps to reduce pain and operative blood loss by reducing vascularity. Restoration of alignment is important and long-term results are not adversely affected.

Post-traumatic arthritis may be complicated by existing scars, poor soft tissue compliance, ligamentous injury, bone loss, deformities and stiffness. Low-grade underlying infection should be ruled out. Preoperative inflammatory markers should be checked and intraoperative cultures obtained. The use of antibiotic-loaded cement is helpful.

Saleh KJ, Sherman P, Katkin P, Windsor R, Haas S, Laskin R, Sculco T. Total knee arthroplasty after open reduction and internal fixation of fractures of the tibial plateau: a minimum 5-year follow-up study J Bone Joint Surg Am 2001;83(8):1144–8. 15 knees following tibial plateau fractures. 38.6 months follow up. 3 had deep infection, 3 required manipulation for stiffness and two had patellar tendon rupture.

Ipsilateral hip fusion should be converted to hip arthroplasty before knee replacement. Conversion to hip arthroplasty in itself may resolve knee pain due to malalignment. A higher rate of stiffness requiring manipulation is reported if knee arthroplasty is performed with an ipsilateral hip fusion without converting to hip arthroplasty beforehand.

Rittmeister M, Starker M, Zichner L. Hip and knee replacement after longstanding hip arthrodesis. Clin Orthop 2000;371:136–45. Total 18 patients underwent knee replacement with or without conversion of hip fusion to hip arthroplasty followed by knee replacement. Patients who were converted had better functional score and outcome.

For patients with juvenile rheumatoid arthritis, total knee replacement is a reasonable option. Despite the relatively young age of these patients, functional demand on the knee arthroplasty is often low and it is therefore worthwhile considering knee arthroplasty.

Palmer DH, Mulhall KJ, Thompson CA, Severson EP, ERG Santos, Saleh KJ. Total knee arthroplasty in juvenile rheumatoid arthritis. J Bone Joint Surg Am 2005;87(7):1510–4. 8 patients, 15 knees, average age 16.8 years, 15.5 year follow up. Three revised, all had improvement in pain and function. Seven were wheelchair bound before surgery and 6 were able to walk at last follow up.

Complications in Knee Arthroplasty

Infection

Infection in knee replacements is disappointing for the surgeon and the patient. Multiple steps can be taken to reduce the prevalence. A meticulous approach to preoperative assessment and preparation, operation room functioning, operative technique and postoperative care is needed.

Preoperative antibiotics are used as standard and are administered prior to start of surgery. Cement with gentamicin is also helpful to reduce infection risk.

Factors that predispose a patient to infection are summarised in Table 14.26.

Deep infection is defined as infection in the subfascial plane and/or intra-articular infection. The presence of a discharging sinus tract indicates chronic deep infection. The risk of deep infection in knee arthroplasty is less than 1%, but is higher in revision surgery (up to 6%).

Blom AW, Brown J, Taylor AH et al. Infection after total knee arthroplasty. J Bone Joint Surg Br 2004:86(5);688–91. Vertical laminar flow, occlusive clothing, chlorhexidine lavage. 931 primary total knees and 69 revisions. 6.5 year follow up. 1% primary and 5.8% revisions had deep infection.

Diagnosis of infection is based on MSIS criteria (see Hip replacement - infection)

Table 14.26 Factors predisposing to infection in joint replacement surgery

Preoperative factors	Operative factors	Postoperative factors
Immunocompromise	Poor soft tissue envelop	Persistent wound discharge
Diabetes	Prolonged surgical time	Low haematocrit
Rheumatoid disease	Breakdown of sterility	Blood transfusion
Malnutrition	Inadequate skin prep	Poor nutrition
Impaired circulation	Damage to skin vascularity	
Smoking		
Obesity		
Steroid use		
Concurrent infection elsewhere		

Clinical Features

The clinical features of infection are pain (constant or night pain); a warm, red and swollen knee; pain on movement; and a discharging wound, cellulitis or sinus.

Diagnosis

ESR is non-specific for infection. CRP normally returns to normal 3–4 weeks after surgery. A persistently raised CRP, or rising levels following operation raise suspicion of postoperative infection. A combination of raised CRP and ESR is helpful in diagnosis of infection. MSIS criteria are employed for diagnosis.

Greidanus NV, Masri BA, Garbuz DS et al. Use of erythrocyte sedimentation rate and c reactive protein level to diagnose infection before revision total knee arthroplasty. J Bone Joint Surg Am 2007; 89:1409–16. 151 knees for revision of which 45 were infected. Sensitivity of ESR is 0.93 and specificity 0.83. For CRP, sensitivity is 0.91 and specificity 0.86.

X-rays can reveal loosening and bone resorption. Radiologic changes occur late in the course of infection.

Tc-99 Bone scan shows increased uptake. Bone scans are of limited use within the 1st year because of bone remodelling changes. Increased uptake in all three phases is suggestive of infection. While cell labeled scans are specific for infection.

Aspiration or synovial biopsy is the most useful test to detect the infecting organism preoperatively. Antibiotics should be stopped 2 weeks prior to aspiration/biopsy to improve diagnostic yield and reduce false negatives.

Intraoperative frozen section with greater than 5 PMN (polymorphonuclear cells) per high power field is suggestive of infection. This has 84% sensitivity and is 99% specific.

Intraoperative deep samples provide definitive evidence of infecting organism. Preoperative antibiotics should be withheld until samples have been obtained at the time of revision surgery.

Treatment

Debridement, Antibiotics and Implant Retention (DAIR) can salvage about 25% joints if performed within 4 weeks of the onset of infection. This involves open debridement, synovectomy and polyethylene liner exchange. The femoral and tibial components are not removed. Prerequisites for DAIR are a well fixed prosthesis, no immune deficiency in the host and an organism sensitive to available antibiotics which can be used over a long term.

Arthroscopic debridement is of questionable efficacy, although some reports have shown good results using multiple portal arthroscopy and debridement of the interface.

Established infection is treated with revision surgery. Either single or two-stage revision surgery may be performed. Two-stage revision surgery is the preferred option, although single stage surgery may be performed in the case of a sensitive organism, adequate soft tissue cover and healthy host.

Haleem AA, Berry DJ, Hanssen AD. Mid to long term follow up of two stage reimplantation for infected total knee arthroplasty. Clin Orthop 2004;428:35–39. 94 patients, 96 knees. All had antibiotic spacer and antibiotic loaded cement. 7.2 year follow up. 16% required reoperation—9% for recurrent infection and 6% for aseptic loosening. Average time for reoperation for reinfection after revision was 1 year.

Hart WJ, Jones RS. Two stage revision of infected total knee replacements using articulating cement spacers and short term antibiotic therapy. J Bone Joint Surg Br 2006;88(8):1011–5. 48 patients managed by articulating spacer and short term parenteral antibiotics after first stage. Infection eradicated in 42 out of 48. Protracted iv antibiotics may not be necessary.

For two stage revisions, the first step is extensive debridement, removal of all components and insertion of static or articulating spacer.

Articulated spacers maintain soft tissue quality and movement and improve outcome. PROSTALAC is Prosthesis of Antibiotic Loaded Acrylic Cement. It is loosely cemented as an articulating spacer and allows preservation of soft tissue envelop and joint mobility in the interval between first and second stage. The antibiotic provides a high local concentration, otherwise unachievable through intravenous administration. Alternatively, a standard knee implant can be loosely cemented using cement with a high concentration of antibiotics.

Arthrodesis is an option in patients with failed reconstruction, poor soft tissue cover or infection with resistant organisms. Arthrodesis helps to control infection and provides a stable knee.

Resection arthroplasty has extremely poor results and is only for the non-ambulatory medically unfit patient. Transfemoral amputation is the last resort.

Wound Problems

In presence of existing scars, the most lateral longitudinal incision should be used as long as it does not compromise access. A gap of 7 cm between longitudinal scars is advisable. Greater vascular supply comes from the medial side and hence the lateral flap has lesser vascularity.

The use of tissue expanders has been successful prior to knee surgery if there is a concern about the adequacy of skin for achieving closure. A plastic surgery consultation is helpful in multiply revised, scarred knees with questionable skin flap vascularity.

Patellofemoral Problems

Patellar clunk occurs due to formation of a fibrous nodule on the deep surface of quadriceps tendon at the superior pole of the patella. The nodule catches on the intercondylar box of a cruciate substituting femoral component causing pain and a 'clunk' sensation. Treatment is with flexion–extension exercises or arthroscopic debridement of the nodule. A superolateral portal is employed for easy access and to avoid scratching the femoral component.

In metal-backed patellar components, loosening of the patellar component may be caused by avascular necrosis of the patella, deficient bone, patellar fracture, subluxation of the patella, a malpositioned component or failure of ingrowth. Failed metal-backed components may be associated with dissociation of the metal plate or the polyethylene, leading to metal–metal contact and accelerated failure of the joint.

Acute open repair is advised for extensor mechanism rupture (quadriceps tendon or patellar tendon rupture), but the results may be unsatisfactory with residual extensor lag.

Patellar fractures are predisposed by:

- Avascular necrosis due to medial parapatellar arthrotomy, with lateral release leading to damage to the superior lateral and medial genicular arteries.
- Inaccurate resection of the patella.
- A too thick or too thin patella after resurfacing.
- An oversized femoral component .
- Maltracking of the patella.
- Use of patellar components with a single central peg.

The classification of patellar fractures is shown in Table 14.27.

Treatment can be non-operative if the component is not loose and the extensor mechanism is competent. The vascular supply of the patella is impaired after knee replacement and this contributes to poor healing of patellar fractures. Open reduction and internal fixation is associated with a high failure rate. Partial patellectomy and extensor mechanism repair is an option.

Problems of patellar maltracking are summarised in Fig. 14.39.

CT scans can help to accurately assess any internal rotation of the femoral or tibial component.

At the time of surgery, patellar tracking should be checked in a full range of flexion–

Table 14.27 Classification of patellar fractures

Type	Description
I	Fractures do not involve the implant–cement interface
II	Fractures involve the implant–cement interface or extensor mechanism
III	Inferior pole fractures
IIIa	Associated patellar tendon rupture
IIIb	No rupture of the patellar tendon
IV	Fracture dislocation of the patella

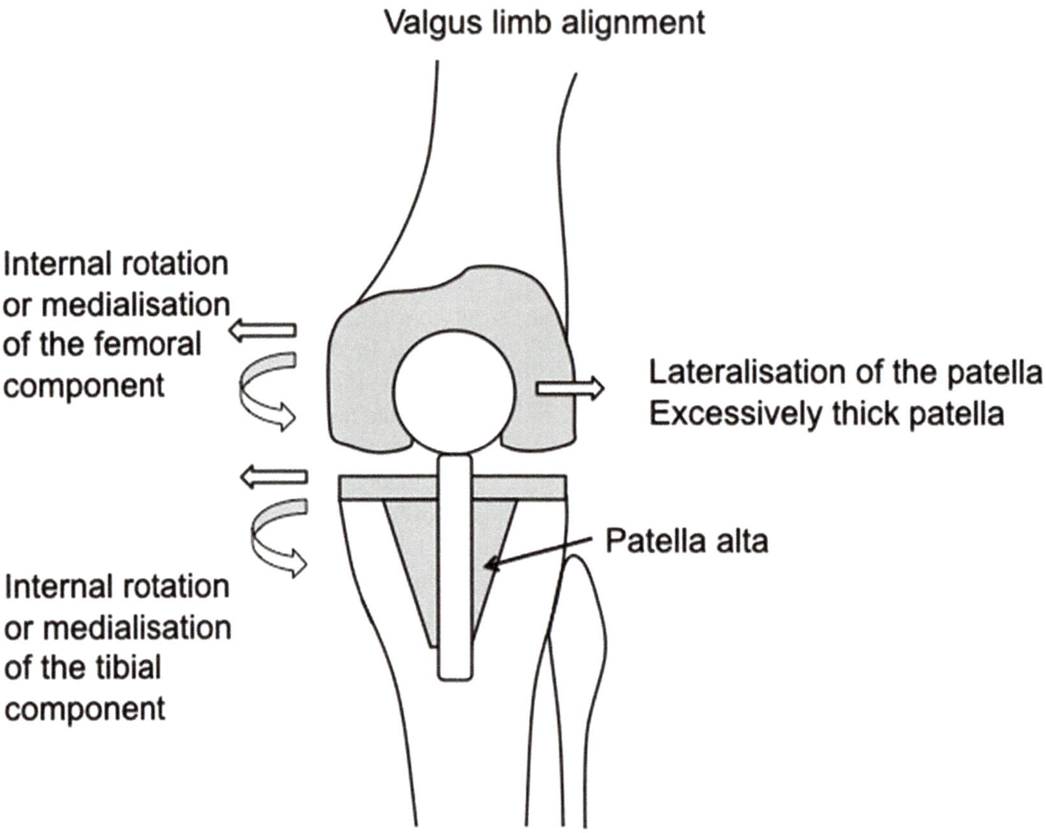

Fig. 14.39 Causes of patellar maltracking in knee replacements

extension with 'no-thumb' technique: it should not be necessary to apply external pressure on the patella to maintain the patella in the trochlear groove.

If the patellar tracking is not satisfactory, alignment and rotation of the femoral and tibial components should be checked. A tight lateral retinaculum can be released, but the release will not compensate for a malaligned femoral or tibial component.

Persistent patellofemoral instability will cause anterior knee pain or a feeling of 'giving way'. Evaluation is with plain X-rays including a sunrise (skyline) view and CT scan. CT scanning is accurate in assessing femoral or tibial component malrotation.

Treatment is based on underlying cause of instability. Options are vastus medialis obliquus exercises, lateral release with vastus medialis obliquus advancement, tibial tubercle transfer or revision of components. The underlying cause has to be addressed.

Venous Thromboembolism

The current NICE guidelines recommend chemical thromboprophylaxis for 2 weeks following knee replacement surgery in addition to mechanical prophylaxis.

Bjornara BT, Gudmundsen TE, Dahl OE. Frequency and timing of clinical thromboembolism after major joint surgery. J Bone Joint Surg Br. 2006;88(3):386–91. 13 year period, 5607 patients, Hip and knee replacement, LMWH was given as prophylaxis. 2.7% had symptomatic venous thromboembolism, 1.1% had pulmonary embolism. 1.5% had DVT. Risk for thromboembolism lasted for 3 months after hip surgery and for 1 month after knee surgery.

Periprosthetic Fracture

Distal femoral supracondylar fractures related to knee replacements are predisposed by osteoporosis, rheumatoid disease, steroid use, a stiff knee preoperatively and anterior femoral notching.

Biomechanical studies on notching of the anterior femoral cortex have shown a 40% reduction in torsional strength of the bone. However, in a clinical study of over 1000 patients, there was no association of notching and supracondylar femoral fracture.

There are many classification systems. One such system is shown in Fig. 14.40.

Nonoperative (cast bracing or cast) can be considered for minimally displaced fractures with a stable prosthesis in good alignment.

Surgical stabilisation options are lateral locking plate, intramedullary nail or distal femoral replacement.

The nail is not suitable for cruciate-substituting femoral components that have a box to house the cam and post mechanism. Some 'open box' designs may be amenable to nailing.

External fixation carries risks of pin site infection. Antegrade nailing may be an option for more proximal fractures.

Revision knee arthroplasty or distal femoral replacement is an increasingly popular treatment for

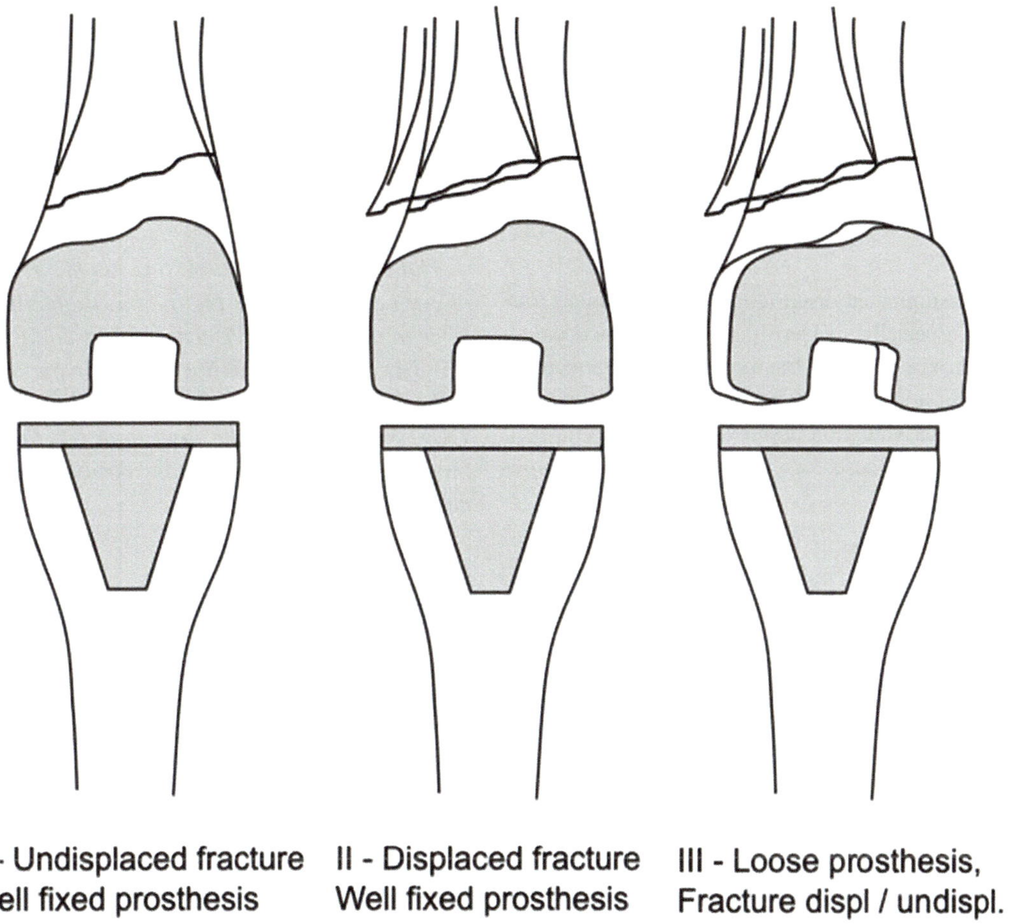

Fig. 14.40 Rorabeck and Taylor classification for distal femoral periprosthetic fractures (displ: displaced; undispl: undisplaced)

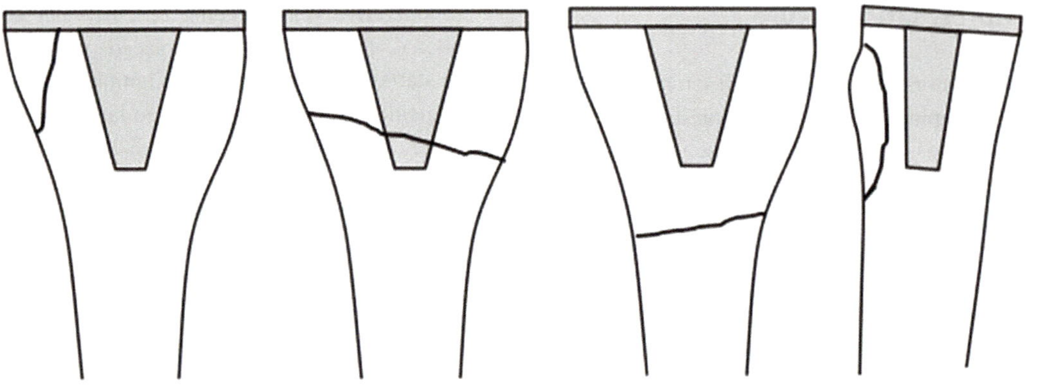

Fig. 14.41 Proximal tibial fractures after knee replacement

Table 14.28 Sub-classification of proximal tibial fractures

Subtype	Description
A	With stable components
B	With loose tibial component
C	Intraoperative fractures

the comminuted distal femoral periprosthetic fracture, especially in elderly patients with osteopenia.

Proximal tibial fractures generally occur in association with stemmed tibial components. Their classification is shown in Fig. 14.41.

Each of these four types have three subtypes (Table 14.28).

Vascular Injury

Intraoperative major vascular injury necessitates immediate vascular repair. In an extremity with a compromised vascular supply or previous bypass graft, the use of a tourniquet should be avoided.

Nerve Injury

Correction of severe valgus can cause a stretch injury to the peroneal nerve. If detected postoperatively, any compressive bandages should be removed and the knee flexed to relax the nerve. Generally, recovery is good.

Stiffness

Open arthrolysis may improve stiffness following TKR. Revision surgery is indicated for persistent stiffness, especially to improve fixed flexion deformity.

Hutchinson JR, Parish EN, Cross MJ. Results of open arthrolysis for the treatment of stiffness after total knee replacement. J Bone Joint Surg Br 2005;87(10):1357–60. 13 patients, open arthrolysis done for stiffness following TKR. Mean ROM improved from 55 to 91°. Mean time between TKR and arthrolysis was 14 months.

Instability After Total Knee Replacement

Instability can be patellofemoral or tibiofemoral. Tibiofemoral instability is described in the next section

Loosening and Wear

Loosening and wear are long-term problems. Loosening is more common in constrained prostheses due to a higher load transfer to the cement–bone interface.

Instability After Total Knee Replacement

Patellofemoral instability is described previously—see Fig. 14.39.

Tibiofemoral instability can be flexion instability, varus-valgus instability or global instability.

Flexion Instability

Sacrifice of the ACL leads to some degree of anterior instability in all prosthetic knees. This is compensated partly by the dished shape of the insert and a high posterior lip. Posterior instability is due to a poorly functioning PCL in posterior cruciate-retaining implants.

Clinical symptoms include anterior knee pain, 'giving way' and effusion. Patients experience difficulty in climbing stairs or standing up from a sitting position. On examination, the posterior drawer and quadriceps active tests are positive.

Flexion instability can be caused by a loose flexion gap at the time of surgery, damage to PCL at time of surgery or late attrition rupture of the PCL.

Symptomatic posterior instability in cruciate-retaining knees can be managed by revising to a thicker insert, or revision of the femoral component to cruciate substituting and using a posterior stabilised insert.

In posterior stabilised knees (cruciate substituting), excess flexion laxity can cause 'cam jump'. This is dislocation of the cam anterior to the post of the polyethylene insert. Reduction and bracing is the initial treatment for cam dislocation. Recurrent cam dislocation requires revision surgery.

Varus Valgus Instability

Varus valgus instability is due to incompetence of the medial or lateral collateral ligament. Patients present with pain, effusion and 'giving way'. Clinically, collateral laxity is evident and stress radiographs are helpful.

Treatment is by revising to a more constrained implant or to a hinged knee. In primary knees, ligament repair or advancement may be an option. Hinged knees have limited long-term survival and hence a semiconstrained option is preferable, if possible.

Global Instability

Global instability is a combination of varus valgus and AP instability. It is usually seen in patients with marked polyethylene wear, component migration, poor quadriceps function, rheumatoid arthritis or collagen vascular disease. It requires revision to a hinged knee implant.

Long Term Results of Total Knee Replacement

Knee replacement has demonstrated excellent long term survival.

Rodricks DJ, Patil S, Pulido P, Colwell CW Jr. Press fit condylar design total knee arthroplasty. 14–17 year follow up. J Bone Joint Surg Am 2007;89(1):89–95. 160 knees, 15.8 year follow up, mean age 70.5 years. Survival rate with revision as end point was 97.2%. Radiolucent lines did not correlate with loosening.

Ritter MA. The anatomic graduated component total knee replacement. A long term evaluation with 20 year survival analysis. J Bone Joint Surg Br 2009;91:745–9. Nonmodular metal backed tibia with compression molded poly, 97.8% 20 year survival.

Unicompartmental Knee Replacement

Unicompartmental knee replacement (UKR) is an alternative to TKR when the arthritis primarily involves either the medial or the lateral tibiofemoral compartment. It is usually performed on the medial side due to the more common pattern of medial arthritis and with more predictable long-term results.

Unicompartmental knee replacement has several advantages over total knee replacement:

- Preserved cruciate ligaments give relatively normal kinematics.
- UKR can be performed through a limited incision and gives faster recovery and shorter hospital stay.
- A better flexion range is achievable.

There are some prerequisites for medial UKR (as applied to mobile bearing Oxford UKR):

- Correctable varus.
- Flexion to 110° or more.
- Fixed flexion deformity of less than 15°.
- Intact ACL.
- Intact lateral compartment.
- Noninflammatory arthritis.

On radiography, the standing AP view will show the loss of medial joint space and a varus alignment of the knee. Stress radiographs will show the varus is correctable. On the lateral radiograph, the erosion on the medial tibial plateau should be predominantly anterior, implying an intact ACL. Invisibility of the lip of the posterior articular surface indicates a dysfunctional ACL.

An intact ACL is a requirement for mobile bearing medial unicompartmental replacements. A fixed bearing unicompartmental replacement may be considered in the ACL deficient knee, but the adverse effect of an absent ACL is not fully understood.

Wear of the polyethylene in mobile bearing unicompartmental replacements has been reported to be very low.

Kendrick BJ et al. Polyethylene wear of mobile bearing unicompartmental knee replacement at 20 years. J Bone Joint Surg Br 2011;93(4):470–5. RSA (radiostereometric analysis) of 13 knees at 20 years. Annual wear rate 0.022 mm/year in phase 2 implants. .

Results

Pandit H, Jenkins C, Barker K, Murray DW. The Oxford medial unicompartmental knee replacement using a minimally invasive approach. J Bone Joint Surg Br 2006;88(1):54–60. 688 Phase III medial uni knees. 100% follow up. 9 out of 688 were revised. 1% required another procedure—MUA/arthroscopy/debridement. Survival at 7 years 97.3%. Mean flexion 133°.

Ackroyd, Newman et al. Survivorship of the St Georg Sled medial unicompartmental knee replacement beyond 10 years. J Bone Joint Surg Br 2006;88(9):1164–8. 203 implants, mean 14.8 years after surgery. 7.9% had been revised at 13 years. Survivorship to 20 years was 85.9% and at 25 years was 80%.

Price AJ, Dodd CA, Svard UG, Murray DW. Oxford medial unicompartmental knee arthroplasty in patients younger than 60 years of age. J Bone Joint Surg Br 2005;87(1):1488–92. 10 year survival 91% in patients under 60 years.

Pandit H et al. Minimally invasive Oxford phase 3 unicompartmental knee replacement: results of 1000 cases. J Bone Joint Surg Br 2011;93(2):198–204. 1000 patients, mean follow up 5.6 years. 10 year survival 96% for implant related reoperations. Progression of arthritis in lateral compartment 0.9%, bearing dislocation 0.6% and revision for unexplained pain 0.6%.

Combined ACL Reconstruction and Unicompartmental Knee Replacement

In patients with an ACL-deficient knee and medial compartmental arthritis, a combination of ACL reconstruction and UKR is an option.

Pandit H, Beard DJ, Jenkins C, Murray DW. Combined Anterior Cruciate Reconstruction and Oxford unicompartmental knee arthroplasty. J Bone Joint Surg 2006;88(7):887–92. 15 patients with combined unicompartmental knee replacement and ACL reconstruction were matched with 15 patients with Unicompartmental replacement and intact ACL. 2.5 year follow up. No difference in Oxford score or functional knee score between the two groups.

Survival of Unicompartmental Replacements

Conversion of UKR to TKR should be considered in patients with ongoing pain in the medial compartment or progression of arthritis in the remaining compartments in the knee.

Data from the New Zealand Joint Registry have shown that TKR after UKR has a four times higher revision rate compared to primary TKR.

Pearse AJ, Hooper GJ, Rothwell A, Frampton C. survival and functional outcome after revision of a Unicompartmental to a total knee replacement. J Bone Joint Surg Br 2010;92:508–512. 4284 Uni, 236 revised. 205 had total knee and 31 had a further uni. The total knee replacement patients after uni had a revision rate of 1.97 per 100 component years. The Uni to Uni revisions had the worst results with 6.67 revision per 100 component years, and this was 13 times the revision rate for primary total knee replacement.

Patellofemoral Replacement

TKR is an effective treatment for patellofemoral arthritis with satisfactory results in up to 90% patients. However, it is a more extensive operation for patients with isolated patellofemoral joint arthritis compared to patellofemoral joint replacement (PFJR). The PFJR allows maintenance of normal tibiofemoral kinematics.

Patellofemoral joint reaction force is 3.3 times body weight at 60° flexion and 7.8 times body weight at 130° flexion.

Replacement of the patellofemoral joint is more commonly indicated in women, and this may be related to higher incidence of patellar maltracking problems. Subtle maltracking may lead to patellofemoral arthritis, even though overt patellar instability may not have manifested.

Table 14.29 Indications and contraindications for patellofemoral joint replacement

Indications	Contraindications
Selected patients with arthritis localised to the patellofemoral compartment Treatment of trochlear dysplasia	Tibiofemoral arthritis Inflammatory arthritis Significant maltracking of the patella or an excess Q angle (relative contraindication) Patellar instability FFD > 10°

Replacement of the patellofemoral joint comprises an 'all poly' patellar button and a cobalt chrome trochlear component. The indications and contraindications are listed in Table 14.29.

For patellofemoral replacement, pain should be localised to the anterior compartment.

A high Q angle should be addressed through a realignment procedure prior to arthroplasty.

ACL deficiency is not a contraindication.

AP, lateral and skyline radiographs are obtained. The skyline view is more useful for diagnosing patellofemoral arthritis and to assess the position of the patella in the trochlea. MR scans are helpful to document the condition of the patellofemoral articulation and the loss of cartilage.

The following factors should be considered when choosing a patellofemoral implant:

- Sagittal radius of the curvature.
- Proximal extent of the trochlear flange.
- Medio-lateral width of the implant.
- Degree of constraint.

Results

First generation patellofemoral replacements implants were highly conforming and had narrow, deep trochlear components. Modern, second generation implants have overcome these design problems and patellar tracking is more predictable and reproducible.

The early results following patellofemoral replacement in carefully selected patients are encouraging. Long term problems relate to loosening, and progression of arthritis in the remaining knee, requiring conversion to total knee replacement.

Ackroyd CE, Chir B. Development and early results of a new patellofemoral arthroplasty. Clin Orthop 2005;436:7–13. 306 arthroplasties in 240 patients, 2 year follow up for 124 and 5 year follow up for 33 knees. No deterioration in pain or function. Disease progression in tibiofemoral joint in 5% requiring revision in 3.6%. Persistent anterior pain in 4%.

Ackroyd CE, Newman JH, Evans R. The Avon patellofemoral arthroplasty. Five year survivorship and functional results. J Bone Joint Surg Br 2007;89:310–5. 109 knees in 85 patients. No loosening. 95.8% survival with revision as the end point. 80% success rate at 5 years based on pain score. 28% had radiological progression of arthritis.

Complications of PFJR include patellar maltracking, instability, loosening and need for conversion to total knee replacement in the event of progression of arthritis.

Results of total knee replacement after patellofemoral replacement are comparable to results of primary total knee replacement.

Lonner JH, Jasko JG, Booth RE Jr. Revision of a failed patellofemoral arthroplasty to a total knee arthroplasty. J Bone Joint Surg Am 2006;88(11):2337–42. Results of total knee replacement are not compromised after a failed patellofemoral replacement.

Bilateral Knee Replacement

Bilateral knee replacement is advocated if there is advanced arthritis in both knees. More importantly, a significant bilateral flexion deformity should be addressed by a bilateral simultaneous knee replacement to prevent recurrence of deformity after unilateral knee replacement. The safe time is considered to be either within the same anaesthetic, or after a gap of 4–6 weeks even though there is evidence to the contrary.

Forster MC, Bauze AJ, Bailie AG, et al. A retrospective comparative study of bilateral total knee replacement staged at a 1-week interval. J Bone Joint Surg Br 2006;88: 1006–10. Three groups—bilateral knee replacement under same anaesthetic, bilateral knee at 1 week interval in same admission, bilateral knee under separate admission. No difference in the three groups.

Computer-Aided Knee Replacement

The use of computer-aided surgery is becoming increasingly common in knee replacements to achieve better alignment compared with conventional jigs. Malalignment is a known factor leading to early failure of knee replacement.

Bathis H, Perlick L, Tingart M. Alignment in total knee arthroplasty. A comparison of computer assisted surgery with the conventional technique. J Bone Joint Surg Br 2004;86(5):682–7. Prospective study. 80 patients, mechanical axis was better in computer assisted group (96% versus 78% within 3° varus/valgus).

In presence of significant femoral bowing, conventional instruments can introduce malalignment of the mechanical axis. Computer navigation aligns the femoral component in relation to the position of the femoral head, and is unaffected by femoral bowing.

Gender Specific Knee Replacement

Gender specific total knee replacements have a narrower femoral component for female patients. Clinical difference in outcome is debatable.

Kim YH, Choi Y, Kim JS. Comparison of standard and gender specific posterior cruciate retaining high flexion total knee replacements: a prospective randomized study. J Bone Joint Surg Br 2010;92(5):639–45. 138 female patients had a standard knee on one side and a gender specific knee on the other side. Mean follow up 3 years. No difference in clinical outcome.

High Flex Knees

Patients with a high degree of flexion prior to knee replacement are likely to achieve high flexion following knee replacements. This is depen-

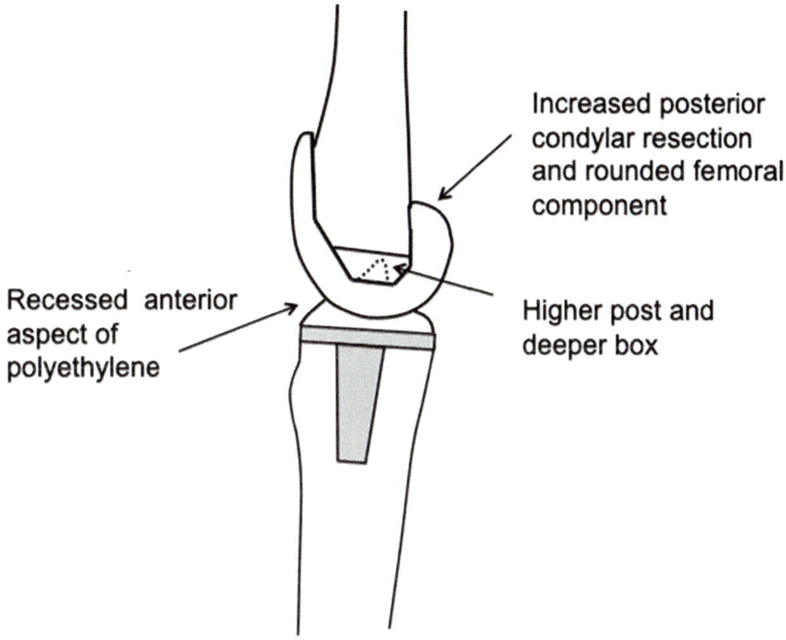

Fig. 14.42 Features of high flex knee design

dent on the ability of the prosthetic knee to allow safe high flexion. In standard posterior stabilised knees, the post on the polyethylene may dislocate from the box in the femoral component—which is known as 'cam jump'. High flex knee prostheses have certain design features, which allow deep flexion safely (Fig. 14.42).

(a) The post on the polyethylene is higher and the box cut in the femoral component is deeper, reducing the risk of cam jump.
(b) The posterior condylar resection on the femur is greater and the femoral component is thicker and more rounded at the posterior flange, which prevent the sharp edge of the tip of posterior femoral flange contacting the polyethylene. The polyethylene contacts a rounded flange on the femur posteriorly in high flexion.
(c) The anterior aspect of the polyethylene is recessed in the midline, avoiding impingement of the patellar tendon against the polyethylene in high flexion.

Revision Knee Arthroplasty

Indications for revision total knee arthroplasty are aseptic loosening, infection, instability, stiffness or periprosthetic fractures.

Malaligned femoral or tibial components can lead to accelerated wear, patellar instability, tibiofemoral instability or restricted ROM.

A painful knee replacement may be due to loosening, infection or instability.

The success rate of revision surgery is 25% if the cause of the pain is not evident preoperatively. Every effort must be made to determine the cause of failure of existing prosthesis and have a clear plan on the objective of revision surgery.

Preoperative Assessment

The history and examination focuses on identifying the specific problem. The hip and spine are potential sites of referred pain. Assessment should consider medical co-morbidities, functional status, skin condition, extensor mechanism, ROM, instability, alignment and neurologic and vascular status.

Radiographs can help to determine the underlying problem. Full-length leg films are useful to check the limb alignment. The extent of bone loss is frequently underestimated on plain radiographs; oblique views help in visualising the bone loss in relation to the femoral condyles. Rotational malalignment and osteolysis is demonstrated well on CT scanning. Gallium and Tc-99 bone scans are sometimes used to detect septic or aseptic loosening.

Laboratory tests are primarily aimed at detecting infection and include CRP and ESR.

Knee aspiration should be under strict asepsis and is useful for preoperative determination of any infecting organism. Synovial biopsy has a higher predictive value than aspiration. Antibiotics therapy reduces the positivity of culture results, and if possible, antibiotics should be stopped 2 weeks prior to aspiration/biopsy.

A good preoperative workup to assess the problems in a problem knee was suggested by Vince (Table 14.30).

If the above conditions are met, revision surgery is unlikely to help. On the same basis, these are the parameters that should be assessed before embarking on revision knee replacement.

Vince KG. The problem total knee replacement. Bone Joint J 2014;96(11) Suppl A;105–11.

Table 14.30 Requirement for functional knee replacement

No Infection
Intact extensor mechanism
Reasonable range of flexion and extension
Stability
Centrally located patella
Sound fixation
No fracture
Components intact

Reconstruction Sequence in Revision Knee Surgery

A useful strategy in reconstruction is to follow a stepwise approach:

1. Restore the tibial articular surface.
2. Restore the flexion gap. Correct sizing of the femoral implant, adjusting the rotation of the femoral component and soft tissue releases are performed at this stage.
3. Match the extension gap to the flexion gap. This may require distal translation of the femoral component and the use of augments and stems to support the femoral component.

Bone Defects in Revision Total Knee Arthroplasty

The final and most accurate assessment of bone loss can be made once the existing components have been removed. Table 14.31 and Fig. 14.43 outline the Anderson Orthopaedic Research Institute classification of bone loss.

Table 14.31 The Anderson Orthopaedic Research Institute classification of bone loss

Defect	Description
Type 1 (F1 and T1)	Healthy cancellous bone present to support the components Preserved metaphyseal bone distal to the femoral epicondyles (F1) and proximal to the fibular head (T1) Preserved level of joint line No osteolysis or component migration
Type 2 (F2 and T2)	Subsidence and migration of component Osteolysis at margins of component If only one femoral condyle or one side of the tibial plateau is involved, the defect is classified as F2A or T2A When both femoral condyles or both sides of the tibial plateau are involved, the defect is classified F2B or T2B
Type 3 (F3 and T3)	Large areas of osteolysis and gross migration of components Femoral epicondyles flare away from the femur Bone loss extends proximally to the femoral epicondyles or distally to the fibular head

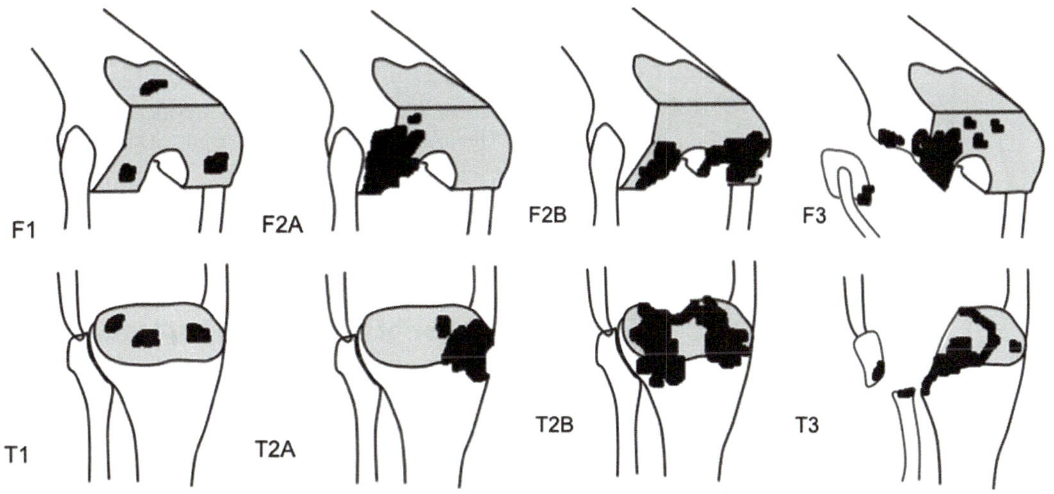

Fig. 14.43 Diagrammatic representation of the AORI classification

Management of Bone Defects

Contained defects (<15–20% of the cut surface of the distal femur or proximal tibia) can be managed with an autogenous bone graft from the resected tibial plateau. Cement can be used to fill small, contained defects.

Uncontained defects of the tibia that are less than 3 mm can be managed with an undercut and use of a thicker polyethylene. For those greater than 3 mm, metal augmentation blocks or wedges may be used.

The development of metaphyseal sleeves (Fig. 14.44) has improved the management of bone defects.

Agarwal S, Neogi DS, Morgan-Jones R. Metaphyseal sleeves in revision total knee arthroplasty: Minimum 7-year follow-up study. The Knee 2018;25:1299–307. 104 knee revisions, mean follow up 95 months, 6.7% revision for aseptic loosening.

Uncontained defects of the femur require augmentation or cemented revision implants. Increasing distal resection of the normal femoral condyle will result in an elevated joint line.

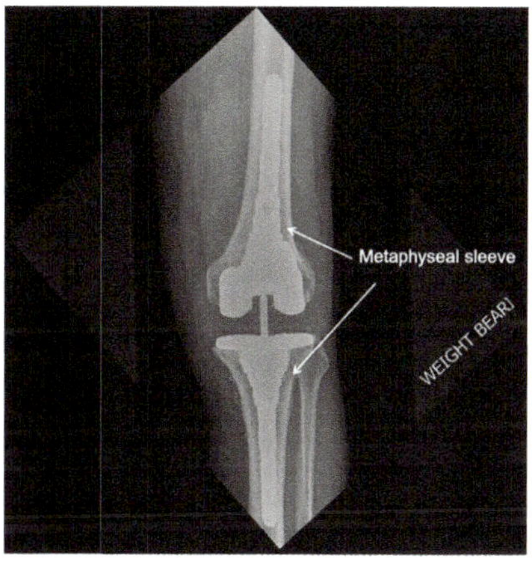

Fig. 14.44 Metaphyseal sleeves in revision knee replacement. The use of metaphyseal tibial sleeves to restore the level of the tibial tray in a patient with circumferential proximal tibial bone loss from previous revision knee arthroplasty. The sleeve fits over the stem and is coated with hydroxyapatite ceramic. Note the level of the proximal tibial bone in relation to the head of the fibula

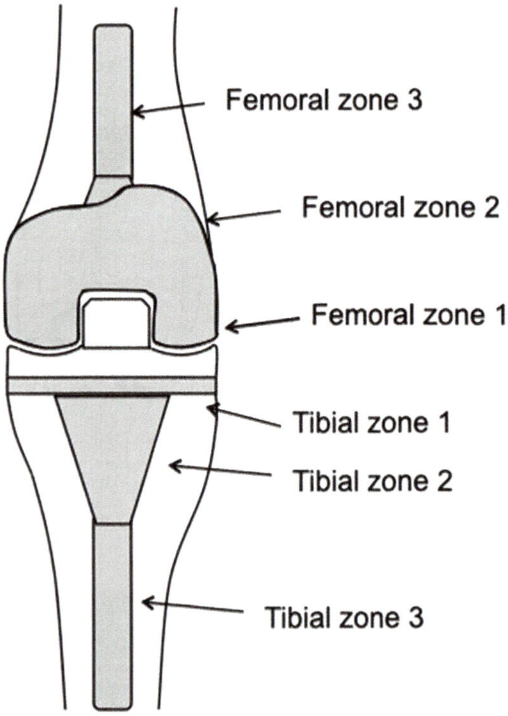

Fig. 14.45 The concept of zonal fixation in revision knee replacement

Stemmed Implants

Both cemented and cementless stems are used. The stems achieve fixation in the metaphysis and diaphysis in situations where adequate support for the implant is lacking at the cancellous surface.

Very wide canals are better managed by cemented stems to avoid inserting a large-diameter cementless stem. Metaphyseal fixation is also easier with cemented stems. Larger defects require longer stems and if fixation in the diaphysis is considered, cementless stems may be advantageous.

The zonal concept designates fixation on the cancellous surface as zone 1, metaphyseal fixation as zone 2 and diaphyseal fixation as zone 3 (Fig. 14.45). In revision situation, where zone 1 is compromised, fixation is achieved in zone 2, and where zone 2 is compromised as well, fixation is achieved in zone 3.

Table 14.32 The hierarchy of knee replacement implants

All 4 ligaments functioning	Unicompartmental replacement, patellofemoral replacement
Absent ACL	Cruciate preserving knee
Absent ACL and PCL	Posterior stabilised knee
Absent ACL, PCL, LCL	Varus valgus constrained knee
Absent MCL	Hinged knee

The Use of Constrained Implants

Constrained implants are available to compensate for ligamentous laxity. Constraint and augmentation are considered as two separate issues. A patient with incompetent MCL will require a hinged implant regardless of any bone loss. A patient with extensive bone loss (F2B or T2B) may require stemmed and sleeved components, but only a posterior stabilised insert if the collaterals are functioning. Less constraint is preferable to more constraint wherever possible.

The hierarchy of knee replacement prosthesis is shown in Table 14.32.

Further Reading

Ackroyd CE, Chir B. Development and early results of a new patellofemoral arthroplasty. Clin Orthop. 2005;436:7–13.

Ackroyd CE, Newman JH, Evans R. The Avon patellofemoral arthroplasty. Five year survivorship and functional results. J Bone Joint Surg Br. 2007;89:310–5.

Agarwal S, Neogi DS, Morgan-Jones R. Metaphyseal sleeves in revision total knee arthroplasty: Minimum seven-year follow-up study. Knee. 2018;25:1299–307.

Bae DK, Yoon KH, Kim HS, Song SJ. Total knee arthroplasty in stiff knees after previous infection. J Bone Joint Surg Br. 2005;87(3):333–6.

Bal BS, Haltom D, Aleto T, Barrett M. Early complications of primary total hip replacement performed with a two incision minimally invasive technique. Surgical technique. J Bone Joint Surg Am. 2006;88(Suppl 1):221–33.

Barrack RL, Mulroy RD, Harris WH. Improved cementing techniques and femoral component loosening in young patients with hip arthroplasty. A 12 year radiographic review. J Bone Joint Surg Br. 1992;74(3):385–9.

Bassett RW. Results of 1000 Performance knees: cementless versus cemented fixation. J Arthroplasty. 1998;13(4):409–13.

Bathis H, Perlick L, Tingart M. Alignment in total knee arthroplasty. A comparison of computer assisted surgery with the conventional technique. J Bone Joint Surg Br. 2004;86(5):682–7.

Berend ME, Ritter MA, Meding JB, et al. Tibial component failure mechanism in total knee arthroplasty. Clin Orthop. 2004;428:26–34.

Berger RA. Total hip arthroplasty using the minimally invasive two incision approach. Clin Orthop. 2003;417:232–41.

Berry DJ, von Knoch M, Schleck CD, Harmsen WS. The cumulative long term risk of dislocation after primary Charnley total hip arthroplasty. J Bone Joint Surg Am. 2004;86(1):9–14.

Berry DJ, von Knoch M, Schleck CD, Harmsen WS. Effect of femoral head diameter and operative approach on risk of dislocation after primary total hip arthroplasty. J Bone Joint Surg Am. 2005;87(11):2456–63.

Bert JM, McShane M. Is it necessary to cement the tibial stem in cemented total knee arthroplasty? Clin Orthop. 1998;356:73–8.

Bjornara BT, Gudmundsen TE, Dahl OE. Frequency and timing of clinical thromboembolism after major joint surgery. J Bone Joint Surg Br. 2006;88(3):386–91.

Blom AW, Brown J, Taylor AH, et al. Infection after total knee arthroplasty. J Bone Joint Surg Br. 2004;86(5):688–91.

Blom AW, Astle L, Loveridge J, Learmonth ID. Revision of an acetabular liner has a high risk of dislocation. J Bone Joint Surg Br. 2005;87(12):1636–8.

Blomfeldt R, Törnkvist H, Ponzer S, Söderqvist A, Tidermark J. Comparison of internal fixation with total hip replacement for displaced femoral neck fractures. Randomised, controlled trial performed at four years. J Bone Joint Surg Am. 2005;87(8):1680–8.

Burnett RS, Haydon CM, Rorabeck CH, Bourne RB. Patella resurfacing versus non resurfacing in total knee arthroplasty. Clin Orthop. 2004;428:12–25.

Callaghan JJ, Katz RP, Johnston RC. One stage revision surgery of the infected hip. A minimum 10 year follow up study. Clin Orthop. 1999;369:139–43.

Callaghan JJ, Templeton JE, Liu SS, Pedersen DR, Goetz DD, Sullivan PM, Johnston RC. Results of Charnley total hip arthroplasty at a minimum of thirty years. A concise follow-up of a previous report. J Bone Joint Surg Am. 2004;86(4):690–5.

Carrington NC, Sierra RJ, Gie GA, Hubble MJW, Timperley AJ, Howell JR. The Exeter universal cemented femoral component at 15 to 17 years. An update on the first 325 hips. J Bone Joint Surg Br. 2009;91:730–7.

Chambers IR, Fender D, McCaskie AW, Reeves BC, Gregg PJ. Radiological features predictive of aseptic loosening in cemented Charnley femoral stems. J Bone Joint Surg Br. 2001;83(6):838–42.

Chang CW, Lai KA, Yang CY, Lan SM. Early mechanical complications of a multidirectional mobile bearing total knee replacement. J Bone Joint Surg Br. 2011;93(4):479–83.

Chee YH, Teoh KH, Sabnis BM, Ballantyne JA, Brenkel IJ. Total hip replacement in morbidly obese patients with osteoarthritis: results of a prospectively matched study. J Bone Joint Surg Br. 2010;92(8):1066–71.

Chiu FY, Lin CF, Chen CM, Lo WH, Chaung TY. Cefuroxime-impregnated cement at primary total knee arthroplasty in diabetes mellitus: A prospective, randomised study. J Bone Joint Surg Br. 2001;83(5):691–5.

Daniel J, Ziaee H, Kamali A, Pradhan C, Band T, McMinn DJ. Ten year results of a double heat treated metal on metal hip resurfacing. J Bone Joint Surg Br. 2010;92(1):20–7.

Darrith B, Courtney PM, Della Valle CJ. Outcomes of dual mobility components in total hip arthroplasty: a systematic review of the literature. Bone Joint J. 2018;100(1):11–9.

De Haan R, Pattyn C, Gil HS. Correlation between inclination of the acetabular component and metal ion levels in metal on metal hip resurfacing replacement. J Bone Joint Surg Br. 2008;90:1291–7.

DeLee J, Charnley J. Radiological demarcation of cemented sockets in total hip replacement. Clin Orthop. 1976;121:20–32.

Della Valle CJ, Berger RA, Rosenberg AG, Galante JO. Cementless acetabular reconstruction in revision total hip arthroplasty. Clin Orthop. 2004;420:96–100.

De Smet K, Campbell PA, Gill HS. Metal on Metal resurfacing. A consensus from the advanced hip resurfacing course, Ghent, June 2009. J Bone Joint Surg Br. 2010;92:335–6.

DeSouza RM, Parsons NR, Oni T, Dalton P, Costa M, Krikler S. Metal ion levels following resurfacing arthroplasty of the hip. Serial results over a ten year period. J Bone Joint Surg Br. 2010;92(12):1642–7.

Dowsey M, Liew D, Stoney JD, Choong PF. The impact of preoperative obesity on weight change and outcome in total knee replacement. J Bone Joint Surg Br. 2010;92:513–20.

Duncan CP, Masri BA. Fractures of the femur after hip replacement. Inst Course Lect. 1995;44:293–304.

Ekelund J. Trochanteric osteotomy for recurrent dislocation of total hip arthroplasty. J Arthroplasty. 1993;8(6):629–32.

Fender D, Harper WM, Gregg PJ. Outcome of Charnley total hip replacement across a single health region in England: the results at five years from a regional hip register. J Bone Joint Surg Br. 1999;81(4):577–81.

Fender D, Harper WM, Gregg PJ. Outcome of Charnley THR across a single health region in England. J Bone Joint Surg Br. 2006;88(10):1293–8.

Forster MC, Bauze AJ, Bailie AG, et al. A retrospective comparative study of bilateral total knee replacement staged at a one-week interval. J Bone Joint Surg Br. 2006;88:1006–10.

Gill TJ, Sledge JB, Müller ME. The Burch-Schneider anti-protrusio cage in revision total hip arthroplasty: indications, principles and long term results. J Bone Joint Surg Br. 1998;80:946.

Glehr M, Friesenbichler J, Hofmann G, Bernhardt GA, Zacherl M, Avian A, Windhager R, Leithner A. Novel biomarkers to detect infection in revision hip and knee arthroplasties. Clin Orthop Relat Res. 2013;471(8):2621–8.

Glyn Jones S, Pandit H, Kwon YM. Risk factors for inflammatory pseudotumour formation following hip resurfacing. J Bone Joint Surg Br. 2009;91:1566–74.

Goddard NJ, Mann HA, Lee CA. Total knee replacement in patients with end stage hemophilic arthropathy—25 years results. J Bone Joint Surg Br. 2010;92(8):1085–9.

Goetz DD, Bremner BR, Callaghan JJ, Capello WN, Johnston RC. Salvage of a recurrently dislocation total hip prosthesis with use of a constrained acetabular component. J Bone Joint Surg Am. 2004;86(11):2419–23.

Greidanus NV, Masri BA, Garbuz DS, et al. Use of erythrocyte sedimentation rate and c reactive protein level to diagnose infection before revision total knee arthroplasty. J Bone Joint Surg Am. 2007;89:1409–16.

Gruen TA, McNeice GM, Amstutz HC. "Modes of failure" of cemented stem-type femoral components: a radiographic analysis of loosening. Clin Orthop Relat Res. 1979;141:17–27.

Gupta S, Augustine A, Horey L, Meek RM, Hullin MG, Mohammed A. Electrocautery of the patellar rim in primary total knee replacement: beneficial or unnecessary. J Bone Joint Surg Br. 2010;92(9):1259–61.

Haleem AA, Berry DJ, Hanssen AD. Mid to long term follow up of two stage reimplantation for infected total knee arthroplasty. Clin Orthop. 2004;428:35–9.

Hart WJ, Jones RS. Two stage revision of infected total knee replacements using articulating cement spacers and short term antibiotic therapy. J Bone Joint Surg Br. 2006;88(8):1011–5.

Hart AJ, Sabah S, Henckel J, Lewis A, Cobb J, Sampson B, Mitchell A, Skinner JA. The painful metal on metal hip resurfacing. J Bone Joint Surg Br. 2009;91:738–44.

Herrera A, Martínez AA, Cuenca J, Canales V. Management of type III and IV acetabular deficiencies with the longitudinal oblong revision cup. J Arthroplasty. 2006;21:857–64.

Hommel H, Perka C, Kopf S. The fate of Baker's cyst after total knee arthroplasty. Bone Joint J. 2016;98:1185–8.

Howell SM, Shelton TJ, Hull ML. Implant survival and function ten years after kinematically aligned total knee arthroplasty. J Arthroplasty. 2018;33:3678–84.

Hsieh PH, Shih CH, Chang YH. Treatment of deep infection of the hip associated with massive bone loss: two stage revision with an antibiotic-loaded interim cement prosthesis followed by reconstruction with allograft. J Bone Joint Surg Br. 2005;87(6):770–5.

Hutchinson JR, Parish EN, Cross MJ. Results of open arthrolysis for the treatment of stiffness after total knee replacement. J Bone Joint Surg Br. 2005;87(10):1357–60.

Kellgren JH, Lawrence JS. Radiological assessment of osteoarthrosis. Ann Rheum Dis. 1957;16:494–502.

Kendrick BJ, et al. Polyethylene wear of mobile bearing unicompartmental knee replacement at 20 years. J Bone Joint Surg Br. 2011;93(4):470–5.

Kiernan S, Hermann KL, Wagner P, Ryd L, Flivik G. The importance of adequate stem anteversion for rotational stability in cemented total hip replacement. Bone Joint J. 2013;95(1):23–30.

Kim YH, Choi Y, Kim JS. Comparison of standard and gender specific posterior cruciate retaining high flexion total knee replacements: a prospective randomized study. J Bone Joint Surg Br. 2010;92(5):639–45.

Kim YH, Kim JS, Park JW, Joo JH. Comparison of total hip replacement with and without cement in patients younger than 50 years of age: the results at 18 years. J Bone Joint Surg Br. 2011;93(4):449–55.

Kunutsor SK, Whitehouse MR, Blom AW, Beswick AD; INFORM Team. Re-infection outcomes following one- and two-stage surgical revision of infected hip prosthesis: a systematic review and meta-analysis. PLoS One. 2015;10(9):e0139166.

Kunutsor SK, et al. One- and two-stage surgical revision of peri-prosthetic joint infection of the hip: a pooled individual participant data analysis of 44 cohort studies. Eur J Epidemiol. 2018;33(10):933–46.

Kuzyk PRT, Saccone M, Sprague S, Simunovic N, Bhandari M, Schemitsch EH. Cross linked versus conventional polyethylene for total hip replacement: a meta-analysis of randomized controlled trials. J Bone Joint Surg Br. 2011;93(5):593–600.

Kyriacou S, Pastides PS, Singh VK, Jeyaseelan L, Sinisi M, Fox M. Exploration and neurolysis for the treatment of neuropathic pain in patients with a sciatic nerve palsy after total hip replacement. Bone Joint J. 2013;95:20–2.

Lee BP, Berry DJ, Harmsen WS, Sim FH. Total hip arthroplasty for the treatment of an acute fracture of the femoral neck. J Bone Joint Surg Am. 1998;80(1):70–5.

Lingaraj K, Teo YH, Bergman N. The management of severe acetabular bone defects in revision hip arthroplasty using modular porous metal components. J Bone Joint Surg Br. 2009;91:1555–60.

Lonner JH, Jasko JG, Booth RE Jr. Revision of a failed patellofemoral arthroplasty to a total knee arthroplasty. J Bone Joint Surg Am. 2006;88(11):2337–42.

Lubbeke A, Garavaglia G, Barea C, Stern R, Peter R, Hoffmeyer P. Influence of patient activity on femoral osteolysis at five and ten years following hybrid total hip replacement. J Bone Joint Surg Br. 2011;93(4):456–63.

Maloney W, Paprosky W, Engh CA, Rubash HE. Surgical treatment of pelvic osteolysis. Clin Orthop Rel Res. 2001;393:78–84.

Malviya A, Walker LC, Avery P, Osborne S, Weir DJ, Foster HE, Deehan DJ. The long term outcome of hip replacement in adults with juvenile idiopathic arthritis: the influence of steroids and methotrexate. J Bone Joint Surg Br. 2011;93(4):443–8.

Maniar RN, Navaneedhan G, Ranvir S, Maniar AR, Dhiman A, Agrawal A. What is the normal trajectory of interleukin-6 and C-reactive protein in the hours and days immediately after TKA? Clin Orthop Relat Res. 2019;477(1):41–6.

Masri BA, Meek RM, Duncan CP. Periprosthetic fractures: evaluation and treatment. Clin Orthop. 2004;420:80–95.
McCalden RW, Charron KD, MacDonald SJ, Bourne RB, Naudie DD. Does morbid obesity affect the outcome of total hip replacement. An analysis of 3290 THRs. J Bone Joint Surg Br. 2011;93(3):321–5.
Meek RM, Greidanus NV, McGraw RW, Masri BA. The extensile rectus snip exposure in revision of total knee arthroplasty. J Bone Joint Surg Br. 2003;85(8):1120–2.
Meermans G, Konan S, Das R, Volpin A, Haddad FS. The direct anterior approach in total hip arthroplasty. A systematic review of the literature. Bone Joint J. 2017;99:732–40.
Mont MA, Rifai A, Baumgarten KM, Sheldon M, Hungerford DS. Total knee arthroplasty for osteonecrosis. J Bone Joint Surg Am. 2002;84(4):599–603.
Namba RS, Inacio MC, Paxton EW, Ake CF, Wang C, Gross TP, Marinac-Dabic D, Sedrakyan A. Risk of revision for fixed versus mobile bearing primary total knee replacement. J Bone Joint Surg Am. 2012;94(21):1929–35.
Nicoll D, Rowley DI. Internal rotation error of the tibial component is a major cause of pain after total knee replacements. J Bone Joint Surg Br. 2010;92(9):1238–44.
Ogonda L, Wilson R, Archbold P, Lawlor M, Humphreys P, O'Brien S, Beverland D. A minimal incision technique in total hip arthroplasty does not improve early postoperative outcomes. A prospective, randomised, controlled trial. J Bone Joint Surg Am. 2005;87(4):701–10.
Palmer DH, Mulhall KJ, Thompson CA, Severson EP, Santos ERG, Saleh KJ. Total knee arthroplasty in juvenile rheumatoid arthritis. J Bone Joint Surg Am. 2005;87(7):1510–4.
Pandit H, Jenkins C, Barker K, Murray DW. The Oxford medial unicompartmental knee replacement using a minimally invasive approach. J Bone Joint Surg Br. 2006a;88(1):54–60.
Pandit H, Beard DJ, Jenkins C, Murray DW. Combined anterior cruciate reconstruction and Oxford unicompartmental knee arthroplasty. J Bone Joint Surg. 2006b;88(7):887–92.
Pandit H, et al. Minimally invasive Oxford phase 3 unicompartmental knee replacement: results of 1000 cases. J Bone Joint Surg Br. 2011;93(2):198–204.
Park JW, Kim YH. Simultaneous cemented and cementless total knee replacement in the same patient. J Bone Joint Surg Br. 2011;93(11):1479–86.
Partridge DG, Winnard C, Townsend R, Cooper R, Stockley I. Joint aspiration, including culture of reaspirated saline after a 'dry tap', is sensitive and specific for the diagnosis of hip and knee prosthetic joint infection. Bone Joint J. 2018;100(6):749–54.
Parvizi J, Morrey BF. Bipolar hip arthroplasty as a salvage treatment for instability of the hip. J Bone Joint Surg Am. 2000;82(8):1132–9.
Parvizi J, Hanssen AD, Spangehl MJ. Total knee arthroplasty following proximal tibial osteotomy: risk factors for failure. J Bone Joint Surg Am. 2004;86(3):474–9.
Pearse AJ, Hooper GJ, Rothwell A, Frampton C. survival and functional outcome after revision of a unicompartmental to a total knee replacement. J Bone Joint Surg Br. 2010;92:508–12.
Pellici PM, Bostrom M, Poss R. Posterior approach to total hip replacement using enhanced posterior soft tissue repair. Clin Orthop. 1998;355:224–8.
Philips JE, Crane TP, Noy M. The incidence of deep prosthetic infections in a specialist orthopaedic hospital. A 15 year prospective survey. J Bone Joint Surg Br. 2006;88(7):943–8.
Pilling RWD, Moulder E, Allgar V, Messner J, Sun Z, Mohsen A. Patellar resurfacing in primary total knee arthroplasty. A meta-analysis. J Bone Joint Surg Am. 2012;94(24):227–8.
Price AJ, Dodd CA, Svard UG, Murray DW. Oxford medial unicompartmental knee arthroplasty in patients younger than 60 years of age. J Bone Joint Surg Br. 2005;87(1):1488–92.
Putnis SE, Wartemberg GK, Khan WS, Agarwal S. A literature review of total hip arthroplasty in patients with ankylosing spondylitis: perioperative considerations and outcome. Open Orthop J. 2015;9:483–8.
Ritter MA. The anatomic graduated component total knee replacement. A long term evaluation with 20 year survival analysis. J Bone Joint Surg Br. 2009;91:745–9.
Rittmeister M, Starker M, Zichner L. Hip and knee replacement after longstanding hip arthrodesis. Clin Orthop. 2000;371:136–45.
Rodricks DJ, Patil S, Pulido P, Colwell CW Jr. Press fit condylar design total knee arthroplasty. 14 to 17 year follow up. J Bone Joint Surg Am. 2007;89(1):89–95.
Saleh KJ, Sherman P, Katkin P, Windsor R, Haas S, Laskin R, Sculco T. Total knee arthroplasty after open reduction and internal fixation of fractures of the tibial plateau: a minimum five-year follow-up study. J Bone Joint Surg Am. 2001;83(8):1144–8.
Schereurs BW, Keurentjes JC, Gardeniers JW, et al. Acetabular revision with impacted morsellised cancellous bone grafting and a cemented acetabular component: a 20- to 25-year follow-up. J Bone Joint Surg Br. 2009;91:1148–53.
Schmalzreid TP, Amstutz HC. Update on nerve palsy associated with total hip replacement. Clin Orthop Relat Res. 1997;344:188–206.
Schreurs BW, Bolder SB, Gardeniers JW. Acetabular revision with impacted morsellised cancellous bone grafting and a cemented cup. A 15-20 year follow up. J Bone Joint Surg Br. 2004;86(4):492–7.
Sexton SA, Yeung E, Jackson MP, Rajaratnam S, Martell JM, Walter WL, Zicat BA, Walter WK. The role of patient factors and implant position in squeaking of ceramic on ceramic total hip replacements. J Bone Joint Surg Br. 2011;93(4):439–42.
Shetty AA, Slack R, Tindall A, James KD, Rand C. Results of Hydroxyapatite coated (Furlong) total hip replace-

ment: a 13-15 year follow up. J Bone Joint Surg Br. 2005;87(8):1050–4.
Shimmin AJ, Back D. Femoral neck fractures following Birmingham hip resurfacing: a national review of 50 cases. J Bone Joint Surg Br. 2005;87(4):463–4.
Shimmin AJ, Walter WL, Esposito C. The influence of the size of the component on the outcome of resurfacing arthroplasty of the hip: a review of literature. J Bone Joint Surg Br. 2010;92(4):469–76.
Silva M, Luck JV Jr. Long-term results of primary total knee replacement in patients with hemophilia. J Bone Joint Surg Am. 2005;87:85–91.
Smith TO, Aboelmagd T, Hing CB, MacGregor A. Does bariatric surgery prior to total hip or knee arthroplasty reduce postoperative complications and improve clinical outcomes for obese patients. Bone Joint Surg. 2016;98:1160–7.
Sporer SM. The use of structural distal femoral allografts for acetabular reconstruction. J Bone Joint Surg Am. 2005;87:760–5.
Steele RG, Hutabarat S, Evans RL, Ackroyd CE, Newman JH. Survivorship of the St Georg Sled medial unicompartmental knee replacement beyond ten years. J Bone Joint Surg Br. 2006;88(9):1164–8.
Trikha SP, Singh S, Raynham OW, Lewis JC, Mitchell PA, Edge AJ. Hydroxyapatite ceramic coated femoral stems in revision hip surgery. J Bone Joint Surg Br. 2005;87(8):1055–60.
Vendittoli J, Lavigne M, Girard J, Roy AG. A randomised study comparing resection of acetabular bone at resurfacing and total hip replacement. J Bone Joint Surg Br. 2006;88(8):997–1002.
Verlinden C, Uvin P, Labey L, Luyckx JP, Bellemans J, Vandenneucker H. The influence of malrotation of the femoral component in total knee replacement on the mechanics of patellofemoral contact during gait: an in vitro biomechanical study. J Bone Joint Surg Br. 2010;92(5):737–42.
Vince KG. The problem total knee replacement. Bone Joint J 2014;96(11) Suppl A;105–11.
Wasielewski RC, Cooperstein LA, Kruger MP, Rubash HE. Acetabular anatomy and the transacetabular fixation of screws in total hip arthroplasty. J Bone Joint Surg Am. 1990;72(4):501–8.
Whiteside L, Arima J. The anteroposterior axis for femoral rotational alignment in valgus knee arthroplasty. Clin Orthop. 1995;321:168–72.
Workgroup Convened by the Musculoskeletal Infection Society. New definition for periprosthetic joint infection. J Arthroplasty. 2011;26:1136–8.
Wroblewski BM, Siney PD, Fleming PA. Charnley low-frictional torque arthroplasty in patients under the age of 51 years. Follow-up to 33 years. J Bone Joint Surg Br. 2002;84(4):540–3.
Wroblewski BM, Siney PD, Fleming PA. Wear of the cup in Charnley LFA in the young patient. J Bone Joint Surg Br. 2004;86(4):498–503.
Yi PH, Cross MB, Moric M, Sporer SM, Berger RA, Della Valle CJ. The 2013 Frank Stinchfield Award: diagnosis of infection in the early postoperative period after total hip arthroplasty. Clin Orthop Relat Res. 2014;472(2):424–9.

Nerve Injuries and Neuromuscular Disorders

15

Sanjeev Agarwal

Nerve Injury

The spinal nerves are formed by union of the dorsal (sensory) and ventral (motor) roots (Fig. 15.1). These nerves supply dermatomes and myotomes, respectively, as segmental nerves or through the formation of plexus—as in the limbs.

There are 31 spinal nerves: eight cervical, 12 thoracic, five lumbar, five sacral and one coccygeal. There are also 14 sympathetic nerves, which exit with the 12 thoracic and the first two lumbar nerves.

Individual axons are surrounded by endoneurium. Groups of axons are organized in fascicles which are bound by perineurium. The perineurium forms the blood-nerve barrier. Blood vessels run in between the fascicles and groups of fascicles are bound by the epineurium, which is the outer covering of the nerve (Fig. 15.2).

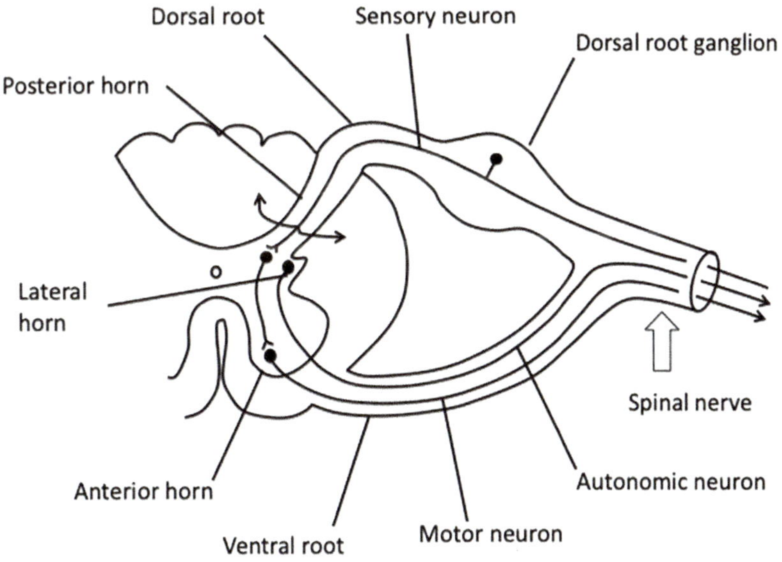

Fig. 15.1 Formation of the spinal nerve

S. Agarwal (✉)
University Hospital of Wales, Consultant Orthopaedic Surgeon, Cardiff, UK

S. Agarwal (ed.), *Current Orthopaedic Practice*, https://doi.org/10.1007/978-3-030-78529-1_15

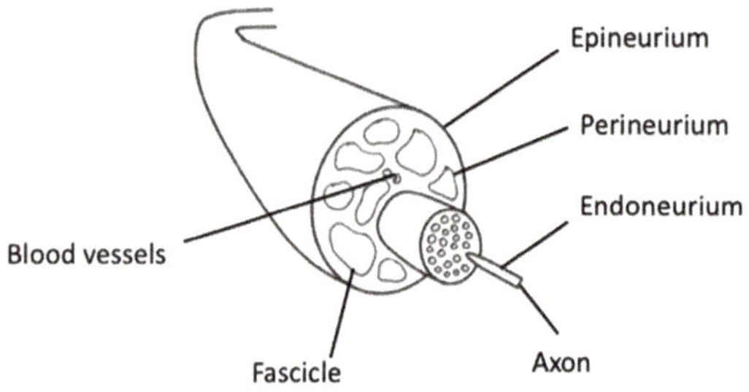

Fig. 15.2 Internal structure of a peripheral nerve

Nerve Degeneration and Regeneration

Injury to a nerve induces changes distal to the injury, proximal to the injury and in the cell body.

Injury to an axon results in Wallerian degeneration in the stump distal to the injury. This was first described by Waller in 1862. This starts within a few hours and can continue for 3 months.

The production of axoplasmic calcium is increased, and the axoplasm and cytoskeleton are broken down. The debris is cleared within 4 weeks. Schwann cells start dividing within 3 days and form cytoplasmic processes. The process is detailed in Fig. 15.3.

Proximal to the injury, retrograde or primary degeneration ensues. This extends only to the first node of Ranvier. This process is similar to Wallerian degeneration. It starts within 48 h and takes 3 weeks to complete.

The axonal cell body swells and undergoes chromatolysis. The nucleus migrates to the periphery of the cell.

Axonal growth starts within 24 hours of injury, and continues at a pace of 1–2 mm/day. Establishing a link with the regenerating axon distally leads to progression of healing and fibre maturation (Fig. 15.4). The presence of intact tubes (endoneurium) guides the axons along the tract. Neurites that fail to make a distal connection die off, or form neuromas.

Irreversible motor end plates degeneration occurs after 12–18 months. Hence re-innervation should be completed within this time frame. Sensory re-innervation can occur after a longer time frame.

Presence of neurilemma in peripheral nerve fibres is essential for regeneration. Central nerve system fibres lack neurilemma, and hence do not regenerate.

Classification of Nerve Injuries

Seddon proposed the first widely used classification of nerve injuries in 1943 (Table 15.1).

In 1951, Sunderland proposed a more detailed and useful classification, dividing the nerve injuries into five groups (Table 15.2).

Grade I nerve injury is equivalent to neurapraxia in the Seddon classification. The injury is a temporary focal conduction defect. The axon in intact, there is no Wallerian degeneration and recovery is complete within 12 weeks. The first modality to recover is sympathetic function, followed by pain and temperature. Proprioception and motor function are the first to be affected and the last to recover.

Tinel's sign (paraesthesia in distribution of nerve on percussion at site of injury) is present in all injuries where there is an anatomical damage (grades 2–5). Tinel's sign is progressive in grades 2 and 3, where there is some continuity of the nerve and spontaneous recovery, and not progressive in grade 4 and 5, unless nerve repair is undertaken.

In grade 2 nerve injury disruption of the axon leads to Wallerian degeneration, but the intact endoneurial tube helps in near-complete recovery. Neuron death in proximal injuries is the cause of some loss of function in this type. Tinel's sign is present and advances distally and the 'motor march' is evident. This means proximal muscles regain function earlier than distal muscles, as regeneration progresses distally in the nerve.

Disruption of the endoneurium in grade 3 injuries causes disorganisation of axonal growth and some loss of function is expected.

The epineurium is intact in grade 4 nerve injury. Tinel's sign is present at the site of injury, but does not progress unless the nerve is repaired successfully. Grade 5 injuries carry little hope of

Fig. 15.3 Sequence of changes following nerve injury

Nerve injury

↓

Wallerian degeneration - both the axon and myelin distal to the injury degenerate. Proximal segment degenerates back to the adjacent node of Ranvier

↓

Schwann cells phagocytose axonal and myelin debris, leaving empty endoneurial tubes

↓

Macrophages enter the area and lead to proliferation of Schwann cells

↓

Schwann cells fill empty endoneurial tubes in longitudinal columns called bands of Bungner

↓

Axon regenerates from the most distal node of Ranvier in the form of dozens of nodal sprouts

↓

Neurotropic and neurotrophic signals guide the sprouts towards the distal nerve stump

↓

Axonal sprouts join with motor or sensory receptors. Pruning of nonconnected sprouts occurs. Some axonal sprouts which do not reach an endoneurial tube may form neuromas

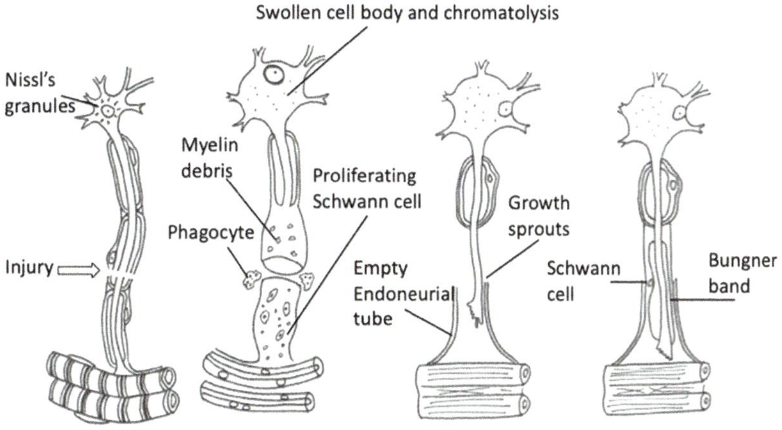

Fig. 15.4 Wallerian degeneration and regeneration of axonal sprouts

Table 15.1 Seddon classification of nerve injuries

Grade	Features
Neurapraxia	Physiological disruption of the nerve, potentially with localised disruption of the myelin sheath. Complete recovery can be expected in 12 weeks after this type of nerve injury
Axonotmesis	The axon is disrupted and there is distal Wallerian degeneration. The endoneurium and the Schwann cell are preserved and good functional recovery is possible
Neurotmesis	Severance of the endoneurial tube and the Schwann cell, and disruption of axons. The perineurium and the epineurium are also disrupted. Recovery is variable and nerve repair is indicated to restore continuity

Table 15.2 The Sunderland classification of nerve injuries

Grade	Description
I	Disruption of myelin; physiological dysfunction
II	Disruption of myelin and axon
III	Disruption of myelin, axon and endoneurium
IV	Disruption of myelin, axon, endoneurium and perineurium
V	Disruption of myelin, axon, endoneurium, perineurium and epineurium

recovery without surgical repair and functional loss is complete without treatment.

The drawback with Sunderland classification is the lack of any test to differentiate types 2–4. This differentiation is based on histology. Additionally, most injuries can be a combination of different types of injuries.

A sixth degree was described by McKinnon, where a part of the nerve is transected and the remaining part suffers an injury of varying degree. This can result in a neuroma-in-continuity.

Evaluation of Nerve Injury

The first step in diagnosis is to record a detailed history and conduct a full physical examination. The history will explain the mechanism of nerve injury, associated injuries, coexisting medical conditions and degree of neurologic involvement. In longstanding nerve injury, evidence of recovery is an important factor with prognostic implications.

Metabolic disorders, collagen diseases and malignancies can cause nerve dysfunction and should be elicited in the history.

The examination of each nerve elicits sensibility in the autonomous distribution, and examination of specific muscles innervated by the nerve. Injuries to the muscle may cause loss of sensation, and this should be differentiated from paralysis due to nerve injury.

Motor deficit indicates a lower motor neuron lesion with atonic paralysis. The grading of muscle strength is shown in Table 15.3.

Because of overlap of sensory distribution between cutaneous nerves, the autonomous area of any particular nerve is examined to determine loss of sensory innervation. This is the zone supplied solely by the nerve.

Surrounding the autonomous zone is the intermediate zone, which is the generally accepted anatomical distribution of the nerve. The intermediate area will demonstrate some loss of sensation in the event of a nerve injury.

The maximal zone is beyond the intermediate zone, and indicates the entire distribution of the nerve. If the surrounding nerves are blocked and the nerve is stimulated, the area where sensations are perceived is known as the maximal area.

In addition to sensory and motor deficit, autonomic loss results in loss of sweating in the distribution of the nerve. Sweat droplets can be observed with an ophthalmoscope or checked with the iodine starch test. The presence of sweating indicates continuity of autonomic innervation.

Table 15.3 Grading of muscle strength

Grade	Description
0	Complete paralysis
1	Muscle flicker
2	Muscle contraction with gravity eliminated
3	Muscle contraction against gravity
4	Muscle contraction against gravity and resistance
5	Normal muscle contraction

Tinel's sign is elicited by percussion along the course of the nerve from distal to proximal, and checking for tingling in the distribution of the nerve. The presence of Tinel's sign indicates axonal regeneration, while distal advancement of Tinel's sign indicates progression of axonal regeneration along the course of the nerve. Sunderland grade 2 and 3 injuries are characterised by a progressive Tinel's sign, as are grade 4 and 5 injuries after repair. Tinel's sign is present and does not progress along the nerve if repair is not undertaken in grades 4 and 5. Grade 1 injuries do not exhibit Tinel's sign, as there is no axonal injury or regeneration.

Other features of a nerve injury are a lack of wrinkling of the skin in water, which is known as pilomotor response. Changes in cutaneous circulation cause vasodilation for 2–3 weeks, followed by vasoconstriction.

Table 15.4 Grading of recovery from the British Medical Research Society and Medical Research Council

Sensory recovery		Motor recovery	
Grade	Description	Grade	Description
S0	Absence of sensibility in the area	M0	No contraction
S1	Recovery of deep cutaneous pain	M1	Perceptible contraction in proximal muscles
S2	Partial recovery of superficial cutaneous pain and touch	M2	Perceptible contraction in proximal and distal muscles
S3	Recovery of superficial cutaneous pain and touch; absence of over-response	M3	Power against resistance in proximal and distal muscle groups
S4	Recovery of two-point discrimination	M4	Synergistic and independent movements possible
S5	Complete recovery	M5	Complete recovery

Nerve Recovery

Nerve recovery following injury follows a specific sequence. Pain and temperature sensation are the first to recover, followed by touch and the perception of 30 Hz vibration, moving touch, constant touch, 256 Hz vibration and finally stereognosis. Perception of touch is determined with Semmes Weinstein monofilaments.

A grading system for sensory recovery has been proposed by the British Medical Research Society (Table 15.4), while motor recovery is graded by the Medical Research Council. Recovery is tested in the autonomous area of the nerve.

Investigations

Electromyography

Electromyography studies are helpful in evaluating nerve injuries. A needle electrode is inserted into the muscle. Normal muscle does not show any activity at rest. In denervated muscle, fibrillation potentials on needle insertion appear on an electromyogram at 8–14 days and spontaneous potentials are evident after 2–4 weeks. Fibrillations persist until reinnervation or muscle atrophy.

Polyphasic motor unit potentials on voluntary activity are a sign of reinnervation.

Nerve Conduction Studies

Nerve conduction studies involve placing an electrode on the skin overlying the nerve and measuring the response from the muscle. The distance between the stimulating and recording electrode is divided by the time between stimulus and response, giving the velocity of conduction.

For motor nerves, the muscle is stimulated through the nerve. The response time is noted. The stimulating electrode is moved closer to the distal end and again the response time is noted. The ratio of the distance between the two points of stimulation and the difference in latency time gives the conduction velocity between these two points.

In the event of significant axonal injury, Wallerian degeneration in the distal segment will impair the amplitude of evoked potentials within 5–10 days. The presence of normal conductivity in the distal segment 10 days following injury indicates a good prognosis.

Somatosensory Evoked Potential

The somatosensory evoked potential (SSEP) is checked by stimulation of the sensory nerve and measuring potentials on the scalp. It is useful for spinal-cord monitoring during spinal surgery.

Management of Nerve Injuries

In severely injured patients, the management of nerve injuries follows after advanced trauma life management guidelines and patient resuscitation.

In open injuries, wound management is undertaken and primary repair of the nerve is preferred if possible. Primary repair is accomplished within a few hours of injury.

If there is a delay in achieving repair because of medical reasons, associated injuries or lack of skilled personnel, repair can be accomplished within 7 days and wound management is carried out as standard. Repair within 7 days is known as delayed primary repair. Beyond 7 days, repair is classified as secondary repair.

Closed nerve injuries are observed for signs of recovery while maintaining the range of motion of joints and preventing contractures.

Nerve palsy that develops following the manipulation of a fracture should be explored to rule out entrapment.

Nerve Repair

Nerve repair is undertaken as soon as possible after a diagnosis of nerve injury, and with the availability of expertise and equipment.

The surgery is performed under general or regional anaesthesia with tourniquet control. Magnification with loupes or an operating microscope is essential. The preparation of the extremity should allow for the incision to be extended to gain exposure if required. A nerve stimulator is helpful to determine the need for neurolysis of a neuroma-in-continuity.

In patients undergoing secondary repair, the orientation of the two nerve ends may be difficult and the arrangement of the fascicles is matched on either side.

The technique for nerve repair can be epineurial or fascicular. There is no proven advantage of one over the other. In epineurial repair, the epineurium of one end is sutured to the corresponding epineurium of the other end. It remains the gold standard. The fascicles and blood vessels are matched on either end to ensure correct rotational orientation. The suture material used is 6-0 to 10-0.

Fascicular repair involves repair of the perineurium. It potentially provides more accurate repair as long as the fascicles are matched. The presence of suture material within the substance of the nerve may interfere with regeneration and inaccurate matching of fascicles leads to a poor result.

Fascicle matching can be conducted with intraoperative nerve stimulation, which requires the patient's cooperation. Immunohistochemical identification can be performed in the first few days after nerve injury. This technique relies on detecting acetylcholinesterase in motor axons and carbonic anhydrase in sensory axons. It requires excision of some nerve tissue from the two ends and some processing time, but does not depend on patient cooperation.

Reversed interposition nerve grafting is helpful in patients with a significant gap. Commonly used donor nerves are the sural nerve and the medial and lateral cutaneous nerves of the forearm (Table 15.5).

Nerve tubes or axonal guidance channels have been used to guide the regenerating axons across a gap. These are arteries or veins from the patient used as a conduit, or synthetic materials such as collagen, silicon, PGA (polyglycolic acid), PLA (poly lactic acid). The use of such channels is still developing and PGA has good results for small and medium defects.

Autografts are better than conduits for gaps greater than 3 cm. Interfascicular nerve graft was described by Millesi and vascularised nerve grafts were described by Taylor and Ham. Vascularised grafts are useful in areas with scarred recipient bed.

The harvested nerve grafts undergo Wallerian degeneration and only act as a physical conduit for passage of axonal sprouts.

Results of Nerve Repair

The following factors influence the results of nerve repair:

- Age—older patients have worse outcomes following nerve repair.
- Tension on the repair site—the gap between nerve ends determines the tension of the repair. Prior to repair, the nerve has to be resected to the level of undamaged fasciculi. Extensive nerve damage may require more resection and with more resection, the arrangement of the fasciculi within the nerve changes between the two ends, making repair less successful. The gap can be minimised by nerve mobilisation or transposition, positioning the joint to relieve tension on the nerve or, in rare events, shortening the bone or nerve grafting.
- Use of nerve graft. Coaptation has better results compared to nerve grafting.
- Timing of repair—early repair is associated with better outcomes. However, repair should be undertaken only when adequate facilities and expertise are available and the patient has been resuscitated and stabilised.
- Level of injury—proximal injuries have a less favourable outcome compared with distal injuries.
- Quality of repair—the quality is determined by the condition of the nerve ends, repair without tension, preservation of the blood supply and accurate apposition of the fascicles.
- Experience of the surgeon—experience directly correlates with outcomes.

Table 15.5 Donor nerves for nerve grafting

Nerve	Length of graft obtained (cm)	Anatomy
Sural nerve	30–40	Adjacent to the short saphenous vein
Medial cutaneous nerve of the forearm	18–20	Adjacent to the basilic vein Good scar Minimal scar problems The anterior branch or both the anterior and posterior branches can be used
Lateral cutaneous nerve of the forearm	8	Along the ulnar border of the brachioradialis Leaves a prominent scar
Nerves for supplying the third web space	24	Useful for median nerve injury Expendable nerves
Dorsal cutaneous branch of the ulnar nerve	–Variable	For ulnar nerve injury
Terminal branches of the anterior interosseous nerve	–Variable	To reconstruct digital nerves No sensory or motor morbidity

Neuroma-in-Continuity

In neuroma-in-continuity, the neuroma is dissected and the damaged nerve fascicles identified.

A simpler technique is to use a nerve stimulator proximal and distal to the injury site to identify the electrically silent sensory and motor fibres, and then use a nerve graft to reconstruct them. This avoids dissection of the neuroma and reduces the risk of injury to the lesser injured fibres.

Complex Regional Pain Syndrome

Complex regional pain syndrome (CRPS) is an abnormal sympathetic response in a limb following an injury. Other terms used to describe this or similar conditions include reflex sympathetic dystrophy (RSD), causalgia, algodystrophy and Sudeck's atrophy.

Patients suffer pain, stiffness, hyperalgesia (increased sensitivity to painful stimulus), allodynia (pain on gentle touch), discolouration, increased sweating and osteoporosis). Vasomotor instability (VMI) and swelling may be seen. The pain is not localised to the distribution of a particular peripheral nerve.

Initial phase is dry, red, warm extremity which turns to cold, sweaty, swollen appearance with time. The pain is out of proportion to what is expected following the injury. Late phase is evidenced by limb atrophy, thin skin, loss of hair, pitted nails and joint contractures.

Radiological changes are local osteoporosis and increase uptake on bone scan.

Common sites affected are hands, feet, knees, shoulder and elbows. Rarely the hip can be involved. CRPS) may present after knee replacement surgery. A psychological cause has been proposed but not consistently proven.

Two types of CRPS have been described (Table 15.6)

The diagnosis is largely clinical and can be supported with radiological findings.

Treatment is with reassurance, analgesia and careful physical therapy. Nonsteroidal anti-inflammatory drugs are more useful and immobilisation should be avoided. Centrally acting analgesics like amitryptiline, gabapentin or carbamazepine can be tried). Other options are desensitization of peripheral nerve with capsaicin, transcutaneous nerve stimulator or dorsal column stimulator. Continuous passive motion may be helpful in the knee.

Stellate ganglion blocks have been reported as effective in upper limbs and surgical sympathectomy can be considered for patients in whom blocks have transient efficacy.

Surgery for release of contractures, or amputation are best avoided.

Table 15.6 Types of CRPS)

Type I	Without an associated nerve injury. This is also known as RSD
Type II	Occurs in association with a peripheral nerve lesion. This is also known as causalgia

Atkins RM. Complex regional pain syndrome. Aspects of Current management. JBJS Br 2003;85:1100–6.

Entrapment Neuropathies

Pronator Teres Syndrome

Pronator teres syndrome describes compression neuropathy of the median nerve along its course in the anterior aspect of the elbow joint. The nerve can be compressed by the ligament of Struthers, lacertus fibrosus, between the two heads of pronator teres or at the fibrous origin of the flexor digitorum superficialis (Fig. 15.5).

Abnormal anatomy, repeated activity or trauma can predispose to this condition.

Patients typically complain of aching in the forearm after activity. Palmar cutaneous branch of the medial nerve is involved, which differentiates this from carpal tunnel syndrome.

Depending on the muscle involved in compression, pain can be reproduced by resisted pronation (indicates the pronator teres), resisted flexion and supination (indicates the lacertus fibrosus) or resisted PIP joint flexion of the fingers (indicates the flexor digitorum superficialis band).

Nerve conduction studies can aid diagnosis and treatment is through avoidance of activity or surgical release. Surgical release should cover all potential sites of compression.

Anterior Interosseous Nerve syndrome

Anterior interosseous syndrome describes compression of the anterior interosseous branch of the median nerve under the pronator teres.

The presenting features are aching in the forearm and a weak pinch. There is no sensory deficit. Patients are unable to touch the tips of their index finger and thumb together due to a weak flexor pollicis longus (FPL) and flexor digitorum profundus (FDP). Weakness of the pronator quadratus is evident by weak pronation in maximal flexion, which neutralizes pronator teres.

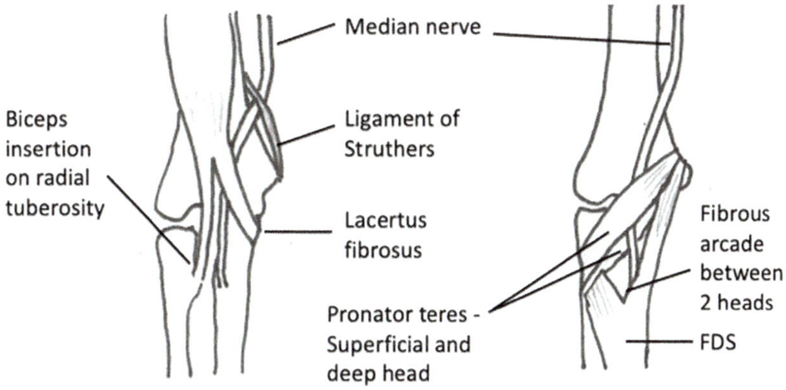

Fig. 15.5 Sites of entrapment of median nerve

Viral brachial neuritis (Parsonage Turner syndrome) may cause transient anterior interosseous nerve palsy. Associated shoulder pain is a feature in this situation. Rupture of the FPL in rheumatoid patients (Mannerfelt syndrome) is a differential diagnosis.

Splintage of the elbow at 90° flexion may help in some patients. Release of the deep head of the pronator teres alleviates the symptoms.

Cubital Tunnel Syndrome

Cubital tunnel syndrome is the second commonest nerve entrapment seen by hand surgeons.

Entrapment of the ulnar nerve at the elbow can be due to medial epicondyle fractures, bony spurs or entrapment under the origin of the flexor carpi ulnaris (FCU) muscle. Arcade of Struthers is the hiatus in the medial intermuscular septum where the ulnar nerve passes from the anterior to the posterior compartment; and is a potential site of entrapment. The ulnar nerve traverses the cubital tunnel where the Osborne ligament forms the roof of the tunnel, connecting the medial epicondyle to the olecranon. Sometimes, this fascia is replaced by the anconeus epitrochlearis muscle. The nerve can also be commonly trapped in the fascia between the two heads of FCU (Fig. 15.6).

The sensory component leads to reduced sensation in the ulnar aspect of the hand. Signs of ulnar motor deficit are wasting of the interossei (evident in the first dorsal interosseous), wasting of the flexor carpi ulnaris and the ulnar part of the FDP. Weak adduction of the thumb (Froment's sign) causes flexion of the IP joint of the thumb on resisted adduction. This is through the action of FPL substituting for weak adductor pollicis.

In Wartenberg's sign, the patient is asked to adduct all fingers. The little finger drifts into abduction due to weakness of the third palmar interosseous.

Tinel's sign may be positive around the elbow and ulnar clawing may be present. Ulnar clawing is reduced if the ulnar half of the FDP is weak—for instance in a high ulnar nerve lesion. An ulnar nerve injury near the elbow (high lesion) denervates the ulnar half of FDP, hence the degree of clawing is less.

Nerve conduction studies (conduction speed under 50 m/s are suggestive of nerve lesion) are helpful in diagnosis.

Night splintage in 45° flexion can be tried. Release of the ulnar nerve is performed within the tunnel without anterior transposition. Endoscopic release has not been shown to be superior to open release.

Caliandro P, La Torre G, Padua R, Giannini F, Padua L. Treatment for ulnar neuropathy at the elbow. Cochrane Database Syst Rev 11(11) 2016 Nov. No evidence to support operative vs nonoperative treatment. Transposition of the nerve is associated with more wound infections. Endoscopic surgery causes more haematomas.

Ulnar Tunnel Syndrome

Ulnar tunnel syndrome describes compression of the ulnar nerve in Guyon's canal. Guyon's canal

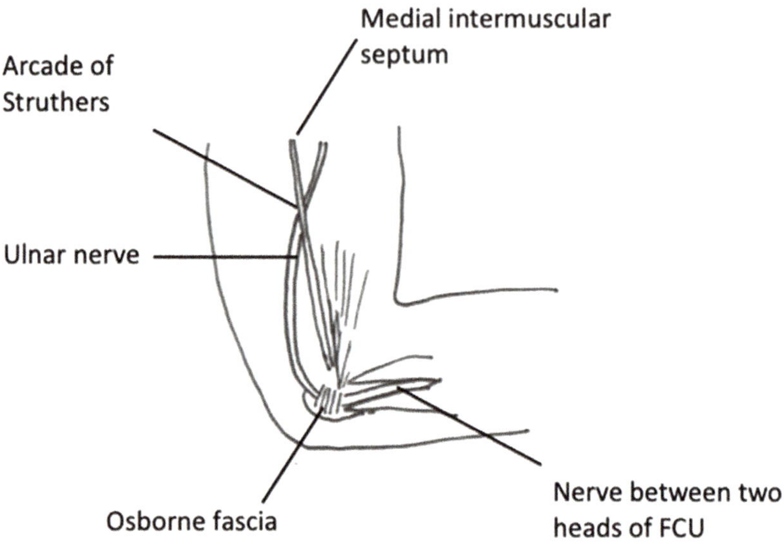

Fig. 15.6 Sites of entrapment of ulnar nerve

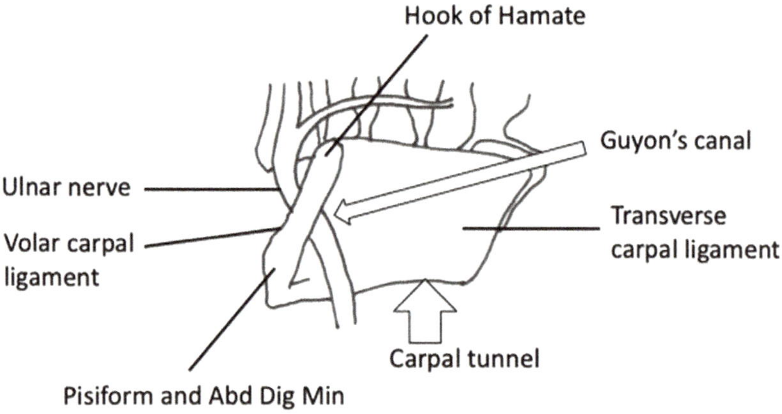

Fig. 15.7 Guyon's canal right wrist

lies in the ulnar side of the carpal tunnel on the volar side of the wrist . It contains the ulnar nerve and artery (Fig. 15.7).

Guyon's canal is formed between the pisiform and the hook of hamate. The floor is the transverse carpal ligament and the roof is the volar carpal ligament (Fig. 15.5). The nerve can be compressed by ganglions (commonest cause), fractures of the hook of hamate, lipomas, ulnar artery thrombosis or arthritis of the pisotriquetral joint. Other causes include chronic related injury (handlebar palsy), risk of vibration (hypothenar hammer syndrome), or in sportsmen.

Shea and McClain (Fig. 15.8) subdivided lesions of the ulnar nerve in the Guyon's canal into three types. Type I involves both sensory and motor components, type II is pure motor loss and Type III is pure sensory loss.

Clinically, the sensory branch of the ulnar nerve is spared and the ulnar clawing is marked because FDP innervation is intact. Phalen's and Tinel's signs may be positive. Froment's sign and Wartenberg's sign are positive in motor involvement.

Splinting can help to relieve symptoms.

Surgical treatment is decompression of the nerve or excision of the hook of hamate.

Radial Nerve Palsy

Radial nerve may be involved in humeral shaft fractures. Pressure on the nerve while intoxicated with the arm hanging over the armrest of a chair is known as 'Saturday night palsy'. Involvement of the nerve in the spiral groove will lead to weakness of brachioradialis, extensor carpi radialis brevis (ECRB) and extensor carpi radialis longus (ECRL) along with sensory loss and weakness of extensor compartment muscles.

Most closed radial nerve injuries recover (neurapraxia). Indications for exploration are open fractures or nerve palsy after fracture reduction. Nerve conduction studies can be undertaken at 6 weeks after closed injury if no recovery is evident.

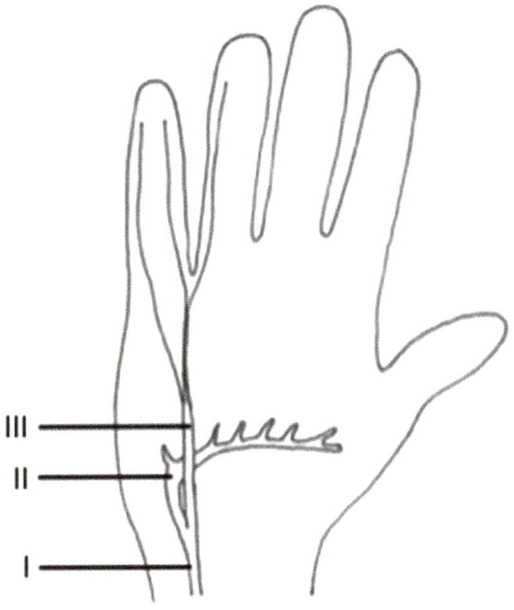

Fig. 15.8 Shea and McClain types of neurological loss in ulnar tunnel syndrome

Posterior Interosseous Nerve Compression Syndrome

The posterior interosseous branch of the radial nerve (PIN) can be compressed along its course by the origin or distal border of the supinator muscle, the origin of the extensor carpi radialis brevis or the arcade of Frohse. Arcade of Frohse is known as the supinator arch and is the proximal margin of superficial part of Supinator (Fig. 15.9). Leash of Henry is a group of vessels at the level of the radial neck which can lead to compression of the PIN.

PIN supplies the ECRB and posterior compartment of the forearm. There is also a sensory branch to the dorsal wrist capsule, but no cutaneous sensory innervation.

Other potential causes are elbow dislocation, dislocation or excision of the radial head or rheumatoid arthritis of the elbow.

Fig. 15.9 The arcade of Frohse

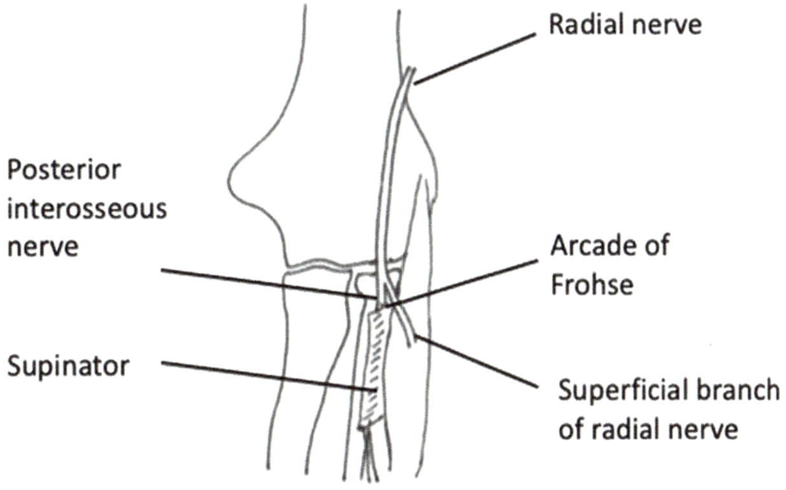

Symptoms are related to motor deficit and aching in the posterior compartment of the forearm. The symptoms are worse after activity. Clinical signs are weak wrist extension and radial deviation of the wrist on extension. The extensor carpi radialis longus deviates the wrist to the radial side on extension and escapes denervation because it is supplied by the radial nerve above the level of the supinator.

Surgical decompression of the nerve is recommended.

Radial Tunnel Syndrome

This is also due to compression of the posterior interosseous nerve and causes aching in the extensor compartment of the forearm. Characteristically, there is no motor deficit. Patients have tenderness over the extensor mechanism about 5 cm distal to the lateral epicondyle and pain over the origin of the extensor carpi radialis brevis on resisted extension of the middle finger.

The site of tenderness and nerve conduction studies help differentiate this condition from tennis elbow.

Surgical release is recommended when non-operative measures fail. Results are not as good as those with PIN compression syndrome.

Wartenberg Syndrome

Wartenberg syndrome is compression neuropathy of the superficial sensory branch of the radial nerve. The site of compression is between brachioradialis and ECRL. Common symptoms are pain, altered sensation on the dorsal and radial aspect of hand. Patients do not have motor deficit and local steroid injection may help to resolve symptoms. Surgical release may be required.

Brachial Plexus Injury

The brachial plexus is predominantly formed from five nerve roots—from the fifth cervical to first thoracic spinal nerves (Fig. 15.10). The fourth cervical or the second dorsal root may contribute.

Injuries to the brachial plexus are usually traction injuries from motor vehicle accidents; motorbike accidents account for a significant per-

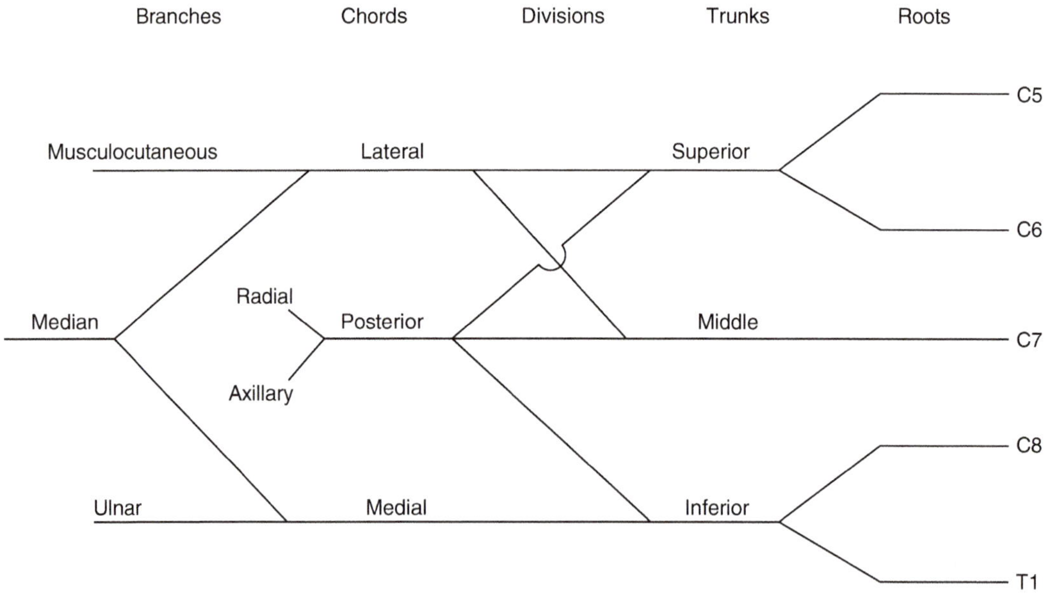

Fig. 15.10 Diagrammatic representation of the main branches of the brachial plexus

centage of cases. Distraction of the head away from the shoulder stretches the upper roots, while violent abduction of the arm leads to traction injury to the lower roots.

Classification

Brachial plexus lesions are classified by Leffert into five types—supraclavicular (75% of all injuries); infraclavicular; postanaesthetic; radiation injury and obstetric palsy.

Supraclavicular lesions are further divided into preganglionic (where the roots are avulsed from the cord) or postganglionic (where the injury is at the level of the root or the trunks). In preganglionic the injury is proximal to the dorsal root ganglion on the sensory side and at the level of rootlets from the anterior horn cell.

Preganglionic injuries imply a permanent loss of the root and the axons and carry a poor prognosis. In postganglionic (infraganglionic) injuries, patients have associated sensory loss. These injuries may be amenable to repair.

Based on anatomic location, plexus injuries can be supraclavicular, retroclavicular or infraclavicular.

Evaluation

A local examination is performed for swelling and bruising, and a detailed neurological examination of sensory and motor loss is performed to document the injury. Tinel's sign, if detectable, should be documented to monitor progress.

The C5 and C6 root can be tested by shoulder abduction and elbow flexion. C7 is for triceps while C8 and T1 can be tested by hand function.

A cutaneous axon reflex response differentiates preganglionic from postganglionic palsy. A scratch on the skin with histamine results in an axonal wheal-and-flare formation if nerve innervation is intact. In preganglionic injury, the flare is present and the wheal is absent. In postganglionic injury, the wheal and vasodilation are present but the flare is absent.

The long thoracic nerve and the dorsal scapular nerve arise from the roots. Dysfunction of these nerves indicates an injury that is proximal to their origin.

A feature of lower preganglionic injury is Horner's syndrome. Patients with Horner's syndrome have ipsilateral ptosis (drooping of the upper eyelid), miosis (pupillary constriction), anhydrosis (loss of sweating on the side of the face) and enophthalmos (sunken eye).

Specific Injury Patterns

Erb's palsy involves trauma to the C5, C6 and C7 roots. It is characterised by shoulder adduction and internal rotation, elbow extension and forearm pronation. Sensory loss corresponds to the roots involved. Obstetric palsy often has an Erb's pattern.

Klumpke's palsy involves trauma to the C8 and T1 roots. The wrist and finger flexors are weak.

Imaging

A plain radiograph of the cervical spine will detect any fracture/subluxation. A high diaphragm on a chest radiograph may indicate a phrenic nerve palsy.

MR neurogram or a CT myelogram is helpful to assess root avulsions.

Nerve conduction studies and electromyography are important to diagnose specific injury patterns. These are undertaken 3–4 weeks following the injury.

Treatment

Brachial plexus injuries often involve high energy impact, and there may be associated injuries to the spinal cord or vessels of the upper limbs. These should be assessed and managed based on advanced trauma life support protocol.

Surgery should be planned within 3 months of injury. Longer delay compromises outcome. The maximum window is 18–24 months, beyond which neuromuscular end plates lose function.

The techniques for dealing with brachial plexus injury are direct repair, nerve grafting or neurotisation.

Direct suture repair is also known as intraplexal repair. It is possible for postganglionic lesions. Autogenous nerve grafts are used to bridge the gap. The repair can be augmented with fibrin sealants to achieve a stronger repair. Nerve grafting follows standard techniques. The use of vascularised nerve grafts has not shown significant benefit over that of non-vascular nerve grafts. Shorter grafts have better outcomes compared to longer grafts.

Root avulsions cannot be repaired. In this situation, local nerves not arising from the plexus, can be diverted to help the patient achieve some function. The spinal accessory nerve is transferred to suprascapular nerve for shoulder abduction and rotator cuff function. The intercostal nerves can be transferred to the musculocutaneous nerve to gain elbow flexion.

The order of priorities when restoring function is elbow flexion, shoulder stabilisation, hand sensation, wrist extension, finger flexion and intrinsic function.

Shoulder abduction can be restored by transfer of the trapezius to the deltoid. The latissimus dorsi can be transferred posteriorly to function as external rotator of the shoulder. Shoulder fusion is an option for stabilising the shoulder.

The pectoralis minor is used for elbow flexion via the biceps.

Neurotisation, or distal nerve transfer, involves transferring a functioning motor nerve to the denervated muscle. A nerve that supplies a synergistic muscle will be able to restore function more quickly to a denervated muscle and hence avoid muscle atrophy. For instance, the ulnar nerve fibres in the upper arm can be transferred to the musculocutaneous nerve to restore elbow flexion (Oberlin procedure). Many other intraplexal or extraplexal transfers have been described, based on whether the donor nerve is part of the brachial plexus.

Contralateral C7 root transfer is a technique where the C7 root of the normal side is harvested and brought across the midline to the affected side. The root is connected to the lateral cord or the posterior cord to regain proximal muscle function.

Gu YD, Zhang GM, Chen DS, Yan JG, Cheng XM, Chen L. Seventh cervical nerve root transfer from the contralateral healthy side for treatment of brachial plexus root avulsion. J Hand Surg 1992;17:518–21.

Recovery from brachial plexus injury can take 18 months or more. Ongoing research into reconnection of nerve root avulsions to the spinal cord may improve outcomes for preganglionic injuries.

Neuromuscular Disorders

The diagnosis of neuromuscular disorders begins with an accurate history, family history and clinical examination. Measurement of serum creatinine phosphokinase and aldolase levels is helpful. Nerve conduction studies, electromyography and nerve and muscle biopsies are further tests that will help to establish a diagnosis.

Creatinine phosphokinase levels are checked. A muscle biopsy is performed, with tissue obtained from involved but functioning muscle at the musculotendinous junction and sent for both light and electron microscopy. A nerve biopsy is conducted at the sural nerve.

In myopathy, the amplitude and duration of muscle action potential is reduced, while the frequency is increased on electromyography testing. In neuropathy, the changes are reversed: the frequency is reduced, while the amplitude and duration are increased. Myotonic dystrophy is characterised by a 'dive-bomber' sound on needle insertion into the muscle. This indicates a reduced frequency, duration and amplitude of action potentials.

Nerve conduction studies are normal in muscle diseases, but will be affected in neuropathies.

Duchenne Muscular Dystrophy

DMD is inherited as a sex-linked recessive trait. Approximately 70% of patients have a family history, and the remaining cases occur as a result of spontaneous mutation. DMD is far more common in men, but can occur in women with Turner syndrome. The site of the mutation is the Xp21 region of the X chromosome.

Mutation in the dystrophin gene, located on the short arm of the X chromosome, leads to the synthesis of an unstable protein that is rapidly degraded. As a result, the muscle fibres are replaced by fat and fibrous tissue.

Clinically, children with DMD meet their milestones within the 1st year, but walking is often delayed. Children tend to walk on their toes and have frequent falls. The disease becomes more apparent around the ages of 3–6 years.

The calf muscles feel enlarged and firm due to fatty and fibrous infiltration (pseudohypertrophy). The tibialis posterior muscle retains strength till later stages, while other muscles lose power; this causes an equinovarus deformity of the foot.

The gait is a wide-based, circumduction gait and there is increased lumbar lordosis.

The Gower test is performed by asking children to stand from a squatting position. Children will use their arms to support themselves when standing up from a squatting position due to proximal muscle (gluteal) weakness in the lower limbs. Child rises by 'walking up' his thigh with his hands. Gluteal muscles are involved early in the disease.

The Meryon test indicates a lack of shoulder stability when children are lifted with one arm around the chest. If the shoulder muscles have normal strength, children will contract their shoulder muscles to increase stability. Affected children are unable to do this.

Sinus tachycardia and right ventricle hypertrophy may be present. Most patients are wheelchair bound by 12 years and survival beyond 20 years is unusual.

The diagnosis is supported by elevated creatinine phosphokinase levels (>100 times normal) and DNA analysis. Muscle biopsy showing absence of dystrophin protein is diagnostic.

Creatinine phosphokinase levels are highly elevated in patients with Duchenne muscle dystrophy (DMD) and can be 200 times normal in children with DMD in the 1st year of life. The levels decline later as muscle tissue is replaced with fibrous tissue. Creatinine phosphokinase levels are also elevated in women carrying the DMD gene and are an important diagnostic tool. The levels rise after activity, and this rise is higher in women who carry the DMD gene than in those who do not.

Treatment

The principal aim of treatment is to keep children mobile for as long as possible. Surgical intervention is indicated when mobility declines due to contractures.

Flexion and abduction contractures of the hip, flexion contractures of the knee and equinovarus contractures of the foot are seen. These are addressed by multiple-level tenotomies and bracing.

It is easier to maintain mobility with early interventions than to restore mobility after it has declined due to contractures. Walking should be resumed immediately after surgery. A little equinus is helpful for ambulation and should not be fully corrected. Transfer of the tibialis posterior anteriorly is an option to avoid progression of equinovarus deformity.

Scoliosis is a major problem. Spinal deformity should be addressed in the early stages before significant pulmonary and cardiac compromise arise. Posterior dorsolumbar fusion is performed with instrumentation and facet joint fusion at all levels. The fusion can be extended to the pelvis to avoid pelvic obliquity progressing.

Becker's Muscular Dystrophy

Becker's dystrophy is a milder form of DMD. The underlying process is similar to DMD, except that there is some intracellular dystrophin. The level of functional dystrophin determines the severity of the disease.

The incidence is one in 30,000 male births and transmission is sex-linked recessive. The symptoms and signs present around the age of 7 years and survival into the fourth or fifth decade of life is common.

Treatment is aimed at correcting contractures and maintaining mobility.

Emery–Dreifuss Muscular Dystrophy

Emery–Dreifuss muscular dystrophy is a sex-linked recessive disorder. The presentation is in the second decade of life with equinus of the ankle, flexion contracture of the elbow, extension contracture of the neck and tightness of the lumbar paravertebral muscles.

Cardiac abnormalities are often seen and may be asymptomatic. These should be actively investigated and treated. There is a high incidence of sudden cardiac death due to these abnormalities.

Management requires correction of Achilles contractures and stretching for neck and back contractures.

Facioscapulohumeral Muscular Dystrophy

Facioscapulohumeral muscular dystrophy is an autosomal dominant condition with weakness of the facial and shoulder muscles.

Weakness of the facial muscles means that patients are unable to whistle, purse their lips or wrinkle their brow. Shoulder muscle weakness causes a winged scapula and weak shoulder abduction.

The responsible gene is located on chromosome 4. Early childhood onset is associated with marked symptoms and the child is confined to a wheelchair by the age of 8–9 years. Onset in the teenage age or later has a more gradual course. Eventually, patients develop muscle weakness in the lower extremities.

Creatinine phosphokinase is normal. Scapulothoracic fusion is an option to stabilise the shoulder joint.

Myotonic Dystrophy

Myotonic dystrophy is an autosomal dominant condition characterised by muscle weakness and an inability of muscle to relax after contraction. Transmission can be autosomal recessive.

Patients have a tent-shaped mouth, dull expression, temporal baldness, hyperostosis of the skull, gonadal atrophy, dysphasia and dysarthria. Hip dysplasia, scoliosis and clubfoot may be associated with myotonic dystrophy. Clubfoot deformities are often resistant to treatment and talectomy may be needed. Cardiac abnormalities may be present, along with compromised respiratory function.

Charcot–Marie–Tooth Disease

Charcot–Marie–Tooth disease (CMTD; also known as peroneal muscle atrophy) is an autosomal dominant neuromuscular disorder causing progressive muscle atrophy and loss of proprioception. Inheritance can be X-linked or autosomal recessive. DNS testing reveals duplication of gene for PMP 22 (peripheral myelin protein 22) on chromosome 17.

Onset of CMTD is usually within the first two decades of life. Patients present clinically with foot weakness, metatarsal pain, clawing of the toes and high-arched feet. Balance is impaired and spinal ataxia may be present. The foot deformity progresses to cavovarus. Muscle atrophy gives the appearance of 'stork legs'.

The rigidity of the foot deformity is assessed by the Coleman Block test (see Chap. 17). A detailed neurological examination is conducted for muscle strength and sensory impairment. Patients may have acetabular dysplasia and scoliosis and these should be specifically examined.

Radiographs of the foot are obtained in a weight-bearing position to document the degree of forefoot adduction and cavus.

Treatment of the cavovarus deformity should be instituted early, before the deformity is fixed. Soft tissue releases may be combined with metatarsal osteotomy in the early stages, while fixed deformities require triple arthrodesis.

The tibialis posterior can be transferred anteriorly to augment weak ankle dorsiflexors where the varus deformity is not fixed.

For claw toes, the Jones procedure can be performed. This involves transfer of the long toe extensors to the metatarsal necks and fusion of the interphalangeal joints. Hibbs procedure involves transfer of the toe extensors to the middle cuneiform in patients with weak ankle dorsiflexion.

Variants of Charcot–Marie–Tooth Disease

Variants of CMTD are summarised in Table 15.7.

CMTD is discussed in more detail in Chap. 6.

Spinal Muscle Atrophy

Spinal muscle atrophy is an autosomal recessive (chromosome 5) degeneration of the anterior horn cells. It results in progressive weakness and areflexia, but sensory function is preserved.

Table 15.7 Variants of Charcot–Marie–Tooth disease (CMTD)

Variant	Inheritance	Age of onset	Features
Roussy Levy syndrome	Autosomal dominant	Infancy	CMTD features with static hand tremor
Dejerine–Sottas syndrome	Autosomal recessive or dominant	Infancy	Pes cavus, sensory loss in all four limbs, clubfoot, scoliosis
Refsum disease	Autosomal recessive	Childhood or puberty	Hypertrophic neuropathy, ataxia, areflexia, retinitis pigmentosa, distal sensory and motor loss in hands and feet
Neuronal CMTD	Autosomal dominant	Middle age	Affects mainly the ankle and foot muscles

Three different types of spinal muscle atrophy are recognised, based on the age of onset (Table 15.8):

The infantile form is known as Werdnig–Hoffman disease, while the juvenile form is Kugelberg–Welander disease.

As the primary abnormality is in the anterior horn cell the muscles show denervation, but nerve conduction studies are normal. A fine tremor and fasciculation of the tongue may be apparent. Weakness is predominantly of the proximal muscles. Serum creatinine phosphokinase levels are normal.

Evans, Drennan and Russman proposed a classification based on function (Table 15.9).

Patients with the acute infantile form have a poor prognosis and limited survival. Juvenile disease can lead to joint contractures and coxa valga. Hip instability should be managed with corrective proximal femoral osteotomy. Scoliosis is a disabling feature in the juvenile form and is managed by bracing or posterior fusion. Compromise of respiratory function is a significant risk factor.

Friedrich's Ataxia

Friedrich's ataxia is an autosomal recessive condition resulting in spinocerebellar degeneration. The frataxin gene on chromosome 9 is the underlying cause. Onset is in childhood or puberty. The

Table 15.8 Types of Spinal muscle atrophy

Type I, acute infantile	Severe generalised weakness in infants aged less than 6 months, leading to respiratory failure
Type II, chronic infantile	Begins within the first 2 years of life, but tends to remain static over many years
Type III, juvenile	Gradual onset in childhood and a progressive course

Table 15.9 Functional classification of spinal muscle atrophy

Type I	Never able to sit independently and does not have head control
Type II	Has head control and can sit, but cannot walk
Type III	Has limited walking use bracing
Type IV	Can walk and run before onset of weakness

Table 15.10 Summary of neuromuscular disorders

Disorder	Inheritance	D/R	Key features
Duchenne Muscular Dystrophy	X linked	R	Proximal muscle weakness, Gower's sign, High CK, absence of dystrophin. Wheelchair bound by teenage
Becker's dystrophy	X linked	R	Milder form of DMD. Some dystrophin present
Emery–Dreifuss dystrophy	X linked	R	Equinus of the ankle, flexion contracture of the elbow, extension contracture of the neck. Check for cardiac abnormalities
Facio-scapulo-humeral dystrophy	Auto	D	Weakness of the face and shoulder muscles. Scapulothoracic fusion considered. Eventual weakness in lower limbs
Myotonic dystrophy	Auto	D	Muscles unable to relax. Hip dysplasia, scoliosis and clubfoot
Charcot–Marie–Tooth disease	Auto	D (R)	Cavovarus foot, spinal ataxia. Tibialis posterior transfer, metatarsal osteotomies or triple arthrodesis
Spinal muscle atrophy	Auto	R	Anterior horn cells degenerate. Muscle weakness, preserved sensation
Friedrich's ataxia	Auto	R	Ataxia, areflexia and positive Babinski sign. Unable to walk by teenage. Foot deformities require tenotomy or fusion

clinical triad is ataxia, areflexia and a positive Babinski reflex. Mobility declines and most patients are unable to walk by their teenage years. Associated features are cardiomyopathy, nystagmus, pes cavus and scoliosis. Areflexia manifests as loss of ankle and knee deep-tendon reflexes.

Surgical intervention is needed for foot deformities. These are managed with tenotomies of the long toe flexors and Achilles tendon, or by triple arthrodesis for correction of the cavovarus deformity. Scoliosis can be managed non-operatively in the case of mild curves and by posterior instrumentation and fusion for severe curves. Most patients are wheelchair bound by late teens. Survival is usually to the fifth decade.

A summary of neuromuscular disorders is presented in Table 15.10.

Further Reading

Atkins RM. Complex regional pain syndrome. Aspects of current management. JBJS Br. 2003;85:1100–6.

Caliandro P, La Torre G, Padua R, Giannini F, Padua L. Treatment for ulnar neuropathy at the elbow. Cochrane Database Syst Rev. 2016;11(11).

Gu YD, Zhang GM, Chen DS, Yan JG, Cheng XM, Chen L. Seventh cervical nerve root transfer from the contralateral healthy side for treatment of brachial plexus root avulsion. J Hand Surg. 1992;17:518–21.

Imaging

16

Sridhar Kamath and Jyoti Bansal

Several imaging modalities are available for musculoskeletal disorders. Each modality has a specific role in management. Multimodality imaging is often required in the diagnostic process.

Plain Films

Plain films (X-rays) are the mainstay of imaging in various orthopaedic disorders. They offer a quick and easy way of obtaining the necessary information in the majority of orthopaedic patients. The main drawback is the radiation dose, although this is often minimal when imaging the extremities, or in comparison to Computed Tomography (CT). Plain films are also used in the postoperative period to assess healing and detect implant-related complications.

Computed Tomography

Computed tomography relies on ionising radiation and is a popular orthopaedic imaging modality. It has benefited tremendously from advances in computer software and the development of thinner slice thicknesses. It is now possible to post-process the data in a multitude of ways, the most common of which is multi-planar reformatting. This refers to the reconstruction of data in any desirable plane, most common of which are often the sagittal and coronal planes. Curved reformats are also possible and are used, for example, in patients with scoliosis for imaging of the spine.

CT has a higher spatial resolution than Magnetic Resonance Imaging (MRI). However, it offers relatively poor contrast resolution and is inferior to MRI for evaluating soft tissues. CT is a much quicker scan than MRI and is, therefore, less susceptible to artefacts in patients who are unable to keep still. Furthermore, it allows for a faster turnover of patients. CT scanners have a shorter bore and are therefore better tolerated by claustrophobic patients.

Due to the high-quality imaging, CT scans are increasingly used in the diagnostic work-up, especially in trauma patients (Fig. 16.1). Furthermore, metallic artefacts from implants can be significantly reduced with the newer CT machines and software packages. This allows much greater visualisation and interpretation of the pathology. CT is also used to aid biopsy of deep-seated lesions and in performing joint injections, such as for the sacroiliac and thoracic facet joints. The major drawback of CT is its reliance on ionising radiation.

Common applications of CT in musculoskeletal disorders are-

- Trauma, especially fractures of the spine, pelvis, tibial plateau, ankle, calcaneum and midfoot.

S. Kamath · J. Bansal (✉)
University Hospital of Wales, Cardiff, UK

S. Agarwal (ed.), *Current Orthopaedic Practice*, https://doi.org/10.1007/978-3-030-78529-1_16

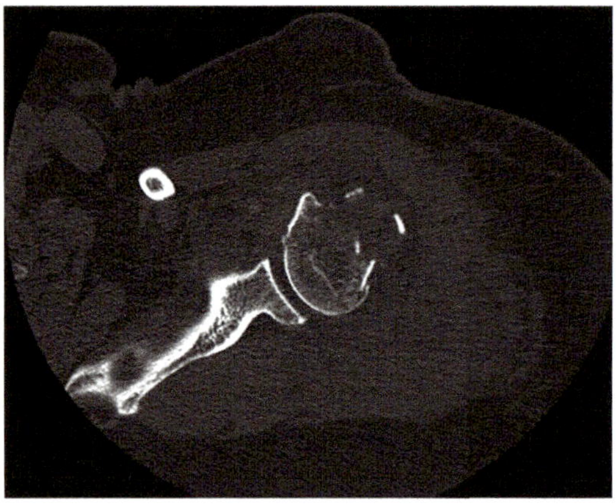

Fig. 16.1 An axial computed tomography scan of the left shoulder demonstrating a comminuted proximal humeral fracture

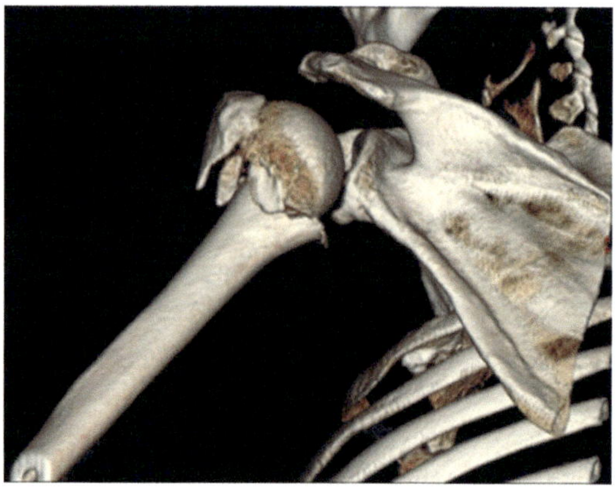

Fig. 16.2 A volume-rendered three-dimensional CT reconstruction of the same proximal humeral fracture

- Postoperative evaluation to assess complications, state of bone fusion, periprosthetic fractures and prosthesis failure.
- Pre-operative planning to aid surgery such as before complex spinal reconstruction or correction
- Assessment of bone lesions, such as, an osteoid osteoma.
- Deep-seated soft tissue lesion biopsy or bone biopsy.
- Guided injections and nerve root blocks.

Dual Energy CT (DECT) is a relatively newer technology that uses X-ray beams of two separate energies to obtain the images. This enables the computer to study the attenuation property of the tissue (or matter) at different X-ray energy levels and therefore, selectively enhance or reduce the effects of specific materials in the body such as iodine or calcium. DECT, therefore, can produce better contrast images and also non-contrast images from a single study (therefore, reducing the dose). It can be used to differentiate tissues of different chemical composition, for example, a gouty tophus from a calcific deposit. It is also helpful in generating better metal artefact reduction images and to potentially detect marrow oedema in the bones.

Some software packages enable three-dimensional (3D) reconstruction of images, including volume rendering and surface reconstructions (Fig. 16.2). Such programs are particularly useful for giving the surgeons a 3D overview of complex fractures and complex spinal abnormalities. It is also possible to 'ghost-out' structures to make fracture lines more clearly visible.

Magnetic Resonance Imaging

The use of MRI has rapidly grown in clinical practice.

MRI scan is acquired by placing the patient in a strong magnetic field, which aligns the nuclei of elements with odd atomic numbers (mostly hydrogen) in the body along the magnetic field. This becomes the steady-state in the magnetic field, and a radiofrequency (RF) pulse is then applied in this steady-state. After the RF pulse is switched off, the steady-state returns to equilibrium with the release of energy in the form of an RF signal, which is detected with the receiver coil.

The above-described 'spin-echo' technique gives T1- and T2-weighted images, depending on the time of application of the RF pulse (TR, repetition time) and the timing of signal acquisition (TE, echo time). Different tissues in the body have different T1 and T2 relaxation times: liquids have long T1 and T2 times, while fat has low T1 and T2 values. Varying the TE and TR times can, therefore, vary the T1 or T2 weighting of images.

Field strength indicates the strength of the magnet. In clinical practice, commonly used MR scanners have field strengths of 1–1.5 Tesla, which allow shorter imaging time and thinner slices compared to older scanners. Also, 3 Tesla scanners are becoming more common in clinical practice. Low-field-strength magnets of 0.3 Tesla have an open configuration and are convenient for imaging claustrophobic patients and extremities such as the elbow and wrist.

MRI is usually performed in at least two and possibly three orthogonal planes.

Commonly used sequences in clinical practice are T1, T2, proton density and STIR (Short Tau Inversion Recovery). The appearance of fluid or fat in different sequences is shown in Table 16.1.

T1 Sequence

Short TE and TR times give a T1-weighted sequence. In this, water returns a low signal and fat returns a high signal. This is a rapidly acquired sequence that provides excellent anatomical detail. Fat, sub-acute haemorrhages and proteinaceous fluids are bright, while fluid is dark. T1-weighted images are generally considered good for looking at bone marrow. However, they are not as good for detecting bone or soft tissue oedema. T1 imaging following gadolinium administration (see later) is often used as a problem-solving tool.

T2 Sequence

Long TE and TR times give a T2-weighted image that is excellent for demonstrating pathological conditions which lead to increased water content—such as oedema, inflammation, infection and tumours. One way to remember this is with the mnemonic 'World War 2'—water is white on T2.

Table 16.1 The tissue appearances in various MRI sequences

	T1	T2	PD	T1/T2/PD with fat-suppression (FS)	STIR
Fluid	Dark	Bright	Bright	Bright	Bright
Fat	Bright	Bright	Bright	Dark	Dark

Proton Density Sequence

Proton-density sequences use a short TE and long TR. This sequence is a mix of T1 and T2, with contrast intermediate between T1- and T2-weighted images. This sequence is used in the assessment of menisci and other structures as part of routine knee protocols. It is often used with fat suppression to increase contrast.

Fast-Spin Echo Sequence

This is an accelerated method of acquiring T2 and proton-density images and is generally referred to as a 'fast' or 'turbo' technique. Fat remains bright on fast or turbo T2 and therefore fat-suppressed sequences are often used to highlight water-containing tissues such as inflammation or tumour. This sequence also reduces artefacts from metal prostheses and can be employed if previous instrumentation is present.

STIR Sequence

A STIR sequence is a specialised spin-echo sequence that suppresses fat from the images, making fluid-containing lesions more conspicuous. This is a very sensitive technique to detect soft tissue and marrow pathology and particularly useful to obtain uniform fat suppression in larger patients.

T2* (Gradient-Echo T2)

This is faster T2 sequence with fluid bright as in the usual spin-echo T2 sequence. It is particularly good for imaging the ligaments, articular cartilage and fibrocartilage. The advantage of this sequence is that very thin sections can be obtained, which are useful for 3D volume reconstruction. However, this sequence is degraded significantly by metal because of susceptibility artefacts.

Fast-Spin Echo

This is an accelerated method of acquiring T2 and proton-density images and is generally referred to as a 'fast' or 'turbo' technique. Fat remains bright on fast or turbo T2 and therefore fat-saturated sequences are often used. This sequence also reduces artefacts from metal prostheses and should be employed if previous instrumentation is present.

Gadolinium-Enhanced Scans

Gadolinium administration is used to delineate an abscess or to differentiate between cystic and solid masses, and viable and necrotic tissue, among other uses. T1-weighted sequencing with fat suppression is usually used when gadolinium is administered, making the pathology stand out.

MR Arthrography

MR arthrography involves MR scanning after the intra-articular injection of gadolinium, clearly demonstrating intra-articular structures. This technique is especially useful in assessing glenoid and acetabular labrum in the context of shoulder instability and femoroacetabular impingement. MR arthrography is also useful in the characterisation of hyaline cartilage and osteochondral defects.

Whole-Body MRI

With improvement in MRI scanner and coil technology, we are now able to obtain images of the entire body and the bony skeleton without the need for patient or coil repositioning. This technique is very useful in the context of multifocal disease especially to detect metastasis, myeloma lesions or multifocal inflammatory foci. Whole-body MRI is replacing plain film skeletal survey in the diagnosis of myeloma.

Contraindications to MRI

The following objects are contraindicated within the MRI scanning room: intracerebral aneurysm clips, cardiac pacemakers, defibrillators, biostimulators, internal hearing aids and metallic orbital foreign bodies. However, many of the newer generations of cardiac pacemakers and defibrillators are now MRI compatible.

Relative contraindications are first-trimester pregnancy, middle-ear prosthesis and penile prosthesis. There is often confusion among clinicians with regards to the safety of orthopaedic implants in an MRI scanner: orthopaedic implants including prosthetic joints, screws, plates and rods can be scanned, but steel implants cause artefacts. Titanium devices produce significantly less artifacts. Metallic external fixators should not be scanned.

Common Applications

Common applications of MRI in musculoskeletal disorders are:

- Spine pathology, like, back pain and sciatica.
- Knee joint evaluation—meniscus and cruciate ligament tears (Fig. 16.3), hyaline cartilage defects.
- Shoulder joint evaluation—rotator cuff tear, anterior or posterior dislocation.
- Wrist—triangular fibrocartilage complex and intrinsic ligament tears.
- Soft tissues and bone neoplasms—to characterise and define the extent of lesions.
- Avascular necrosis.
- Osteomyelitis (including, discitis).
- Arthritis.
- Bone-marrow pathology.

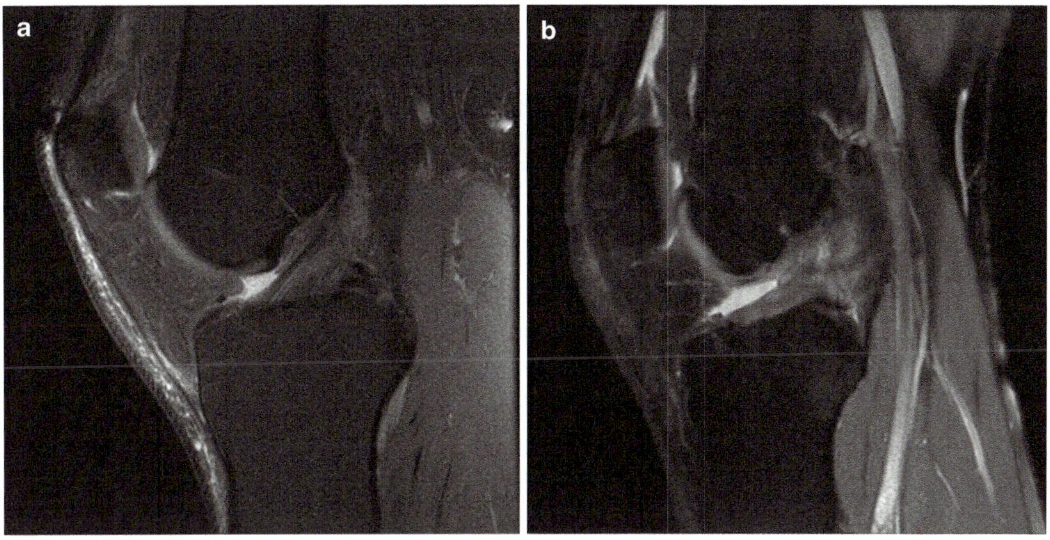

Fig. 16.3 Fat-suppressed sagittal proton-density image of the knee demonstrating (**a**) a normal and (**b**) ruptured anterior cruciate ligament

Ultrasound

Musculoskeletal ultrasound (US) imaging is widely used for a variety of conditions. Compared with MRI, US is less expensive and more patient-friendly, avoiding the claustrophobia sometimes experienced by patients during MR examination. Its real-time and dynamic nature can direct examiners towards the symptomatic area, allowing them to focus on the relevant abnormality. The dynamic capability allows examiners to observe pathologic movements in tendons, bursae or joints with continuous patient feedback. MR and US are often used as complementary imaging modalities to help solve the problem.

However, the US is operator dependent and the US images are often difficult to interpret for others. MR and US are often used as complementary imaging modalities to help interpretation. Another limitation of the US is the dependence of the quality of images on the body habitus. It is not particularly useful in obese patients because of poor beam penetration of high-frequency probes.

Ultrasound offers advantages over CT when used for interventions because it does not use ionising radiation or contrast. US guidance decreases the inaccuracy rate of blind injections into the knee or shoulder joint, which can approach 30% in some instances.

Common Applications

Ultrasound is commonly used to evaluate tendon pathology, especially the rotator cuff tendons. Many studies have been performed on this subject and sensitivity can approach 100% for full-thickness tears, with lower sensitivity for partial-thickness tears. The Achilles tendon is another well-defined structure imaged with diagnostic US. Dynamic US imaging allows small tendon tears become more apparent. This technique can also be used to detect biceps, peroneal or posterior tibialis tendon subluxation.

Diagnostic US can also be used for imaging ligaments such as the ulnar collateral ligament of the elbow; the anterior talofibular and calcaneofibular ligaments of the ankle; and the medial and lateral collateral ligaments of the knee. When combined with dynamic stress imaging, US is a particularly useful modality to identify medial collateral ligament tears or laxity. It is not good for detecting intra-articular knee pathology such as meniscal or cruciate ligaments as ultrasound doesn't travel through bone.

Ultrasound is also an excellent imaging modality for detecting small joint effusions and to guide interventions such as joint aspiration or injection. Doppler US can detect increased blood flow in the synovium and therefore, diagnose active synovitis of inflammatory or infectious aetiology. US is useful for early detection of synovitis or erosion in inflammatory arthropathy such as rheumatoid arthritis, resulting in early treatment and disease modification.

Labral tears of the shoulder and hip are best diagnosed with MRI, but diagnostic US can be used if the defect extends to the peripheral margin of the joint and if it is associated with ganglion formation. The portability, ease of use and high spatial resolution of the US make it an excellent tool for imaging muscular injuries and superficial nerves.

Another vital utility of ultrasound in the musculoskeletal field is its ability to diagnose and differentiate soft tissue lumps and tumours. It is usually the first investigation of choice to ascertain the nature of any soft tissue lump as it can easily diagnose benign lumps such as lipomas and ganglion cysts. It is also useful to diagnose and guide further management in more malignant looking soft tissue lesions such as sarcomas.

Common applications of US in musculoskeletal disorders are:

- Shoulder—rotator cuff pathology.
- Assessment of soft tissue lumps and bumps.
- Tendinosis or tenosynovitis, especially around the ankle and wrist (Fig. 16.4).
- Infection—assessment of joint effusion, soft tissue collection.
- Guided injections.
- Guided biopsy or drainage.

Radioisotope Bone Scan

Radioisotope bone scanning involves the use of radiopharmaceuticals, the most common of which is 99m-Technetium (99m-Tc) attached to a tracer, methylene diphosphonate (MDP). When injected intravenously, this tracer is 'taken up' preferentially by the bone and incorporated into the surface of its calcium hydroxyapatite crystals of the bone to produce insoluble calcium phosphate complexes. The 99mTc emits Gamma rays, which is then detected by the Gamma Camera and computer projects it as a 'hot spot'.

An isotope bone scan thus can provide 'functional' imaging, as the complexes accumulate in areas with increased blood flow or increased bone turnover. Osteoblastic lesions are apparent due to increased bone turnover, while lytic lesions are usually visible due to the surrounding rim of reactive bone. Bone uptake is demonstrated on whole-body views and spot views of the region of interest acquired 2–4 h after injection (delayed phase). In a three-phase bone scan, images are obtained not only in the delayed phase (showing osteoblastic activity), but also in the 'blood flow' (early) and 'blood pool' (intermediate) phases. The three-phase bone scan is commonly used to investigate bone infection, trauma and reflex

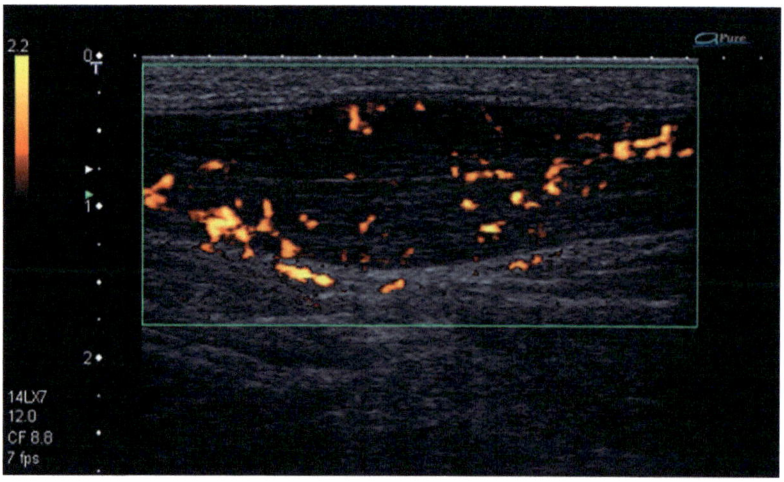

Fig. 16.4 An ultrasound image demonstrates Achilles tendinosis

sympathetic dystrophy. The first (blood flow) phase involves a dynamic flow study, with images obtained every 2–3 s for 30 s following injection. Imaging in this phase indicates the vascularity of the lesion. The second phase (blood pool) is obtained at 5 min, and reflects extracellular fluid uptake within the bone due to changes in capillary permeability.

A positive bone scan in all three phases can suggest an acute lesion of less than 4 weeks with an increased blood flow, whereas a scan positive in only delayed images suggests an abnormality with increased osteoblastic activity. Tc scans help differentiate septic from aseptic loosening in joint replacements. In septic loosening, there is increased uptake in all three phases, while aseptic loosening will lead to increased uptake predominantly in the delayed phase.

SPECT and SPECT/CT

Conventional planar bone scan imaging provides a two-dimensional projection of a 3D source of activity. SPECT, however, which involves taking projection images at many angles in a tomographic fashion, and is, therefore, able to accurately project the source of activity. This method allows removing the activity from overlying or underlying tissues, which would otherwise obscure the image at the required depth of interest.

SPECT scanning improves visualisation and localisation of the uptake (hot spot). It is particularly useful for accurately visualising the area of uptake in more complex anatomical areas such as the posterior elements of vertebrae.

Hybrid imaging combines the functional images obtained with an isotope scan with the anatomical information obtained from CT, thereby overcoming the drawbacks of both modalities. SPECT with CT correlation (SPECT-CT), for example, maybe useful in assessing anterior knee pain, and can demonstrate patellofemoral osteoarthritic change, patellar enthesopathy or osteochondral bone bruising. In assessing painful scoliosis, it can demonstrate the precise location of osteoblastoma.

Common causes of 'hot spots' on a bone scan are as follows:

- Trauma and stress fractures.
- Previous arthroplasty—can be positive for up to 3 years.
- Malignant tumours and metastasis.
- Arthritis.
- Loosening in hip and knee prosthesis
- Infections—osteomyelitis.
- Paget's disease.
- Fibrous dysplasia.
- Benign tumours.
- Bone infarction.
- Soft tissue uptake due to an infection, inflammation or tumour.

Common Applications

In patients with bone tumours/malignancy, bone scanning is used to detect metastasis for staging, assess areas of bone pain with negative radiographs, determine response to treatment, assess the ribs and sternum (which are difficult to assess with plain radiographs) and detect other sites of involvement (Fig. 16.5).

The term 'super scan' indicates widespread skeletal disease and is often seen in diffuse metastatic bone disease or metabolic bone disease. This results in diffuse and 'uniform' increased isotope uptake in the skeleton, rather than localised hot spots, and can give a false impression of normal skeletal uptake. The kidneys and bladder, which are normally visualised in bone scans due to isotope excretion, are not well visualised in a super scan. This is commonly termed 'absent kidney sign'.

Positron Emission Tomography

Positron emission tomography (PET) is another form of highly sensitive metabolic imaging in nuclear medicine. It depends on the detection of gamma rays emitted when the positron emitted by the radionuclide tracer collides with the electron indirectly by a positron-emitting radionuclide

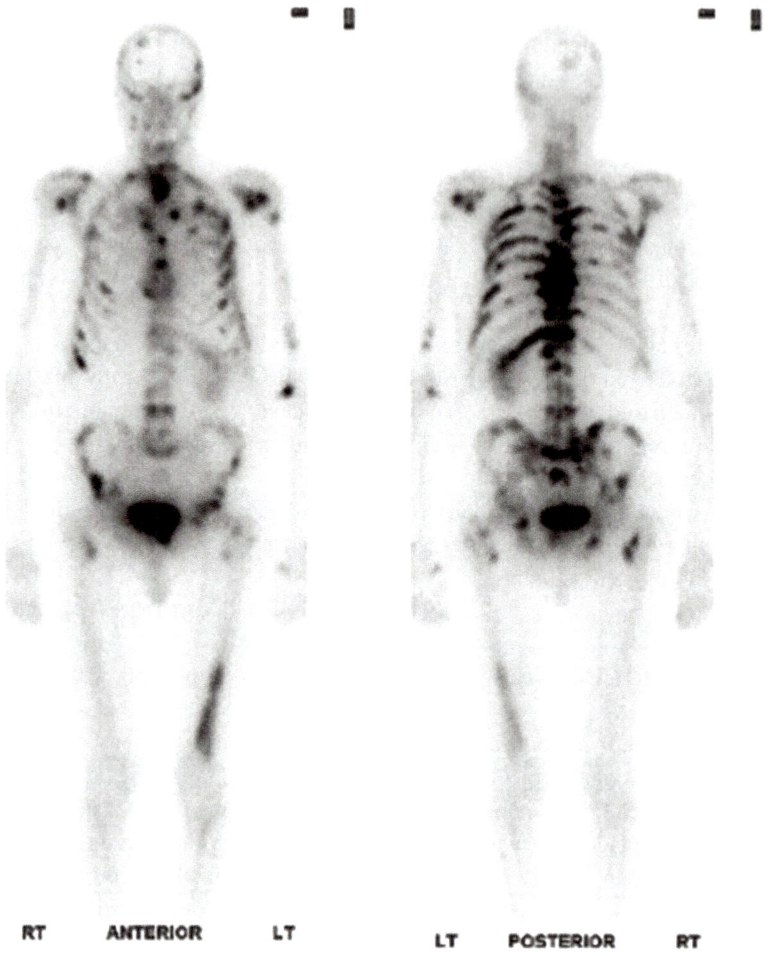

Fig. 16.5 Whole-body planar bone scan (in delayed phase) demonstrates widespread bony metastasis in a patient with prostate cancer

(tracer). The most commonly used tracer is [18F]-2-fluoro-2-deoxy-d-glucose (FDG). FDG, as a glucose analogue, is taken up by high-glucose-using metabolically active cells such as brain, heart and cancer cells. Malignant cells concentrate this radionuclide tracer and retain it until radioactive decay, which is detected by the camera. As a result, FDG-PET can be used for the diagnosis, staging and monitoring of cancers.

Common indications for PET imaging are:

- Head and neck malignancies for detection of the primary lesion.
- Differentiating scar tissue from recurrent disease.
- Monitoring response to treatment.

Clinical Examination

17

Wasim Khan and Matthew Seah

Shoulder Assessment

History

The history is an essential component of the evaluation of shoulder pain. Age, handedness, occupation and leisure activities are relevant information in the assessment of upper limb problems. The main symptoms include pain, instability, stiffness, weakness, and mechanical symptoms such as catching or locking of the joint. Associated medical problems may influence treatment decisions.

Distinguishing between an acute and a chronic problem is helpful in diagnosis. For example, a history of acute trauma to the shoulder with the arm abducted and externally rotated strongly suggests shoulder subluxation or dislocation and possible glenoid labral injury. In contrast, chronic pain and loss of passive range of motion may be associated with frozen shoulder or tears of the rotator cuff.

Pain may be localised or diffuse. Night pain is a feature of frozen shoulder, cuff tears, glenohumeral arthritis, infection and tumours. Sudden severe pain may point to resolving calcific tendonitis or acute brachial neuritis (Parsonage Turner syndrome). A painful arc in 60–120° abduction indicates impingement.

For patients presenting with instability of the shoulder, it is important to obtain a comprehensive history regarding the nature of the shoulder injury. For first-time dislocators, patients may describe a single traumatic event involving the shoulder that resulted in immediate symptoms. Patients with recurrent instability may complain of several dislocation/subluxation events or limitations/apprehension due to the history of recurrent instability events. Thus, additional information regarding the mechanism of injury, such as the nature of the injury, the direction of force placed on the shoulder, and the direction of perceived instability must be elucidated in order to accurately characterize shoulder instability.

It is important to note whether or not the patient required reduction in the Emergency Department (or other hospital setting), or if it was successfully self-reduced, or reduced in the field. Patients may be able to detail if the injury was a dislocation or a subluxation. The number of recurrences should be assessed as well. Finally, the level of activity required to cause instability is important. This will provide information regarding the severity of the soft tissue or bony damage in the shoulder. Clinicians should also determine if the shoulder instability has a voluntary component, as these patients often demonstrate poor response to surgical stabilization.

W. Khan (✉) · M. Seah
Addenbrooke's Hospital, Cambridge, UK
e-mail: wasimkhan@doctors.org.uk;
ms2340@cam.ac.uk

S. Agarwal (ed.), *Current Orthopaedic Practice*, https://doi.org/10.1007/978-3-030-78529-1_17

Examination

Examination of the shoulder involves inspection, palpation, assessment of range of motion, and the performance of various special maneuvers depending on the presenting complaint.

Inspection

The shoulders are fully exposed to allow visualization of the anterior, posterior, and lateral aspects. Inspect the skin for ecchymosis and for rash and redness, which may suggest cellulitis. The presence of a scar may indicate previous trauma or surgery. Atrophy of the musculature may be the result of a chronic tear of the rotator cuff or of neurologic impairment. The acromioclavicular joint should also be visualized. Elevation of the clavicle may represent an acromioclavicular injury.

Palpation

Begin with palpation of the sternoclavicular joint and assess for tenderness, deformity, or increased movement in the affected shoulder as compared with the unaffected shoulder.

Continue to palpate, moving from the proximal to the distal clavicle and paying particular attention to the acromioclavicular joint and the acromioclavicular ligament. Acute tenderness in this region may represent an acromioclavicular sprain or acromioclavicular joint separation. In patients with a history of chronic pain, tenderness in this region may suggest osteoarthritis.

Next, palpate the acromion and the subacromial space. Tenderness in this region may suggest subacromial impingement or injury of the supraspinatus tendon. Subacromial impingement is caused by compression of the rotator cuff, the subacromial bursa, and other soft-tissue structures between the humeral head and the undersurface of the acromion.

Palpate the biceps tendon and the muscle in the bicipital groove. Tenderness may indicate bicipital tendinopathy. Again, note any differences between the affected and unaffected shoulders. In bicipital tendinopathy, the patient may have tenderness in both shoulders. Pain may increase on palpation of the affected shoulder if bicipital tendinopathy is present.

Range of Motion

Evaluate the range of motion in forward flexion, abduction, external rotation, and internal rotation. If the patient has full pain-free active range of motion, there is no need to assess the passive range of motion. However, if the patient does not have full range of motion, assistance should be provided. Loss of active and passive ranges of motion in all planes, especially during external rotation, is characteristic of adhesive capsulitis, but it may also represent advanced osteoarthritis of the glenohumeral joint.

The sensation of pain on active abduction of the arm between 60 and 100° may be associated with a rotator cuff injury. Pain in this region during both active and passive abduction suggests subacromial impingement.

Range of motion can be evaluated individually or in compound movements. For example, the Apley scratch test is another useful maneuver to assess shoulder range of motion. Abduction and external rotation are measured by having the patient reach behind their head and touching the superior aspect of the opposite scapula. Conversely, internal rotation and adduction of the shoulder can be examined by having the patient reach behind their back and touching the inferior aspect of the opposite scapula.

Assessment of the Rotator Cuff

The muscles of the rotator cuff are the supraspinatus, infraspinatus, teres minor, and subscapularis. The supraspinatus muscle allows abduction of the arm. Test its function using the empty-can test. Have the patient abduct the arms to 90°, with palms facing the floor. Then ask the patient to rotate the arms forward, so the thumbs point downward — as if the patient were emptying a can of liquid. Apply downward pressure on the arms, and ask the patient to resist the pressure. Weakness in the affected shoulder as compared with the unaffected shoulder may indicate injury of the supraspinatus, possibly caused by overuse, tendinopathy, or a tear.

The infraspinatus and teres minor each contribute to external rotation of the arm. These muscles can be tested simultaneously. Have the patient flex the elbow to 90°, with the upper arm positioned at the patient's side. As you apply resistance, ask the patient to rotate the arm outward. Weakness in the affected shoulder may indicate a tear or tendinopathy in the infraspinatus or teres minor. It is important to stabilize the patient's elbow with your hand during this examination. Weakness or pain in the affected shoulder suggests injury of the infraspinatus.

The subscapularis allows internal rotation of the shoulder. Test this muscle with the Gerber's lift off test. Place the patient's hand on the patient's lower back and ask him or her to rotate the shoulder inward, against resistance. Inability to lift the hand off the back may indicate a tear or tendinopathy in the subscapularis.

Subacromial Impingement

Inflammation of the subacromial bursa can lead to pain and limited range of motion, especially when the patient is performing overhead maneuvers. The Hawkins–Kennedy test is used to assess for subacromial impingement. Have the patient flex the elbow to 90°. Elevate the patient's shoulder to a 90°, forward-flexed position and then internally rotate the arm. Pain with this maneuver may indicate subacromial impingement.

An additional test for subacromial impingement is Neer's test. To perform this test, rotate the patient's arm internally and raise (forward flex) it. If the maneuver is painful, the test is positive and may indicate subacromial bursitis.

Assessment of the Acromioclavicular Joint

The cross-body adduction test, also known as the crossover test, is used to evaluate the acromioclavicular joint. Adduct the patient's arm across the body. Pain in the region of the acromioclavicular joint may indicate sprain, separation, or osteoarthritis.

Testing for Instability

To test for anterior shoulder instability, place the patient in the supine position. Abduct the patient's arm to 90° and then flex the elbow to 90°. Apply pressure to externally rotate the shoulder further. If this maneuver induces a sense of instability or fear (or the appearance of apprehension), the test is considered to be positive. Next, apply pressure to the shoulder, pressing in a posterior direction. If this force alleviates symptoms, then the relocation test is positive and constitutes another indication of shoulder instability. In a patient with suspected anterior shoulder instability, perform this test gently, and limit the force applied so as not to dislocate the shoulder while conducting the test.

Assessment of the Biceps

Inflammation of the tendon of the long head of the biceps can cause anterior shoulder pain. Use Speed's test to assess the biceps by extending the patient's elbow, supinating the forearm, and then flexing the arm forward while applying opposing force. If the patient has pain in response to this maneuver, bicipital tendinopathy may be the cause. The Yergason's test can also be done to evaluate the biceps. Flex the patient's elbow to 90° and supinate the forearm against resistance. Pain with this maneuver suggests bicipital tendinopathy.

Provocative tests provide a more focused evaluation for specific problems and are typically performed after the history and general examination have been completed. Once the location, quality, radiation, and aggravating and relieving factors of the shoulder pain have been established, the possibility of referred pain should be excluded. Neck pain and radicular pain extending below the elbow are often subtle signs of a cervical spine disorder that is mistaken for a shoulder problem.

Tests for evaluation of painful shoulder are summarised in Table 17.1 and tests for shoulder instability are summarised in Table 17.2.

Table 17.1 Tests for evaluation of painful shoulder

Test	Scope of test	Technique	Positive
Pain provocation tests			
Cross-body adduction	ACJ pathology	Arm in 90° elevation, adduction of elevated arm toward contralateral shoulder	Pain during adduction
Neer	Subacromial impingement	Elbow in extension, internal rotation by examiner, then passive elevation by examiner while stabilizing scapula	Pain during passive abduction
Painful arc	Subacromial Impingement	Examiner brings shoulder in full abduction	Pain between 60° and 120° abduction
Hawkins	Subacromial impingement	Arm in 90° elevation, elbow in 90° flexion, examiner stabilizes elbow and brings arm into internal rotation	Pain during internal rotation
Yocum	Subacromial impingement	Elbow in flexion, hand on contralateral shoulder, patient elevates elbow without raising ipsilateral shoulder	Pain while elevating elbow
Yergason	Bicipital tendonitis	Arm by the side and elbow to 90°. The patient starts in full pronation and is asked to supinate against resistance	Pain in the bicipital groove
Speed	LHB or biceps/labral complex pathology	Elbow is flexed to 30° with supination and the patient is asked to flex against resistance	Pain in the bicipital groove
Strength tests			
Drop arm	Supraspinatus muscle	Arm in 90° abduction, slow descent of arm	Immediate drop of arm accompanied by pain
Dropping sign	Infraspinatus muscle	Shoulder in 90° abduction, elbow in 90° flexion, full external rotation by examiner	Unable to maintain position of external rotation
Gerber (lift-off test)	Subscapularis muscle	Hand of affected arm on back, elbow in 90° flexion, patient is asked to lift hand off the back	Unable to lift arm toward posterior direction
Composite test for pain or weakness			
External rotation resistance	Infraspinatus muscle	Elbow in 90° flexion, examiner applies pressure proximal to wrist against external rotation	Pain or muscle weakness on application of pressure
Full can	Supraspinatus muscle	Elbow in extension, arms in 90° abduction, 30° horizontal adduction, and 45° external rotation, thumb points upward, patient resists downward pressure (proximal from elbow) from examiner	Pain or muscle weakness while resisting downward pressure
Empty can (Jobe)	Supraspinatus muscle	Arm in 90° abduction, 30° horizontal adduction, and 90° internal rotation, elbow extended, thumb pointing toward floor, patient resists downward pressure (proximal from elbow) from examiner	Pain or muscle weakness or while resisting downward pressure

Table 17.2 Summary of shoulder tests for instability

Test	Patient position	Procedure	Inference
Anterior instability			
Drawer	Sitting	Stand behind patient Push humeral head in centre of glenoid Push forwards and backwards Normally—slight anterior translation is possible as well as about half of head diameter posterior translation	Anterior instability
Sulcus	Sitting or standing	Pull hand down in ER	Sulcus below acromion—inferior instability
Fulcrum	Supine, 90° abduction	Extend and externally rotate arm (Apprehension test) Push back on head—more ER possible (Relocation test) Push head anteriorly—less ER possible (Augmentation test)	Anterior instability
Crank or apprehension test	Sitting	90° abduction, ER causes apprehension Test in 45° abduction—for middle glenohumeral ligament	Anterior instability
Posterior instability			
Jerk test	Sitting	IR, flex to 90°, axially load humerus and move arm horizontally	Jerk indicates posterior instability
Push–pull	Supine	90° abduction, 30° flexion Pull wrist up and push proximal humerus down	Apprehension indicates posterior instability

Tests for Anterior and Posterior Instability

Elbow Assessment

History

Age, handedness, occupation and level of function are relevant information in the assessment of the patient who presents with upper limb pathology. It is also important to exclude referred pain from proximal pathology: the lateral aspect of the elbow is formed by the C5 dermatome, the anterior aspect by C6, the inner aspect by T1–T2 and posteriorly by C7. Other pathologies to consider include instability, tendinopathy, nerve entrapment/compression syndromes, and trauma.

Examination

Inspection

The patient should be examined from the front for the carrying angle, and from the side to look for a flexion deformity. Inspection may reveal diffuse or local swelling: arthritis causes a more generalized effusion, whereas other lesions (bursitis and tendinitis) may give rise to more localized swelling. There may also be associated findings such as scars, skin erythema, muscular atrophy, psoriatic plaques or rheumatoid nodules.

Palpation

Palpation of the elbow joint begins at the lateral supracondylar ridge which is readily palpable. Examination should extend down the ridge to the lateral epicondyle, common extensor origin and lateral collateral ligament.

The radio-capitellar joint line should be palpated as tenderness here may indicate an articular injury. The sulcus formed by the infra-condylar recess between the lateral condyle and radial head may be less apparent in the presence of a joint effusion. The radial head should also be examined in relation to the capitellum in all positions of the elbow.

Table 17.3 Features of common elbow pathologies

Diagnosis	Tests
Lateral epicondylitis	Resisted wrist extension causes pain locally (lateral epicondyle) Resisted middle-finger extension causes pain locally Passive volar flexion of the wrist with the elbow extended and pronated elicits pain locally Weak pinch grip between the thumb and middle finger Local anaesthetic injection can help the diagnosis
Medial epicondylitis	Tenderness at the medial epicondyle Pain on resisted wrist flexion Passive extension of the wrist and elbow causes pain Clenching the fist causes pain Local anaesthetic injection helps to relieve the symptoms
Pronator syndrome	Causes diffuse forearm pain; sensory median nerve changes may be present Tinel's sign is positive at the elbow for the median nerve Resisted pronation for 60 s reproduces pain Resisted elbow flexion and supination reproduces pain Resisted middle finger flexion at the proximal interphalangeal joint (PIPJ) reproduces pain
Impingement	Impingement can be present in the posterior or anterior compartment of the elbow Osteophytic changes at the tip of the olecranon suggest posterior impingement Pain may occur on hyperextension in the fully extended elbow Anterior impingement is due to osteophytes on the coronoid or radial head
Varus instability	Flex elbow to 30°, with full IR at the shoulder. Varus stress is applied and the gap between the capitellum and the radial head is assessed
Valgus instability	Flex the elbow to 30°, hold the patient's forearm between the arm and the trunk and apply valgus force. The milking test was described by O'Brien—fully flex the elbow, hold the thumb so that the forearm is fully supinated and apply valgus force to the elbow
Posterolateral rotatory instability (LCL damage)	A lateral pivot shift test is performed in the supine position, with the shoulder and elbow flexed to 90°. A valgus and axial force is applied to the elbow and the elbow is slowly extended. This causes apprehension and at 40°, the ulna reduces with a clunk. The clunk may not always be evident, but the test is positive if the patient feels apprehension
Posterolateral rotatory draw test	The elbow is flexed to 90° and supinated. AP Anteroposterior translation force is applied and instability assessed. The test is repeated in 30° flexion

Movements

Functionally important movements such as the patient being able to reach behind their head or bring their hand to their mouth should be evaluated as part of a routine screening examination.

The passive movements (flexion/extension/supination/pronation) are used to examine the inert structures: the joint, the capsule, the capsular ligaments and the bursae. It is also clear that, by passively testing the elbow, one also indirectly stretches or pinches muscular and tendinous structures. The range of motion is ascertained and the feeling of the end point noted.

In passive flexion of the elbow, the normal end-feel is one of tissue approximation as the muscles of the forearm come in contact with the brachial muscles at an angle of about 140°. The normal end-feel in passive extension is hard and bony, caused by the olecranon coming into contact with the posterior aspect of the humerus, and by tightening of the anterior capsule of the joint. As the forearm now lies in line with the upper arm, the angle of extension is 0°. This is increased in hyper-extension of the elbow. Full passive supination is approximately 85° from the mid-prone position. Together with passive pronation, this movement tests the integrity of the upper radioulnar joint. Pain at the end of the range may also be a localizing sign in tendinitis of the insertion of the bicipital tendon on to the radial tuberosity, because of pinching of the tendon between the radial tuberosity and the ulna.

Clinical features of common elbow pathologies are summarised in Table 17.3.

Wrist Assessment

History

A focused history will guide subsequent clinical examination. Hand dominance, occupation, previous injuries and level of function should be asked about, and attention should be paid to any pain, stiffness, weakness or clicking. The location of the pain is a strong guide towards the diagnosis, and this helps focus the clinical examination.

Examination

Inspection

Look at the hand and wrist, paying particular attention to skin condition, swelling (e.g. over ECU tendon, first extensor compartment), masses (e.g. ganglion, rheumatoid nodules) muscle atrophy (e.g. of the thenar eminence) and deformity (e.g. Z thumb). Diagnoses such as rheumatoid arthritis or a Madelung deformity should be obvious at this stage of the examination.

Palpation

Tenderness, instability, crepitus, and clicking are elicited by palpation. It is important to consider the dorsal and volar surface anatomy during palpation. For example, De Quervain's tenosynovitis manifests as pain/swelling over the first dorsal compartment; intersection syndrome as tenderness between the first and second compartments. Pulses of the radial and ulnar artery are palpated and sensation in the distribution of the median, ulnar, and superficial radial nerves is checked.

Movements

The wrist has multiple points of articulation, which produce a variety of movements including flexion, extension, radial and ulnar deviation, pronation and supination which should be compared with the contralateral side. Flexion and extension originate from the radiocarpal and midcarpal joints and loss of this motion suggests pathology in these joints. Supination and pronation occur at the distal radioulnar joint and pathology at this joint leads to decreased rotation. In addition to assessing movements in isolation, a useful measure of combined functional motion is the 'dart throwing motion'.

It is important to remember that proximal pathology may present with hand symptoms. An examination of the cervical spine, shoulder or elbow should be carried out if required. A summary of wrist examination is presented in Table 17.4.

Hand Assessment

History

The patient's age, hand dominance and occupation are elicited as part of the clinical history. If the patient has had an injury, the exact mechanism as well as prior treatments are recorded. Prior surgical procedures, infections, medications, and therapy also are noted. After this background information is obtained, the patient is questioned specifically regarding the involved hand and extremity, including a pain interview. Open-ended questions about the present signs and symptoms are included to determine what the patient is not able to do now that he or she could do before the injury or what brought the patient to the surgeon or therapist. Questions related to the history of present illness allow the clinician to develop a hypothesis about the level of irritability. Low irritability is defined as minimal to no pain at rest, transient pain with movement, and symptoms that are not easily provoked. Highly irritable conditions present with resting pain, higher pain levels with activity, and decreased mobility.

As with other systems, the patient's social history should be obtained. What is his support system? How well do the patient and his family understand the injury and required care? What are his interests? The patient's economic status may also influence ability to comply with therapy and follow-up care. If the patient is working, information should be gathered about his job description, physical demands, or essential functions, and the last date worked even if the injury

Table 17.4 Special tests for wrist examination

Test	Procedure	Notes
Finkelstein test	Adduction of the thumb and ulnar deviation of the wrist causes pain	De Quervain's tenosynovitis
Scapholunate instability		
Kirk Watson	Place fingers dorsally over the scapholunate ligament and thumb on the scaphoid tubercle on the volar aspect. Apply pressure on the tubercle and move wrist from ulnar to radial deviation The scaphoid subluxes dorsally as the thumb prevents it from flexing	
Scaphoid thrust test	In the same position as Kirk Watson, pressure is applied to the scaphoid tubercle in slight radial deviation and dorsal dislocation of the scaphoid is palpated	
Scaphoid lift	lunate is stabilised and the scaphoid is lifted volar and dorsally	
Midcarpal instability		
Radiocarpal and midcarpal drawer test	Holds forearm with one hand and the metacarpals with other hand. Distraction and then volar/dorsal translating force is applied. Then the distal hand is moved proximally to the proximal carpal row and the test is repeated	Not very specific
Midcarpal shift test	The forearm is stabilized and the examiner places a thumb over the capitate dorsally and pushes down, along with ulnar deviation of the wrist	If a clunk felt as wrist ulnar deviates, the test is a positive test
Pivot shift pattern	The elbow is placed on a firm surface and with the forearm fully supinated. Pressure is applied on the dorsoulnar aspect of the carpus and the wrist is ulnar deviated	A normal wrist goes into less supination as the capitate engages the lunate
Lunotriquetral instability		
Reagan ballottement test	The lunate is fixed between the thumb and index finger of one hand, and the triquetrum is held between the thumb and index finger of the other hand and displaced dorsally and volarly	Pain indicates a positive test
Shear test	The examiner places a thumb on the dorsum of the lunate and pushes pisiform from the volar side	Pain on pressing indicates lunotriquetral instability
Compression test	The examiner presses over the ulnar snuff box between the extensor carpi ulnaris (ECU) and the flexor carpi ulnaris distal to the ulnar styloid	This loads the triquetrohamate and triquetrolunate joints eliciting pain
Pisotriquetral arthritis		
Grind test	The pisiform is compressed in a radial and ulnar direction between the thumb and index finger	Pain in the local area is a positive test
Distal radioulnar joint		
Compression test	Supination and pronation while compressing the distal radioulnar joint	Pain indicates DRUJ pathology
Piano key test	The forearm is stabilised and pressure applied over the distal ulna	Increased excursion indicates dorsal subluxation (instability)
Radioulnar drawer test	The radius is stabilised, and the ulna held between the thumb and index finger and moved dorsally and volarly	Comparison is made with the other side

is not work-related. This information may indicate the presence of risk factors associated with the injury. Therapists and surgeons can use these data to outline a plan of care that incorporates appropriate modified-duty work, if available, and the use of work-oriented tasks in the clinic to keep the patient on track to return to full duty.

Examination

Inspection and Palpation

Observations include how patients position or use their hands and the digital cascade or resting posture of the hand. Skin color and the presence of any swelling should be noted and compared with the opposite extremity.

Scars, which indicate previous surgery or trauma, should be described. Chronic skin lesions, ulcerations, non-healing wounds, or swelling should also be noted. Inspection of the nail complex and paronychium can reveal pitting, spots, or brittle nail plates. These findings may indicate systemic disease, nutritional deficiencies, or chronic nail infections.

Movements

Have patients flex their fingers and oppose the thumb, observing for normal range of motion, abnormal movements, rotational deformity, or scissoring of the digits with flexion, and any limitation of full flexion.

Both extrinsic and intrinsic motor function of the hand should be assessed. Abnormalities in the motor examination can result from musculotendinous problems or neurological conditions and these can often be differentiated by tenodesis effect. When the musculotendinous units are intact, wrist extension will produce finger flexion and wrist flexion will produce finger extension. With loss of motion from neurological injury, there will be a normal pattern of tenodesis. When this motion is altered, it indicates a disruption of the musculotendinous units. Lack of tenodesis motion can indicate transection of the tendon or musculotendinous junction.

Extrinsic Muscles

The extrinsic flexors are evaluated with the palm up and the fingers extended, testing the joint on which the tested tendon inserts.

The flexor pollicis longus (FPL) is tested by blocking the metacarpophalangeal (MCP) joint of the thumb and assessing active flexion of the interphalangeal (IP) joint.

The flexor digitorum superficialis (FDS) is assessed by blocking the flexor digitorum profundus (FDP) of adjacent digits and asking the patient to flex the proximal interphalangeal (PIP) joint. Because the FDPs have a common muscle belly (at least for middle, ring, and little fingers), blocking adjacent digits will eliminate FDP flexion and require isolated contraction of FDS. This is completed for all four fingers. Weak or absent FDS function in the little finger can be a normal variant.

The FDP is assessed by blocking flexion of the PIP joint and asking the patient to flex the distal interphalangeal (DIP) joint, isolating the only muscle that flexes the DIP joint. The extrinsic extensors are evaluated with the hand flat on the table, palm down. The tendons are palpated during the following maneuvers. The wrist extensors should be assessed with the fingers closed into the palm, whereas finger extrinsic extensors are assessed by asking the patient to extend the fingers.

The abductor pollicis longus and extensor pollicis brevis are assessed by abducting the thumb away from the hand and extending the MCP joint against resistance.

The extensor carpi radialis longus and brevis are assessed by wrist extension and radial deviation against resistance.

The extensor pollicis longus is assessed by lifting the thumb up from the table. It is possible to have IP extension through interconnections with extensor pollicis brevis, but only an intact, functioning extensor pollicis longus will allow the thumb to be elevated off the table.

Having the patient lift the fingers off the table actively and against resistance assesses the function of the extensor digitorum communis, extensor indicis, and extensor digiti quinti muscles. The intrinsic muscles flex the MCP and extend the IP joints, so the MCP joints should be extended to eliminate the intrinsic contribution to PIP extension. The ring finger is difficult to independently elevate because of the interconnection (juncturae) between adjacent tendons. The arm can be elevated from the table and strength against resistance can be evaluated. This is important because a patient may have the ability to extend a finger with a complete laceration of the tendon proximal to the juncturae as the extension occurs through the adjacent tendon.

With forearm pronation, the extensor carpi ulnaris muscle lies along the ulnar aspect of the ulna, so it is assessed by extension and ulnar deviation.

Intrinsic Muscles

This begins with flexion of the MCP joints and extending the PIP joints.

Then, the MCP joints are extended and the fingers are abducted to test dorsal interossei (D-AB). Adduction of fingers tests the palmar interossei (P-AD). Opposing the thumb to the tip of the little finger assesses thenar muscle function. Adducting the thumb against the index finger assesses the adductor pollicis muscle.

Intrinsic tightness is evaluated by comparing the amount of IP flexion with the MCP joints extended and flexed. This is known as the Bunnell test and is considered positive when PIP joint flexion is limited while the MCP joint is passively extended.

Thumb

The thumb has motion in multiple planes. Radial abduction is the motion of the thumb away from the palm in the plane of the hand and is a result of function of the abductor pollicis longus. Palmar abduction is the motion of the thumb at a 90° angle to the hand, into the plane of the palm. Opposition is a combination of palmar abduction, pronation, and flexion. This movement occurs through the thenar muscles. Circumduction is the ability to rotate the thumb in a circular manner through radial and palmar abduction.

Spine Assessment

History

Spinal pathology affects patients of all ages. A thorough history and examination of the axial skeleton and associated neurology can accurately diagnose several pathologies and direct the requesting of appropriate imaging. The generic spine examination follows the Apley approach of look, feel, move and special tests.

In the history, prior to examining a patient, you will have very likely elicited many salient points that will help guide your examination. Infection, trauma, tumour and inflammatory arthropathy can affect the spine in patients of all ages; however, the age of the patient significantly narrows the differential diagnosis (Table 17.5).

Table 17.5 Common spinal presentations at different stages of life

Children
Scoliosis
Spondylolisthesis
Infection
Adolescents
Scheuermann's kyphosis
Scoliosis
Infection
Young adult
Mechanical back pain
Prolapsed intervertebral disc
Spondylolisthesis
Fracture
Ankylosing spondylitis
Infection
Middle aged
Mechanical back pain
Osteoarthritis
Spinal stenosis
Paget's disease
Spinal metastases
Infection
Elderly
Myelopathy
Osteoarthritis
Osteoporosis
Osteomalacia
Spinal metastases
Spinal stenosis

Examination in Standing

It is vital to adequately expose the patient to assess the alignment of the spine in both the sagittal and coronal planes. When the head is centred over the pubic symphysis in stance in the coronal plane and over the femoral heads in the sagittal plane, the spine is said to be balanced. This head position, in relation to the pelvis, is optimal for normal function in life. If patients have a spinal deformity which displaces their head, they may compensate for the deformity by flexing a hip or knee to bring the head back over the optimal centre of gravity (compensating for the deformity). Typically, with increasing age, due to a loss of disc hydration and height, humans become increasingly kyphotic (head in front of femoral heads in sagittal plane). It is possible to compensate for this mechanical disadvantage by increasing lumbar lordosis and by flexing the hips and knees (compensated sagittal imbalance). When these measures are exhausted, sagittal imbalance becomes increasingly evident on inspection and results in increasing disability. Kyphosis, for example due to ankylosing spondylitis, is encountered in children; however, coronal plane deformities predominate in this age group. Idiopathic scoliosis is the most common diagnosis. Inspection may assist in assessment of the severity of the deformity, and provides the clinician with an opportunity to observe features that are associated with non-idiopathic aetiologies.

Scoliosis is a three-dimensional deformity characterized by vertebral rotation. Asking the patient to bend forward from the hips while inspecting from behind (Adam's forward bend test) gives a better appreciation of the curvatures and allows easy comparison of each side of the patient's posterior trunk. Thoracic curvatures are associated with rib prominences, while lumbar curves can result in waistline asymmetry. Shoulder balance is assessed by comparing acromial or scapular height. Asymmetry of the top of the pelvis or the 'dimples of Venus' indicates pelvic obliquity. The obliquity of the pelvis can be due either to a leg length discrepancy, or could be driven by the spinal deformity. It is important to measure true leg length formally in patients with scoliosis. If there is a leg length discrepancy, the scoliosis may be compensatory for the difference in limb length. In such patients, asking them to sit on the examination couch, or placing an appropriately sized block under the short leg will correct the scoliosis. Severe spinal deformities are associated with an inability of other portions of the spine to compensate and result in displacement of the thorax and head. This is referred to as truncal decompensation. Truncal shift is when the chest is deviated laterally beyond a line subtended up from the lateral extent of the pelvis. 'Listing' is when there is deviation of the vertebra prominens from a vertical line centred on the sacrum. To identify listing clinically, hold a piece of string with a weight attached to the free end, against the C7 spinous process. If the string does not overlie the natal cleft, listing is present.

Palpation

The spinous process of each vertebra should be palpated for tenderness, steps or masses, working from the occiput all the way down to the coccyx. Steps in the spinous processes may suggest a spondylolisthesis. The facet joints on each side of the spine are palpated and tenderness is suggestive of facet joint pathology, which is usually due to degenerative disease.

Movement

While the patient is still standing, Schoeber's test can be performed to measure lumbar flexion. Make a mark at the level of the posterior superior iliac spines or dimples of Venus and a further mark 10 cm proximal to this. On forward bending the space between the two marks should increase by at least 5 cm. The range of spinal movements should also be documented. To assess other cervical spine movement, the patient is asked to put their chin on their chest, look up to the ceiling, put their ear onto their shoulder and look over their shoulder. Rotation of the thoracic spine is best tested with the patient seated to eliminate rotation at the pelvis, with their arms held up at shoulder height so you can use them as a goniometer. In the lumbar spine ask the patient to touch their toes and slide their hand down the side of each leg and then lean backwards as far as they can.

Neurological Examination

A full neurological examination of the limbs should be undertaken and muscle power should be graded using the Medical Research Council (MRC) Grade of 0–5. Sensation should be graded as 0—absent, 1—altered, 2—normal. A useful aide memoir is the American Spinal Injury Association (ASIA) chart which details the muscles to be tested and where to assess sensation.

The full assessment is completed with examination of the perianal region for sensation and a digital rectal examination to assess resting anal tone, and voluntary anal contraction. The vascular status of the patient's upper and lower limbs should also be assessed. A summary of the special tests is given in Table 17.6.

Table 17.6 Special test for spine examination

Cervical spine	
Spurling's manoeuvre	Performed to investigate cervical radiculopathy due to disc herniation. The neck is hyperextended, flexed laterally and rotated to the side of the suspected lesion. Reproduction of symptoms suggests cervical radiculopathy
Lhermitte's sign	Pain or paraesthesia in a lower limb on flexion of the neck
Thoracic outlet syndrome	
Adson's test	Head is extended and rotated to the affected side. The radial pulse is obliterated on deep inspiration
Roos test	The shoulder is abducted to 90° and the elbows flexed to 90°. The shoulder is braced back and the patient asked to extend and flex the fingers. Reproduction of pain is a positive test
Lumbar spine	
Straight leg raise (SLR)	With the patient supine elevate the leg, with an extended knee, if positive there will be radicular pain. The pain is usually reproduced at 30–70° of hip flexion. It causes tension on the L5 and S1 nerve roots, causing the pain
Lasegue's sign	The pain felt on SLR is exacerbated by dorsiflexing the ankle. Suggestive of spinal nerve compression
Bowstring test	The pain felt on SLR is relieved by flexing the knee and then exacerbated by applying pressure to the popliteal fossa. Suggestive of spinal nerve compression
Crossover sign	Perform a SLR on the contralateral side to the pathology and the patient experiences pain down the leg that remains on the examination couch. Highly suggestive of spinal nerve compression
Femoral stretch test	Lie the patient prone and flex the knee. A positive test is when there is resultant anterior thigh pain and this is caused by tension on the L2, L3 and L4 nerve roots

Hip Assessment

History

An accurate history is important as patients may variably refer to symptoms in various anatomical locations as 'hip' pain.

With any hip joint problem, the clinician should look closely for predisposing factors. For example, femoro-acetabular impingement is a recognized cause of joint problems in young adults. Often, the cause may be multi-factorial including age, type of sport, and joint morphology. Mechanical symptoms such as locking, catching or popping may also feature in the presenting complaint and this finding may indicate an unstable lesion inside the joint, but it is important to note that many painful intra-articular problems never demonstrate this finding, and popping and clicking can occur due to many extra-articular causes, most of which are normal.

There are characteristic features of the history that often indicate a mechanical hip problem. These characteristics are helpful in localizing the hip as the source of trouble, but are not specific for the type of pathology. Straight plane activities such as straight ahead walking or even running are often well tolerated, while twisting manoeuvres such as simply turning to change direction may produce sharp pain, especially turning towards the symptomatic side which places the hip in internal rotation. Sitting may be uncomfortable, especially if the hip is placed in excessive flexion. Rising from the seated position is especially painful and the patient may experience an accompanying catch or sharp stabbing sensation. Symptoms are worse with ascending or descending stairs or other inclines. Entering and exiting a car is often difficult with accompanying pain, because the hip is in a flexed position along with twisting manoeuvres. Difficulty with shoes and socks may simply be due to pain or may reflect restricted rotational motion and more advanced hip joint involvement.

In addition, the following items must be documented: previous consultations; surgical interventions; past injuries; childhood or adolescent hip disease; ipsilateral knee disease; history of inflammatory arthritis; and risk factors for osteonecrosis. Factors related to the patient's social history that can affect the blood supply to the femoral head are reviewed and family medical history should also be taken into account. Any treatments to date should be explored. A detailed account of current functional limitations is helpful. A history of sports and recreational activities can help determine the type of injury and also guide the treatment, considering the patient's goals and expectations.

Examination

As with previous systems, the history assists the surgeon in performing an appropriately directed clinical examination.

Inspection

Inspection for hip problems starts in the standing position, followed by assessment of gait and finally examination on the examination couch.

The most important aspect of inspection is stance and gait. The patient's posture is observed in both the standing and seated position. Any splinting or protective maneuvers used to alleviate stresses on the hip joint are noted. While standing, a slightly flexed position of the involved hip and concomitantly the ipsilateral knee is common. In the seated position, slouching or listing to the uninvolved side avoids extremes of flexion. While the patient is standing, it is important to observe for abnormalities such as pelvic tilt, muscle wasting and leg length discrepancy.

In an antalgic gait, the patient has a short stance and leans to the affected side. Typically, the stance phase is shortened and hip flexion appears accentuated as extension is avoided during this phase. Varying degrees of abductor lurch may be present as the patient attempts to place the center of gravity over the hip, reducing the forces on the joint. In a short-leg gait, the centre of gravity shifts to the short side in stance. In addition, the centre of gravity drops. In a Trendelenburg gait, the patient drops his/her pelvis on the opposite side, and lurches to the same side. In a gluteus maximus gait, there is forward thrust of the pelvis and backward thrust of the trunk.

Examination in Supine Position

Limb lengths should be recorded as a routine part of the assessment, and true limb length should be measured from the anterior superior iliac spine to the medial malleolus. In the presence of limb shortening, it is important to remember Galeazzi's test (to identify if the shortening is coming from the femur or tibia). Special tests to measure shortening include Bryant's triangle (measures supratrochanteric shortening), Nelaton's line (line from the ischial tuberosity to the anterior superior iliac spine—the tip of the greater trochanter normally lies below this line) and Schoemaker's line (this is a line from the greater trochanter to anterior superior iliac spine projected onto the abdomen from both sides—the lines should normally meet in the midline above the umbilicus).

The range of motion of the hip should be accurately recorded in a consistent and reproducible fashion. While reduced range of motion itself is rarely an indication for arthroscopic intervention, decreased range is often a good indicator of the extent of disease and response to treatment.

The degree of flexion and the presence of a flexion contracture are determined by using the Thomas test. Maximal extension of the uninvolved hip stabilizes the pelvis, eliminating the contribution of pelvic tilt in recording flexion of the involved hip. Conversely, maximal flexion of the uninvolved hip locks the pelvis and allows assessment for a flexion contracture of the involved hip. Flexing the hip 90° and then internally and externally rotating the joint is an easy, reproducible method for recording rotational motion.

Knee Assessment

History

The patient's description of knee pain is helpful in focusing the differential diagnosis, including its onset (rapid or insidious), location (anterior, medial, lateral, or posterior knee), duration, severity, and quality (e.g., dull, sharp, achy). Aggravating and alleviating factors also need to be identified. If knee pain is caused by an acute injury, the surgeon needs to know whether the patient was able to continue activity or bear weight after the injury or was forced to cease activities immediately.

The patient should be asked about mechanical symptoms, such as locking, popping, or giving way of the knee. A history of locking episodes suggests a meniscal tear. A sensation of popping at the time of injury may suggest ligamentous injury. Episodes of giving way are consistent with some degree of knee instability and may indicate patellar subluxation or ligamentous rupture.

The timing and amount of joint effusion are important clues to the diagnosis. Rapid onset of a large, tense effusion suggests rupture of the anterior cruciate ligament or fracture of the tibial plateau with resultant haemarthrosis, while a slower onset (24–36 h) of a mild to moderate effusion is consistent with meniscal injury or ligamentous sprain. Recurrent knee effusion after activity is consistent with meniscal injury.

Specific details of the injury are important e.g. if the patient sustained a direct blow to the knee, if the foot was planted at the time of injury, if the patient was decelerating or stopping suddenly, if there was a twisting component to the injury, and if hyperextension occurred. Anterior force applied to the proximal tibia with the knee in flexion (e.g., when the knee hits the dashboard in an automobile accident) can cause injury to the posterior cruciate ligament. The medial collateral ligament is most commonly injured as a result of direct lateral force to the knee; this force creates a valgus load on the knee joint and can result in rupture of the medial collateral ligament. Conversely, a medial force that creates a varus load can injure the lateral collateral ligament. Non-contact forces also are an important cause of knee injury. Quick stops or turns create significant deceleration forces that can cause ligamentous injury. Sudden twisting or pivoting motions create shear forces that can injure the meniscus.

A history of knee injury or surgery is important. The patient should be asked about previous attempts to treat knee pain, including the use of medications, supporting devices, and physical therapy. The physician also should ask if the patient has a history of gout, pseudogout, rheumatoid arthritis, or other degenerative joint disease.

Examination

Examination of the knee starts in the standing position, followed by walking, and finally examination in the supine position.

On standing, the inspection is done from the front, side and back. The limb alignment, foot positioning, swelling around the knee, flexion or recurvatum deformity, varus or valgus deformity, quadriceps and calf wasting, skin changes, scars, and deformities of the feet are recorded.

The gait pattern is assessed. Specifically, antalgic gait, foot drop gait and any thrust should be noted. Thrust is accentuation of deformity (varus or valgus) on weight bearing or stance phase of gait.

Inspection in Supine Position

The painful knee should be compared with the asymptomatic knee and inspected for erythema, swelling, bruising, and discoloration. The musculature should be symmetric bilaterally. The knee is then palpated and checked for pain, warmth, and effusion.

Point tenderness should be sought, particularly at the patella, tibial tubercle, patellar tendon, quadriceps tendon, and joint lines. Moving the patient's knee through a short arc of motion helps identify the joint lines. Range of motion should be assessed by extending and flexing the knee as far as possible.

Patellofemoral tracking is assessed by observing the patella for smooth motion while the patient contracts the quadriceps muscle. The presence of crepitus should be noted during palpation of the patella.

The quadriceps angle (Q angle) is determined by drawing one line from the anterior superior iliac spine through the center of the patella and a second line from the center of the patella through the tibial tuberosity. A Q angle greater than 15° is a predisposing factor for patellar subluxation (i.e., if the Q angle is increased, forceful contraction of the quadriceps muscle can cause the patella to sublux laterally).

A summary of knee ligament tests is shown in the Table 17.7.

Foot and Ankle Assessment

History

Common presenting complaints include pain, swelling, deformity, stiffness, instability and/or abnormal gait.

Ask the patient to finger point to the exact site of the maximum pain. If the pain is diffuse and not localized to one spot, try to identify the area/side of maximum discomfort. Ask about the radiation of pain and quality or nature of it (sharp, dull or burning), whether it is related to weight bearing (degenerative changes, stress fracture or Inflammatory conditions like plantar fasciitis), radiation, severity, functional disturbance, duration, pattern (constant/intermittent), aggravating factors (walking distance, walking on flat or uneven floor; going up and down the stairs; relation with shoes), and any alleviating factors (rest, analgesia, preferred type of foot wear). Common pathologies related to sites of pain are presented in a table below.

The chronicity and the severity of the pain can help to establish whether there is an element of central sensitization where by the patient becomes more sensitive and experiences more pain with less provocation. Factors like sleep deprivation and depression can drive central sensitization. Finally, it is important to clarify what is the patients' belief about their foot pain.

Enquire about the duration and when the patient or their family member first noticed the deformity, which area it involves, is it progressing, and whether it associated with other symptoms (for example, skin ulcer, pain, recurrent infection, rapid wear of shoes, or cosmetic).

It is important to establish whether swelling, if present, is localized to one area or the whole leg or ankle, whether it is unilateral or bilateral, associated with activities, as well as the frequency and the duration of swelling. Generalized bilateral swelling that involves the whole foot and ankle is usually related to more systematic pathology, such as cardiac or renal problems. Swelling which includes the area only around the ankle joint may be related to the tibio-talar joint (for example, degenerative changes or inflammatory arthropathy). On other hand, localized swelling is more likely to result from a specific local pathology. As an example, swelling anterior to the distal fibula may indicate chronic injury of the anterior tibiofibular ligament (ATFL) and swelling posterior to the distal fibula may indicate peroneal tendon pathology. Acute painful or painless swelling with or without the deformity of the mid foot could result from Charcot neuropathy.

In a patient with ankle instability, it is important to determine when the first episode of instability or sprain occurred, how often it happens and what can precipitate it. History of trauma with details of immediate symptoms and treatment, surgery, injections or infection should be identified.

It is important to look out for 'red flags' symptoms such as night sweating, temperature or weight loss, which may be related to an infection or neoplasm. Neurological symptoms like numbness, limb weaknesses or burning sensation are usually related either to spinal problem or peripheral neuropathy. Table 17.8 shows a quick diagnosis summary of common foot pathologies.

Table 17.7 Knee examination tests.

Test	Technique	Positive result	Comments
Anterior cruciate ligament			
Lachman	Hold knee in 15–30° of flexion Attempt to pull tibia forwards while holding femur stationary with other hand	Anterior laxity (with/without firm end point)	Most sensitive test for ACL injury
Anterior drawer	Flex hip to 45° and knee to 90° Stabilise foot with pressure directed towards exam table Hold proximal end of the tibia and pull forward	Increased laxity suggests ACL injury	
Rotary drawer	As above with external or internal rotation		An anterior drawer that is increased in 30° ER and decreased in 15° IR indicates anteromedial instability. An anterior drawer that is increased in 15° ER and decreased in 30° IR indicates anterolateral instability
Pivot shift	Valgus force and IR is applied to the knee, and the knee is flexed from an extended position	If the tibia reduces back on flexing around 20–30°, this indicates ACL deficiency	The prerequisites for a pivot shift test are an intact MCL, intact ITB and the knee not locked (full extension possible). The ITB passes posteriorly as the knee flexes, causing the tibia to reduce in flexion. Instability is increased if the hip is abducted as this relaxes the ITB
Posterior cruciate ligament			
Posterior sag	The patient flexes both hips and both knees to 90°. Normally, the tibial plateau is 1 cm anterior to the femoral condyle. A comparison is made with the contralateral side	Posterior sag with regards to the femur	Assess before performing anterior drawer test
Posterior drawer	As with anterior drawer but posteriorly-directed force applied to tibia	Posterior displacement	
Medial/lateral collateral ligaments			
Varus/ valgus stress	Instability is checked in 30° flexion to relax the posterior capsule and the cruciate ligaments	Increased laxity on valgus stress indicates MCL laxity while increased laxity on varus stress indicates LCL laxity	
Meniscal injury			
McMurray	In the supine position, the knee is flexed and the examiner places an index finger and thumb on the medial and lateral joint line. The other hand applies axial load and rotation in varying flexion	Pain on the medial joint line in ER indicates medial meniscus pathology, while pain on the lateral joint line in IR indicates lateral meniscal pathology	
Posterolateral corner injury			
Reverse pivot shift	Valgus, ER stress and flex–extend knee and the tibia reduces	The lateral tibial plateau reduces from a posterior subluxed position	This indicates injury to the PCL, LCL or arcuate complex
Dial test	Patient prone and knees flexed. ER compared	ER increased at 30° flexion—posterolateral corner injury ER increased at 90° flexion—posterolateral corner plus PCL injury	

Table 17.8 Common foot pathologies

Site of pain	Common pathologies
Anterior ankle pain	Degenerative disease Impingement Ankle joint capsule injury
Medial pain (inferior to medial malleolus)	Sinus tarsi syndrome Subtalar degenerative changes Tarsal coalition of mid facet Spring ligament or deltoid ligament pathology Tibialis posterior pathology or medial impingement
Posteromedial pain	Tibialis posterior tendinitis Tarsal tunnel syndrome
Posterior pain	Achilles tendonitis Os trigonum pathology Posterior impingement
Posterolateral pain	Peroneal tendon pathology
Lateral pain	Distal fibula fracture ATFL injury Lateral impingement Sinus tarsi syndrome Subtalar pathology Calcaneal fracture malunion
Heel pain	Plantar fasciitis Calcaneal stress fracture Entrapment of first branch of lateral plantar nerve Tarsal tunnel syndrome Plantar fascia rupture
Midfoot pain	Degenerative disease/ post-traumatic arthritis Tarsal bones stress fracture Ligament injury Insertional tendinopathy of peroneal brevis
Forefoot pain	Metatarsalgia Morton neuropathy Stress fracture Freiberg disease MTPJ synovitis
Forefoot pain—big toe	Hallux valgus/rigidus Inflamed bunion Sesamoiditis/sesamoid fracture
Forefoot pain—lesser toes	Hammer toes Claw toes Bunionette

Examination

The examination begins by inspecting the patient shoes and pattern of wear, which may indicate abnormal contact of the foot with the ground. Early lateral, proximal, and mid shoe wear, indicates a supination deformity; wear on the medial border indicates a pronation deformity. Orthoses (including insoles) or walking aids should be noted.

Examination in a Standing Position

With the patient standing, assess the alignment of the lower limbs. In particular look for any excessive varus or valgus knee deformity. Inspect the alignment of the spine in case of scoliosis, and look for any pelvic tilt. Inspect for any thigh or calf muscles wasting. Look from the side for the feet arches (is there any pes cavus or pes planus), any swelling or scars. Inspect for any big toe deformity (hallux valgus, hallux valgus interphalangeus or hallux varus), lesser toes deformity (mallet toe, hammer toes, claw toes). In a normal ankle, the heel pad should not be visible on the medial side during inspection from the front. If this is visible, there is likely a degree of pes cavus. It is important to compare both sides as a false-positive sign may be caused by a very large heel pad or significant metatarsus adductus.

Inspect the ankle from the back for any bony bumps like calcaneal boss. In a normal foot you should not be able to see more than fifth and fourth toes when you look at it from behind. If there were more toes visible, this so-called "too many toes" sign can indicate an increased heel valgus angle.

Ask the patient to stand on tiptoes and both ankles should turn into varus. This indicates normal subtalar movement and, in case of flat feet, if a medial arch forms on standing on tiptoes then this is a flexible pes planus.

Observing the gait from the front and the back helps to assess the shoulder and pelvic tilt. Look for hip movements, knee movements, initial contact, three rockers, stride length and cadence. The patient should then be asked to walk on his/her tiptoes, then heels, inner borders and finally the outer borders of the feet.

Examination in a Sitting Position

By this stage, the surgeon should have a fair idea of the possible diagnoses and the examination can be directed accordingly. The patient should be sat on the examination couch, with the legs hanging loosely from the side. Raise the bed so the patient's foot is at the level of the examiner's hand, and sit on a chair opposite the patient.

Start with meticulous inspection of the sole then the rest of the foot. Look for skin discoloration, scars, ulcers, lack of hair (circulatory changes), nail health, any skin thickening (callosity), hard/soft corns and any signs of infection. Palpation should be systematic and followed by an examination of the range of movement (both active and passive).

Palpation of the ankle should be systematic, and include the:

1. Anterior joint line
2. Lateral gutter and lateral ligaments
3. Syndesmosis
4. Posterior joint line
5. Medial ligament complex
6. Medial gutter

Palpation of the hindfoot and midfoot should include the following structures:

Lateral (from Distal to Proximal)

1. Styloid process of fifth metatarsal
2. Groove in the cuboid for Peroneus Longus tendon (just posterior to 1)
3. The peroneal tubercle (a small lateral extension of the calcaneus, separating the peroneus longus & brevis tendons)
4. Sinus tarsi—soft tissue depression just anterior to the lateral malleolus. (Sinus tarsi is filled with EDB & fat pad & ligaments)
5. Talar dome (made prominent by plantarflexing ankle)

Medial (from Proximal to Distal)

1. First metatarso-cuneiform joint.
2. Navicular tubercle—most obvious bony prominence in front of medial malleolus (insertion of Tibialis Posterior tendon)
3. Head of talus—felt just behind the navicular, by everting & inverting the midfoot.
4. Sustentaculum tali—one fingerbreadth below medial malleolus (serves as an attachment for the spring ligament & supports the talus)
5. Medial malleolus.

The examination is completed with the forefoot, paying particular attention to the first metatarsal head, first MTPJ and the remainder of the metatarsal heads.

This will be followed by passive dorsiflexion: As the patient is already sitting, the knee is flexed to 90° then repeat the test with knee straight (Silfverskiold test). Keep the foot in a neutral position (0° of inversion and eversion), hold the back of the leg with one hand and use the palm of the other hand to push the sole of the examined foot. Now move the palm of the hand to the dorsum of the examined foot to produce the passive plantar flexion.

It is important to note that supination and pronation are triplanar movements. Supination is the combination of inversion, plantarflexion and adduction. Pronation is the combination of eversion, dorsiflexion and abduction.

Inversion

Place one hand over the back of the leg and use your other hand to grasp the calcaneus between index finger and thumb and use your forearm to fully dorsiflex and lock the talus in the ankle. Rotate the calcaneus in a medial direction to test for inversion and move your hand in a lateral direction to test for eversion.

Midfoot Movements

Stabilize the calcaneus and talus with one hand and use the other hand to move the foot medially to test for adduction). Move the foot laterally to test for the abduction. It is also important to examine the motion of midfoot (transverse tarsal joint) on sagittal plane (especially for patients with end stage ankle arthritis). The motion of first TMT joint should be examined as well (for patients with hallux valgus or flexible flatfoot).

Forefoot Movements (Metatarsophalangeal and Interphalangeal Joints)

You should test the movement in each joint separately. If there is any deformity, try to find whether it is correctable or not (for example, a fixed flexion deformity).

The examination of muscular function and the special tests should be the next step of the assessment (Table 17.9).

Table 17.9 Special tests for ankle examination

Test	Structure	Technique
Anterior drawer	Lateral ligament complex	The leg hangs loosely off the table. The examiner holds the patient's leg just above the ankle joint with one hand. The examiner uses the other hand to hold the ankle in plantar flexion and tries to gently to pull the ankle forward—anterior translation. Look at the skin over the anterolateral dome of the talus to watch for anterior motion of the talus with this maneuver—sulcus sign.
Inversion stress test	Stability of lateral ankle ligaments	The knee is flexed to 90°. With one hand perform the inversion stress test by pushing the calcaneus and talus into inversion while holding the leg from the medial side with the other hand. The test is positive when there is excessive inversion and/or pain.
Calf compression or "squeeze" test	Syndesmotic injury	The leg hangs loosely off the table—knee flexed. The examiner uses both hands to squeeze the midpoint of the tibia and fibula. Pain caused by this maneuver indicates syndesmotic injury.
Coleman block test	To assess the flexibility of the hindfoot, i.e., whether the cavus foot is caused by the forefoot or the hindfoot	A block is placed under the lateral border of the patients foot. The medial forefoot is allowed to hang over the side. The first metatarsal will be able to drop below the level of the block, i.e., eliminate the contribution by the first ray. With a flexible hindfoot, the heel will fall into valgus or neutral, termed forefoot-driven hindfoot varus. In case of rigid hindfoot or hindfoot-driven hindfoot varus, the heel will remain in varus and no correction will happen
Silfverskiold test	Differentiate between a tight gastrocnemius and a tight soleus muscle	The leg hangs loosely off the table—knee flexed. Dorsiflex the ankle to the maximum. Patient should then extend their knee. Repeat the ankle dorsiflexion—if there was more ankle dorsiflexion with the knee flexed then there is gastrocnemius tightness.

18 Surgical Approaches

Sanjeev Agarwal

Shoulder: Deltopectoral Approach

Indications

Indication are shoulder arthroplasty, open stabilisation, cuff repair, fixation of proximal humeral fractures.

Position of Patient

Beach chair position.

Incision

Incision starts at the coracoid process and extends distally along the deltopectoral groove (Fig. 18.1). The cephalic vein can be retracted medially or laterally. The proximal end can be curved laterally along the anterior border of the lateral third of the clavicle.

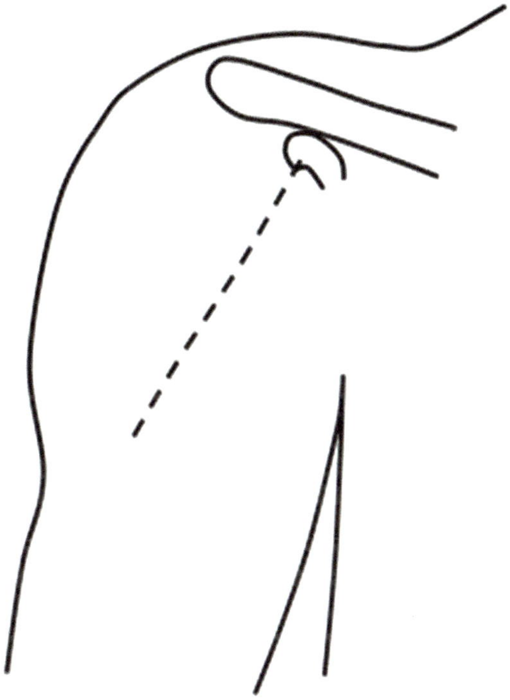

Fig. 18.1 Incision for deltopectoral approach

Plane

The plane is between the deltoid and pectoralis major. Blunt dissection between these muscles exposes the clavipectoral fascia which is divided.

The subscapularis is divided between stay sutures if a shoulder replacement is intended. Haemostasis is needed for transverse circumflex humeral vessels at the lower border of subscapularis. For fracture fixation, muscle attachments are preserved.

S. Agarwal (✉)
University Hospital of Wales, Consultant Orthopaedic Surgeon, Cardiff, UK

S. Agarwal (ed.), *Current Orthopaedic Practice*, https://doi.org/10.1007/978-3-030-78529-1_18

Extension

The deltoid can be elevated off the lateral third of the clavicle. The superficial and deep fascia of the deltoid should be preserved, and can be used to reattach the deltoid to the clavicle. The tip of the coracoid process can be removed and retracted medially with the conjoint tendon for added exposure.

Distally, the deltoid insertion on the deltoid tuberosity can be released and will reattach to bone spontaneously. The brachialis can be split to expose the humeral shaft.

Structures at Risk

The cephalic vein, musculocutaneous nerve, brachial plexus and axillary vessels are at risk. The musculocutaneous nerve is at risk of neurapraxia from retraction of the conjoint tendon, especially when the tip of the coracoid has been osteotomised.

Shoulder: Anterosuperior Approach

Indications

Indications are rotator cuff repairs and fixation of greater tuberosity fractures.

Position of Patient

Beach chair position.

Incision

Incision is from the anterolateral margin of the acromion towards the coracoid process (Fig. 18.2).

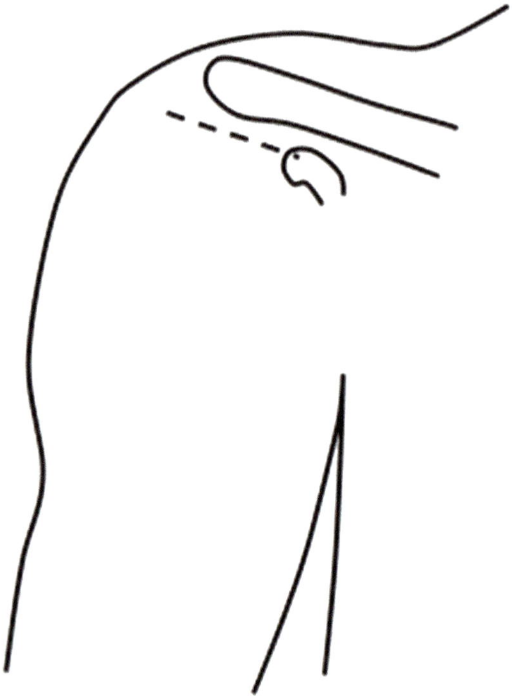

Fig. 18.2 Incision for anterior approach to shoulder

Plane

There is no true internervous plane. The deltoid fibres are split.

Structures at Risk

The axillary nerve is approximately 7 cm distal to the lateral margin of acromion.

Shoulder: Lateral Approach

Indications

Indications are rotator cuff repair, fixation of greater tuberosity fractures, and insertion of humeral intramedullary rod.

Position of Patient

Supine position with a pad under the shoulder to elevate.

Incision

Incision is from the tip of the acromion distally (Fig. 18.3).

Plane

There is no internervous plane. The deltoid fibres are split.

Structures at Risk

The axillary nerve is approximately 7 cm distal to the lateral margin of acromion.

Shoulder: Posterior Approach

Indications

Fixation of posterior rim fractures of the glenoid or recurrent posterior instability of shoulder.

Position of Patient

Lateral position.

Incision

Incision is along the spine of the scapula, extending to the posterolateral border of the acromion (Fig. 18.4).

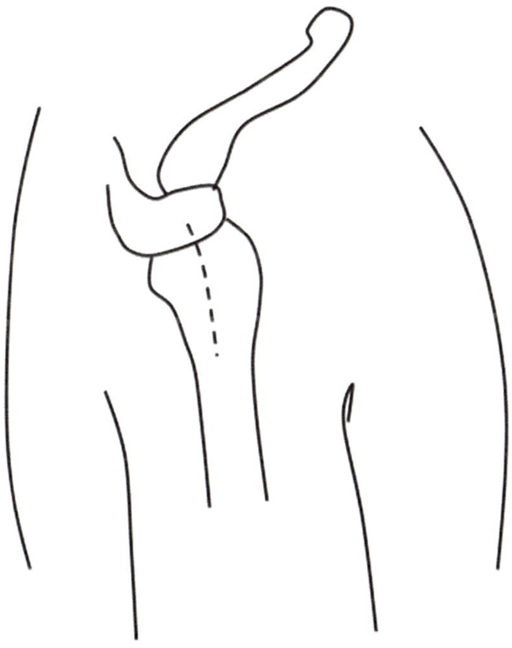

Fig. 18.3 Incision for lateral approach to shoulder

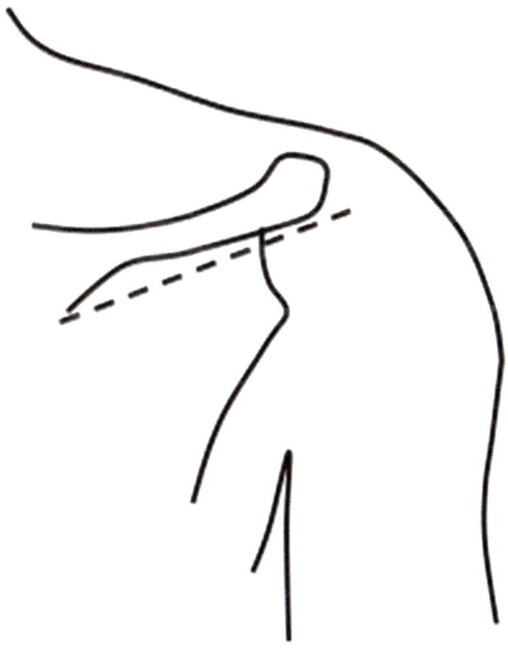

Fig. 18.4 Posterior approach to shoulder

Plane

The deltoid fibres are split or detached from the spine of the scapula. The plane is between the teres minor and infraspinatus. Teres minor is retracted inferiorly and infraspinatus is retracted superiorly.

Structures at Risk

The axillary nerve runs in the quadrilateral space inferior to the teres minor. The suprascapular nerve is at risk of traction injury through retraction of the infraspinatus.

Humerus: Anterior Approach

Indications

For exposure of the anterior aspect of humerus for internal fixation of fractures, treatment of tumours or treating humerus infections.

Position of Patient

Supine with the arm abducted on arm table.

Incision

The incision runs along the line from the coracoid tip to the deltoid insertion. Distally, it can be extended along the lateral border of the biceps brachii stopping short of the flexor crease of elbow (Fig. 18.5).

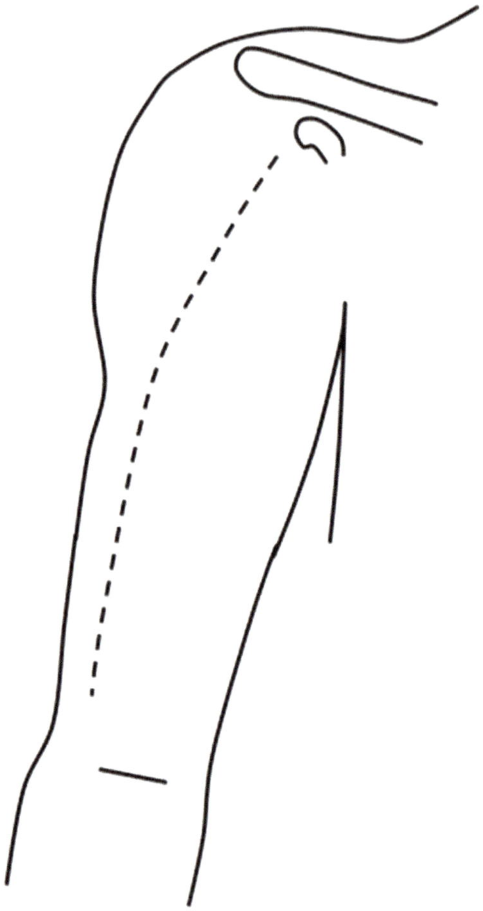

Fig. 18.5 Incision for anterior approach to humerus

Plane

Proximally, the plane is between the deltoid and the pectoralis major. Distally, it lies between the medial and the lateral half of the brachialis. The biceps is retracted medially and the brachialis is split longitudinally.

Structures at Risk

The radial nerve and axillary nerve are at risk. The dissection should be subperiosteal to avoid radial nerve injury. The lateral half of brachialis protects the radial nerve in the lower part of the approach. The anterior humeral circumflex artery may have to be ligated as it crosses the operative field.

Humerus: Posterior Approach

Indications

Fractures of the lower half of the humerus, treatment of tumours or humerus infections, exploration of radial nerve.

Position of Patient

Lateral with the arm across the chest, or prone position.

Incision

Longitudinal incision is used along the midline posteriorly. The incision can be curved round the olecranon distally to extend into proximal forearm for elbow fracture fixation.

Plane

The triceps is split in line with fibres. The long and lateral head are encountered first and are retracted to medial and lateral side respectively. The medial head of triceps is deeper and can be split longitudinally with minimal denervation.

Structures at Risk

Radial nerve, profunda brachii artery and ulnar nerve are at risk. The radial nerve separates the medial and lateral heads of triceps. It is identified at the proximal end of the spiral groove and protected throughout the procedure.

An olecranon osteotomy can be combined with this approach to expose the distal end of humerus for fixation of intercondylar fractures.

Lateral Approach to the Distal Humerus

Indication

Exposure of the lateral condyle of humerus.

Position of Patient

Supine with arm across the chest.

Incision

Curved incision is applied overlying the lateral epicondyle (Fig. 18.6).

Plane

In the lower arm, the plane is between the triceps and brachioradialis. The brachioradialis is reflected anteriorly.

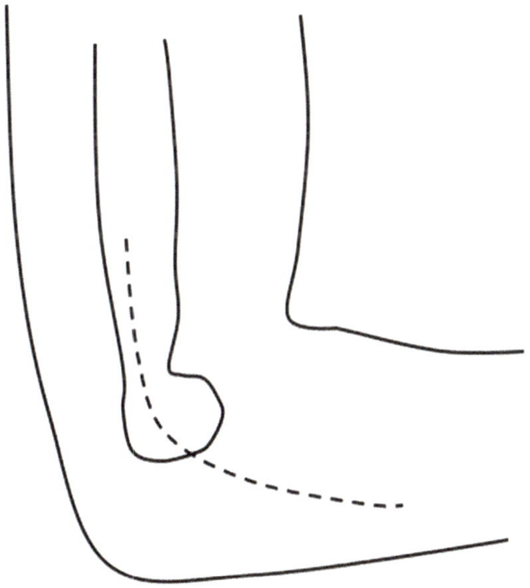

Fig. 18.6 Lateral approach to elbow

Structure at Risk

The radial nerve is at risk proximally.

Elbow: Posterior Approach—Transolecranon

Indication

Intercondylar fractures of the humerus.

Position of Patient

Lateral, with the arm across the chest.

Incision

Posterior midline incision is used, avoiding the tip of the olecranon.

Plane

The ulnar nerve is identified and protected. An olecranon osteotomy is performed to elevate the triceps from the distal humerus and expose the joint.

The osteotomy is predrilled, chevron shaped and aimed at the bare area on the olecranon surface (Fig. 18.7). The starting point is 2 cm distal to the tip of olecranon. Chevron shape allows rotational stability and the chevron points distally. The osteotomy can be fixed securely with a combination of an intramedullary, partially threaded cancellous screw and a tension-band wire. Alternatively, a standard tension band wiring can be done.

Structures at Risk

Ulnar, median and radial nerves, and the brachial artery.

Elbow: Medial Approach

Indications

Fixation of coronoid fractures, removal of loose bodies.

Position of Patient

Supine with the arm abducted and externally rotated.

Incision

Incision is on the medial aspect of elbow, centred on the medial epicondyle.

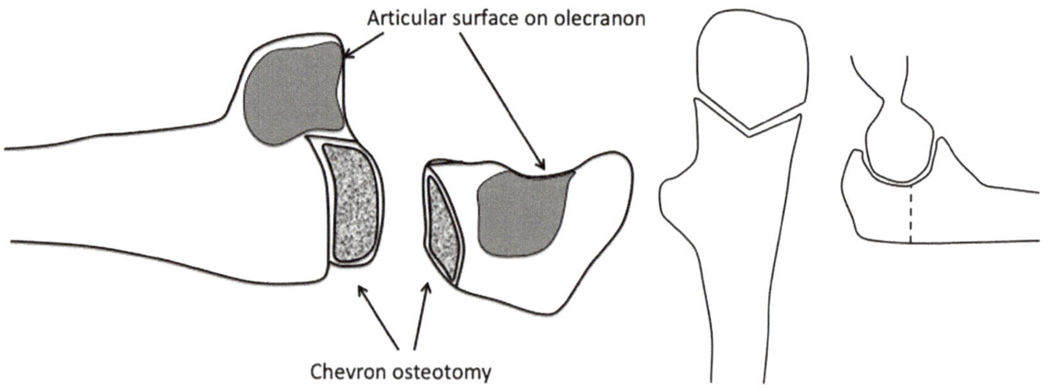

Fig. 18.7 A chevron osteotomy of olecranon

Plane

Proximally, the plane lies between the brachialis and triceps. Distally, it is between the brachialis and pronator teres.

Structures at Risk

Median and ulnar nerves.

Elbow: Posterolateral Approach

Indications

Excision or replacement of the radial head.

Position of Patient

Supine with the arm across the chest.

Incision

Curved incision from the posterior aspect of lateral epicondyle extending medially to the proximal ulna (Fig. 18.8).

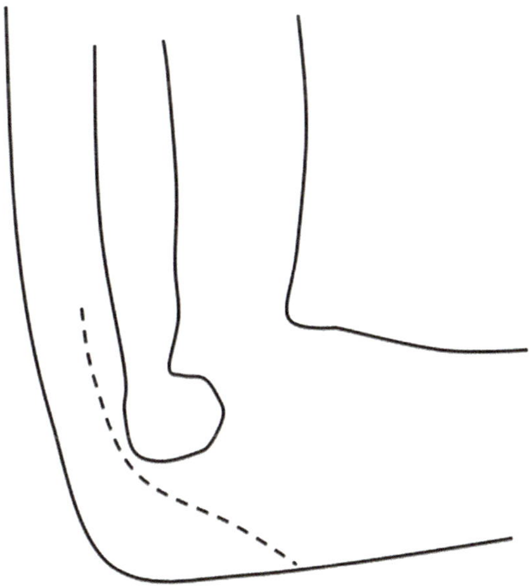

Fig. 18.8 Posterolateral approach to elbow

Plane

Between the anconeus and extensor carpi ulnaris. The forearm is pronated to protect the posterior interosseous nerve.

Structures at Risk

Posterior interosseous and radial nerves.

Forearm: Anterior Approach for Radius

Indications

Fixation of fractures of the radius, radial osteotomy, tumour excision.

Position of Patient

Supine with the arm on arm board.

Incision

Along a line from the lateral border of the bicipital aponeurosis to the radial styloid (Fig. 18.9)

Plane

The brachioradialis lies on the lateral side of the approach, with the pronator teres on the medial side in the proximal part. Distally, the approach is between the brachioradialis and flexor carpi radialis. The pronator teres and pronator quadratus are incised on the radial border and reflected medially to expose the radius.

Structures at Risk

Superficial radial nerve (on the deep surface of the brachioradialis), posterior interosseous nerve (in the proximal end of the approach) and the radial artery. Recurrent radial vessels may be

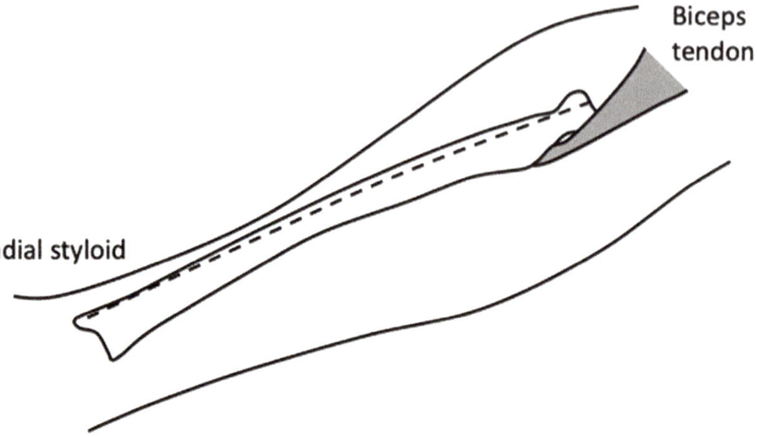

Fig. 18.9 Anterior approach to radius

encountered in the proximal extent of the approach.

Posterior Approach to the Radius

Indications

Reduction and fixation of fractures, osteotomy, or approach to the posterior interosseous nerve.

Position of Patient

Supine with the arm on arm board.

Incision

Along a line joining the lateral epicondyle of the humerus to Lister's tubercle on the dorsum of the distal radius (Fig. 18.10).

Plane

In the proximal part of the approach, the plane is between the extensor carpi radialis brevis and the extensor digitorum. This plane is easier to define in the lower part of the incision. Distally, the plane lies between the extensor carpi radialis brevis and the extensor pollicis longus.

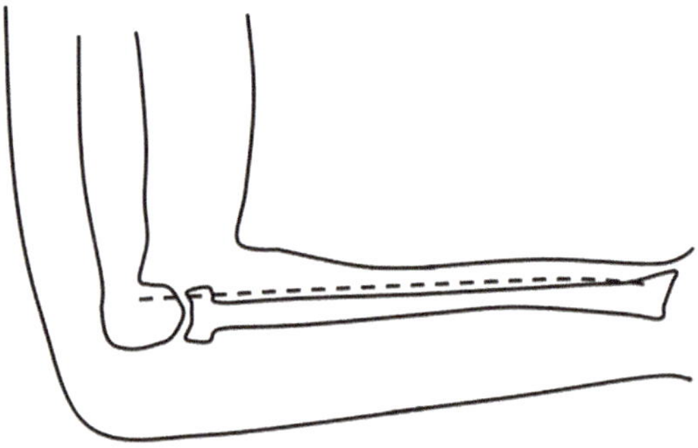

Fig. 18.10 Posterior approach to radius

Structures at Risk

The posterior interosseous nerve is at risk in the proximal extent of the approach.

Approach to the Ulna

Indications

Reduction and fixation of fractures of the ulna, ulnar osteotomy.

Position of Patient

Supine with the arm across the chest.

Incision

Along the subcutaneous border of the ulna.

Plane

Between the extensor carpi ulnaris and the flexor carpi ulnaris.

Structures at Risk

The ulnar artery is close to flexor carpi ulnaris.

Dorsal Approach to the Wrist

Indications

Extensor tendon repair, wrist fusion, fixation of distal radius fractures, proximal row carpectomy and wrist synovectomy.

Position of Patient

Supine with the forearm pronated.

Incision

A longitudinal incision on the dorsum of the wrist in the midline.

Plane

The approach is made between the extensor carpi radialis longus and the extensor carpi radialis brevis.

Structures at Risk

Superficial branches of the radial nerve.

Volar Approach to the Wrist

Indications

Fixation of distal radius fractures, access to the medial nerve and flexor tendons in the wrist, and for drainage of infections in the midpalmar space.

Position of Patient

Supine with an arm board.

Incision

The incision runs from the ulnar side of palmaris longus along the thenar crease in the palm (Fig. 18.11). At the level of the wrist flexor crease, the incision curves towards the ulna to avoid crossing the wrist crease at a right angle.

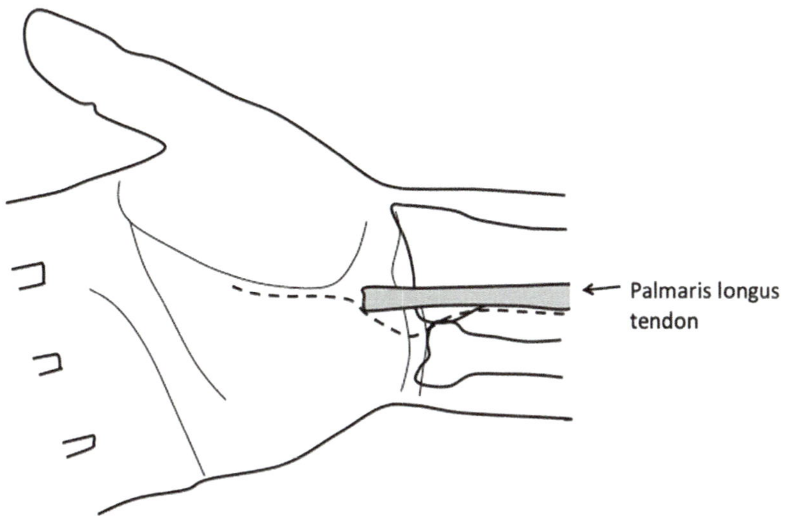

Fig. 18.11 Volar approach to wrist

The incision in the carpal tunnel is made on the ulnar side of the median nerve to protect the motor branch of the median nerve.

Plane

There is no true internervous plane.

Structures at Risk

Palmar cutaneous branch of the median nerve, ulnar vessels and nerve, radial vessels and the median nerve.

Volar Approach to the Scaphoid

Indication

Bone grafting of scaphoid nonunion, and excision of radial styloid.

Position of Patient

Supine with the forearm supinated on arm board.

Incision

Curved incision lateral to the flexor carpi radialis towards the scaphoid tuberosity (Fig. 18.12).

Plane

There is no true internervous plane.

Structure at Risk

Radial artery.

Dorsal Approach to the Scaphoid

Indications

Scaphoid fractures and non-union, excision of radial styloid.

Position of Patient

Supine with the arm pronated.

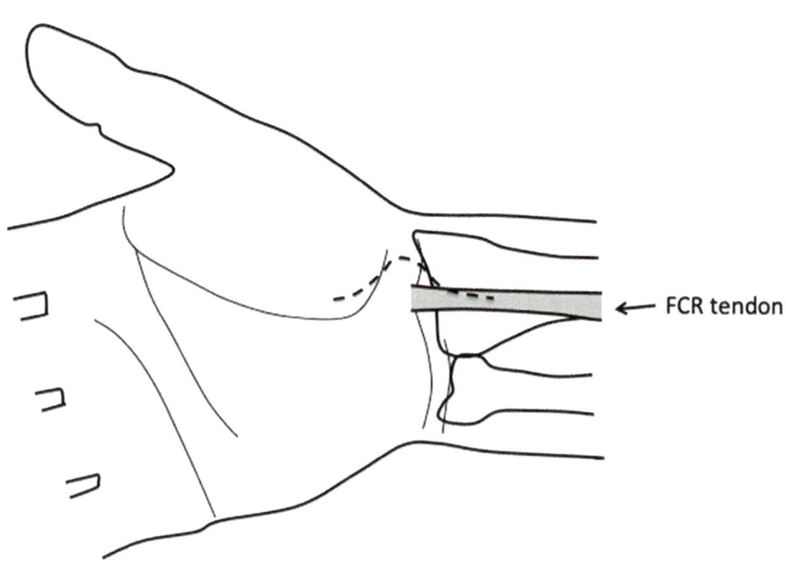

Fig. 18.12 Volar approach to scaphoid

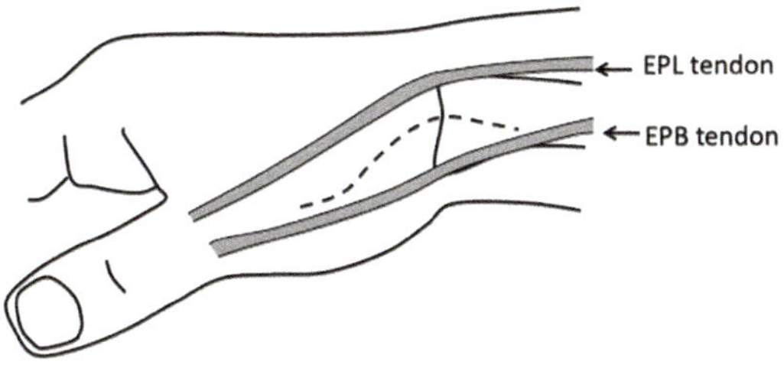

Fig. 18.13 Dorsolateral approach to scaphoid

Incision

Curved incision on the dorsolateral aspect of the scaphoid centred on the anatomical snuff box (Fig. 18.13). The approach is between the tendon of extensor pollicis longus and extensor pollicis brevis.

Plane

There is no true internervous plane.

Structures at Risk

Branches of the superficial radial nerve.

Pelvis: Ilioinguinal Approach

Indications

Anterior column exposure for acetabular fracture fixation.

Position of Patient

Supine on radiolucent table, urinary catheter in situ.

Incision

Curved incision along the inguinal ligament from the midline extending 5 cm beyond the anterior superior iliac spine.

Plane

There is no true internervous plane.

The external oblique muscle is divided in line with the fibres protecting the spermatic cord/round ligament in a sling at the medial extent. The transversus abdominis and the internal oblique muscles are divided on exposing the posterior wall of the inguinal canal.

The inferior epigastric artery runs medial to the deep inguinal ring and should be identified and ligated. The lateral cutaneous nerve is often divided in the lateral part of the incision.

Three slings are passed. The first goes round the spermatic cord (in males) or the round ligament (in females). The second sling goes around the femoral vessels. The third sling goes around the iliopsoas tendon and femoral nerve. Access to the pelvis is obtained by retraction of these slings.

Structures at Risk

Femoral nerve, femoral vessels, inferior epigastric artery, lateral cutaneous nerve, spermatic cord and urinary bladder.

Hip: Anterior (Iliofemoral or Smith–Petersen) Approach

Indications

Surgery for congenital dislocation of the hip, hip arthrodesis, rarely hip arthroplasty.

Position of Patient

Supine with a sandbag under the ipsilateral buttock.

Incision

The incision starts from the middle of the iliac crest. At the anterior superior iliac spine, it curves distally aiming for lateral border of patella

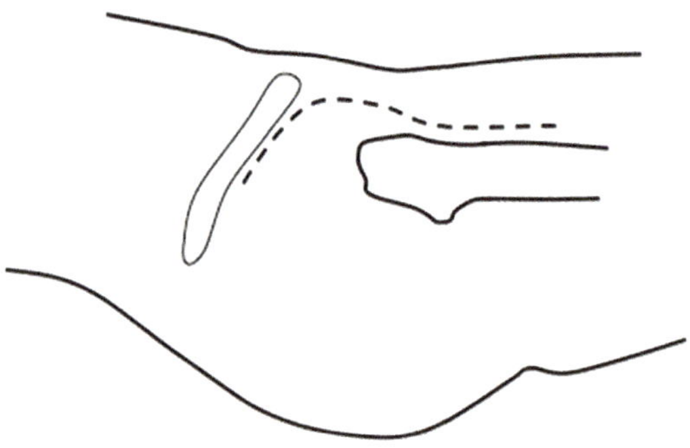

Fig. 18.14 Smith Peterson approach

(Fig. 18.14). A part of the approach may be used instead of full exposure as dictated by surgical need.

Plane

Between the sartorius and tensor fascia lata and then between the rectus femoris and glutei—medius and minimus. The rectus can be detached from the ilium for access.

The approach gives good access to the anterior acetabulum but limited access to the posterior acetabulum

Structures at Risk

Ascending branch of the lateral circumflex femoral artery and branches of the lateral cutaneous nerve of the thigh.

Hip: Anterolateral (Watson–Jones) Approach

Indications

Hip arthroplasty or washout of hip joint infections

Position of Patient

Supine with a sandbag under the ipsilateral buttock

Incision

Centred over the tip of the greater trochanter, curving posteriorly

Plane

Between the tensor fascia lata and gluteus medius. The anterior third of the gluteus is reflected off the greater trochanter.

The approach causes minimal bleeding and there are no significant structures at risk. The main limitation is limited access to the posterior acetabulum

Structures at Risk

Ascending branch of the lateral circumflex femoral artery

Hip: Direct Lateral (Hardinge) Approach

Indications

Hemiarthroplasty and total hip replacement, hip revision surgery, rarely hip resurfacing.

Position of Patient

Supine with a sandbag under ipsilateral buttock or, more commonly, lateral position.

Incision

Centred on tip of trochanter, curving posteriorly in the proximal part.

Plane

There is no true internervous plane. The abductors are split, and the anterior third is reflected anteriorly along with the vastus lateralis.

A significant advantage of this approach is the low dislocation rate (0.3%) reported with hip replacements. However, poor healing of abductors to the trochanter, or injury to superior gluteal nerve can cause a postoperative limp in up to 10% of patients. Exposure of the acetabulum is often limited.

Structures at Risk

There are no major structures at risk, but abductor muscle weakness postoperatively is a problem.

Hardinge K. The direct lateral approach to the hip. J Bone Joint Surg Br 1982;64:17–19.

Hip: Posterior (Moore or Southern) Approach

Indications

This approach can be used for most hip operations, including replacements, resurfacing, tumour surgery and hip revisions.

Position of Patient

Lateral position

Incision

Curved incision centred over the tip of the greater trochanter. The proximal half is parallel to the fibres of the gluteus maximus, while the distal half is parallel to the femur (Fig. 18.15).

Plane

The gluteus maximus is split in line with the fibres. The short external rotators and capsule are detached as a flap from the femur.

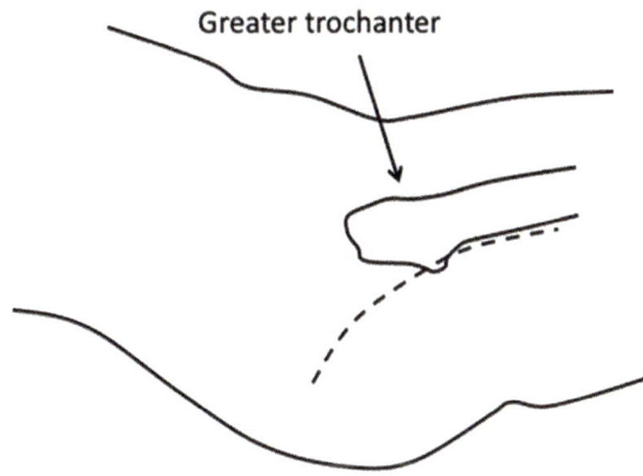

Fig. 18.15 Posterior approach to hip

The advantages are preservation of abductors, ability to extend, and lower heterotopic ossification.

The potential disadvantage is a higher dislocation rate if the capsule is not adequately repaired. With an enhanced repair of capsule to bone, the dislocation rate is comparable with that of the direct lateral approach.

Pellicci PM, Bostrom M, Poss R. Posterior approach to total hip replacement using enhanced posterior soft tissue repair. Clin Orthop Relat Res 1998;355: 224–8. A reduction in the dislocation rate from 6.2% to 0.8% if the capsule is repaired to bone.

Structures at Risk

Inferior gluteal vessels and sciatic nerve.

For fixation of posterior column fractures of the acetabulum, the same approach can be extended proximally up to posterior superior iliac spine (Kocher Langenbeck approach). Gluteus maximus is split and iliotibial band is incised. The gluteus medius is elevated by blunt dissection from the outer aspect of the ilium. The short rotators and the capsule do not always have to be taken down for acetabular fracture fixation. The superior gluteal vessels can be at risk if the gluteus medius is retracted proximally.

Trochanteric Slide

Indications

Hip replacement, hip infections

Position of Patient

Supine or lateral

Incision

Centred on tip of greater trochanter

Plane

The abductors and the vastus are not detached but a sliver of bone is taken off from the greater trochanter. The approach avoids damage to abductors and injury to superior gluteal nerve. The exposure can be limited.

Structures at Risk

Trochanteric anastomosis. Non-healing of the trochanter is a potential problem.

Trochanteric Osteotomy (Charnley)

Indications

Hip replacement

Position of Patient

Supine or lateral

Incision

Centred on tip of greater trochanter

Plane

The abductors are not detached. Osteotomy is performed in line with the superior border of the neck of the femur using a Steinman pin inserted in line with the superior border of the neck (Fig. 18.16). Classically, a Gigli saw is used to create a chevron for accurate approximation for fixation.

The approach avoids damage to the abductors and gives an excellent exposure. Potential problem is trochanteric non-union with resultant pain or a limp.

Structures at Risk

Superior gluteal nerve due to retraction

Wroblewski BM, Shelley P. Reattachment of the greater trochanter after hip replacement. J Bone Joint Surg Br 1985;67:736–40.

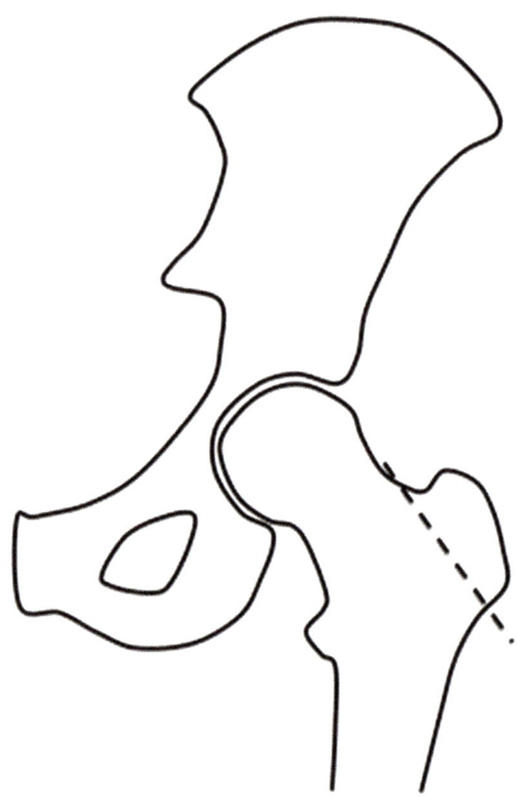

Fig. 18.16 Plane of trochanteric osteotomy

Extended Trochanteric Osteotomy

Indications

Extensile exposure for hip replacement, revision surgery

Position of Patient

Supine or lateral

Incision

The abductors are not detached. The length of the osteotomy is planned preoperatively and the lateral third of the proximal femur is osteotomised. The osteotomy narrows distally to avoid a stress fracture at the end of the osteotomy (Fig. 18.17). The lateral fragment is reattached using cerclage wiring.

Plane

The approach avoids damage to the abductors and injury to the superior gluteal nerve. Good exposure of the femoral canal makes it easier to remove components and cement from the femur. Acetabular exposure is also facilitated.

Non-union of the osteotomy fragment is rare. Eccentric reaming and femoral fracture have been reported.

Structures at Risk

Injury to perforators is possible during exposure. The sciatic nerve can be at risk when cabling the fragment.

Younger TI, Bradford MS, Magnus RE, Paprosky WG. Extended proximal femoral osteotomy. A new technique for femoral revision arthroplasty. J Arthroplasty 1995;10:329–38.

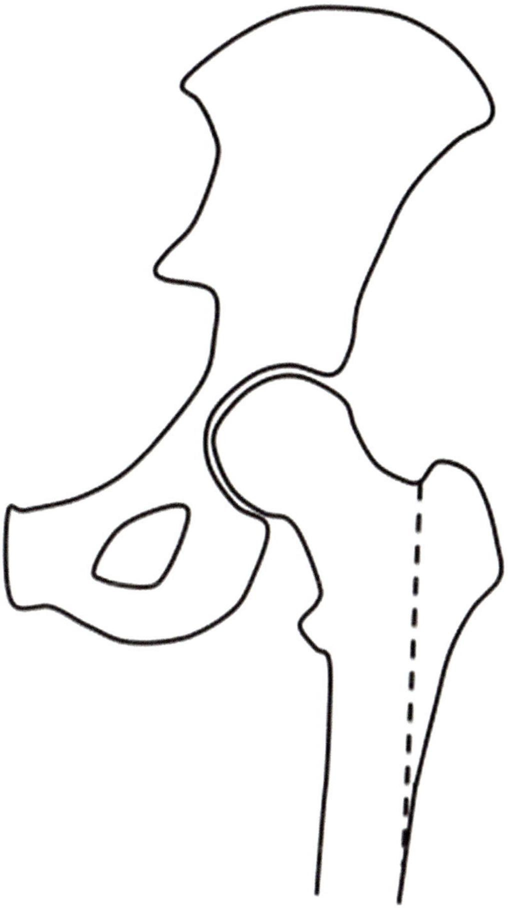

Fig. 18.17 Plane of extended trochanteric osteotomy

Minimally Invasive Hip Replacement

Various approaches have been described, which essentially use a part of conventional approaches to perform the arthroplasty. The approach can be posterior, direct lateral or through a Smith–Peterson approach. Potential advantage is faster recovery and shorter hospital stay. The approach gives limited access and can have a long learning curve for surgeons.

Two-Incision Hip Replacement

This approach is based on making two separate incisions: one to insert the acetabular component and the other to insert the femoral component. Each incision is around 5 cm in size and does not involve cutting any muscles. The intermuscular plane is used for access.

Despite initial widespread enthusiasm, there have been concerns about the benefits of minimally invasive surgery in terms of early results and long term problems.

Ogonda L, Wilson R, Archbold P, et al. A minimal-incision technique in total hip arthroplasty does not improve early postoperative outcomes. A prospective, randomized, controlled trial. J Bone Joint Surg Am 2005; 87: 701–10. 219 patients were randomised to surgery through a short (≤10 cm) or standard (16 cm) incision. The short-incision approach offered no postoperative benefit in terms of blood loss, pain score, walking ability, cement mantle quality, component placement or hospital stay.

Direct Anterior Approach (DAA) Hip Replacement

The direct anterior approach for hip has been used for over 100 years in various forms. It has recently become popular for hip replacement for a perceived benefit in early discharge, faster rehabilitation and reduced dislocation risk. The DAA is essentially similar to the vertical limb of the Smith Peterson approach.

Indications

Hip replacement surgery

Position of Patient

Supine

Incision

Longitudinal incision along the tensor fascia lata muscle.

Plane

Between tensor fascia lata and rectus femoris.

Structures at Risk

Branches of lateral circumflex femoral vessels are coagulated. Intraoperative femoral fracture and damage to lateral cutaneous nerve are other risks. Fluoroscopy is needed to check component positioning.

Malek IA, Royce G, S. U. Bhatti SU, Whittaker JP, S. P. Phillips SP, Wilson IRB, JR, Starks I. A comparison between the direct anterior and posterior approaches for total hip arthroplasty the role of an 'Enhanced Recovery' pathway. Bone Joint J 2016;98(6):754–60. 265 DAA and 183 posterior approach patients compared. No difference in clinical outcome. DAA group had higher femoral fracture rate.

Knee: Medial Parapatellar Approach

This is the most commonly used approach to the knee. It allows full and extensile access.

Indications

Total knee replacement, fixation of proximal tibial and patellar fractures, patellectomy, synovectomy.

Position of Patient

Supine. Using a lateral support and foot rest, the knee can be maintained in a flexed position with minimal assistance.

Incision

A longitudinal, straight midline incision.

Plane

There is no internervous plane. Deep dissection involves a medial parapatellar arthrotomy dividing the quadriceps tendon. The patella can be everted if required.

Proximally, the quadriceps tendon can be divided transversely to aid exposure (quadriceps snip). Distally, the tibial tubercle can be divided and reflected laterally.

Structures at Risk

The infrapatellar branch of the saphenous nerve is often divided. This can lead to neuroma formation along the scar.

Knee: Posterior Approach

Indications

Repair of bony avulsion of the posterior cruciate ligament, access to the posterior capsule, excision of cyst / tumours from posterior aspect of knee.

Position of Patient

Prone

Incision

Curved incision starting from the superolateral aspect over the biceps femoris tendon, curving across the popliteal fossa and downwards medially and inferiorly (Fig. 18.18).

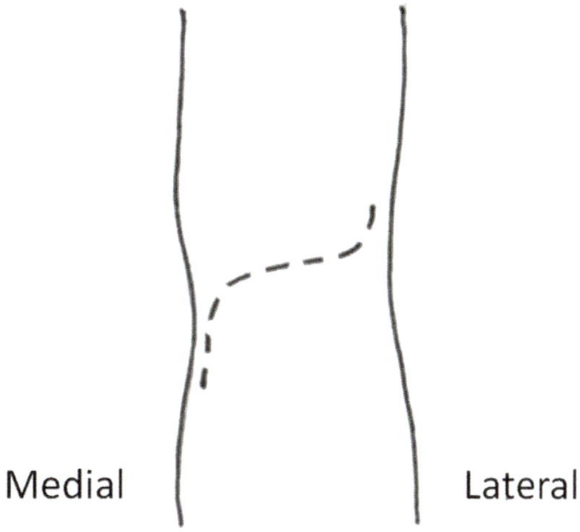

Fig. 18.18 Incision for posterior approach to the knee

Plane

There is no internervous plane. The fascia of the popliteal fossa is divided medial to short saphenous vein. The medial sural cutaneous nerve runs alongside the short saphenous vein and can be used as a guide to locate the tibial nerve.

The muscles forming the boundary of the popliteal fossa are retracted for access. The popliteal artery gives off five genicular arteries. One of these may have to be divided to enable retraction of the neurovascular bundle.

Structures at Risk

Medial sural cutaneous nerve, peroneal vessels, tibial and common peroneal nerve.

Knee: Medial Approach

Indications

Access to the medial collateral ligament, fixation of medial tibial plateau fractures.

Position of Patient

Supine. The hip is externally rotated and abducted and the affected knee is flexed.

Incision

Begins proximal to the adductor tubercle and curves anteriorly and distally.

Plane

There is no internervous plane. Deep dissection can be carried out anterior or posterior to the medial collateral ligament.

Structures at Risk

Infrapatellar branch of the saphenous nerve, medial inferior genicular artery, saphenous vein.

Knee: Lateral Approach

Indication

Lateral ligament repair.

Position of Patient

Supine with a sandbag under the ipsilateral buttock. The knee is flexed to 90°.

Incision

Curved incision on the lateral aspect with the proximal part parallel to the femur and the distal part parallel to the tibia.

Plane

The plane lies between the iliotibial band and the biceps femoris. The fascia between these can be incised to gain access to the joint. The arthrotomy can be made anterior or posterior to the lateral collateral ligament.

Structures at Risk

Lateral popliteal nerve, lateral meniscus, popliteus tendon, lateral superior genicular artery.

Tibia: Posterolateral Approach

Indications

Internal fixation of fractures, posterolateral bone grafting of delayed union or non-union.

Position of Patient

Lateral with the operated leg up.

Incision

Along the lateral border of the gastrocnemius.

Plane

Between the posterior and lateral compartments. The plane lies between the gastrosoleus and the flexor hallucis longus on the medial side and the peroneal muscles on the lateral side.

Structures at Risk

The branches of peroneal artery may need to be ligated. The posterior tibial artery and tibial nerve are separated from the plane of dissection by the flexor hallucis longus.

Ankle: Anterior Approach

Indications

Ankle arthrodesis or replacement, drainage of septic arthritis, fixation of pilon fractures.

Position of Patient

Supine.

Incision

Longitudinal incision between the two malleoli. An alternative approach is along the tibialis anterior tendon.

Plane

The tendon of the extensor hallucis longus is retracted medially along with the neurovascular bundle. The plane is between the extensor hallucis longus and the extensor digitorum longus.

Structures at Risk

Branches of the superficial peroneal nerve, the deep peroneal nerve and the anterior tibial artery.

Ankle: Posteromedial Approach

Indication

Access to the medial malleolus.

Position of Patient

Supine with the hip externally rotated or lateral with the non-operated leg up.

Incision

Midway between the medial malleolus and the Achilles tendon (Fig. 18.19).

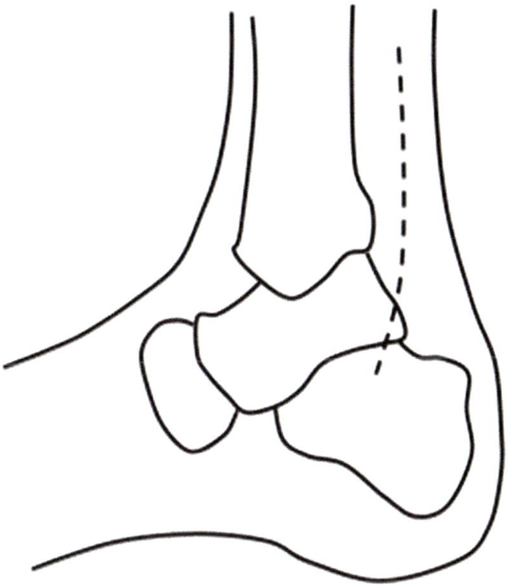

Fig. 18.19 Posteromedial approach to ankle

Plane

The dissection can be performed between the flexor hallucis longus and the peronei, or the flexor hallucis longus and the flexor digitorum longus. The FHL can be identified as it has muscle fibres at this level. The posteromedial structures including the neurovascular bundle can be retracted anteriorly to expose the posterior aspect of tibia and the ankle joint.

Structures at Risk

Posterior tibial artery, tibial nerve.

Ankle: Posterolateral Approach

Indications

Fixation of the posterior malleolus, fusion of the subtalar joint.

Position of Patient

Prone.

Incision

Midway between the lateral border of the Achilles tendon and the lateral malleolus (Fig. 18.20).

Plane

Between the peroneus brevis and the flexor hallucis longus.

Structures at Risk

Short saphenous vein, sural nerve.

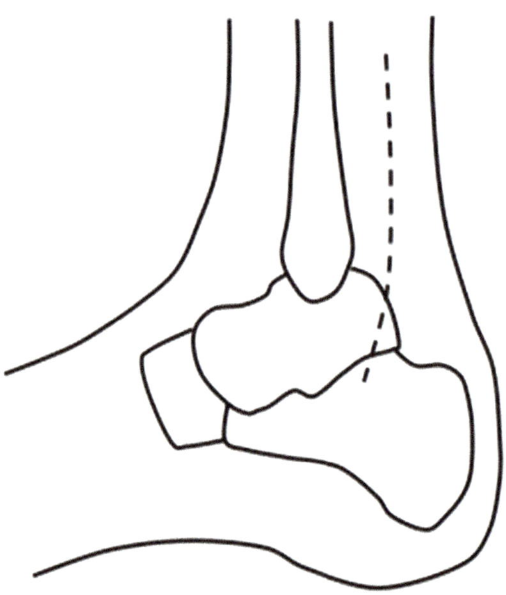

Fig. 18.20 Posterolateral approach to ankle

Lateral Approach for Triple Arthrodesis

Indications

Approach to the talocalcaneal joint, calcaneocuboid joint and talonavicular joint.

Position of Patient

Supine with a sandbag under the ipsilateral hip.

Incision

From the tip of the lateral malleolus, over the sinus tarsi and curving medially (Fig. 18.21). The distal end of incision is at the base of fourth metatarsal.

Plane

Between the peroneus tertius and the peroneus longus / brevis tendons.

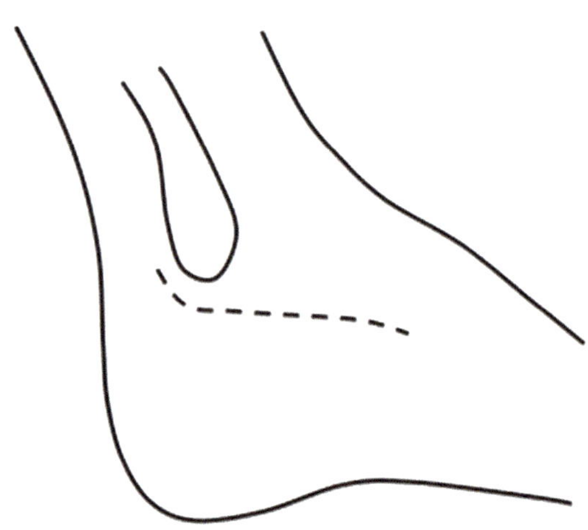

Fig. 18.21 Incision for lateral approach for triple arthrodesis

Structures at Risk

Dorsalis pedis artery and the deep peroneal nerve.

Further Reading

Hardinge K. The direct lateral approach to the hip. J Bone Joint Surg Br. 1982;64:17–9.

Malek IA, Royce G, Bhatti SU, Whittaker JP, Phillips SP, Wilson IRB, Jr., Starks I. A comparison between the direct anterior and posterior approaches for total hip arthroplasty the role of an 'Enhanced Recovery' pathway. Bone Joint J. 2016;98(6):754–60.

Ogonda L, Wilson R, Archbold P, et al. A minimal-incision technique in total hip arthroplasty does not improve early postoperative outcomes. A prospective, randomized, controlled trial. J Bone Joint Surg Am. 2005;87:701–10.

Pellicci PM, Bostrom M, Poss R. Posterior approach to total hip replacement using enhanced posterior soft tissue repair. Clin Orthop Relat Res. 1998;355:224–8.

Wroblewski BM, Shelley P. Reattachment of the greater trochanter after hip replacement. J Bone Joint Surg Br. 1985;67:736–40.

Younger TI, Bradford MS, Magnus RE, Paprosky WG. Extended proximal femoral osteotomy. A new technique for femoral revision arthroplasty. J Arthroplasty. 1995;10:329–38.

Index

S. Agarwal (ed.), *Current Orthopaedic Practice*, https://doi.org/10.1007/978-3-030-78529-1

D

G

Q

R

U

GPSR Compliance

The European Union's (EU) General Product Safety Regulation (GPSR) is a set of rules that requires consumer products to be safe and our obligations to ensure this.

If you have any concerns about our products, you can contact us on ProductSafety@springernature.com

In case Publisher is established outside the EU, the EU authorized representative is:

Springer Nature Customer Service Center GmbH
Europaplatz 3
69115 Heidelberg, Germany

Batch number: 10731391

Printed by Printforce, the Netherlands